MANUAL
OF
EQUINE
EMERGENCIES

MANUAL OF EQUINE EMERGENCIES

Treatment & Procedures

JAMES A. ORSINI, DVM, Diplomate ACVS
Associate Professor of Surgery
University of Pennsylvania
School of Veterinary Medicine
New Bolton Center
Kennett Square, Pennsylvania

THOMAS J. DIVERS, DVM, Diplomate ACVIM, ACVECC
Professor of Medicine
Department of Clinical Sciences
New York State College of Veterinary Medicine
Cornell University
Ithaca, New York

W.B. SAUNDERS COMPANY
A Division of Harcourt Brace & Company

Philadelphia   London   Toronto   Montreal   Sydney   Tokyo

W.B. SAUNDERS COMPANY

A Division of Harcourt Brace & Company

The Curtis Center
Independence Square West
Philadelphia, Pennsylvania 19106

Library of Congress Cataloging-in-Publication Data

Orsini, James A.
Manual of equine emergencies: treatment and procedures / James A. Orsini, Thomas J. Divers.—1st ed.

p.   cm.

ISBN 0–7216–2425–1

1. Horses—Diseases.   2. Veterinary emergencies.   I. Divers, Thomas J.
II. Title.

SF951.077   1998

636.1′0896025—dc21   97–35784

Permissions: Dr. Naylor holds the copyright to the tables and charts in his chapter.

MANUAL OF EQUINE EMERGENCIES:
TREATMENT AND PROCEDURES   ISBN 0–7216–2425–1

Contributors

Michael A. Ball, DVM
Lecturer, Department of
   Pharmacology, New York State
   College of Veterinary Medicine,
   Cornell University, Ithaca, New
   York
   Organ System Examination:
   Gastrointestinal Emergencies and
   Other Causes of Colic

Thomas J. Divers, DVM,
Diplomate ACVIM, ACVECC
Professor of Medicine, Department of
   Clinical Sciences, New York State
   College of Veterinary Medicine;
   Cornell University, Ithaca, New
   York

   Organ System Examination:
   Gastrointestinal Emergencies and
   Other Causes of Colic; Liver
   Failure; Hemolytic Anemia;
   Nervous System; Reproductive
   System; Respiratory; Urinary;
   Shock and Systemic Inflammatory
   Response Syndrome; Temperature-
   Related Problems; Pharmacology
   and Toxicology

Robin D. Gleed, BVSc, MRCVS,
DVA, Diplomate ACVA
Associate Professor of
   Anesthesiology, Cornell University,
   Ithaca, New York
   Anesthesia for Field Emergencies
   and Euthanasia

Robert B. Hillman, AB, DVM,
MS
Senior Clinician Emeritus, New York
   State College of Veterinary

Medicine, Cornell University,
   Ithaca, New York
   Organ System Examination:
   Reproductive System

Kent A. Humber, DVM, MS,
Diplomate ACVIM
STAT Veterinary Laboratory, Rancho
   Santa Fe, California
   Cytology

Nita L. Irby, DVM, Diplomate
ACVO
Lecturer, Cornell University, New
   York State College of Veterinary
   Medicine, Cornell University,
   Ithaca, New York
   Organ System Examination:
   Ophthalmology

Cynthia A. Jackson, DVM,
Diplomate ACVIM
Postdoctoral Fellow, Michigan State
   University, East Lansing, Michigan
   Organ System Examination:
   Nervous System

J Edward Kirker, BS, RPh
Pharmacy Director, Department of
   Clinical Sciences, New York State
   College of Veterinary Medicine,
   Cornell University, Ithaca, New
   York
   Pharmacology and Adverse Drug
   Reactions

Christine Kreuder, VMD
Staff Veterinarian, C.R.O.W. Wildlife
   Hospital, Sanibel, Florida

*Emergency Medical and Surgical
Principles and Procedures*

**Richard A. Mansmann, VMD,
PhD**

Owner, Central Carolina Equine
  Practice, Apex, North Carolina

Disaster Medicine

**James N. Moore, DVM, PhD,
Diplomate ACVS**

Professor and Department Head,
  Department of Large Animal
  Medicine, University of Georgia
  College of Veterinary Medicine,
  Athens, Georgia

*Organ System Examination:
Gastrointestinal Emergencies and
Other Causes of Colic*

**P. O. Eric Mueller, DVM, PhD,
Diplomate ACVS**

Assistant Professor of Surgery,
  Department of Large Animal
  Medicine, University of Georgia
  College of Veterinary Medicine,
  Athens, Georgia

*Organ System Examination:
Gastrointestinal Emergencies and
Other Causes of Colic*

**Jonathan M. Naylor, PhD,
Diplomate ACVIM, Diplomate
ACVN**

Professor, Department of Veterinary
  Internal Medicine, Western College
  of Veterinary Medicine, University
  of Saskatchewan, Saskatoon,
  Saskatchewan, Canada

*Nutritional Guidelines for the
Injured Horse*

**James A. Orsini, DVM,
Diplomate ACVS**

Associate Professor of Surgery,
  University of Pennsylvania School
  of Veterinary Medicine, New
  Bolton Center, Kennett Square,
  Pennsylvania

*Emergency Medical and Surgical
Principles and Procedures;
Organ System Examination:
Musculoskeletal; Reproductive
System; Appendices*

Jonathan E. Palmer, VMD

Associate Professor of Medicine,
  Graham French Neonatal Section,
  Connelly Intensive Care Unit,
  University of Pennsylvania School
  of Veterinary Medicine, New
  Bolton Center, Kennett Square,
  Pennsylvania

*Neonatology; Foal
Cardiopulmonary Resuscitation*

**Virginia B. Reef, BS, DVM,
Diplomate ACVIM**

Professor of Medicine in the Widener
  Hospital, University of
  Pennsylvania College of Veterinary
  Medicine; Chief, Section of Sports
  Medicine and Imaging, Director of
  Large Animal Cardiology and
  Ultrasonography, New Bolton
  Center, Kennett Square,
  Pennsylvania

*Organ System Examination:
Cardiovascular*

Mary C. Smith, DVM

Associate Professor, Department of
  Clinical Sciences, New York State
  College of Veterinary Medicine,
  Cornell University, Ithaca, New
  York

Toxicology

**Ted S. Stashak, DVM, MD,
Diplomate ACVS**

Professor of Surgery, Department of
  Clinical Sciences, Colorado State
  University School of Veterinary
  Medicine and Biomedical Sciences,
  Fort Collins, Colorado

*Organ System Examination:
Integumentary*

Ann Townsend Sturmer, AAS, LVT
Veterinary Technician, Cornell University, Ithaca, New York

Anesthesia for Field Emergencies and Euthanasia

Larry J. Thompson, DVM, PhD, Diplomate ABVT
Clinical Toxicologist, Diagnostic Laboratory, College of Veterinary Medicine, Cornell University, Ithaca, New York

Toxicology

Wendy E. Vaala, VMD, Diplomate ACVIM
Staff Veterinarian, Mid-Atlantic Equine Medical Center, Ringoes, New Jersey

Neonatalogy; Foal Cardiopulmonary Resuscitation

Pamela Wagner Von Matthiessen, DVM, MD, Diplomate ACVS
Wright State University School of Medicine, Dayton, Ohio

Organ System Examination: Musculoskeletal

Preface

The idea of the first text dedicated to equine emergency therapy stemmed from our long interest in emergency and critical care medicine and the realization that there was no similar text available for the equine clinician. It is our goal to provide the most up-to-date information available regarding current diagnostics and therapeutics in equine emergency medicine. We have added many new diagnostics and treatments not yet documented because we believed the evidence was strong enough from use in other species (especially humans), and from personal experience with the horse, to be included in this edition. We are particularly grateful to our colleagues who have generously provided information and ideas for the book. The distinguished contributors are to be congratulated for their excellent presentations. We also thank W.B. Saunders Company for permitting us the editorial liberties to make the last-minute additions to keep the book current.

It has been our intent to list equipment and laboratory specifications so that diagnostic procedures, sample collection, laboratory testing, and treatments could be accomplished more easily. We have also included a list of manufacturers and laboratory phone numbers that we believe are correct at the time of printing but, undoubtedly, will change over time.

Finally, we made the book easy to use, durable, and reasonably priced in the hope that it will become your irreplaceable partner in any emergency. We hope you find the book useful in reducing the stress involved in treating emergencies. We appreciate any comments and/or suggested changes that should be incorporated in future editions.

THOMAS J. DIVERS
JAMES A. ORSINI

Acknowledgments

We thank and acknowledge the invaluable help of many colleagues, students, and fellow workers who contributed so much to the publication of this first edition. Indeed, without the tireless efforts of so many there would be no book. Listed below are only a small number of the many individuals that offered their support and loyalty in its completion and our professional development and for this we are very grateful.

Roy V.H. Pollock, DVM, PhD for his early input and suggestions; Mary Alice Malone and Lawrence and Vonnie Steinbaum for their support and friendship; Drs. Doug Byars, Lisle George, Robert H. Whitlock, and Willard H. Daniels for their professional support and friendship; the Noble and McIlvain Families for providing a quiet place to work; Students: Vered Bar, John MacGregor, Diane Simpson, Corrina Snook, Ric Zappala; Drs. William Jackson, Dana King; Philip Ashley for the clear and precise medical illustrations; Stephanie Donley, Denise LeMelledo, Edna Dick, and the staff at W.B. Saunders for their outstanding editorial and professional guidance. We are particularly indebted to Margie Schwartz, Joyce Reyna, and Debbie Lent for their superior editorial skills, proofreading, manuscript revision, and organizational skills, making this book clear and rich in its presentation.

JAMES A. ORSINI
THOMAS J. DIVERS

Contents

Color Plates follow the Table of Contents.

SECTION 1
Emergency Medical and Surgical Principles and Procedures, 1

SECTION 2
Organ System Examination, Neonatology, Shock, and Temperature-Related Problems, 93

SECTION 3
Laboratory Tests, 549

SECTION 4
Pharmacology and Toxicology, 565

SECTION 5
Management of Special Problems, 637

SECTION 6
Appendices, 665

Index, 721

A complete listing of section contents can be found on the first page of each section.

FIGURE 31–1. *A,* Four weeks before this photo, a 3-year-old Warmblood stallion sustained iatrogenic blunt trauma to the eye. Consolidating subretinal hemorrhage is visible at the left, with resolving peripapillary retinal and choroidal edema. *B,* One year after injury, a classic "butterfly" lesion is evident (peripapillary choroidal atrophy and scarring).

FIGURE 31–2. Eye of a 2-year-old Thoroughbred colt with severe subconjunctival emphysema secondary to dorsal orbital rim fracture involving the frontal sinus.

FIGURE 31–3. Severe corneal stromal ulceration, with severe keratomalacia, hypopyon, and early corneal neovascularization. The cornea did not retain fluorescein stain prior to referral. A V-shaped tear in the loose corneal epithelium, evident dorsally, occurred during the examination.

FIGURE 31–4. Eye of a 4-month-old Thoroughbred filly with a 5-mm-diameter superficial corneal ulcer of 3 days' duration. The lesion developed an acute increase in edema, a change in contour, and a mucoid appearance, indicating active keratomalacia. *Staphylococcus aureus* was cultured.

FIGURE 31–5. Eye of a 12-year-old Thoroughbred gelding with a severe corneal ulcer of 8 days' duration. A toothed forceps is being used to elevate the malacic cornea for debridement with small scissors.

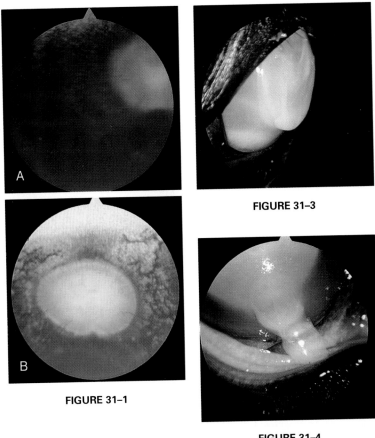

FIGURE 31–1

FIGURE 31–3

FIGURE 31–4

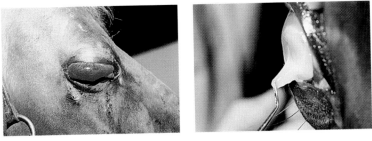

FIGURE 31–2

FIGURE 31–5

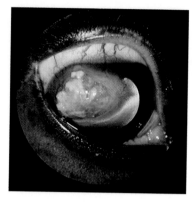

FIGURE 31–6

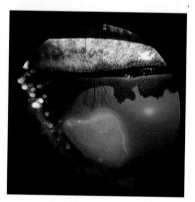

FIGURE 31–7

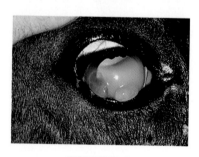

FIGURE 31–8

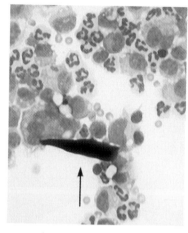

FIGURE 38–1

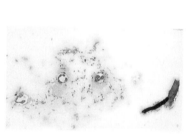

FIGURE 38–2

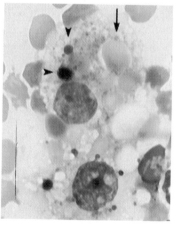

FIGURE 38–3

FIGURE 31–6. Eye of a 12-year-old Thoroughbred mare with an 8-week history of a superficial corneal ulcer that began in the ventrotemporal perilimbal cornea and gradually progressed centrally.

FIGURE 31–7. Eye of a 9-month-old Thoroughbred filly with a 10-day history of corneal disease that began as a superficial erosion in the dorsotemporal perilimbal cornea. Photo illustrates the caseous, white surface exudate and severe corneal neovascularization.

FIGURE 31–8. Severe corneal edema with bullae formation in the right eye of a weanling Thoroughbred filly. She was one of 18 Thoroughbred weanlings from a group outbreak of acute unilateral or bilateral corneal edema (mild to extremely severe), some cases of which involved concurrent retinal detachments. An etiology was not conclusively determined.

FIGURE 38–1. Peritoneal fluid (400 X). A mixture of nondegenerate neutrophils and macrophages. One eosinophil is present. The arrow points to a keratin flake (rolled-up squamous epithelial cell). A small number of erythrocytes are present in the background.

FIGURE 38–2. Peritoneal fluid (400 X). Ruptured intestine.

FIGURE 38–3. Peritoneal fluid (1000 X). Macrophages containing erythrocytes (arrow) and hemosiderin pigment (arrowheads). The cells demonstrate erthrocytophagia and provide evidence of hemorrhage into the sample site.

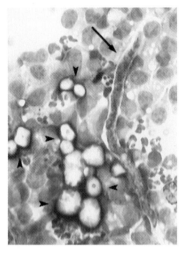

FIGURE 38–4

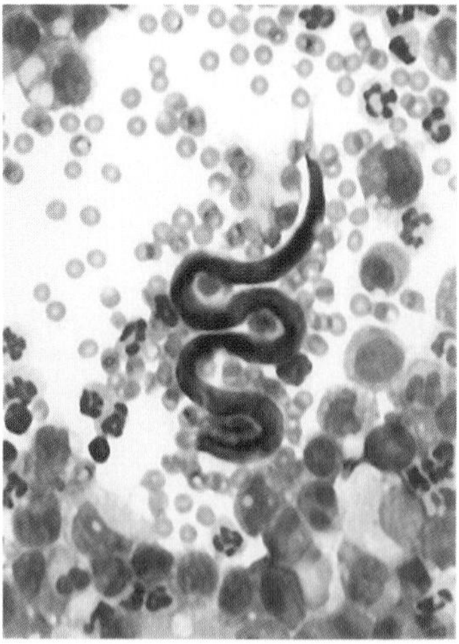

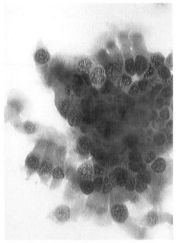

FIGURE 38–6

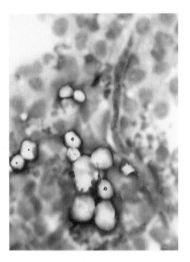

FIGURE 38–5

FIGURE 38–7

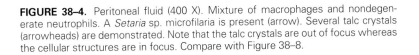

FIGURE 38–4. Peritoneal fluid (400 X). Mixture of macrophages and nondegenerate neutrophils. A *Setaria* sp. microfilaria is present (arrow). Several talc crystals (arrowheads) are demonstrated. Note that the talc crystals are out of focus whereas the cellular structures are in focus. Compare with Figure 38–8.

FIGURE 38–5. Peritoneal fluid (400 X). Same microscopic field as Figure 38–7; however, the focus has been changed to show the three-dimensional depth and central nidus of the talc crystals.

FIGURE 38–6. Peritoneal fluid (400 X). *Setaria* sp. microfilaria. A mixture predominantly of macrophages, along with nondegenerate neutrophils and erythrocytes, is present.

FIGURE 38–7. Transtracheal aspirate (400 X). A sheet of normal ciliated columnar epithelial cells.

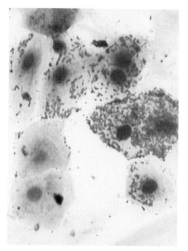

FIGURE 38–8

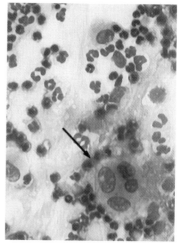

FIGURE 38–10

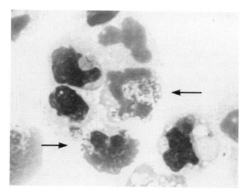

FIGURE 38–9

FIGURE 38–8. Transtracheal aspirate (400 X). Keratinized squamous epithelial cells with large numbers of a mixed population of adherent extracellular bacteria. The pink material in the background is mucus. This is compatible with oropharyngeal contamination of the sample.

FIGURE 38–9. Transtracheal aspirate (1000 X). Degenerate neutrophils containing intracellular bacteria (cocci in pairs and rods). Note the swollen appearance of the nuclear chromatin (karyolysis) and the more eosinophilic staining character compared with nondegenerate neutrophils. Cytoplasmic vacuolization is a common feature. The diagnosis is septic suppurative inflammation.

FIGURE 38–10. Transtracheal aspirate (1000 X). Increased numbers of neutrophils, abundant mucus, and pulmonary macrophages are present. One multinucleate giant cell (arrow) is demonstrated. No microorganisms are present. The diagnosis is suppurative inflammation. The presence of multinucleate giant cells indicates chronicity. The sample is compatible with chronic obstructive pulmonary disease (COPD).

Emergency Medical and Surgical Principles and Procedures

PART I: General Diagnostic and Therapeutic Procedures **2**
   1. Blood Collection 2
   2. Medication Administration 6
   3. Intravenous Catheter Placement 12
   4. Intraosseous Infusion Technique 15
   5. Bacterial, Fungal, and Viral Infection Diagnoses 17
   6. Biopsy Techniques 21
   7. Endoscopy Techniques 30

PART II: Respiratory System **34**
   8. Nasotracheal and Orotracheal Tube Placement 34
   9. Transtracheal Aspiration and Bronchoalveolar Lavage 36
  10. Nasal Oxygen Insufflation 40
  11. Assisted Ventilation 41
  12. Tracheotomy 44
  13. Paranasal Sinus Trephination 46
  14. Thoracocentesis and Chest Tube Placement 50

PART III: Gastrointestinal System **53**
  15. Nasogastric Tube Placement 53
  16. Abdominocentesis and Peritoneal Fluid Analysis 55
  17. Cecal Trocharization 59

PART IV: Genitourinary System **61**
  18. Urinary Tract Catheterization 61

PART V: Musculoskeletal System **64**
  19. Local Anesthesia for the Diagnosis of Lameness 64
  20. Arthrocentesis and Synovial Fluid Analysis 77

PART VI: The Eye **81**
  21. Fluorescein Staining 81
  22. Nasolacrimal Duct Cannulation 82
  23. Subpalpebral Catheter Placement 83

PART VII: Central Nervous System **86**
  24. Cerebrospinal Fluid Collection 86

PART I

General Diagnostic and Therapeutic Procedures

1 Blood Collection

James A. Orsini and Christine Kreuder

VENIPUNCTURE

Blood collection from a vein is a routine procedure performed commonly during patient examination. Many diagnostic tests require either whole blood or serum and specific additives to prevent coagulation (Table 1–1).

> The **external jugular vein** is most accessible and is easily found within the jugular groove along the ventral aspect of the neck. The vein is safely punctured in the cranial half of the neck where muscle (omohyoideus muscle) interposes between the vein and the underlying carotid sheath containing the carotid artery. The vein distends rapidly with firm pressure applied near the thoracic inlet. Stroking the vein distally causes motion waves higher up, which is helpful if the distended vein is not easily seen.

Equipment

- 20–25-gauge, ⅝–1.5-inch Vacutainer[1] needle (or a 10-ml syringe and 20-gauge needle for fractious individuals)
- Vacutainer cuff
- appropriate Vacutainer tube(s)

Procedure

- Screw the protected, short end of the needle into the Vacutainer cuff.
- Distend the vein and swab the venipuncture site with alcohol.
- Align the needle parallel with the vein in the direction against the blood flow.

---

[1]Vacutainer needles, cuffs, and blood tubes. Becton-Dickinson Vacutainer Systems, Rutherford, NJ 07070.

TABLE 1–1. **Blood Tubes for Diagnostic Procedures**

Vacutainer Tube-Top Color	Additive	Analysis Possible
Red or red/black	None	Chemistry studies; viral antibody studies; cross match*
Purple	Na EDTA	Hematology studies—CBC platelet count Immunohematology; Coombs' test; fluid cytology; cross match*
Green	Na heparin	Chemistry studies; blood gases
Yellow	Acid citrate Dextrose	Cross-match; blood typing
Blue	Na citrate	Coagulation studies—fibrinogen, PT, PTT, AT III
Gray	Na fluoride K oxalate	Glucose

Na, sodium; EDTA, ethylenediaminetetraacetic acid; K, potassium; PT, prothrombin time; PTT, partial thromboplastin time; AT III, antithrombin III.
*Both required.

- Insert the needle through the skin at a 45° angle and then redirect it in a parallel direction once the vein lumen has been entered.
- Attach the Vacutainer by pushing the cover of the tube onto the short protected needle in the Vacutainer cuff. The vacuum draws blood into the tube to the appropriate level. If additional tubes are needed, switch tubes while leaving the needle and cuff in place.

> The **transverse facial vein** in the head is commonly used in adults and/or nonfractious individuals to sample very small volumes of blood for a packed cell volume (PCV) or total solids (TS) determination. The vein runs transversely beneath the facial crest and above the transverse facial artery.

Equipment

- 22–25-gauge, ⅝–1-inch needle
- 3-ml syringe
- appropriate Vacutainer or hematocrit tube(s)

Procedure

- Swab the area beneath the facial crest with alcohol.
- Align the needle perpendicular to the skin beneath the facial crest, and thrust through the skin until bone is encountered.
- Attach the syringe and withdraw the needle while aspirating until the needle is in the vein lumen.

- A Vacutainer needle and tube may also be used to collect blood.

Other sites for venipuncture include (Fig. 1–1):

- The **superficial thoracic vein** located in the cranial and ventral third of the thorax caudal to the point of the elbow
- The **cephalic vein** on the medial aspect of the forelimb
- The **medial saphenous vein** on the medial aspect of the hindlimb

If the sample is collected in a syringe, immediately transfer it to a Vacutainer tube because the sample begins to clot as soon as it is drawn. Push the needle through the cover of the Vacutainer tube and let the vacuum aspirate the blood from the syringe. Actively pushing blood into the tube damages the blood cells. Mix the anticoagulant into the sample by gently rotating the tube upside down several times. The sample should last for several hours if properly mixed and kept cool. Serum should be separated from whole blood by centrifugation if the sample is to sit for longer than several hours, to prevent hemolysis. Hemolysis has a significant effect on many parameters, such as calcium (increased), chloride (decreased), creatine (increased), alkaline phosphate (increased), and lactate dehydrogenase (increased). Slides for a differential are best made soon after the sample is taken.

Complications

A **hematoma** often forms if a large-gauge needle is used, or if the vein is excessively traumatized and continues to leak blood from the venipuncture site. *Keeping the head elevated and applying direct pressure to the puncture site minimizes this complication.*

Thrombosis of the vein is an uncommon complication that may occur if the vascular endothelium is damaged from repeated venipuncture. **Septic thrombophlebitis** occurs if the site becomes infected.

ARTERY PUNCTURE

Most commonly performed for blood gas analysis, which is an excellent indicator of respiratory and metabolic status. Several arteries are suitable for sampling (see Fig. 1–1).

The **carotid artery** is accessible in the caudal third of the neck.

Equipment

- 20- or 25-gauge, $5/8$–1.5-inch needle
- heparinized plastic syringe
- gauze sponges soaked in alcohol
- green top (heparin) Vacutainer tube

Procedure

- The carotid pulse is palpable within the jugular groove. The carotid artery lies slightly dorsal and immediately deep to the jugular vein.
- Clean the area thoroughly with alcohol and gauze. While palpating the

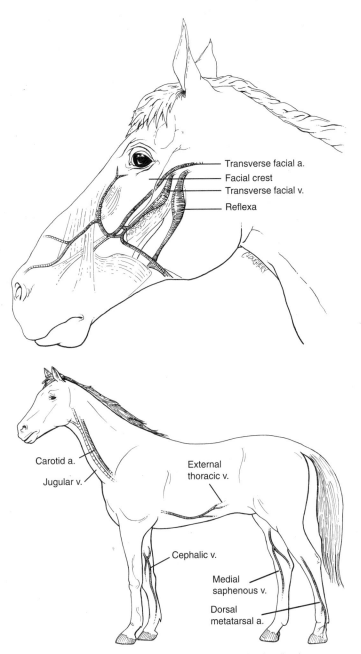

FIGURE 1–1. Veins and arteries used for blood collection.

pulse, puncture the artery with the needle. If the artery has been punctured, bright red blood flows rapidly from the needle.

■ Attach a syringe and aspirate a sample. Remove air from the syringe immediately. If blood gas analysis is desired, it should be performed within minutes or the sample should be placed in a heparin Vacutainer tube and cooled.

■ As soon as the needle is withdrawn, apply digital pressure over the puncture site with a gauze sponge for several minutes.

Other sites for artery puncture include:

The **facial artery,** as it courses from under the mandible to the facial crest, is easily punctured in a heavily sedated or anesthetized patient.

The **dorsal metatarsal artery,** which courses laterally and distally from the cranial aspect of the proximal metatarsus, is the preferred site in recumbent foals.

The transverse facial artery lies caudal to the lateral canthus of the eye (Fig. 1–1).

Complications

As with venipuncture, the most common complication is **hematoma** formation:

Use the smallest-gauge needle possible to minimize vessel trauma, and apply pressure to the artery until bleeding ceases.

Local skin infiltration of 2% local anesthetic directly over the site for needle puncture improves patient compliance and thus decreases trauma to the vessel wall.

2 Medication Administration

James A. Orsini and Christine Kreuder

Multiple routes of administration exist for equine pharmaceuticals. Each route affects the pharmacokinetics of a drug. The pharmaceutical package insert describes the routes available and is a valuable source of information.

ORAL DRUG ADMINISTRATION

The oral route is the most convenient route of administration and creates the fewest complications. This route is ideal for client/owner drug administration. Drugs with an oral preparation come in tablets, granules, powders, suspensions, and pastes.

Many horses eat powders, granules, and crushed tablets mixed with a palatable food (sweet feed, pellets, chopped apples, and applesauce).

For finicky or anorectic individuals, an alternative is to mix the powder or dissolve the tablets in water and administer with a dose syringe.[1] The addition of molasses, syrup, or baby carrot food increases palatability and therefore encourages acceptance by the patient. Medications in paste or suspension form should be administered as follows:

- Proper restraint of the head is necessary.
- Make sure the mouth is cleared of food.
- The dose syringe should be carefully placed between the buccal mucosa and the molars and angled over the tongue. Gently grasping the tongue and pulling it forward and out of the way before placing the syringe in the mouth helps ensure that the medicine remains in the mouth.
- Spread the medicine evenly over the back of the tongue and dispense slowly to encourage swallowing.

Administration via **nasogastric tube** is useful for horses that refuse to be dosed in the preceding manner or that need delivery of a large volume of medication. Nasogastric tubing also ensures that the entire dose is received.

- See section on placement of a nasogastric tube (p. 53).
- Medication is easily delivered with a large 400-ml dose syringe[2] that fits on the end of most nasogastric tubes.
- After administering the medication, deliver a dose syringeful of water, then air, to ensure that all the drug has cleared the tubing.
- Leave the syringe attached or kink the tube when removing to reduce the chances of aspiration.

Complications

The complete dose often is not delivered unless administered via nasogastric tube.

Some drugs are inactivated in the stomach of herbivores, so make sure that the drug is for oral delivery in horses.

This route results in high drug levels in the gastrointestinal tract and can alter the normal bacteria flora, causing diarrhea or colic.

INTRAMUSCULAR ADMINISTRATION

Intramuscular administration typically causes slower absorption than the intravenous route, creates lower peak blood levels, and permits less frequent administration. As with oral administration, many owners are comfortable administering drugs intramuscularly. Several large muscle masses are suitable for drug administration (Fig. 2–1):

- Small volumes (10 ml or less) may be administered in the neck in the indented triangular space that lies above the cervical vertebrae, below the nuchal ligament, and a handsbreadth in front of the cranial border of the scapula.

---

[1]Dose syringe with catheter tip (60 or 35 ml). Monoject, Sherwood Medical, St. Louis, MO 63103.

[2]400-ml nylon dose syringe. J.A. Webster, Inc., 86 Leominster Road, Sterling, MA 01564-2198; (800) 225-7911.

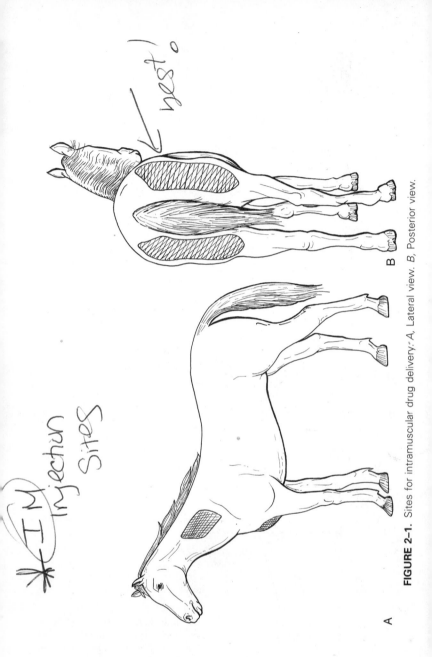

FIGURE 2–1. Sites for intramuscular drug delivery. *A,* Lateral view. *B,* Posterior view.

- The lower half of the semitendinosus and semimembranosus muscles are suitable for large volumes. Proper restraint of the horse is needed, and the individual dispensing the drug should stand as close to the horse's side as possible to avoid personal injury.
- Large volumes may be administered in the pectoral muscles (pectoralis descendens) between the front limbs.

Procedure

- Clean site with an alcohol- or chlorhexidine-soaked swab until dirt is removed.
- Use a 1.5-inch, 22-, 20-, 19-, or 18-gauge needle (depending on the viscosity of the medicine to be delivered).
- Quickly thrust the needle through the skin up to the hub.
- Attach the syringe with the drug and aspirate to ensure that the needle is not in a vessel.
- Ideally, no more than 5–10 ml should be administered at any one site. For large volumes, the needle may be redirected without leaving the skin after each 5–10 ml aliquot.
- When dosing must be repeated, rotate between muscle groups to avoid repeated trauma to any one muscle.

Complications

Abscess formation is an occasional complication. Clean the skin thoroughly before injecting and choose a site that is easily drained if this complication occurs.

Muscle **soreness,** in particular neck soreness, is fairly common and is related to drug irritation and associated inflammation, the volume administered, and the site of administration. Sites in high-motion areas should be avoided. Avoid repeated **intramuscular** injection in foals.

Severe **drug reactions** may occur if certain drugs are accidentally placed in a vessel (procaine penicillin G).

INTRAVENOUS ADMINISTRATION

This route provides immediate high blood levels of the drug but typically requires more frequent administration. Medication must be administered very slowly (at a rate of approximately 1 ml per 5 seconds) or diluted in sterile water or saline, especially if the particular drug is known to cause any type of adverse reaction.

The external jugular vein is most commonly used for medication delivery. The vein should be punctured only in the cranial third of the neck. See section on blood collection (Fig. 1–1) for location of this and other accessible veins.

Equipment

- alcohol-soaked gauze
- 18-, 19-, or 20-gauge, 1.5-inch needle
- syringe with medication

Procedure

- Clean site with an alcohol wipe until dirt is removed.
- Ideally, the syringe should be detached from the needle. While the vein is held off below the venipuncture site, align the needle directly over the vein, pointing against blood flow.
- Thrust the needle through the skin and into the vein. Blood fills the hub of the needle if the needle is in the vein. If blood is pulsing out of the needle, an artery may have been accidentally entered, and the needle must be redirected. Venipuncture is also commonly performed with the syringe and needle attached, but experience is required to ensure that medication is not accidentally administered into an artery.
- Once the needle has been properly placed, attach the syringe to the needle without changing the needle position. Always check correct placement of the needle by drawing back on the syringe and confirming a flashback of blood in the syringe before injecting the solution. Recheck the position of the needle between delivery of each 5 ml.
- Frequent and long-term administration of intravenous drugs requires an indwelling catheter to reduce trauma to the vein and increase patient cooperation. See intravenous catheter placement (p. 12).

Complications

CAUTION: Accidental **intra-arterial** injection is **life-threatening** with most substances. Using a large-bore needle and puncturing the vein with the needle detached increases the likelihood of detecting arterial puncture (Chapter 39).

Accidental delivery of a caustic substance (phenylbutazone, thiopental, and so on) outside of the vein can cause **necrosis** and **sloughing** of the surrounding skin.

Thrombosis and **infection** of the vein are uncommon. The risk increases with frequent venipuncture, especially if the medication is known to be irritating to the vessel lumen.

TOPICAL ADMINISTRATION

Medication may be placed topically on the skin, eyes, and mucous membranes and within body cavities (intravaginal, intrauterine, intracystic, intramammary, and intrarectal) for a direct local effect. Drugs meant for topical use are special preparations in ointments, creams, pastes, sprays, and powders. Possible systemic effects should be considered since many drugs are absorbed systemically. Certain oral medications (metronidazole/aspirin) may be made into solution and delivered per rectum in patients that are NPO.

RECTAL ADMINISTRATION

Used for drugs to produce local or systemic effects. Absorption is inconsistent but can be useful in patients unable to take medication by mouth (e.g., postoperatively).

Drugs can be suspended in 1–2 oz of water and introduced rectally by way of a soft feeding tube and 60-ml syringe.

TRANSDERMAL/CUTANEOUS ADMINISTRATION

Use of dosage form in which the drug is incorporated in a stick-on patch and applied to an area of thin skin is increasing in clinical practice—drugs include fentanyl, scopolamine, nitroglycerin, and estrogen.

INTRASYNOVIAL ADMINISTRATION

The decision to administer drugs intra-articularly should be made with consideration of the potential complications of altering the intra-articular environment. Direct intrasynovial administration naturally creates very high drug levels in a joint compared with the systemic route and is commonly used for therapy of degenerative joint disease and infectious arthritis. Medications to be injected intra-articularly should be carefully evaluated for their potential to cause irritation or inflammation. It is safest to use only drugs specifically labeled for intra-articular use. Certain acids or bases may be modified by the addition of a buffering solution before intrasynovial injection. Sites for intra-articular injection and the relevant anatomy are discussed in the section on intrasynovial anesthesia (p. 64).

INTRATHECAL ADMINISTRATION

This route of drug administration is used only to achieve direct spinal analgesia, perform myelography, or treat meningoencephalitis. Medication is placed directly into the subarachnoid space. See CSF collection for equipment needs, procedure, and potential complications (p. 86).

EPIDURAL ADMINISTRATION

Epidural drug administration is used for anesthesia for urogenital surgery and/or analgesia. Medications injected into the epidural space include local anesthetics (lidocaine, mepivacaine, and bupivacaine) and alpha$_2$-adrenergics (xylazine) and narcotics (morphine). The sacrococcygeal interspace or the first and second coccygeal interspaces (more common) are sites for epidural entry.

Equipment

- stocks for restraint
- twitch and/or sedation (detomidine/xylazine and butorphanol tartrate)
- clippers
- material for sterile scrub
- sterile gloves
- 2% local anesthetic, 5-ml syringe, and 22-gauge, 1-inch needle
- 18-gauge, 10.2-cm-thick walled Tuohy needle; 18-gauge Teflon epidur' catheter with stylet or 18-gauge 1½-inch needle
- 12-ml syringe (sterile)

Procedure

- Restrain horse in stocks. Sedate using xylazine, 0.2 to 1.1 mg/kg butorphanol, 0.01 to 0.1 mg/kg IV to effect.

- Clip and prepare aseptically an area over the first coccygeal interspace.
- The first coccygeal interspace (Co_1–Co_2) is the first palpable depression on the midline caudal to the sacrum.
- A bleb of 2% bupivacaine (Carbocaine) is injected subcutaneously to desensitize the skin.
- A stab incision is made through the skin to facilitate passage of the epidural needle. An 18-gauge (Periflex[3]) Tuohy needle is inserted on the midline into the interspace and directed cranially and ventrally at a 45° angle to the rump. Entry into the epidural space is confirmed by a loss of resistance to passage of the needle. Correct placement of the needle is confirmed by the ability to inject 5–10 ml of air without resistance.
- An 18-gauge, polyethylene epidural catheter (Accu-Bloc Periflex[3]) is threaded through the Tuohy needle into the epidural space and secured to the skin for repeated drug administration.
- If an 18-gauge 1½-inch hypodermic needle is used, a stab incision is not required.

Complications

Incomplete block due to congenital membranes, adhesions from previous epidural procedures, location of the epidural catheter or needle in the ventral epidural space, or escape of the epidural catheter tip through the intervertebral foramen.

---

[3]Burrow Accu-Bloc Periflex, 18-gauge polyethylene epidural catheter. Burrow Medical Inc., 824 Twelfth Avenue, Bethlehem, PA 18018; (800) 359-2439.

3 Intravenous Catheter Placement

James A. Orsini and Christine Kreuder

Intravenous catheters are placed for the administration of large volumes of fluids and/or frequent dosages of intravenous medications. The size and catheter-type required depend on its intended use. Large-gauge, 5-inch catheters (14-, 12-, or 10-gauge) are used to administer intravenous fluids rapidly in the adult. Bilateral jugular vein catheters may be used for rapid, large-volume fluid replacement in severely dehydrated patients. The large-bore catheters are more likely to cause thrombophlebitis, cellulitis, or both. A 16-gauge, 5-inch catheter may be used if IV access is required only for frequent dosing of medications. A 16-gauge, 5-inch catheter is also appropriate for foals. Catheters are available for short-term[1] and long-term[2] use. Short-term catheters may be left in for a maximum of 3 days, whereas long-term catheters may be maintained for up to 2 weeks. The jugular vein is most accessible for catheter placement. If the jugular vein cannot be used, the cephalic vein and lateral thoracic vein are also suitable for catheterization.

NOTE: The following technique applies to simple over-the-needle catheter placement. Guidewire catheters[3] are also available in longer length and for long-term use. Instructions for placement accompany the product.

Equipment

- material for a sterile scrub
- clippers
- sterile gloves
- appropriate over-the-needle catheter
- heparinized saline flush (2000 units of heparin in 500 ml of saline)
- 2-0 nonabsorbable suture
- rapid-acting glue (cyanoacrylate)
- 20- or 35-ml syringe and 18-gauge needle filled with heparinized saline flush
- extension set[4] filled with heparinized saline
- intermittent injection cap[5]
- Elasticon roll[6]

Procedure

- Choose an area in the cranial third of the jugular groove to place the catheter.
- Clip and/or shave the area to be surgically prepared.
- Perform a sterile scrub at the area to be catheterized and an area 10–15 cm below where the jugular vein is to be occluded.
- Fill extension set tubing with heparinized saline.
- Put on sterile gloves.
- Remove the protective sleeve on the catheter and loosen the cap on the stylet. The catheter should be touched at the **hub only.**
- Distend the jugular vein using three fingers in the jugular groove distal to the site to be catheterized.

---

[1]Abbocath-T radiopaque FEP Teflon IV catheter. Abbott Hospitals, Inc., North Chicago, IL 60064.

[2]Milacath polyurethane catheter-over-needle. MILA International, Inc., 510 West Sixth Street, Covington, KY 41011; (606) 261-6631.

[3]Guidewire catheters (14- or 16-gauge, 8-inch). Mila International, Inc., 510 West Sixth Street, Covington, KY 41011; (606) 261-6631. Single- and double-lumen styles available.

Central venous catheter (16-gauge, 8-inch). Arrow International, Inc., 3000 Bernville Road, Reading, PA 19605; (610) 378-0131.

[4]Extension set (7-inch or 30-inch). Abbott Laboratories, North Chicago, IL 60064.

Large animal extension set (large-bore, 7-inch). International Win, Ltd., 340 North Mill Road, Suite 6, Kennett Square, PA 19348; (800) 359-4946.

[5]Injection (along with Luer-Lok). Baxter Healthcare Corp., Deerfield, IL 60015.

[6]Elasticon. Johnson and Johnson Medical, Inc., Arlington, Texas 76004-3130.

- Angle the catheter so that it is parallel to the jugular groove and with the flow of blood in the vein.
- Puncture percutaneously at a 45° angle, and advance the catheter and stylet slowly until blood appears at the catheter hub. When it is in the vein, angle the catheter parallel to the jugular groove and advance the catheter and stylet 2 to 5 cm. Then separate the catheter and stylet and slide the catheter down the vein, holding the stylet in place. The catheter should advance without resistance. Remove the stylet.
- Attach the extension set tubing and injection cap.
- Use the syringe with flush to aspirate blood into the extension set to ensure the catheter is in the vein. Blood should flash back easily. Flush the catheter with heparinized saline.
- Use glue (cyanoacrylate) to anchor the catheter hub to the skin.
- Suture the catheter hub to the skin. Care should be taken not to kink the catheter or puncture the jugular vein. Suture the extension set to the skin in several places.
- The extension set may be left exposed for ease of inspection for catheter-associated problems or covered by a sterile dressing and an Elasticon bandage placed around the neck. To deliver fluids, remove the injection cap and attach the extension set to an intravenous administration set.[7]

CATHETER USE AND MAINTENANCE

Replace injection caps daily.

The injection port should be wiped with an alcohol swab prior to needle insertion.

All catheters need to be flushed with 5 to 7 ml of heparinized saline every 4 to 6 hours to prevent blood from clotting in the catheter.

Patency should be checked each time the catheter is flushed and before administration of any medications. Check patency by attaching a syringe filled with heparinized saline and aspirating to achieve a flashback of blood. Then slowly flush in 5 to 7 ml of heparin saline. Failure to achieve a flashback may be due to:

- blood clot in the catheter
- kinking of the catheter or extension set
- loose attachment of the injection cap or extension set

If no flashback is seen, gently flush 5 to 7 ml of heparinized saline into the catheter and then draw back. The catheter needs to be replaced if a flashback is not confirmed.

When administering medication through a catheter, choose an injection port close to the catheter. Clamp off any fluids that are flowing through the catheter. Check for a flashback, then inject 5 ml of heparinized saline before the first drug, between each drug, and after the last drug administered. Certain drugs precipitate when mixed (Chapter 39). Flushing between each drug prevents this complication. Drugs should be administered very slowly, at a rate no faster than

---

[7]Stat large animal IV set (large-bore, 10 feet long). International Win, Ltd., 340 North Mill Road, Suite 6, Kennett Square, PA 19348; (800) 359-4946.

1 ml per 5 seconds. Medications that are known to cause adverse systemic reactions should be administered slower and diluted in saline.

When replacing a catheter, use an alternate vein to minimize phlebitis. If possible, do not catheterize the same venipuncture site until it is healed. Use a long-term catheter if venous access is required for more than 6 days, to avoid trauma to the veins.

Complications

Thrombophlebitis, phlebitis, or **local cellulitis** is a common complication of long-term venous access (catheterization).

Examine the catheter site twice daily for swelling, heat, and pain. A small circle of reactive skin at the site of skin puncture is normal, but any thickening at this site and any associated heat or pain are abnormal and require immediate removal of the catheter. Phlebitis may also cause a fever and an increase or decrease in nucleated cell count.

Phlebitis is usually responsive to local therapy (hot packing, topical dimethyl sulfoxide [DMSO]) but must be monitored closely because complete occlusion of the vein with a septic thrombus, abscess formation, and secondary bacteremia or septicemia may require more aggressive treatment.

Embolization of the catheter may occur if the catheter is accidentally severed or breaks off. This is a very uncommon occurrence if the catheter is examined for holes and kinks and replaced as needed. Chest radiographs can be used to locate the catheter. Surgical retrieval may be necessary if it is in the jugular vein or heart. If in the lung, it usually does not cause a problem.

4 Intraosseous Infusion Technique

James A. Orsini and Christine Kreuder

Intraosseous infusion technique (IIT) is an alternative method for rapid delivery of fluids and medications in the neonatal intensive care patient when IV access is not possible. Access to the central circulation is via the intramedullary vessels in the bone marrow, which do not collapse because of the rigid bony shell that maintains the vascular space. The absorption rate of medications is similar to that of the IV route of administration. IIT has been used in human medicine for patients with cardiac arrest, hypovolemic shock, and circulatory collapse.

Equipment
- material for sterile scrub
- clippers

- sterile gloves
- sedation—xylazine and butorphanol
- local anesthesia—2% mepivacaine (Carbocaine)
- #15 scalpel blade
- #4 (28-mm) Steinmann pin and Jacobs chuck
- 12- or 14-gauge intraosseous needles/Sur-Fast Cook[1] intraosseous needle
- 14-gauge, 0.5-inch stainless steel needle
- heparinized saline
- crystalloid solution/lactated Ringer's solution
- sterile wrap

Procedure

- Sedate foal with xylazine (0.5–1.1 mg/kg IV) and butorphanol (0.01–0.04 mg/kg IV)
- Place foal in right or left lateral recumbency.
- Sterile preparation of intraosseous site on the tibia is the proximal medial one third of bone 3 cm distal to the tendinous (flat area devoid of vessels) band from the semitendinous muscle.
  - □ **CAUTION:** A branch of the saphenous vein crosses the tibia 2 cm distal to the infusion site. The nutrient foramen is 2–3 cm distal to the infusion site near the popliteal line in the center of the tibial shaft.
- Infiltrate skin, subcutaneous tissues, and periosteum with 2% mepivicaine (Carbocaine) over the intraosseous site.
- A small stab incision is made through the skin.
- A #4 Steinmann pin and Jacobs chuck are used to penetrate the tibial cortex by placing the pin at a 90° angle to the bone, using a downward pressing and twisting motion until a loss of resistance is felt.
- Confirm entry site into the medullary cavity by placement of a 14-gauge, 0.5-inch stainless steel needle and aspirate blood and/or marrow contents.
- Flush needle with 5 to 10 ml of heparinized saline.
- The intraosseous needle can be removed after infusion of a maximum of 1 liter of crystallized solution or secured in place. It should be heparinized every 4 to 6 hours to maintain patency.
- A sterile wrap should be placed over the intraosseous site to maintain sterility.

Complications

Subperiosteal or subcutaneous leakage of fluids, malposition of the intraosseous needle resulting in partial occlusion of the needle.

Tibial fractures due to poor needle placement.

Soft tissue swelling, cellulitis, and periosteal reactions are usually transient, lasting up to 60 days.

---

[1]Sur-fast. Cook Critical Care, Inc., Bloomington, Indiana 47401.

5 | Bacterial, Fungal, and Viral Infection Diagnoses

James A. Orsini and Christine Kreuder

Laboratory confirmation of an etiologic agent is often necessary when treating infectious diseases. Bacterial and fungal infections are difficult to distinguish, and bacterial culture and sensitivity results are essential for specific antibiotic therapy. A suspected pathogen may not be isolated owing to improper sample collection, handling procedures, weak virulence of a pathogen relative to the contaminants, and concurrent antibiotic therapy. To interpret results correctly, the clinician must have a working knowledge of the likely pathogens at a particular site, the normal flora associated with the site, common environmental contaminants, and the probability of an accurate laboratory identification. Patient history and physical examination must also be applied to laboratory result interpretation. All samples should be clearly labeled.

Equipment

- The equipment and techniques used for collection of synovial, peritoneal, cerebrospinal, and pleural fluids, transtracheal aspiration, and bronchoalveolar lavage samples are described as separate procedures elsewhere in this manual.

Bacterial Samples

NOTE: The collection and transport system depends on the bacteria suspected (aerobic vs. anaerobic). Anaerobic infection is frequently seen in peritonitis, pleuritis, osteomyelitis, adult pneumonia, and abscesses.

- Culturette collection and transport system[1] for aerobic or facultative anaerobic samples
- Port-A-Cul tube[2] for anaerobic samples
- blood culture bottle[3] for blood samples
- Gram stain and microscope slides

---

[1]Culturette collection and transport system. Becton-Dickinson Microbiology Systems, Cockeysville, MD 21030.
[2]Port-A-Cul tube. BBL Division of Becton-Dickinson, Cockeysville, MD 21030.
[3]Septi-check. BB blood culture bottle. Roche Diagnostic Systems, Nutley, NJ 07110-1199.

Fungal Samples

- sterile vial
- Gram stain and microscope slides

Viral Samples

- Culturette collection and transport system[1]
- viral transport medium[4]
- Vacutainer tubes;[5] plain (red top) and EDTA (purple top) for blood samples. Citrate or heparin tubes may be required for certain viral isolation tests; request information from the diagnostic laboratory.
- icepacks and Styrofoam container for transport

Procedure

Bacterial Samples

- Collect the sample, using sterile technique.
- Culture the site before debridement or manipulation.
- Ideally, the patient shall not have received antibiotic therapy for 24 hours before culture sampling.
- Swabs may be used to culture **abscesses, wounds, pustules,** or sites without fluid.
- Select an abscess or pustule that is intact and uncontaminated.
- Use a sterile #15 scalpel blade to incise the abscess.
- Select the appropriate swab depending on whether aerobic, anaerobic, or both cultures are desired.
- Moisten the swab with the transport media before collecting the sample. Many microbes are very susceptible to desiccation.
- Swab the wall of the abscess or pustule, since the center may be sterile. Culture the deepest, least contaminated part.
- Once the sample is collected, immediately place the swab in the transport media and seal the container. Obligate anaerobes do not survive more than 20 minutes in room air.
- If possible, aspirate fluid from abscesses or pustules using a sterile needle and syringe and submit it to the laboratory.
- Transport fluid samples of **exudate, transtracheal wash** and **BAL** (bronchoalveolar lavage) samples, **synovial fluid, cerebrospinal fluid, pleural fluid,** and **peritoneal fluid** in the syringe used for collection—see individual procedure for method of collection. Remove the air from the syringe and cap the syringe with a sterile needle. If anaerobes are suspected, bend the needle back on itself or place the sample into a Port-A-Cul tube. NOTE: Do **NOT** refrigerate Port-A-Cul samples for anaerobic cultures. Place sample in a blood culture bottle if the samples are not to be analyzed for more than 12 hours. This dilutes the antibacterial factors that naturally occur in these fluids.

---

[4]Viral transport medium is supplied by diagnostic laboratories upon request.
[5]Vacutainer tubes. Becton-Dickinson Vacutainer Systems, Rutherford, NJ 07070.

☐ **Urine** samples degrade rapidly. Transport the sample in a syringe or sterile vial and refrigerate. The sample does not last more than 2 days. See urinary tract catheterization procedure (p. 61) for method of collection. **Request colony counts on isolated organisms.**

☐ **Blood** samples (10 to 20 ml) should be placed directly into special blood culture bottles. Clip the hair and perform a sterile scrub at the venipuncture site. Use a syringe to aspirate the blood and change needles before injecting the blood into the culture bottle. Several cultures taken over a 24-hour period may be indicated if bacterial growth is not obtained initially and bacteremia is highly suspected. Polymerase chain reaction (PCR) testing for organisms in blood (e.g., *Ehrlichia risticii*) is best performed on EDTA samples.

☐ **Feces** may be collected into a clean container. Because the gastrointestinal tract has normal bacterial flora, request isolation of specific species only. If attempting to isolate *Salmonella* species, submit five separate cultures taken 12 hours apart and/or a single sample for PCR. If a delay in processing is expected, place the sample in an enrichment broth[6] for *Salmonella.*

☐ **Uterine** cultures may be collected using a sterile guarded swab[7] with a protective cap. Preferably, the mare is in estrus so the cervix is open. Wash the perineum with antiseptic solution and rinse with water. Use sterile gloves. Place a small amount of sterile lubricating jelly[8] on one hand and insert the gloved, lubricated hand into the vagina. Gently dilate the cervix with one finger and guide the swab into the cervix with the other hand. Once it is in the uterus, push the swab out through the protective cap, obtain a sample, and retract the swab into the guarded sleeve before removing it from the uterus. Break off the swab and place it in a Culturette transport system and moisten the sample.

■ Transport **solid tissue** samples in the smallest sterile container possible. Add sterile saline to the sample to prevent desiccation. Keep the sample refrigerated.

■ Routine samples taken at **necropsy** include lung, liver, lymph nodes, sections of GI tract, gross lesions, and organs suspected because of clinical signs. In individuals dead more than 4 hours, accurate samples cannot be obtained.

■ The sooner the samples are processed, the more accurate the results.

■ Laboratory results may require 3 to 6 days.

■ Use a separate swab to make a slide at the time of collection. Roll the swab onto the slide. Fluids should be spread in a thin layer on the slide; tissue samples should be compressed on the slide and removed to make an impression smear. Allow the slide to air dry, stain with Gram stain. Gram-positive bacteria stain blue or purple, and gram-negative bacteria stain pink or red. Assess bacterial morphology, reaction to Gram stain, relative numbers of each type of bacteria, inflammatory cells, and phagocytosis.

---

[6]Difco. BBL Division of Becton-Dickinson, Cockeysville, MD 21030.

[7]Double-guarded uterine swab. Hartford Veterinary Supply, 9100 Persimmon Tree Rd., Potomac, MD 20854.

[8]KY lubricating jelly. Johnson and Johnson Medical, Inc., Arlington, TX 76004-3130.

Fungal Samples

- Fungal samples are collected the same as bacterial samples. Use syringes and sterile containers for transport.
- **Skin** should be sampled by plucking hairs and performing a skin scrape of the suspected lesion. Use a #10 scalpel blade to scrape the skin at the lesion's edge. Mineral oil placed on the skin minimizes loss of the sample. Submit the hair, skin scrapings, and scalpel blade in a sterile vial.
- Expect laboratory results in 2 to 3 weeks.
- Gram stain should be used to look for evidence of a fungal infection (spores, hyphae, filamentous rows of coccoid cells). This is particularly important for suspected fungal keratitis (Chapter 31).

Viral Samples

- Viral samples should be taken as soon as viral disease is suspected because the highest yield is in the early stages of infection. Sample individuals that are in contact with the sick patient because they are likely to be in an earlier stage of infection.
- Contact the laboratory for information on sample sites, collection, and handling techniques for a specific virus. Also request viral transport media.
- Sites most affected by the infection should be sampled: mucosal vesicles, nasal secretions, transtracheal wash or BAL samples, feces, and so on. Use a moistened swab for sample collection. A fluid sample is preferred. Scraping or biopsy of the lesion is also appropriate.
- Place the sample in viral transport medium and refrigerate as soon as possible. If the sample will not be processed within 4 hours, freeze the specimen and ship in dry ice.
- **Blood** samples are useful since most infections have a viremic stage. Divide 12 to 20 ml of blood into plain Vacutainer tubes (for serum) and 10 ml into EDTA tubes. Do not freeze blood samples for shipment.
- Expect laboratory virus isolation results in 2 to 8 weeks. Fluorescent antibody testing, if available, may speed the diagnosis.
- Paired serum antibody titers may be used to confirm a laboratory diagnosis. Antibody titers should be taken 2–4 weeks apart: acute phase and convalescent phase. A fourfold increase in antibody titer is considered diagnostic of a recent exposure.

6 | Biopsy Techniques

James A. Orsini and Christine Kreuder

Tissue biopsy is often helpful in antemortem diagnosis of disease. The different procedures are sometimes invasive and are therefore used for treatment or prognosis purposes only. Biopsy techniques are discussed for the different tissues.

Note:

- Samples should be sent to a veterinary pathologist or specialist with the appropriate information.
- Biopsies should be less than 1 cm $\times$ 1 cm for proper formalin fixation.
- The formalin to tissue volume ratio is 10:1.
- Do not allow samples to freeze during transport.

SKIN BIOPSY

Skin biopsy is used in cases of undiagnosed skin disease because of treatment failure or persistent clinical signs. Biopsies should be performed early, within 3 weeks, because histopathology is difficult to interpret in chronic cases. Generally, a punch biopsy or a wedge biopsy (elliptical incision) is taken. Punch biopsies are preferred, unless sampling vesicular, bullous, or ulcerative lesions for which a wedge biopsy is more useful.

Equipment

- 6- or 8-mm cutaneous biopsy punch[1] or a #15 scalpel blade for wedge biopsy
- 2% local anesthetic, 25-gauge needle, and 3-ml syringe
- rat-toothed forceps
- Metzenbaum scissors
- needle holders
- sterile gauze sponges
- 2–0 absorbable suture
- 10% buffered formalin

Procedure

- Select areas representative of disease. A biopsy should include the lesion, point of transition, and normal skin.

---

[1]Baker's biopsy punch. Baker Cummins Pharmaceuticals, Inc., Miami, FL 33178; (800) 347-4474.

- Do not wash or scrub the intended sample, to prevent tissue architecture disruption.
- Infiltrate local anesthetic in the subcutaneous tissue beneath the area to be biopsied. Do not inject directly through the intended sample. Mark the area anesthetized.
- **Punch biopsy:** Select the site and rotate the biopsy punch while applying firm pressure until the instrument has cut through the dermis. Because the biopsy is adhered by subcutaneous fat, grasp it with forceps and sever with scissors.
- **Wedge biopsy:** Use a scalpel blade to make an elliptical skin incision and cut the subcutaneous fat with scissors to free the sample.
- **Be careful not to create tissue artifact.**
- Place the sample on a tongue depressor, subcutaneous fat side down, and immerse in formalin. The tongue depressor preserves sample architecture during transport. Michel medium is for immunofluorescence tests and is not a good preservative for histopathology.
- Close the wound with a simple interrupted or cruciate suture pattern. Large wedge biopsies require a two-layer closure.

Complications

Infection is rare; avoid biopsies over joint capsules or contaminated areas. If **dehiscence** occurs, clean daily. Healing is by second intention. *If a large wedge biopsy is in a high motion area, restrict exercise for 1 week to decrease chances of dehiscence.*

BIOPSY OF MASS, NODULE, AND CYST

Cutaneous masses, nodules, and cysts are sampled by aspiration or excisional biopsy. Fine needle aspiration yields a cellular sample and is differentiated cytologically as infectious, allergic, parasitic, or neoplastic. Excisional biopsy requires complete removal of a mass for treatment purposes. Histopathology is used to confirm a diagnosis.

Equipment

For fine needle aspiration:

- 20-gauge, 1- to 1½-inch needle and 20-ml syringe
- microscope slides

For excisional biopsy:

- material for sterile scrub
- 2% local anesthetic
- #10 blade and handle
- rat-toothed forceps
- Metzenbaum scissors
- needle holder and suture scissors
- sterile 4 × 4 gauze sponges
- container with 10% buffered formalin
- 1–0/2–0 absorbable suture

Procedure

Fine Needle Aspiration

- Insert the needle with attached syringe into the center of the mass.
- Aspirate sample material into the needle and not into the syringe barrel.
- Redirect the needle several times without leaving the mass or contaminating the aspirate with normal tissue. If blood contaminates the sample, repeat with a new needle and syringe. Release the negative pressure before withdrawing.
- To make a slide for cytology: disconnect the needle, fill the syringe with air, reattach the needle, and expel the needle contents onto a slide. The aspirate is smeared for blood, or compressed between two slides and pulled apart. Allow the slides to air dry.
- Aspiration of a fluid-filled mass or cyst is performed in a similar manner. Aspirate 1 to 2 ml of fluid and make a smear.
- Stain the slides with Wright or Diff-Quick stain. Send stained and unstained slides to pathologist.

Excisional Biopsy

- Perform a sterile scrub of the mass to be excised. Do not scrub if the surface is important for histologic interpretation.
- Inject local anesthetic into the subcutaneous tissue or use a ring block.
- Make an elliptical incision around the mass and undermine the subcutaneous tissue with scissors.
- Place the tissue in formalin. If the mass is greater than 1 cm, fillet it longitudinally into 1-cm-wide sections.
- Subcutaneous and skin layers are used for closure. A horizontal or vertical mattress pattern relieves tension.
- Restrict exercise to handwalking the patient for 7 to 10 days.

Complications

See earlier Skin Biopsy Complications.

LYMPH NODE ASPIRATE

Fine needle aspiration of enlarged or abnormal lymph nodes is adequate for cytology and can be helpful in differentiating infectious and neoplastic causes of lymphadenopathy. Complications are unusual.

Equipment

- 22-gauge, 1.5-inch needle
- 10-ml syringe
- microscope slides

Procedure

- Stabilize the lymph node with one hand and insert the needle with attached syringe into the center of the lymph node.

- See Fine Needle Aspiration for technique.
- Allow the slides to air dry. Stain slides with Diff-Quick. Send stained and unstained slides to a pathologist experienced in reading equine cytology, as the cytologic diagnosis of lymphosarcoma is difficult in the horse.

RENAL BIOPSY

Biopsy of the kidney is unusual because renal disease is well characterized by serum chemistry and renal function tests. Indications include renal masses and undiagnosed causes of renal failure. Percutaneous renal biopsy entails risk and is performed when the information is likely to affect the outcome. The right kidney is easily viewed by ultrasound, and biopsies should be performed with ultrasound guidance to obtain an accurate sample and decrease the potential for complications. The left kidney is biopsied during rectal palpation using a blind technique or via ultrasound guidance.

Equipment

- sedation (xylazine hydrochloride and butorphanol tartrate)
- 14-gauge, 6-inch biopsy needle[2]
- #15 scalpel blade
- clippers
- material for a sterile scrub
- sterile gloves
- 2% local anesthetic, 25-gauge needle, 3-ml syringe
- rectal sleeve for left kidney biopsy
- sterile sleeve and sterile lubricant for ultrasound guided biopsy of the right kidney
- 10% buffered formalin

Procedure

- Sedate patient to minimize motion during the procedure.

RIGHT KIDNEY ULTRASOUND-GUIDED BIOPSY:

- The right kidney is located between the 15th and 17th intercostal spaces ventral to the lumbar processes.
- Clip the hair over the area and perform a sterile scrub.
- Place the ultrasound transducer in a sterile sleeve and identify a site to sample away from the renal vessels.
- Inject local anesthetic subcutaneously at the site and repeat the sterile scrub.
- With sterile gloved hands, make a stab incision and advance the biopsy needle through the stab incision to the kidney.

---

[2]Tru-Cut biopsy needle. Baxter Healthcare Corp., Pharmaseal Division, Valencia, CA 91355-8900.

- A second person can perform the ultrasound during the biopsy. The needle appears as a hyperechoic line on the ultrasound screen.

NOTE: Be familiar with operation of the selected biopsy unit.
- Place the biopsy specimen in 10% formalin.

LEFT KIDNEY BIOPSY:

- The left kidney is more loosely attached to the abdominal wall and requires stabilization per rectum during the biopsy procedure. Stabilize the kidney per rectum so that it lies against the left flank. Select a percutaneous biopsy site against the flank.
- Skin preparation and biopsy technique are identical to that of the ultrasound-guided biopsy. The kidney must remain motionless during needle placement.

Complications

Infection and **peritonitis** occur if sterile technique is not maintained or if the rectum is perforated. *If rectal tissue or feed material is found, begin systemic antibiotic therapy.* Do not biopsy a suspected renal abscess because of the risk of infection.

Hemorrhage is a serious complication if the needle penetrates the renal artery or vein or one of the accessory arteries entering the caudal pole of the kidney. All patients should be closely monitored for several days using serial packed cell volume (PCV) and total protein (TP) determinations. *A clotting profile should be performed before the renal biopsy.*

Hematuria is not uncommon and generally resolves spontaneously.

LIVER BIOPSY

Percutaneous liver biopsy is a simple procedure indicated in patients with undiagnosed liver disease. Histopathology can often define the liver disease as infectious, toxic, or obstructive/congestive. NOTE: A specific diagnosis is made in a few diseases. Ultrasound should be used to ensure that the biopsy specimen is taken from an affected section of liver.

Equipment

- sedation (xylazine hydrochloride and butorphanol tartrate)
- 14-gauge, 6-inch biopsy needle
- #15 scalpel blade
- clippers
- sterile scrub
- 2% local anesthetic, 25-gauge needle and 3-ml syringe
- sterile gloves
- 10% buffered formalin

Procedure

- Using ultrasound, a portion of the liver is viewed between the 6th and 15th intercostal spaces of the right lower to upper abdomen, respectively. Clip the hair and select a section of liver for biopsy.

- Liver biopsy is performed "blindly" (without ultrasound) from the right 14th intercostal space in a line drawn from the point of the shoulder to the tuber coxae. Occasionally the liver cannot be seen on the right and it is necessary to biopsy the liver, under ultrasound guidance, on the left at the level of the elbow, just caudal to the diaphragm.
- Sedate the patient.
- Clip the hair and perform a sterile scrub at the selected site.
- Infiltrate local anesthetic subcutaneously and perform a second sterile scrub.
- With sterile gloved hands, make a stab incision, insert the biopsy needle into the incision, and advance it in a cranial and ventral direction.
NOTE: Know operation of the biopsy needle before using.
- Place the biopsy in 10% formalin.

Complications

Hemorrhage occurs if the liver disease is affecting the clotting profile. *Assess clotting time before biopsy.* Monitor all patients for signs of hemorrhage for 48 hours after the procedure.

Infection (cellulitis, peritonitis) is unlikely if sterile technique is maintained. Do not biopsy liver abscesses. *Accidental biopsy of the colon mandates antibiotic therapy.*

LUNG BIOPSY

Percutaneous biopsy of the lung is used in patients with diffuse lung disease if radiographs, ultrasound, and bronchoalveolar lavage fail to provide a diagnosis. The procedure is relatively safe and easy to perform.

Equipment

- sedation (xylazine hydrochloride)
- material for a sterile scrub
- clippers
- sterile gloves
- 2% local anesthetic, 22-gauge, 1.5-inch needle, 3-ml syringe
- #15 scalpel blade
- 14-gauge, 15-cm Tru-Cut biopsy needle
- 2–0 nonabsorbable suture on a straight needle
- 10% buffered formalin

Procedure

- Sedation depends on the temperament of the patient.
- The most common site for biopsy, when lung disease is diffuse, is the right 7th or 8th intercostal space. The needle should be placed approximately 8 cm above the level of the olecranon and at the cranial aspect of the rib to avoid the intercostal vessels.

- Clip the hair and perform a gross scrub.
- Infiltrate local anesthetic into the subcutaneous tissue and parietal pleura.
- Perform a sterile scrub at the site for needle puncture.
- With sterile gloved hands, make a stab incision through the skin and muscle.
- Advance the biopsy needle through the skin, muscle layer, and parietal pleura in a cranial and medial direction and continue during end inspiration for an additional 2 cm into lung parenchyma. NOTE: Be familiar with operation of the biopsy unit.
- Place the tissue in formalin.
- Close the skin incision using a simple cruciate pattern.

Complications

A small amount of air may leak into the thorax before suture placement and should not cause a problem. Hemoptysis may occur and is rarely a problem. Fatal tension pneumothorax rarely occurs following a lung biopsy (Chapter 31).

BONE MARROW BIOPSY

Bone marrow biopsy is a useful procedure to determine causes for changes in peripheral blood cell count or cell morphology. The finding of neoplastic or abnormal cells in the circulating blood is an indication for bone marrow biopsy. This procedure differentiates between primary hematopoietic disease (lymphosarcoma, multiple myeloma, myeloproliferative disease) and compensatory marrow changes (iron deficiency anemia, anemia of chronic disease). Bone marrow is analyzed by core aspirate or biopsy. A complete blood count (CBC) drawn at the time of biopsy should be sent with the sample.

Equipment

- sedation (xylazine hydrochloride and butorphanol tartrate)
- material for a sterile scrub
- clippers
- sterile gloves
- 2% local anesthetic, 25-gauge needle, and 3-ml syringe
- #15 scalpel blade
- 15-gauge, 2-inch bone marrow needle[3] for marrow aspirate, or 11-gauge, 4-inch bone marrow needle for marrow biopsy
- 12-ml Luer-Lok syringe with anticoagulant (10% disodium EDTA), Petri dish, and microscope slides if performing an aspirate
- 10% buffered formalin if submitting a biopsy specimen

Procedure

- The sternebrae are most commonly used. The marrow cavity lies just below the periosteum. The tuber coxae is also accessible and is used in individuals less than 4 years of age.

---

[3]Jamshidi disposable bone marrow biopsy/aspiration needle. Baxter Healthcare Corporation, Deerfield, IL 60015.

- Sedation is recommended.
- Infiltrate local anesthetic into the subcutaneous tissue and periosteum.
- Clip the hair and perform a sterile scrub.
- With sterile gloved hands, make a small stab incision.

FOR BONE MARROW ASPIRATE:

- Insert the needle and stylet through the skin and advance to the periosteum. A rotational motion is needed to advance the needle through the cortex and into the marrow cavity.
- Remove the stylet and attach the syringe. Aspirate the bone marrow with negative pressure on the plunger, using short, gentle aspirates. Excessive negative pressure results in contamination with blood.
- Place the sample in a Petri dish and remove the marrow spicules and place them on a microscope slide. A squash smear is made by placing one slide on top of the other and gently pulling apart. Send both stained (Diff-Quick) and unstained slides to the laboratory.

FOR BONE MARROW BIOPSY:

- Insert the biopsy needle through the skin and advance to the cortex with a forceful rotational movement.
- The stylet is removed and the needle is advanced 2 cm.
- A rotational thrust of the needle should detach the specimen; withdraw the needle.
- Use the stylet to push the biopsy out of the needle and into a container with formalin.

Complications

Hemorrhage may occur and is rarely clinically significant unless the patient has thrombocytopenia or another clotting deficiency.

Osteomyelitis is rare.

MUSCLE BIOPSY

Histopathology of muscle samples is useful whenever disease of muscle fibers, neuromuscular junctions, or peripheral nerves is suspected. This is a minor surgical procedure performed in the standing horse. Samples of diseased and normal muscle should be collected. If polysaccharide storage myopathy is suspected, a biopsy of the semimembranosus is required. For motor neuron disease the muscle at the tail head (sacrocaudalis dorsalis medialis) is biopsied.

NOTE: Formalin may not be the preservative of choice, depending on the desired analysis. Contact the pathology laboratory before performing a muscle biopsy for the appropriate preservative.

Equipment

- material for sterile scrub
- clippers
- sterile gloves
- 2% local anesthetic, 25-gauge needle, and 5-ml syringe

- #10 scalpel blade and handle
- Metzenbaum scissors
- tongue depressor
- 0 or 2–0 absorbable and nonabsorbable suture material
- appropriate fixative

Procedure

- Sedation depending on temperament and state of debilitation of patient.
- The sample should be approximately 5 mm wide, 20 mm long, and 5 mm thick and should be longitudinal to the direction of the diseased muscle fibers.
- Clip hair and perform a gross scrub at the biopsy site.
- Infiltrate local anesthetic into the subcutaneous tissue. Do not inject anesthetic into the muscle; this affects histopathology.
- Perform a sterile scrub.
- With sterile gloved hands, incise the skin over the muscle belly. Use blunt dissection to separate the skin from the muscle belly. Remove a muscle sample, using sharp dissection.
- Secure the sample to a tongue depressor with stay sutures to prevent sample shrinkage.
- Suture the incision in two layers, minimizing dead space.

Complications

Infection is uncommon.

ENDOMETRIAL BIOPSY

Endometrial biopsy is a useful tool to evaluate infertility. NOTE: Rule out pregnancy before biopsy to avoid accidental abortion. The procedure is best performed during estrus.

Equipment

- sedation (xylazine hydrochloride and butorphanol tartrate)
- scrub material
- sterile sleeve (shoulder length)
- sterile lubricant[4]
- 70-cm alligator punch[5] (sterile)
- Bouin fixative

Procedure

- Sedation is recommended, with the mare restrained in stocks with a twitch.
- Tie the mare's tail to the side.

---

[4]KY lubricating jelly. Johnson and Johnson Medical, Inc., Arlington, Texas 76004-3130.

[5]Jackson uterine biopsy forceps. Jorgensen Laboratories, Inc., 1450 North Van Buren Ave., Loveland, CO 80538; (970) 669-2500.

- Scrub the perineum with a dilute antiseptic solution (povidone-iodine or chlorhexidine) and rinse with water.
- With sterile gloved arm, digitally dilate the cervix and gently guide the biopsy instrument through the cervix.
- Advance the biopsy instrument into the uterus and with the gloved arm in the rectum, confirm instrument placement.
- Per rectum, depress a portion of the uterine mucosa between the jaws of the biopsy instrument and obtain sample.
- Place sample in fixative and process within 24 hours.

Complications

Abortion if the mare is pregnant at the time of biopsy. *Perform a complete reproductive examination before biopsy.* The cervix should be closed if the mare is pregnant.

   Endometritis if bacterial pathogens are introduced into the uterus.

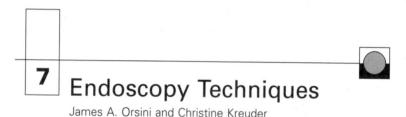

7 Endoscopy Techniques

James A. Orsini and Christine Kreuder

Endoscopy is now performed routinely in equine practice and has become an extremely valuable tool. Endoscopy permits direct examination of the upper and lower airway, esophagus, stomach, duodenum, urethra, and bladder. This procedure may be used to clarify disorders found on radiographic and ultrasound examination and to find lesions that are not detectable by other methods. Samples (biopsies and aspirates) may be obtained transendoscopically for culture, cytology, and histopathology. Regardless of the system examined, endoscopic examination should be performed systematically. A thorough knowledge of the applied anatomy is necessary to "drive" the endoscope and to differentiate normal from abnormal.

   Many of the flexible endoscopes used in equine practice have been designed for use in humans. Flexible endoscopes are either fiberoptic endoscopes or videoendoscopes. Both are easily adapted for procedures in horses. The fiberoptic endoscope is portable and considerably less expensive but produces inferior image quality. The image is viewed through an eyepiece on the endoscope, allowing only one person to view the examination unless adapted for a teaching head. The videoendoscope has excellent image quality that is projected onto a monitor. The examination can be seen by all and can be recorded. The unit is generally not suited for field use because it is not portable. Endoscopes should have a biopsy channel and a system for air and water delivery. The size of the endoscope required depends on the anatomic site examined and the size of the patient. This is addressed under endoscopic examination of each system.

Equipment

- appropriately sized flexible endoscope
  - □ flexible fiberoptic endoscope[1]
  - □ videoendoscope[2]
- saline bowl with warm water
- biopsy forceps, grasping forceps, polypectomy snares, and polyethylene tubing are accessories available with each unit
- 30-ml syringe for transendoscopic aspirates

General Procedure

- Two to three people are required to perform the scopic examinations.
- Sedation and/or a twitch may be needed depending on the patient, and system examined. The patient is best restrained in stocks or in a stall.
- Set up the endoscope to minimize danger to the operators, patient, and equipment.
- Familiarity with the mechanics of the endoscope is necessary. Practice manipulating the tip in all directions and administering air and water by operating the handpiece. Typically, the red button delivers air and the blue button delivers water.
- Lubricate the endoscope with warm water or a small amount of sterile lubricating jelly[3] (avoid the tip of the endoscope).
- Passage of the endoscope is described separately for each system.
- Water delivered to the tip of the endoscope cleans the lens. Air is delivered to dilate collapsed lumens and improve visibility.
- Biopsies are performed by advancing the biopsy instrument through the biopsy channel until it protrudes 2 to 3 cm beyond the tip of the endoscope. Manipulate the instrument to obtain a sample, then withdraw. Place the specimen in appropriate fixative.
- A transendoscopic **aspirate** is performed by passing sterile polyethylene tubing through the biopsy channel until it protrudes 2 to 3 cm beyond the tip of the endoscope. Aspirate a sample using a 30-ml syringe. Administering sterile saline may facilitate aspiration. Place the sample directly onto slides or into an EDTA Vacutainer tube.
- The endoscope should be cleaned with antiseptic solution and rinsed after each use.

ENDOSCOPIC EXAMINATION OF THE AIRWAY

Endoscopy of the airway is indicated in patients with nasal discharge, epistaxis, coughing, dyspnea, dysphagia, facial asymmetry, respiratory noise, or exercise intolerance. This is the method of choice for diagnosing ethmoid hematomas,

---

[1]Flexible fiberoptic endoscopes: 11-mm outer diameter, 100-cm long, 12-mm outer diameter, 160-cm long, and 8-mm outer diameter, 150-cm long. Karl Storz Veterinary Endoscopy—America, Inc., 175 Cremona Drive, Goleta, CA 93117; (800) 955-7832.

[2]Flexible videoendoscopes: GIF 130 gastroscope (9.8-mm outer diameter, 200- or 300-cm long), SIF 100 (11.2-mm outer diameter, 300-cm long), and CF 100 TL (12.9-mm outer diameter, 200- or 300-cm long). Available by special order from Olympus America Inc., 2 Corporate Center Drive, Melville, NY 11747; (516) 844-5000.

[3]KY lubricating jelly. Johnson and Johnson Medical, Inc., Arlington, TX 76004-3130.

laryngeal hemiplegia, epiglottic entrapment, dorsal displacement of the soft palate (DDSP), guttural pouch empyema and mycoses, exercise-induced pulmonary hemorrhage (EIPH), and tracheal trauma or stricture. This procedure may also aid in the diagnoses of paranasal sinusitis and pulmonary infection or abscess.

- The endoscope should be 150 to 200 cm in length and 9 mm in diameter for examination of the lower airway; a 9-mm-diameter unit is the largest that can be safely passed in a foal.
- Do not sedate the patient, if possible, because sedation may affect the function of the pharynx and the larynx. Sedation is recommended for examination of the lower airway to reduce coughing.
- Pass the endoscope into a nostril and systematically evaluate the upper airway structures, taking care not to traumatize the ethmoid turbinates. Maintain visibility during the entire examination. The trachea is entered by passing the scope between the arytenoid cartilages. Tracheal rings will be evident if the scope has been properly placed. Note any abnormal discharge, mucosal inflammation, cysts, or masses.

CAUTION: The scope can retroflex in the pharynx and enter the oral cavity, causing damage to the instrument. Ensure an unobstructed view to prevent this problem.

- Pass the endoscope into the pharynx through either nostril.
- The nasomaxillary opening is located in the caudal middle meatus and can be reached with a 9-mm-diameter scope. Drainage from the paranasal sinuses into the middle meatus may be seen in cases of sinusitis.
- Entering the guttural pouch is aided by using a biopsy instrument or brush as a guide and/or can be performed by passing a Chambers catheter up the opposite nostril and "flipping" open the opposite pouch opening.
- Spray the trachea with 4 to 6 ml of sterile 2% lidocaine through the biopsy channel to decrease coughing if the lower respiratory tract is examined.

ENDOSCOPIC EXAMINATION OF THE GASTROINTESTINAL TRACT

Endoscopy permits examination of the esophagus, stomach, duodenum, rectum, and distal small colon and is the method of choice to confirm gastric and duodenal ulceration.

- The endoscope must be 225–300 cm long to examine fully the stomach and duodenum in adults. A 200-cm endoscope is the minimal length permitting a superficial examination of the stomach in an adult.
- Adults should be fasted for 12 to 24 hours before gastroscopy and weanling foals fasted for 6 to 12 hours. If examining the duodenum, longer fasting periods may be required (24 to 48 hours for adults). Do not fast nursing foals.
- Sedation is generally required.
- See Nasogastric Tube Placement (p. 53) for passage of the endoscope into the esophagus. Confirm entry into the esophagus to prevent damage to the endoscope.
- To prevent damage to the endoscope, a short nasogastric tube may be passed into the proximal esophagus and used as a cannula.

- Insufflation assists passage and examination of the esophagus, cardiac sphincter, and stomach.

ENDOSCOPIC EXAMINATION OF THE URINARY TRACT

- The endoscope should be at least 100 cm in length and 9 mm or less in diameter to examine the urethra and bladder.
- The procedure must be performed using aseptic technique.
- Cold-sterilize the endoscope in Cidex for 30 minutes. Flush the biopsy channel.
- Sedation is recommended in stallions and geldings. Administer 0.4–0.6 mg/kg xylazine, 0.01 mg/kg butorphanol, and 0.02 mg/kg acepromazine (geldings only) IV for restraint and relaxation.
- Perform a sterile scrub of the distal penis and external urethral process, catheterize the bladder, and evacuate the urine. See Urinary Tract Catheterization (p. 61).
- Using sterile gloves, lubricate the length of the endoscope, avoiding the tip.
- Advance the endoscope, using the same technique as for catheterization of the bladder.
- Systematically evaluate the urethra and the bladder, using insufflation to enhance visibility. Insufflation normally causes the urethral vessels to appear engorged.

PART II

Respiratory System

8 | Nasotracheal and Orotracheal Tube Placement

James A. Orsini and Christine Kreuder

Establishing an airway is the first step for a patient exhibiting respiratory distress (cyanotic mucous membranes, respiratory stridor, apnea). Intubation is the most rapid and least invasive method and is performed via the nose or mouth. Tracheotomy is used in those patients with obstruction of the upper airway. Nasotracheal intubation is preferred to orotracheal intubation because it can be performed in the conscious horse and the tube left in place indefinitely, whereas general anesthesia is required for orotracheal intubation. In the anesthetized patient, orotracheal intubation is preferred because a larger endotracheal tube can be used for oxygen supplementation (p. 40) or assisted ventilation (p. 41).

NASOTRACHEAL INTUBATION

Equipment

- sedation (xylazine hydrochloride and butorphanol tartrate)
- appropriately sized nasotracheal tube: adults: 11- to 14-mm internal diameter;[1] foals: 7- to 12-mm internal diameter[2]
- lubricating jelly[3] or warm water
- white tape
- 20-ml syringe

Procedure

- Sedation may be required in the adult. Sedation is generally unnecessary in foals. Suggested adult (physiologically stable) dose: 0.3 mg/kg xylazine and 0.01 mg/kg butorphanol IV. **CAUTION:** Sedation and/or tran-

---

[1]Cuffed endotracheal tubes. Cook Veterinary Products, 127 South Main Street, P.O. Box 266, Spencer, IN 47460; (800) 826-2380.

[2]Cuffed foal nasotracheal tubes. Cook Veterinary Products, 127 South Main Street, P.O. Box 266, Spencer, IN 47460; (800) 826-2380.

[3]KY lubricating jelly. Johnson and Johnson Medical, Inc., Arlington, TX 76004-3130.

quilization in a dyspneic patient may lead to cardiopulmonary depression, increased upper airway resistance, and apnea.

- Lubricate the tube sparingly or place in warm water.
- Reflect the alar fold of the nostril and insert the tube medially along the ventral nasal meatus.
- Extend and elevate the head to permit easier access to the trachea and prevent the tube from being swallowed.
- Advance the tube into the pharynx. DO NOT USE FORCE. If resistance is encountered, rotate and advance. If still meeting resistance, use a smaller-diameter tube.
- Air flow through the tube is confirmed if the tube is correctly placed.
- Use an air-filled syringe to inflate the cuff to the point at which air cannot escape around the tube. **CAUTION:** Do not inflate the cuff past the point where resistance is first encountered.
- Secure the tube by placing tape around the tube end and tying it to the horse's halter.

OROTRACHEAL INTUBATION

Equipment

- drugs for general anesthesia (xylazine hydrochloride and ketamine for adults, diazepam and ketamine for physiologically stable foals)
- appropriately sized orotracheal tube with inflatable cuff[4]
  - ☐ adults: 18- to 28-mm internal diameter
  - ☐ foals: 8- to 11-mm internal diameter
- oral speculum PVC pipe, 5-cm diameter, 4–5 cm long, wrapped with white tape
- lubricating jelly[5]
- 20- or 30-ml syringe, not-Luer-Lok

Procedure

- General anesthesia should be induced if the patient is fully conscious. Recommended dose for adults: 1 mg/kg xylazine IV for sedation, followed by 2 mg/kg ketamine IV. Recommended dose for foals: 0.1 mg/kg diazepam IV **slowly** for sedation, followed by 1 mg/kg ketamine IV **slowly** (p. 42).
  CAUTION: Intubate **as soon as** the patient is recumbent. Equipment for cardiopulmonary resuscitation should be available.
- Dorsiflex the head and pull the tongue out through the interdental space.
- Place the speculum between the lower and upper incisors.
- Sparingly lubricate the endotracheal tube.
- Advance the tube through the center of the speculum. If resistance is encountered, rotate and advance gently. If the patient repeatedly swallows, administer 0.1 mg/kg doses of ketamine IV until swallowing stops; allow 2–3 minutes for effect.

---

[4]Cuffed endotracheal tubes. Cook Veterinary Products, 127 South Main Street, P.O. Box 266, Spencer, IN 47460; (800) 826-2380.

[5]KY lubricating jelly. Johnson and Johnson Medical, Inc., Arlington, TX 76004-3130.

- Air moving through the tube helps confirm placement. The tube should not be palpable in the proximal cervical area.
- Using a 20-ml syringe, inflate the cuff until resistance is encountered.
- General anesthesia is maintained while the orotracheal tube is in place.

Complications

Overinflation of the endotracheal tube cuff can cause **pressure necrosis** of the tracheal mucosa and sloughing. In the most severe cases, tracheal stenosis may result. *Do not inflate the cuff beyond the point where resistance is first met.*

An excessively long tube may terminate in a main stem bronchus with ventilation of only a portion of the pulmonary tree.

Hemorrhage from trauma to nasal mucosa occurs commonly during nasotracheal intubation. Generally, this is clinically insignificant.

9 Transtracheal Aspiration and Bronchoalveolar Lavage

James A. Orsini and Christine Kreuder

TRANSTRACHEAL ASPIRATION

Transtracheal aspiration is a simple, commonly used technique for assessing disease in the lower respiratory tract. The fluid obtained from aspiration is a mixture of secretions and cellular material that has collected in the distal trachea. Cytology of the aspirate determines the type and severity of inflammation and the level of the respiratory tract involved. The upper respiratory tract is host to a large bacterial population, and cultures taken from the nares or guttural pouch are very difficult to interpret. Transtracheal aspiration bypasses the upper respiratory tract and is the best method for obtaining an adequate sample for culture. Tracheal aspirates may also be retrieved through a flexible fiberoptic endoscope biopsy channel, and several protected culture swabs are available to decrease the likelihood of contamination from the pharynx or endoscope. Cultures are reasonably accurate and use of an endoscope allows the clinician to see the area sampled and avoids complications from tracheal puncture.

Equipment

- twitch (sedation is usually unnecessary unless the patient is very young, difficult to restrain, or coughs excessively during the procedure; xylazine hydrochloride (0.3–0.5 mg/kg) with butorphanol tartrate (0.01 mg/kg) IV is recommended for restraint and as a cough suppressant)
- clippers
- material for sterile scrub
- sterile gloves
- 16-gauge through-the-needle catheter[1] with or without a 7-inch extension set[2]
- 60-ml syringe (sterile)
- alternatively, a 12-gauge nondisposable needle and a 5 Fr. polyethylene tubing may be used
- 100-ml sterile 0.9% saline without bacteriostatic agent
- plain and EDTA Vacutainer tubes[3]
- Port-a-Cul culture system[4]

Procedure

- Clip and sterilely prepare a 10-square-cm area on the ventral midline of the middle third of the trachea.
- The trachea should be palpated with sterile gloves and stabilized with one hand.
- The cannula bevel should face downward with the catheter placed through the skin and **between tracheal rings** into the tracheal lumen (Fig. 9–1).
- Feed the catheter down the trachea to the thoracic inlet and remove the stylet. Coughing may cause the catheter to retroflex into the pharynx and become contaminated.
- Attach the syringe and rapidly inject 20–30 ml of sterile saline.
- Aspirate fluid back into the syringe; only a portion of the fluid instilled is retrievable.
- If the sample is inadequate, inject another aliquot of fluid. Do not inject more than 100 ml total. Reposition or slowly withdraw the catheter to assist aspiration.
- Carefully withdraw the catheter after obtaining the sample.
- If the sample appears purulent, infiltrate a local antibiotic subcutaneously at the puncture site. Apply a sterile dressing for 24 hours.

Complications

Catheter laceration and loss into airway. Almost always coughed out within 30 minutes.

Subcutaneous **abscess** or **cellulitis** at site of needle puncture. In severe cases, infection may extend to mediastinum. *Administer systemic antimicrobial*

---

[1]Intracath intravenous catheter placement unit. Deseret Medical, Inc., Becton-Dickinson and Company, Sandy, UT 84070.

[2]7-inch or 30-inch extension set. Abbott Laboratories, North Chicago, IL 60064.

[3]Vacutainer, Becton-Dickinson Vacutainer Systems, Rutherford, NJ 07070.

[4]Port-a-Cul, Becton-Dickinson Microbiology Systems, Cockeysville, MD 21030.

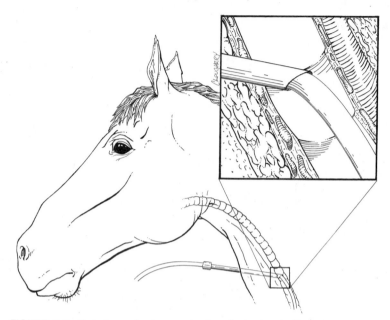

FIGURE 9–1. Techniques for transtracheal aspiration/wash. Through the needle catheter is placed between tracheal rings.

therapy. Hot pack and paint DMSO over the infected site. If needed, incise for drainage.

Subcutaneous **emphysema** around the trachea is common and may result in **pneumomediastinum.** It is rarely a problem unless the individual is in respiratory distress.

Damage to the tracheal rings may result in **chondritis** or **chondroma** formation. **Stenosis** of the tracheal lumen would be the most severe sequela.

BRONCHOALVEOLAR LAVAGE

Bronchoalveolar lavage (BAL) samples the terminal airway and associated alveoli and is an excellent method for evaluating pathology in the most distal portion of the respiratory tract. Since only a limited section of lung may be evaluated and the sample is generally not as suitable for culture, BAL should be performed as an adjunct to transtracheal aspiration. It may be done blind or with endoscopic guidance.

Equipment

- sedation (xylazine hydrochloride and butorphanol tartrate)
- 3-meter BAL catheter[5] **or** 2–3-meter, 9-mm-diameter flexible fiberoptic endoscope[6]

---

[5]Darien microbiological aspiration catheter. Mill-Rose Labs, Inc., 7310 Corporate Boulevard, Mentor, OH 44060; (216) 255-7995.

[6]GIF 130 gastroscope (2 or 3 meters long, 9.8 mm outer diameter). Olympus America Inc., 2 Corporate Center Drive, Melville, NY 11747; (516) 844-5000.

- 2% mepivacaine (Carbocaine) hydrochloride
- sterile 60-ml syringe
- 300-ml sterile 0.9% saline without bacteriostatic agent; warm to body temperature
- plain and EDTA Vacutainer tubes

Procedure

- Sedation is generally required. Recommended doses: 0.4–0.6 mg/kg xylazine with 0.01 mg/kg butorphanol IV.
- If using a BAL catheter, extend the head and gently pass the catheter through the nose and into a terminal airway. Wedge the catheter into the bronchus of a lower lung lobe. The main disadvantage to this procedure is that the location of the catheter is not specifically known.

If using an endoscope, clean the biopsy channel of the endoscope with antiseptic solution and rinse with sterile water. Pass the endoscope (see Endoscopic Examination of the Airway, p. 30) and gently wedge it into the smallest-diameter bronchus.

Infuse 50-ml aliquots of sterile saline until an adequate sample is aspirated. Do not infuse more than 300 ml.

May need to heavily sedate or infuse 5 ml of dilute mepivacaine if excessive coughing occurs.

Place sample into an EDTA Vacutainer tube (purple top) for cytologic analysis.

RESPIRATORY FLUID ANALYSIS

A direct smear of the fluid can be made if the sample appears cellular; otherwise the sample is centrifuged and the centrifugate placed on a glass slide. The slide prep may be air dried and stained with Wright stain. Cytology should include a differential cell count, degenerative status of the cells, and an assessment of a bacterial component. Total cell counts are not meaningful because the density of the cell population varies with the amount of saline retrieved. The differential cell count should be determined, although the aspiration reflects only a small segment of the pulmonary tree in both transtracheal aspiration and bronchoalveolar lavage. A normal BAL, in particular, does not rule out lung disease, as a normal section of lung may accidentally be lavaged.

A normal aspirate contains strands of mucus; columnar epithelial cells and pulmonary alveolar macrophages are the predominant cell types. Lymphocytes may account for 40% of the population in a BAL sample. Neutrophils and eosinophils are normally less than 5% of the differential. A few degenerate neutrophils are normal. Increased numbers of nondegenerate neutrophils are common in chronic obstructive pulmonary disease (COPD), while a large population of degenerate, toxic neutrophils is seen with septic bronchitis or pneumonia. An infectious process is supported by the presence of intracellular bacteria. Squamous epithelial cells, usually seen in rafts or rolled into a cigar shape, indicate either pharyngeal contamination or metaplasia in the lower respiratory tract from chronic irritation or inflammation. Curschmann spirals are coiled mucous plugs from terminal airways, sometimes indicating chronic inflammation. Pulmonary hemorrhage is detected by finding hemosiderin-laden alveolar macrophages. Free bacteria and fungal elements are common in normal samples. For a morphologic description of cell types and their role in disease processes, see Beech (1991).

The transtracheal aspirate should be submitted for aerobic and anaerobic culture. Gram stain is useful in determining antibiotic therapy while awaiting culture results. The significance of the results should be interpreted in conjunction with cytology, since contamination is always a possibility and the normal trachea may contain bacteria.

REFERENCES

Beech J. Equine Respiratory Disorders. Philadelphia, Lea & Febiger, 1991.

Darien BJ, Brown CM, Walker RD, Williams MA, Derkson FJ. A tracheoscopic technique for obtaining uncontaminated lower airway secretions for bacterial culture in the horse. Equine Vet J 1990; 22(3):170–173.

Sweeney CR, Sweeney RW, Benson CE. Comparison of bacteria isolated from specimens obtained by use of endoscopic guarded tracheal swabbing and percutaneous tracheal aspiration in the horse. J Am Vet Med Assoc 1989; 195(9):1225–1229.

10 Nasal Oxygen Insufflation

James A. Orsini and Christine Kreuder

Oxygen administration is more frequently used in the neonatal foal than in the adult horse but is therapeutic for both. Supplementation of oxygen should be based on clinical signs and blood gas analysis. Hypoxia is suspected in patients with pneumonia, neonatal isoerythrolysis, marked blood loss, obstructive pulmonary disease, hypoventilation, and recumbency-associated ventilation/perfusion mismatch. Nasal oxygen insufflation is beneficial in all patients undergoing general anesthesia. Increasing the concentration of oxygen in the inspired air will increase blood PaO_2 levels. Individuals with severe parenchymal involvement may not respond to nasal oxygen administration.

Equipment

- oxygen source (high-pressure oxygen cylinder[1])
- oxygen flowmeter/humidifier[2] (humidifier should be filled with sterile water)

---

[1]High-pressure oxygen cylinder (size E is small and portable). Oxygen supply service is available through local health care companies. Reusable oxygen cylinders are provided.

[2]Flowmeter/humidifier. Breathing Services, Inc., P.O. Box 817, 931 E. Main Street, Ephrata, PA 17522; (800) 732-0028.

- oxygen tubing (2 to 4 meters) to extend from the flowmeter to the patient
- nasal catheter[3]
- 1-inch white tape
- examination gloves
- 2–0 nonabsorbable suture on a straight needle

Procedure

- Attach the humidifier to the flowmeter on the oxygen source.
- Connect the nasal catheter to the oxygen tubing, then connect the oxygen tubing to the humidifier.
- Using the nasal catheter, measure the distance between the nostril and the medial canthus of the eye. This is the approximate distance to the nasopharynx.
- Reflect one nostril and place the catheter along the ventral meatus (the most ventral and medial portion of the nasal passage) and into the nasopharynx.
- Place a butterfly square of tape around the tubing (about 6 cm from the nostril), then reflect the tubing around and suture the tape to the nostril. Gloves are optional but recommended when handling suture material. Tubing may need to be sutured in several places.
- Set the flow of oxygen between 5 and 15 liters per minute, depending on the size and needs of the animal.
- Check the setup frequently (every 2 hours) to ensure tube patency. Replace the nasal catheter daily.

NOTE: This may only increase FiO_2 to $\pm 30\%$. Two catheters and 2 lines may result in an additional increase to $\pm 40\%$.

---

[3]Nasal catheter "Levin tubes" 235200-160. Rusch, Inc., Duluth, GA 30136; (800) 553-5214/50.

11 Assisted Ventilation

James A. Orsini and Christine Kreuder

Assisted ventilation is used in patients with apnea, hypoventilation, or respiratory distress not corrected by placement of an endotracheal tube and oxygen supplementation. Clinical disorders inducing hypoventilation include foal maladjustment syndromes, respiratory disease resulting in decompensation, thoracic injury or disease, diaphragmatic herniation, and botulism. Persistent cyanotic mucous membranes and dyspnea or an arterial pCO_2 greater than 60 mm Hg are strong clinical indicators of hypoventilation and tissue hypoxia. Short-term ventilation is relatively easy, whereas long-term ventilation is expensive and labor intensive, requiring 24-hour nursing care and sophisticated equipment.

NOTE: Unless the patient is semiconscious or unconscious, **general anesthesia** is needed before assisted ventilation. Assisted ventilation can be performed in the standing patient but is not well tolerated. **Endotracheal intubation** (or tracheotomy) must be performed before attempting to ventilate. Placement of a cuffed, wide-diameter orotracheal tube is preferred (see p. 34).

Equipment

- oxygen cylinder[1] with a regulator[2] having a flowmeter and a DISS fitting for a demand valve (small "E" cylinder is portable)
- regulator for E cylinder with BOTH a flowmeter giving 1, 2, 4, 6, 10, 15, and 25 LPM and a DISS connection for a demand valve
- one of the following methods for delivering positive pressure ventilation:
  - ☐ oxygen demand valve[3]
  - ☐ Ambu bag with an adapter for oxygen insufflation[4] (for foals only)
  - ☐ appropriately sized nasogastric tube if the Ambu bag, or an endotracheal tube, is not available

Procedure

- The patient should be intubated and the cuff of the endotracheal tube inflated (p. 34).

Ventilation with a Demand Valve

- Attach the demand valve to the oxygen cylinder.
- Open the tank by turning the valve on the tank regulator counterclockwise.
- Attach the demand valve directly to the endotracheal or tracheotomy tube.
- To assist ventilation, press the button on the demand valve. The demand valve delivers oxygen at 160 L/min. Monitor chest expansion, then release; exhalation occurs passively.
- Generally, **2 to 3 seconds** are required to deliver one breath to an adult—to a foal **significantly** less time. It is safest to watch the chest rise and end inspiration as soon as the chest nears full expansion. **CAUTION:** Do not overinflate the lungs, causing barotrauma. This may readily occur in foals when using a demand valve. Therefore, an Ambu bag is preferred for foal resuscitation.

---

[1]Oxygen supply service is available through local health care companies. Reusable oxygen cylinders are provided.

[2]LSPO2 Regulator 270-020. Allied Health, St. Louis, MO (800) 444-3960

[3]LSP Demand Valve (with 6 ft hose and female DISS fitting) 063-03. (Must specify 160 LPM when ordering. Allied Health, St. Louis, MO (800) 444-3960.

[4]Adult human Ambu bag PMR-2 manual resuscitator (self-inflating bag with accumulator). Breathing Services, Inc., P.O. Box 817, 931 E. Main Street, Ephrata, PA 17522; (800) 752-0028.

- If the chest does not rise, check for leaks and tube placement. Confirm that the esophagus was not accidentally intubated.
- In the adult, deliver **10 to 12 breaths per minute** and in foals, deliver **15 to 20 breaths per minute.**
- The demand valve can also be used to assist ventilation if the patient breathes independently. The demand valve triggers automatically when inspiration begins and shuts off when exhalation begins. This method increases airway resistance and the work of breathing and should be discontinued as soon as the patient is able to breathe room air.
- A full E oxygen cylinder contains ~ 600 liters of O_2 and lasts *ONLY* 15–20 minutes when resuscitating an adult.

Ventilation Using an Ambu Bag in Foals

- Attach the Ambu bag to the endotracheal or tracheotomy tube.
- Place the oxygen insufflation tube (Chapter 35) into the reservoir of the Ambu bag to increase inspired O_2 concentration.
- Open the oxygen tank and turn the flowmeter to 15 L/min.
- Compress the Ambu bag until full expansion of the lungs is achieved.
- Exhalation is passive through a valve on the Ambu bag.
- Administer about **20 breaths per minute.**

Ventilation with a Nasogastric Tube and Demand Valve

- Intubate the patient with a clean, lubricated nasogastric tube (see intubation procedure, p. 34). Do not advance beyond the midcervical area of the trachea.
- Attach the free end of the tube to the oxygen cylinder regulator.
- Open the regulator on the tank to a maximal flow rate.
- Occlude both nares and watch the chest rise to full inflation, which can take up to 8 seconds in an adult, depending on lung compliance. **Do not overinflate the lungs.**
- Once the lungs are inflated, open the nostrils to permit passive exhalation.
- Deliver **10 to 12 breaths per minute** in an adult and **15 to 20 breaths per minute** in a foal.
- The E oxygen cylinder lasts *ONLY* 10–15 minutes at maximal flow.

Complications

Overinflation of the lungs results in barotrauma and injury to the alveoli and, potentially, pulmonary emphysema.

12 Tracheotomy

James A. Orsini and Christine Kreuder

Tracheotomy is performed on an emergency basis when acute respiratory obstruction occurs. This procedure establishes an airway that bypasses the larynx and nasal passages and may be lifesaving if there is an obstruction of the upper respiratory tract. Tracheotomy provides a direct route for manual ventilation regardless of the cause of respiratory distress. Occasionally, tracheotomy is indicated before recovery from laryngeal or nasal passage surgery when respiratory obstruction is anticipated.

Equipment

- clippers
- material for sterile scrub
- 2% local anesthetic, 5–10-ml syringe, and 22-gauge, 0.5-inch needle
- sterile gloves
- #10 scalpel blade and handle
- appropriately sized tracheotomy tube[1]
- 0 nonabsorbable suture on a straight needle

Procedure

- Sedate patient if circumstances permit.
- **LANDMARKS:** The trachea is easily palpated directly on the ventral midline of the neck. Isolate a section of the trachea between the upper and middle third of the neck.
- Clip area and prepare with a sterile scrub.
- Infiltrate 5–10 ml of local anesthetic into the subcutaneous tissue over the trachea. The bleb should be 5 to 7 cm long on the midline.
- With sterile gloves, grasp the trachea and make a 5-cm incision through the skin and subcutaneous tissue with a scalpel blade.
- Bluntly dissect the underlying muscle bellies and retract each laterally until the trachea is found on the midline (Fig. 12–1).
- Incise a tracheal annular ligament **between** two cartilage rings. The incision should be parallel to the cartilage rings and thus perpendicular to the skin incision. The incision should be only long enough to allow

---

[1]Tracheotomy tube (18-mm or 28-mm internal diameter). Jorgensen Laboratories, Inc., 1450 North Van Buren Avenue, Loveland, CO 80538; (970) 669-2500.

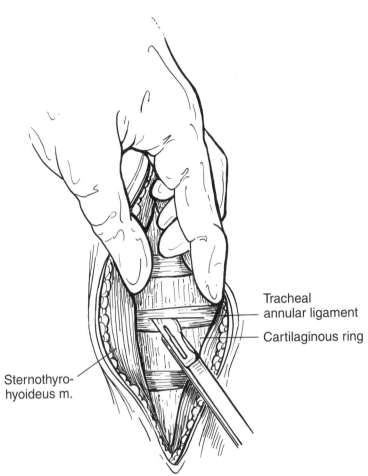

Tracheal
annular ligament

Cartilaginous ring

Sternothyro-
hyoideus m.

FIGURE 12–1. Surgical technique for tracheotomy. Make a vertical incision in the skin, divide the sternothyrohyoideus muscle, and horizontally incise an annular ligament to allow passage of the tracheotomy tube.

passage of the tracheal tube and should not exceed more than a third of the circumference of the trachea (Fig. 12–1).

- Insert the tracheal tube through the incision and suture in place.
- Tracheotomy tubes become obstructed easily and need to be suctioned and cleaned or replaced daily.
- The tube should be large enough to fill the tracheotomy site and should not extend beyond the bifurcation of the trachea to ensure that all lung fields are ventilated.

In a **life-threatening** emergency, sterile technique is abandoned, any sharp object is used to incise in the foregoing manner, and any tube available (stomach tube, garden hose, and so on) may be used to establish an airway initially.

Complications

Wound infection, particularly if sterile technique is not used. The airway is a contaminated environment, and the tracheotomy site should be cleaned several times daily until the wound has healed.

Subcutaneous **emphysema** is likely if air can move around the outside of the tube. The air is a problem only if it carries infection with it or if it dissects along tissue planes, leading to pneumomediastinum, pneumothorax, or both.

Tracheal **stricture** is possible as the tracheal mucosa contracts during healing. Granulation tissue is produced intraluminally and may contribute to luminal narrowing if excessive.

13 Paranasal Sinus Trephination

James A. Orsini and Christine Kreuder

Trephination, or creating a hole in the bone overlying the paranasal sinuses for access to the sinus cavity, is a procedure used for diagnosis and treatment of paranasal sinus disease. Clinical signs suggestive of sinus disease (nasal discharge, facial asymmetry) are frequently supported by abnormal radiographs that help localize the disease to a particular sinus. If radiographs are normal or inconclusive, exploratory sinoscopy of the frontal and caudal maxillary sinuses can be performed through the trephination site. If a bacterial infection is suspected, sinocentesis provides a sample suitable for cytology and culture and sensitivity determinations. Trephination and sinus lavage is the treatment of choice for patients with chronic sinusitis and associated empyema that are refractory to systemic antibiotic therapy.

The **frontal sinus** is dorsal and medial to the orbit. The left and right frontal sinuses are separated by a median septum. The frontal sinus communicates with the caudal maxillary sinus through the frontal maxillary opening. Sinoscopy of both the frontal and caudal maxillary sinuses is most easily performed by trephination of the frontal sinus (Ruggles, 1994).

The **maxillary sinus** is also paired and is rostral and ventral to the orbit. It is divided into rostral and caudal compartments by an incomplete oblique septum. Both compartments communicate with the ventral nasal meatus through the nasomaxillary aperture. Because of its more ventral location, the maxillary sinus is usually the site of greatest fluid accumulation in a sinusitis. Ideally, both compartments should be cultured and lavaged, but lavage of the rostral compartment only may provide satisfactory results.

Equipment

- sedation (xylazine hydrochloride or detomidine)
- clippers
- 2% local anesthetic, 25-gauge, ⅝-inch needle, 3-ml syringe
- material for a sterile scrub
- sterile gloves
- #15 scalpel blade with handle
- The **trephine** used depends on availability and the size of the hole required:
  □ For sinus lavage: 2.5-, 3.2-, or 4.5-mm (³⁄₁₆–0.25-inch) drill bit and drill or 2.0–4.5-mm (⁵⁄₃₂, ³⁄₁₆, or 0.25-inch) Steinmann pin[1] with Jacobs chuck[2]
  □ For passage of a 4-mm endoscope: 6.34-mm Steinmann pin with Jacobs chuck.

FOR SINOCENTESIS AND SINUS LAVAGE:

- intravenous catheter[3] (14-gauge, 2-inch long); remove stylet and cut end so that the catheter is only 0.75-inch long
- 2–0 nonabsorbable suture
- 5-ml syringe
- EDTA (purple top) Vacutainer tube[4] for cytology
- Culturette[5] and/or Port-a-Cul[6] culture systems
- 1 liter of saline with 0.5–1% Betadine and a 30-inch extension set[7] for sinus lavage

Procedure

- May be done in the standing sedated individual or under general anesthesia. For sedation, administer 0.01–0.02 mg/kg detomidine IV **OR** 0.4–0.7 mg/kg xylazine IV.

---

[1]Steinmann pin (size 2.5, 3.2, 4.5, 6.34-mm). Synthes (USA), P.O. Box 1766, 1690 Russell Road, Paoli, PA 19301-0800; (800) 523-0322.

[2]Jacobs chuck. A.J. Buck and Son, Inc., 11407 Cronhill Drive, Owings Mills, MD 21117; (800) 638-8672; (Fax) (301) 581-1809.

[3]Abbocath-T radiopaque FEP Teflon IV catheter (14-gauge, 2-inch long). Abbott Hospitals, Inc., North Chicago, IL 60064.

[4]Vacutainer tubes. Becton-Dickinson Vacutainer Systems, Rutherford, NJ 07070.

[5]Culturette collection and transport system. Becton-Dickinson Microbiology Systems, Cockeysville, MD 21030.

[6]Port-a-Cul tube. BBL Division of Becton-Dickinson and Co., Cockeysville, MD 21030.

[7]30-inch extension set. Abbott Laboratories, North Chicago, IL 60064.

- See Figure 13–1 for trephination sites for each paranasal sinus.
- Choose a trephination site and infiltrate 2 ml of 2% local anesthetic subcutaneously to the periosteum.
- Clip a 5-square-cm area and perform a sterile scrub.
- With sterile gloves, make a 0.5–1.5-cm stab incision (depending on the portal size required).
- Drill a hole in the bone overlying the sinus perpendicular to the bone

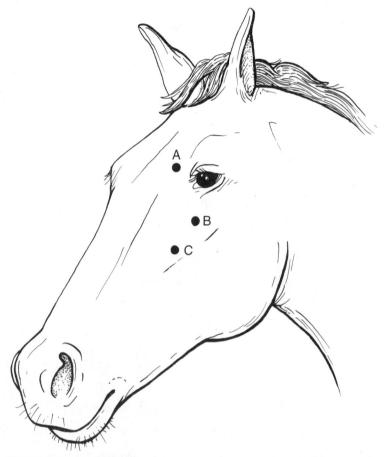

FIGURE 13–1. Sites for paranasal sinus trephination in the adult. *A,* **Frontal sinus.** Draw a horizontal line from midline to the medial canthus of the eye and trephine at a location 1 cm caudal to the midpoint of this line. *B,* **Caudal maxillary sinus.** Trephine at a location 3 cm rostral from the medial canthus of the eye and 3 cm dorsal from the facial crest. *C,* **Rostral maxillary sinus.** Trephine at a location half the distance along a line drawn from the medial canthus of the eye to the rostral end of the facial crest.

surface. **CAUTION:** Be careful not to overdrill the bone and traumatize the sinus cavity. The bone is only a few millimeters thick, and drilling should stop as soon as there is loss of resistance.

FOR SINOCENTESIS AND SINUS LAVAGE:

- Insert the catheter and attempt to seat the injection portal into the bone.
- Attach a 5-ml syringe to the catheter and aspirate fluid in the sinus. If no fluid is obtained, infiltrate 30 ml of warm sterile saline before reaspiration. A sample for cytology should be collected at this time.
- Once a sample is obtained, attach the extension set to the catheter and flush the dilute Betadine solution into the sinus. The saline, along with any purulent exudate, is lavaged out through the nasal passages if the nasomaxillary opening is patent (Merriam, 1993).
- If repeated lavage is required, suture the catheter to the skin. If not, remove the catheter and place several interrupted sutures in the skin. If purulent material has exited from the trephination site, clean the area and place topical antibiotics in the wound before suture placement.

Complications

Wound infection or **abscess** formation at the trephination site. *Lance the abscess or remove the sutures and allow the area to drain and heal by second intention.* Clean aseptically and apply topical antibiotics until healed.

Epistaxis occurs if the sinus mucosa is excessively traumatized during trephination or catheter placement.

REFERENCES

Merriam JG. Field sinusotomy in the management of chronic sinusitis and alveolitis. 39th Annual Convention Proceedings of the American Association of Equine Practitioners, San Antonio, TX, 1993.

Ruggles AJ. Endoscopic examination of the paranasal sinuses in the horse. 22nd Annual Surgical Forum of the American College of Veterinary Surgeons, Washington, DC, 1994.

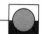

14 Thoracocentesis and Chest Tube Placement

James A. Orsini and Christine Kreuder

Thoracocentesis is the aspiration of fluid from the thoracic cavity and serves both diagnostic and therapeutic functions. It is easily performed in the standing horse and indicated whenever pleural effusion is suspected based on auscultation of the chest, radiographs, and/or ultrasound. Pleural effusion most often accompanies pleuropneumonia, pleural abscessation, and neoplasia. Analysis of pleural fluid differentiates among these problems and can be lifesaving if the effusion compromises respiratory function.

Equipment

- clippers
- material for sterile scrub
- local anesthetic
- 5-ml syringe and 25-gauge, ⅝ inch needle
- sterile scalpel blade (#12) and handle (#3)
- sterile metal teat cannula (2½-4-inch long),[1] or metal bitch urinary catheter (10.5-inch long).[2] Blunt-tipped cannulas are less likely to lacerate the lung
- three-way stopcock[3] or extension set tubing[4]
- 60-ml syringe
- nonabsorbable 0 suture
- chest tube[5] with or without Heimlich one-way valve[6] for repeated drainage
- plain and EDTA Vacutainer tubes[7]
- Port-a-Cul (aerobic/anaerobic) culture system[8]

---

[1]Ideal udder infusion cannula. Butler Company, 5000 Bradenton Ave., P.O. Box 7153, Dublin, OH 43017-0753.

[2]Metal bitch urinary catheter. Jorgensen Laboratories, Inc., 1450 North Van Buren Avenue, Loveland, CO 80538.

[3]Pharmaseal K75 3-way stopcock. Baxter Healthcare Corp., American Pharmaseal Co., Valencia, CA 91355-8900.

[4]Extension set, 7 or 30 inch. Abbott Laboratories, North Chicago, IL 60064.

[5]Thal-Quick chest drainage catheter set (24–36 French, 41-cm long). Cook Veterinary Products, 127 South Main Street, P.O. Box 266, Spencer, IN 47460; (800) 826-2380.

[6]Heimlich chest drainage valve. Cook Veterinary Products, 127 South Main Street, P.O. Box 266, Spencer, IN 47460; (800) 829-6535.

[7]Vacutainer. Becton-Dickinson Vacutainer Systems, Rutherford, NJ 07070.

[8]Port-a-Cul. Becton-Dickinson Microbiology Systems, Cockeysville, MD 21030.

Procedure

- Sedation is usually not necessary unless the patient is intractable. Recommended dosage: 0.3 mg/kg xylazine with 0.01–0.025 mg/kg butorphanol IV.
- Choose a site for thoracocentesis based on auscultation of dull lung fields and radiographic or ultrasound examination. Fluid usually collects ventrally. A common site for thoracocentesis is the lower third of the thorax between the 7th and 8th intercostal space. Both sides of the chest should be aspirated if bilateral effusion is suspected, because in general the healthy horse has an intact mediastinum. **CAUTION:** Avoid the heart when placing the needle ventrally. Ultrasound guidance is recommended for precise needle placement.
- Clip and prepare the site aseptically.
- Inject 5–10 ml of local anesthetic subcutaneously and into the intercostal muscle. Perform a final skin prep.
- Make a stab incision through the skin and fascia at the cranial aspect of the rib to avoid the intercostal vessels and nerves, which are located on the caudal border.
- Use sterile gloves to hold the cannula and attach a three-way stopcock or tubing with the end clamped to prevent pneumothorax if negative pressure exists in the thoracic cavity.
- Insert the cannula into the skin incision and push it through the intercostal muscle. A sudden decrease in tension is felt as the pleural space is entered.
- Attach a 60-ml syringe to the stopcock or tubing. Aspiration should yield fluid if an effusion is present. Rotation or redirection of the cannula is often needed. If fluid is freely flowing, it may be siphoned off into a bucket.
- Keep the tubing or stopcock closed when not removing fluid to prevent aspiration of air and iatrogenic pneumothorax.
- Once fluid is no longer retrievable, place a pursestring suture around the cannula and tighten as the cannula is removed. If septic fluid is removed, infiltrate antibiotics in and around the incision, apply an antiseptic or antibiotic ointment, and bandage the wound.

Chest Tube Placement

Repeated drainage is often necessary, particularly when large volumes of fluid are present or infection is suspected. For these patients, an indwelling human chest tube is required.

- The smallest-size tube should be chosen as long as fibrinous material will pass through.
- Instructions for chest tube placement accompany the product. A one-way valve may be used to maintain negative pressure.
- Use a pursestring suture to attach the tube to the skin and tie the free suture ends around the tube several times in a locking pattern or use rapid-acting glue.
- The tube must be clamped and sealed when not in use.
- The chest tube may be left in place for up to 1 month and is generally

changed every 2–3 days because of fibrinous debris occluding the lumen. Sinus tracts that form around the tube often heal spontaneously after tube removal.

Pleural Fluid Analysis

Only 1–2 ml of straw-colored fluid is retrieved from a normal pleural cavity. Color, opacity, volume, and odor are all useful parameters. Yellow, opaque fluid with fibrinous clots suggests a septic exudate. Foul-smelling effusion is well correlated with anaerobic bacterial colonization. A relatively clear to serosanguineous exudate is occasionally seen in neoplastic processes. Often neoplastic cells are shed into the pleural fluid and can be identified on cytology. Cytology (with a total cell count and differential) and total protein should be performed to classify the effusion definitively. Normal total protein is less than 2.5 gm/dl, and total nucleated cell count is typically less than 8000 cells per μl. Neoplastic disease often has a significant inflammatory component and can mimic an infectious process. Specimens for anaerobic and aerobic cultures should be submitted to the laboratory if an infection is suspected.

Complications

Pneumothorax may occur when air enters the pleural cavity when the cannula is placed too dorsally during thoracocentesis. The thorax normally has negative pressure and, when an effusion has been removed, the thorax should return to negative pressure. *To correct a pneumothorax, aspirate air dorsally in the same manner that fluid is aspirated* (Chapter 33).

Hemothorax may occur if a large vein or artery is punctured during insertion of a cannula. *Avoid the lateral thoracic vein (in the ventral third of the thorax) and always enter along the cranial margin of a rib.*

If the heart is accidentally punctured during cannula placement, **fatal cardiac arrhythmia** may result. *Avoid the cranial/ventral aspect of the thorax and use ultrasound guidance.*

Hypovolemia may occasionally result when large volumes (10–20 liters) are removed by thoracocentesis. Rarely, horses collapse if fluid is removed too rapidly, since fluid shifts from the circulating volume into the thorax. *Fluid therapy should be instituted to replace the volume lost.*

Gastrointestinal System

15 Nasogastric Tube Placement

James A. Orsini and Christine Kreuder

Placement of a nasogastric tube is often required for the administration of large volumes of oral medication. This is also an important diagnostic and therapeutic procedure in the colicky horse. A tube is passed to determine whether fluid has accumulated in the anterior gastrointestinal tract. The fluid is then refluxed in order to relieve the pressure on the stomach and the associated pain. Nasogastric intubation is also necessary in suspected cases of choke to relieve the obstruction in the esophagus. Every clinician develops his or her own technique for passing a nasogastric tube. The following description may be useful to the less experienced.

Equipment

- nasogastric tube (sized appropriately)
- bucket, half-filled with warm water
- 400-ml nylon dose syringe[1]

Procedure

- Soak the nasogastric tube in warm water until it is clean and flexible.
- The individual must be adequately restrained, which may require a chain shank over the nose or under the lip and/or a twitch.
- Stand on the horse's left at the withers, place the right hand over the nose, and use the thumb to reflect the alar fold of the left nostril dorsally. Do not obstruct airflow in the right nostril.
- Use the left hand to guide the tube ventrally and medially into the ventral nasal meatus. The middle nasal meatus lies immediately dorsal and must be avoided.
- Advance the tube slowly and with care. Avoid forcing the tube if excessive resistance is encountered. If the patient is tossing its head, hold the tube in the nostril with the thumb of the right hand.
- The tube encounters a small amount of resistance as it passes over the epiglottis. Most horses swallow the tube immediately. Try to pass the tube

---

[1]400-ml nylon dose syringe. J.A. Webster, Inc., 86 Leominster Road, Sterling, MA 01564-2198; (800) 225-7911.

on the patient's first swallow, because subsequent attempts to stimulate swallowing become progressively more difficult. The end of the tube should remain in front of the epiglottis while waiting for swallowing. Gently bumping the epiglottis with the end of the tube or blowing into the tube to trickle water down the pharynx may encourage some individuals to swallow. If no swallow reflex is elicited, attempt to pass the tube through the other nostril.

- One must be absolutely certain the tube is in the esophagus and not in the trachea. There are several ways to ensure correct placement. All the following must be confirmed before the tube is advanced further and before any medication is delivered:
  □ Some resistance is encountered when the tube moves down the esophagus. The tube passes through the trachea relatively easily, and the tracheal rings may be palpable.
  □ Negative pressure is obtained with suction if the tube is in the esophagus because the lumen is collapsible. Suction on the end of a tube in the trachea does not result in negative pressure.
  □ The end of the tube is seen advancing down the neck to the left of midline. The tube is usually not seen if it is in the trachea. If the tube is not apparent, it must be palpated as it passes through the thoracic inlet or, more likely, as it rests beside the rostral trachea (usually to the left). This is most easily accomplished by gently pushing the trachea dorsally with a hand and palpating the tube in the esophagus with the fingertips of the same hand. This is the most reliable assessment of correct tube placement. A very small percentage of horses have a right-sided esophagus.

- Blowing into the tube facilitates advancement through the cardia into the stomach. Once in the stomach, gas that smells like ingesta is emitted, and blowing on the end of the tube produces an audible bubbling noise. This is final assurance that the tube is indeed in the stomach.

- One should attempt to obtain reflux before administering large volumes of fluid. To obtain reflux, a siphon must be created by establishing a column of water between the stomach and the outside. A syringeful of warm water is administered to fill the tube, a small amount of fluid is aspirated back, the syringe is detached, and the tube end is lowered. Several attempts are usually required before gastric fluid is siphoned off the stomach.

- If no net reflux is obtained, medication warmed to body temperature may be administered into the tube. The tube end is lifted above the patient's head to complete delivery of the medication. Before removal, the tube end should again be lowered to ensure that there is not excessive pressure on the stomach.

- Kink the tube or leave the syringe attached during removal so that fluid does not leak into the pharynx or nasal passages.

A normal horse usually refluxes less than 2 liters of fluid. Measure the amount of fluid pumped into the stomach in order to know how much of the fluid retrieved is reflux. Medication should not be delivered to patients with large volumes of reflux because it is not absorbed and adds to the pressure on the stomach. Excessive reflux indicates ileus, an abnormal secretory process in the anterior gastrointestinal tract (anterior enteritis), or an obstructive process (usually in the small intestine). The volume, appearance, and odor of the fluid are important parameters to assess when treating a horse with colic. Individuals with a large quantity of reflux should have a nasogastric tube left in place and secured to the halter to prevent gastric rupture. Reflux should be repeated every few hours in these cases.

Complications

Accidentally administering a large volume of fluid into the lungs of a patient can be **fatal.** For this reason, one must literally "see, feel, smell, and hear" that the tube is in the correct position.

Hemorrhage from a nostril is an occasional complication. The conchal mucosa is extremely vascular and is easily injured. Almost all nosebleeds eventually stop even though their duration often seems prolonged.

If a nosebleed occurs, rinse the tube and attempt to pass it gently through the other nostril.

A smaller-diameter tube is less likely to damage the mucosa. Also, make sure that the tube has no nicks or sharp edges that would cause mucosal trauma.

If bleeding continues for more than 10–15 minutes or is believed excessive, an intranasal spray of 10 mg phenylephrine hydrochloride diluted in 10-ml of sterile saline can be infused, using a nasal catheter.

16 Abdominocentesis and Peritoneal Fluid Analysis

James A. Orsini and Christine Kreuder

Peritoneal fluid analysis is an excellent measure of gastrointestinal disease. This procedure is indicated whenever a patient presents with acute or intermittent abdominal pain, diarrhea, or chronic weight loss.

Equipment

- twitch (sedation is generally not necessary)
- clippers
- material for sterile scrub
- sterile gloves
- sterile 18–22-gauge, 1.5-inch needles OR metal teat cannula (3.75-inches

long)[1] for foals or metal bitch urinary catheter (10.5 inch long)[2] for larger or obese individuals
- 2% local anesthetic (with 25-gauge needle and 3-ml syringe)
- #15 blade if using a cannula or urinary catheter
- sterile gauze sponge
- EDTA and plain Vacutainer tubes[3] for analysis
- sterile vial, Port-a-Cul culture and transport system[4] or blood culture bottle[5] for culture and sensitivity

Procedure

- Choose an area in the most dependent portion of the abdomen (usually directly on the midline 5 cm caudal to the xiphoid). A right paramedian approach may be used to avoid splenic aspiration.
- Clip or shave the area chosen for abdominocentesis.
- Perform a sterile scrub.
- Place twitch.
- Glove and maintain sterility throughout the procedure.
- While standing next to the patient, insert the needle with a quick thrust through the skin and linea alba. If drops of abdominal fluid are not seen at the needle hub, reposition and rotate the needle or attach a syringe and aspirate. If necessary, place a second needle a few inches from the first to release the negative pressure in the abdomen.
- Ultrasound examination can be used to locate fluid pockets; however, peritoneal fluid can still be obtained even if not seen following ultrasound evaluation.
- If abdominal fluid is not obtained, use a teat cannula or a stainless steel bitch urinary catheter to reach the peritoneal cavity. *A small-diameter teat cannula is recommended for foals because their intestinal wall is thin and easily lacerated.*
  - □ Place a subcutaneous bleb of local anesthesia.
  - □ Make a small stab incision with a #15 blade through skin and subcutaneous tissue.
  - □ To reduce blood contamination from the incision, push the tip of the cannula through a sterile sponge.
  - □ Gently insert the cannula or urinary catheter into the incision. Some force is required to push the blunt-tipped instrument through the linea alba. A marked decrease in resistance is noted once the abdomen is entered.
- Allow the abdominal fluid to drip directly into EDTA Vacutainer tubes with or without culture material.

[1]Ideal udder infusion cannula. Butler Company, 5000 Bradenton Ave., P.O. Box 7153, Dublin, OH 43017-0753.

[2]Metal bitch urinary catheter. Jorgensen Laboratories, Inc., 1450 North Van Buren Avenue, Loveland, CO 80538; (970) 669-2500.

[3]Vacutainer. Becton-Dickinson Vacutainer Systems, Rutherford, NJ 07070.

[4]Port-a-Cul. Becton-Dickinson Microbiology Systems, Cockeysville, MD 21030.

[5]Septi-check, BB blood culture bottle. Roche Diagnostic Systems, Nutley, NJ 07110-1199.

PERITONEAL FLUID ANALYSIS (Table 16–1)

Changes in peritoneal fluid are manifested fairly rapidly after the onset of gastrointestinal disease. In cases of acute obstruction or strangulating obstruction, changes in peritoneal fluid are seen several hours after the onset of clinical signs. More insidious lesions, such as nonstrangulating obstruction, enteritis, and peritonitis, are likely to produce changes in the peritoneal fluid before or concurrent with clinical signs. Inguinal herniation, intussusception, and entrapment of diseased bowel in the omental bursa or epiploic foramen may cause a local peritonitis with normal peritoneal fluid initially.

Normal peritoneal fluid is clear and light yellow. Color and specific gravity are easily assessed and are the most predictive of the severity of the lesion. Normal specific gravity is 1.005 mg/dl. Increased turbidity results from an increased protein and/or cellular content, which may be due to septic peritonitis or inflammation of a bowel segment. The color of the fluid reflects the type of cells present. Cloudy white-to-yellow fluid or exudate represents large numbers of white blood cells, as in septic peritonitis. In an abdominal crisis, segments of bowel become compromised once there is diminished venous and lymphatic drainage from the bowel segment. Initially transudate, red blood cells, and protein leak out of vessels. An elevated total protein level and red cell count in serosanguineous fluid are often the first changes seen. Peritoneal fluid becomes white or yellow as bowel becomes ischemic and necrotic and white blood cells begin to leave the vessels. Necrotic bowel also leaks bacteria and endotoxin, which accelerates chemotaxis of white cells and increases the turbidity and white cell count. Red-brown or green-colored fluid may indicate rupture of the stomach or intestine and may contain plant material. Dark red fluid may be obtained when a vessel or the spleen is entered. Rarely, a hemoperitoneum may result from a ruptured vessel; the sample contains no platelets and may have evidence of erythrophagocytosis. The packed cell volume (PCV) may be compared with a systemic sample to distinguish between a sample from the spleen (PCV is higher) or a vessel (PCV is the same).

A direct smear is made with Wright or Gram stain or both. Cytology should include a white blood cell count and differential and evaluation of cellular degeneration and the presence of bacteria and food particles. White cell counts are normally lower in foals. A moderate amount of blood contamination in the sample (not more than 17%) should not affect any parameters except the number of red blood cells. White cell count and total protein levels are elevated in a patient having undergone abdominal surgery even with manipulation of the intestines only. A sample with increased white cell numbers in which most neutrophils appear toxic and degenerate is evidence of septic peritonitis, even if the sample is taken after a celiotomy.

Complications

Cellulitis or **abscess** formation may occur from a break in sterile technique or removal of septic/purulent peritoneal fluid.

Accidental **enterocentesis** (aspiration of bowel contents) is not uncommon but rarely causes a problem other than sample contamination. *A blunt-tipped cannula decreases the likelihood of bowel puncture. Ultrasound-guided abdominocentesis is useful in foals to prevent intestinal laceration.*

TABLE 16-1. Correlation of Peritoneal Fluid Parameters and Intraperitoneal Disorders

Condition	Appearance†	Total Protein† (gm/dl)	Total Nucleated† Cells/L	Cytology Findings†
Normal	Yellow, clear	<2.0	<7.5 × 10⁹/L	40–80% neutrophils 20–80% mononuclear
Nonstrangulating obstruction	Yellow, clear to slightly turbid	<3.0	3.0–15.0 × 10⁹/L	Predominantly neutrophils (well preserved)
Strangulating obstruction	Red-brown, turbid	2.5–6.0	5.0–50.0 × 10⁹/L	Predominantly neutrophils (degenerate)
Proximal duodenitis-jejunitis	Yellow-red, turbid	3.0–4.5	<10.0 × 10⁹/L	Predominantly neutrophils (well preserved)
Bowel rupture	Red-brown, green, turbid ±/– particulate matter	5.0–6.5	>20.0 × 10⁹/L (20–150 × 10⁹/L)	>95% neutrophils (severely degenerate); intracellular and extracellular bacteria, ± plant matter
Septic peritonitis	Yellow-white, turbid	>3.0	>20.0 × 10⁹/L (20–100 × 10⁹/L)	Predominantly neutrophils (degenerate)
Postceliotomy	Yellow-red, turbid	Variable	Variable	Predominantly neutrophils (slight to moderate degenerate); no intracellular bacteria
Enterocentesis	Brown-green, ±/– particulate matter	Variable	<1.0 × 10⁹	Free bacteria, few cells, plant matter
Intra-abdominal hemorrhage	Dark red	Initially similar to peripheral blood, WBC count increases with time		PCV less than PCV of peripheral blood, erythrocytophagia, few to no platelets

NOTE: Absence of gross or cytologic abnormalities in the peritoneal fluid does not rule out compromised intestine.
PCV, packed cell volume.
†Most common findings; exceptions can occur.

Accidental **splenic aspiration** also causes sample contamination.

Omental herniation may occur in foals following abdominocentesis in the rostral to middle abdomen using a teat cannula. Transect the omentum at or near the body wall, apply an antiseptic cream or ointment, and cover with an abdominal bandage.

REFERENCES

Freden GO, Provost PJ, Rand WM. Re-evaluating the clinical application of abdominal fluid analysis in the equine colic patient. 5th Equine Colic Research Symposium, Athens, Georgia, 1994.

Malark JA, Peyton LC, Galvin MJ. Effects of blood contamination on equine peritoneal fluid analysis. J Am Vet Med Assoc 1992; 201(10):1545–1548.

17 Cecal Trocharization

James A. Orsini and Christine Kreuder

Cecal trocharization is performed for removal of gas from the cecum in patients with cecal tympany. Cecal gas distention is suspected in colicky patients when a ping is heard on simultaneous percussion and auscultation in the right paralumbar fossa and confirmed with rectal palpation. Cecal tympany may be a primary or secondary disorder. Decompression stimulates cecal motility and relieves the pain caused by cecal distention. The procedure helps normalize intra-abdominal pressure and improves venous return and breathing. This procedure is frequently performed in surgical patients before general anesthesia. If the patient is not a surgical candidate, trocharization may resolve colic in simple cases of tympany or certain colonic displacements.

Equipment

- twitch
- clippers
- material for sterile scrub
- 2% local anesthetic, 5-ml syringe, and 22-gauge, 1.5-inch needle
- sterile gloves
- 16-gauge, 5-inch pliable intravenous catheter[1]
- 7-inch extension set[2]
- small cup of tap water

---

[1]Abbocath-T radiopaque FEP Teflon IV catheter. Abbott Hospitals, Inc., North Chicago, IL 60064.

[2]Extension set, 7-inch. Abbott Laboratories, North Chicago, IL 60064.

Procedure

- A twitch may be required if the patient is not sedated. Sedation is generally not necessary.
- Clip an area in the right paralumbar fossa where the ping is best heard.
- Infiltrate 3 to 5 ml of local anesthetic subcutaneously and in the underlying muscle at the trocharization site.
- Perform a sterile scrub.
- Using sterile gloves, insert the catheter and stylet through the skin, subcutaneous tissue, and abdominal muscle. The catheter should remain perpendicular to the skin. Remove the plastic cap on the catheter; if the catheter is in the cecum, gas escapes. When the catheter is in the cecum, remove the stylet.
- Attach the extension set and place the free end in the cup of water. Bubbles are produced as long as gas is being removed from the cecum; suction may be used if available.
- If gas is no longer retrievable, withdraw the catheter; do not attempt to redirect the catheter.

Complications

A low-grade, localized **peritonitis,** which may affect peritoneal fluid parameters, is expected to occur after this procedure. Clinical evidence or subsequent complications are rarely noted. Signs of infection should raise suspicion, however, and be treated promptly with the appropriate therapy. *Injecting antibiotics (ampicillin, neomycin, or gentamicin) through the catheter during removal may minimize this complication.* Repeating the trocharization is **not recommended,** as clinical peritonitis may develop.

A local **cellulitis** and/or **abscess** may occur at the trocharization site. The inflammation is usually self-limiting but should be monitored and treated appropriately.

Genitourinary System

18 Urinary Tract Catheterization

James A. Orsini and Christine Kreuder

Urinary tract catheterization assures an accurate, uncontaminated urine sample in a timely manner. A midstream free catch urine sample is adequate for urinalysis, but is less suitable for culture. Catheterization is also used to perform cystoscopy or urethroscopy.

Equipment

- sedation and/or tranquilization (xylazine hydrochloride, butorphanol tartrate, and acepromazine)
- tail tie for mares
- sterile gloves
- lubricating jelly[1]
- appropriate urinary catheter (sterile)
  □ stallions and geldings—9-mm outer diameter urinary catheter[2]
  □ mares—11-mm outer diameter urinary catheter[3]
- 60-ml catheter-tip syringe[4] (sterile)
- 3 sterile vials for urinalysis, cytology, and culture specimens

Procedure

Male Catheterization

- Stallions and geldings usually require sedation and tranquilization for restraint and extrusion of the penis. (Recommended dose: 0.4 mg/kg xylazine, 0.01 mg/kg butorphanol, combined with 0.02 mg/kg acepromazine IV)

---

[1]KY lubricating jelly. Johnson and Johnson Medical, Inc., Arlington, TX 76004-3130.
[2]Stallion Foley catheter (28 French Foley). Cook Veterinary Products, 127 South Main Street, P.O. Box 266, Spencer, IN 47460.
[3]Mares' urinary catheter. Jorgensen Laboratories, Inc., 1450 North Van Buren Avenue, Loveland, CO 80538; (970) 669-2500. Uterine flushing tube (33 French, 80 cm long). Cook Veterinary Products, 127 South Main Street, P.O. Box 266, Spencer, IN 47460.
[4]Monoject 60-ml syringe with catheter tip. Sherwood Medical, St. Louis, MO 63103.

- Scrub the penis with a dilute antiseptic solution (povidone-iodine or chlorhexidine) and rinse with water.
- Using sterile gloves, minimally lubricate the catheter.
- Stabilize the penis with one hand and gently advance the catheter through the urethral opening.
- The catheter should advance approximately 50–70 cm and glide through the urethra easily until the urethral sphincter is contacted. Injection of 60 ml of air into the urethra may aid passage through the sphincter.
- If urine does not flow freely when the catheter has reached the bladder, gently aspirate using a 60-ml syringe.
- Place samples directly into the sterile vials for urinalysis, cytology, and/ or culture.

Female Catheterization

- Sedation is generally not needed although a twitch is recommended.
- Wrap the tail and pull it to the side.
- Scrub the perineum with a dilute antiseptic solution (povidone-iodine or chlorhexidine) and rinse with water.
- Using sterile gloves, minimally lubricate the catheter.
- Place a hand within the vagina and locate the urethral opening on the floor of the vagina. Insert one finger into the urethra and gently guide the catheter with the other hand.
- The catheter should advance approximately 5 to 10 cm. If urine does not flow freely, aspirate with a 60-ml syringe.
- Place samples in appropriate containers.

URINALYSIS

Urinalysis is useful in the diagnosis of both lower and upper urinary tract disorders. Each sample should be submitted for a complete urinalysis, cytology, and bacterial culture with **colony count**. A urine sample should be examined within 20 minutes of collection or refrigerated immediately. Gross evaluation of equine urine is difficult because of its high mucus content. Pigmenturia is easily seen but must be differentiated from hematuria, hemoglobinuria, and myoglobinuria by microscopic examination.

A urine dipstick is routinely used to determine pH, protein content, glucose, bilirubin, and the presence of pigments. A refractometer is used to determine specific gravity. Specific gravity of adults is normally between 1.008 and 1.045; of foals, between 1.001 and 1.025. Highly concentrated urine is often due to decreased water intake. If urine specific gravity remains isosthenuric (equal to blood specific gravity of 1.010) despite changes in water intake or a water deprivation test, significant renal disease should be suspected.

Normal urine should not contain protein, glucose, or bilirubin. If a dipstick is used, protein may be falsely elevated if the urine is highly concentrated or very alkaline. Protein is detected if there is pigmenturia or inflammation and/or infection in the urinary tract. Absolute (true) proteinuria should be quantitated by mechanical methods and is seen with glomerulonephritis and amyloidosis. Glucosuria occurs in hyperglycemia with normal renal function. If blood glucose is normal, glucosuria is highly suggestive of renal tubular disease. Pigmenturia occurs with myolysis (muscle damage), hemolysis (bilirubinuria and hematuria), cystitis (secondary to urinary calculi), pyelonephritis, and rarely, neoplasia. Normal equine urine is alkaline; adult urine pH is 7.5 to 8.5, foal urine pH is 5.5 to 8.0. Increased acidity is seen with strenuous exercise, metabolic acidosis, and starvation.

Urine cytology is important in differentiating between urinary tract inflammation and infection. Slides should be made from the sample centrifugate, air dried, and stained with Wright or Diff-Quik stain. Five red blood cells and five white blood cells per high powered field ($\times 1000$) is normal. More than 10 red blood cells per field suggests hemorrhage and more than 10 white blood cells per field suggests inflammation. If inflammation is present, a Gram stain should be performed to look for bacteria. Bacteria should not be detected in normal urine if the sample is collected using aseptic technique. Noting bacterial morphology helps in instituting antibiotic therapy before culture results. Casts (cellular debris shed from the renal tubules) indicate renal tubular damage. Calcium carbonate crystals are common and considered within normal limits unless clinical signs suggest the presence of urinary calculi.

Complications

Infection of the lower urinary tract if sterile technique is not followed or if the bladder is atonic.

PART V

Musculoskeletal System

19 | Local Anesthesia for the Diagnosis of Lameness

James A. Orsini and Christine Kreuder

Local anesthesia is a diagnostic tool used to help localize lameness or confirm examination findings. Perineural anesthesia infiltrates the sensory fibers of a nerve and desensitizes specific anatomic regions in a systematic manner. A thorough knowledge of neuroanatomy is required for performance and accurate interpretation of nerve blocks. Intrasynovial anesthesia is more specific and is used to localize lameness within joints, tendon sheaths, and bursas. Anesthesia may be placed directly into a joint, bursa, or tendon sheath and often alleviates intrasynovial pain more completely than nerve blocks.

CAUTION: Trotting a horse after placement of local anesthesia is contraindicated if a fracture is suspected. Radiography is recommended before regional anesthesia in these cases to rule out an incomplete fracture and prevent catastrophic bone failure after desensitization. Local anesthesia may be utilized in the severely lame (grades 4 to 5 out of 5) individual in order to localize the lameness by determining whether weight bearing or soundness at a slow walk is achievable. Stall confinement with or without mild tranquilization is necessary until the effects of the block wear off.

Equipment

- twitch (optional)
- material for sterile scrub
- 2% mepivacaine[1] local anesthetic. Most commonly used because it causes less tissue reaction and has a rapid onset of action, which lasts 60–90 minutes. Lidocaine[2] is also a well-suited local anesthetic. Bupivacaine[3] lasts 4–6 hours and should be used when longer-lasting anesthesia is desired.

---

[1]Carbocaine-V (2% mepivacaine hydrochloride). The Upjohn Company, Kalamazoo, MI 49001.

[2]Anthocaine (2% lidocaine hydrochloride). Anpro Pharmaceutical, Arcadia, CA 91006.

[3]Marcaine (0.5% bupivacaine hydrochloride). Abbott Laboratories. North Chicago, IL 60064.

- sterile disposable 18–25-gauge needles and an assortment of 3- to 60-ml syringes (not Luer-Lok); see the illustrations for exact needle and syringe size required for each block.
- clippers and sterile gloves for intrasynovial procedures

Procedure

Perineural Anesthesia

- See Figures 19–1, 19–2, and 19–3 for sites and landmarks for perineural anesthesia, size of needle recommended, and amount of local anesthesia required. Begin with the most distal block, regardless of suspicions, and move proximally until the lameness is eliminated. Perineural anesthesia is less specific in the proximal limb.
- Scrub injection sites to remove gross contamination and wash hands.
- Place twitch. Sedation or tranquilization is not recommended because both affect interpretation of the block.
- Once the nerve is palpated, place the needle with a quick thrust through the skin, attach the syringe with anesthetic, aspirate to rule out intravascular placement, and inject anesthetic around the nerve. If resistance is encountered, the needle may be in a ligament, tendon, or intradermal tissue and should be repositioned.
- Allow 5–10 minutes before testing skin sensation for anesthesia. Check for deep pain with hoof testers, flexion, and deep palpation.
- Repeat the lameness examination and assess improvement (0–100%).

Intrasynovial Anesthesia

- See Figures 19–4 to 19–10 for sites and landmarks for intrasynovial (intra-articular) anesthesia, size of the needle recommended, and amount of local anesthesia required for each joint.
- Joint blocks may be used in conjunction with perineural anesthesia if only partial relief of the lameness is achieved and a joint is suspected. The technique is similar to that for perineural anesthesia, except sterile technique and patient restraint are essential.
- Clip and shave the site for needle placement.
- Perform a sterile scrub at the site to be injected and the landmarks to be palpated.
- Sterile gloves should be worn to handle the syringe and needle and to palpate the landmarks.
- Use an unopened bottle of local anesthetic. One needle should be used to fill the syringe and another for joint injection. Needles and syringes should remain sterile.
- Place a twitch for restraint.
- Detach the needle from the syringe and place the needle with a quick thrust through the skin. If the needle has been placed successfully, synovial fluid appears at the hub of the needle in most cases. Digital pressure on the joint capsule encourages synovial fluid to flow from the needle. Care should be used in needle placement to prevent articular cartilage and surrounding soft tissue damage.

Text continued on page 76

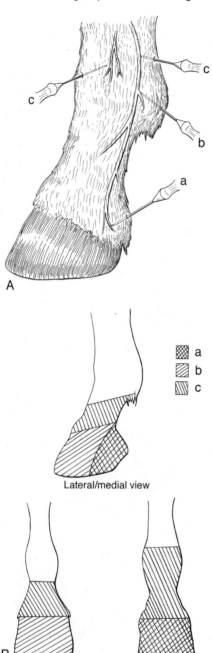

A

Lateral/medial view

Dorsal view   Palmar/plantar view

B

FIGURE 19–1. *A,* Sequential sites for perineural anesthesia of the distal limb.

a. **Palmar digital nerve block** (25-gauge, ⅝-inch needle). The posterior digital nerve runs along the medial and lateral borders of the deep digital flexor tendon. The nerves are easily palpable within a neurovascular bundle—the nerve lies palmar to the digital vein and artery (VAN relationship). Elevate the foot and block the nerve with 2–3 ml of local anesthetic just above the collateral cartilages.

b. **Abaxial sesamoid nerve block** (25-gauge, ⅝-inch needle). The palmar digital nerves are easily palpable on the abaxial surfaces of the sesamoid bones. Hold the limb in a flexed position and deposit 3–4 ml of local anesthetic over each nerve.

c. **Low palmar and palmar metacarpal nerve blocks** (25-gauge, ⅝-inch needle). The palmar nerve runs in the medial and lateral groove between the suspensory ligament and the deep digital flexor tendon. Block the palmar nerve with 3–4 ml of local anesthetic above the level of the bell of the splint bone (to avoid the digital tendon sheath). Block the palmar metacarpal nerve as it emerges distally from the bell of the splint bone with 2–3 ml of local anesthetic. This block may be performed with the limb in a flexed or standing position. Note: The plantar and plantar metatarsal nerves of the hindlimb are blocked in a similar manner. For complete anesthesia of the distal hindlimb, the medial and lateral dorsal metatarsal nerve must be blocked with 2 ml of local anesthetic on either side of the long digital extensor tendon just above the fetlock.

B, Hash marks represent affected area of limb.

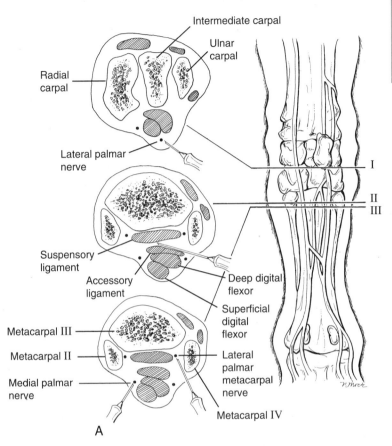

I High palmar nerve block
II High suspensory block
III High palmar and palmar metacarpal nerve block

FIGURE 19–2. Sequential sites for perineural anesthesia of the proximal forelimb.
A, **High palmar and palmar metacarpal nerve blocks** (22-gauge, 1½-inch needle). The palmar nerves lie beneath a dense fascial sheath between the deep digital flexor tendon and the suspensory ligament. Use 3–5 ml of local anesthetic to block the lateral nerve at the level of the distal accessory carpal bone and the medial nerve at the level of the medial splint bone head. A subcutaneous bleb should NOT appear if the fascial sheath has been successfully penetrated. The palmar metacarpal nerves course axially to the splint bones and should be blocked with 3–5 ml of local anesthesia below the head of each splint bone.
CAUTION: Inadvertent anesthesia of the carpal sheath, carpometacarpal joint, or middle carpal joint may occur when one deposits local anesthesia in the palmar carpometacarpal region. As a precaution, a sterile skin preparation and sterile technique should be used when performing these blocks. If a lameness is successfully blocked with anesthesia of this region, anesthesia of the middle carpal joint is indicated to confirm placement of anesthetic.

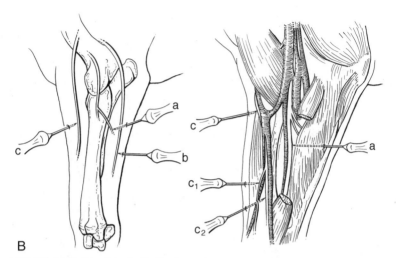

B

FIGURE 19–2 *(Continued)*. B, **Median, ulnar, and medial cutaneous antebrachial nerve blocks** (20- or 22-gauge, 1½-inch needle). Block the median nerve with 10 ml of local anesthetic in the posterior medial aspect of the radius approximately 10 cm proximal to the chestnut (a). Block the ulnar nerve with 8 ml of local anesthetic in the groove between the flexor carpi ulnaris and the ulnaris lateralis muscles, approximately 10 cm proximal to the accessory carpal bone (b). Block the medial cutaneous antebrachial nerve by depositing 5 ml of local anesthetic on either side of the cephalic vein, approximately 10 cm proximal to the chestnut (c). (C₁ and C₂ are cranial and caudal branches of medial cutaneous antebrachial nerve.)

FIGURE 19–3. Sequential sites for perineural anesthesia of the proximal hindlimb.

A, **High plantar (a), plantar metatarsal (b), and dorsal metatarsal (c) nerve blocks** (22-gauge, 1½-inch needle). Landmarks for the hindlimb are similar to those of the forelimb for the high plantar and plantar metatarsal blocks. Both the medial and lateral plantar nerves should be blocked below the level of the head of the splint bones. Block the dorsal metatarsal nerves with 3 ml of local anesthesia on each side of the long digital extensor tendon in the proximal metatarsus.

B, **Tibial and peroneal nerve blocks** (20-gauge, 1½-inch needle). Block the tibial nerve by depositing 15 ml of local anesthetic medially between the deep digital flexor tendon and the calcanean tendon, approximately 10 cm proximal to the point of the hock. Deposit the anesthetic beneath the fascial sheath. Block the peroneal nerve laterally with 10 ml of local anesthetic in the groove between the long and lateral digital extensor muscles, approximately 4 cm proximal to the point of the hock.

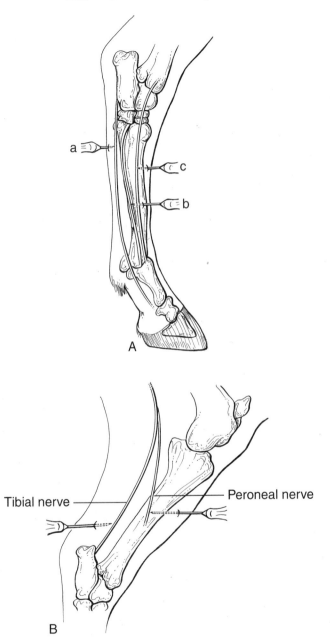

FIGURE 19–3. *See legend on opposite page*

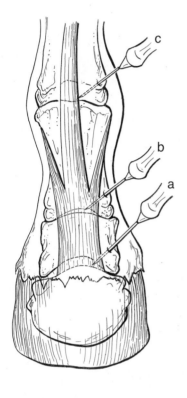

FIGURE 19–4. Intrasynovial anesthesia of the distal limb.

a. **Coffin joint** (20-gauge, 1½-inch needle). Palpate a depression 0.5–1 cm dorsal to the coronary band either medial or lateral to the common digital extensor tendon. With the limb in a weight-bearing position, insert a needle perpendicular to the hoof surface to a depth of 1.5–2.0 cm. Block the joint with 5–8 ml of local anesthetic.

b. **Pastern joint** (20-gauge, 1½-inch needle). Draw a line from the lateral eminence of the first phalanx to midline and insert a needle 1 cm distal to this line and lateral to the common digital extensor tendon. The limb is in a weight-bearing position, and the needle is parallel to the hoof surface. Block the joint with 4–6 ml of local anesthetic.

c. **Fetlock joint** (20-gauge, 1½-inch needle). The palmar pouch is located between the caudal aspect of the cannon bone and the lateral branch of the suspensory ligament. With the limb in a standing or flexed position, insert the needle perpendicular to the limb axis or in a slightly downward direction to a depth of 1.0 cm. Block the joint with 5–8 ml of local anesthetic. The figure demonstrates intrasynovial anesthesia using the dorsal approach, medial or lateral to the common digital extensor tendon.

FIGURE 19–5. *A, B,* Intra-articular anesthesia of the proximal forelimb. **Carpal joints** (20-gauge, 1½-inch). To enter the radiocarpal joint (a), locate the depression between the radius and the radial carpal bone with the carpus flexed. Insert the needle medial to the extensor carpi radialis tendon to a depth of 1 cm. Block the joint with 10 ml of local anesthetic. To enter the intercarpal/middle carpal joint (b), locate the depression between the radial carpal bone and the third carpal bone. Insert the needle medial to the extensor carpi radialis tendon and block the joint with 10 ml of local anesthetic. The carpometacarpal joint communicates with the intercarpal joint.

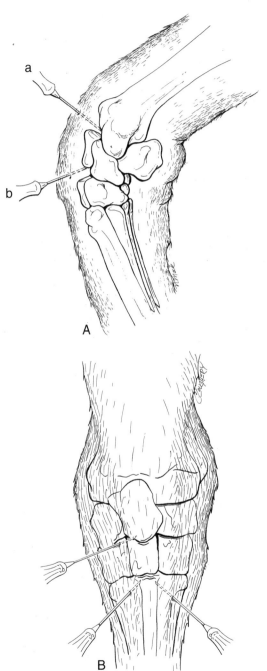

FIGURE 19–5. *See legend on opposite page*

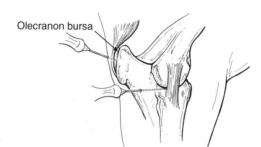

FIGURE 19–6. Elbow joint (20-gauge, 1½-inch). The elbow joint is palpable between the lateral humeral epicondyle and the radial tuberosity. Insert the needle caudal to the lateral collateral ligament in a horizontal direction to a depth of 2–3 cm. Block the joint with 20 ml of local anesthetic.

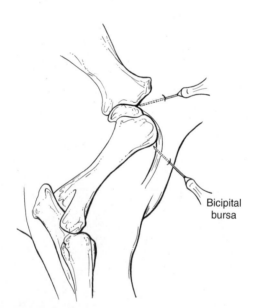

FIGURE 19–7. Scapulohumeral joint (18-gauge, 5-inch needle). Palpate a notch between the anterior and posterior portions of the lateral humeral tuberosity (point of the shoulder). Direct the needle in a horizontal and slightly caudomedial direction to a depth of 8–10 cm. Block the joint with 20 ml of local anesthetic.

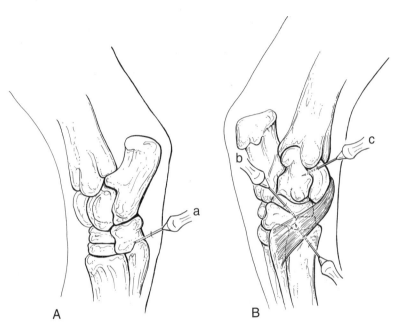

A   B

FIGURE 19–8. *A, B,* Intra-articular anesthesia of the proximal hind limb. **Tarsal joints** (20-gauge, 1½-inch needle). To enter the tarsometatarsal joint (a), palpate a small depression proximal to the head of the lateral splint bone. Insert the needle in a horizontal and slightly downward and anterior direction to a depth of 2–3 cm. Block the joint with 4–6 ml of local anesthetic. Enter the distal intertarsal joint (b) by inserting a needle distal to the anterior aspect of the cunean tendon on the medial aspect of the hock. Block the joint with 4–6 ml of local anesthetic. The tibiotarsal joint (c) is entered on either side of the saphenous vein 2–3 cm below the medial malleolus. Insert the needle to a depth of 1–2 cm and block the joint with 10–15 ml of local anesthetic. The tibiotarsal joint communicates with the proximal intertarsal joint.

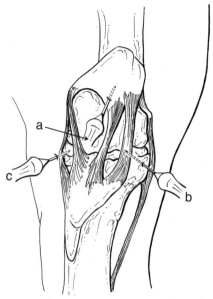

FIGURE 19–9. Stifle joint (18-gauge, 1½–3-inch needle). Access the femoropatellar joint by inserting a needle between the middle and medial patellar ligaments approximately 2–3 cm above the palpable proximal tibial crest (a). Direct the needle horizontally to a depth of 4–5 cm. Block the joint with 40–50 ml of local anesthetic. Enter the lateral femorotibial joint posterior to the lateral patellar ligament and above the proximal edge of the tibia (b). Insert the needle to a depth of 1–2 cm and block the joint with 20–30 ml of local anesthetic. Access the medial femorotibial joint between the medial patellar and medial femorotibial (collateral) ligament and above the palpable proximal tibia (c). Insert the needle horizontally to a depth of 2–3 cm and block the joint with 20–30 ml of local anesthetic.

1

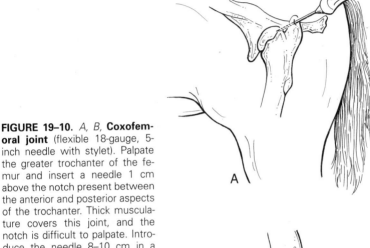

FIGURE 19–10. *A, B,* **Coxofemoral joint** (flexible 18-gauge, 5-inch needle with stylet). Palpate the greater trochanter of the femur and insert a needle 1 cm above the notch present between the anterior and posterior aspects of the trochanter. Thick musculature covers this joint, and the notch is difficult to palpate. Introduce the needle 8–10 cm in a slightly downward and anterior direction. Block the joint with 40 ml of local anesthetic.

- Synovial fluid should be collected and analyzed. (See arthrocentesis procedure, p. 77.)
- Once the needle is in place, attach the syringe and rapidly inject anesthetic. There should be very little resistance to injection. If resistance is encountered, detach the syringe and redirect the needle without exiting the skin. Holding onto the hub of the needle with one hand and injecting with the other facilitates rapid detachment of the syringe should the patient move.
- Allow 20–30 minutes before assessing the effect.
- Repeat the lameness examination and assess improvement (0–100%).
- For distal limbs, place an alcohol-soaked wrap over the injection site.

EVALUATING THE RESULTS OF LOCAL ANESTHESIA

The limitations of local anesthesia for the diagnosis of lameness need to be well understood if this method is to be used accurately. Determining which structures have been desensitized by a particular block is sometimes difficult because of variation in nerve supply. Assessing skin sensation does not always reflect the presence of deep pain. Many individuals retain skin sensation over the dorsal aspect of the distal limb while deeper structures are adequately anesthetized. Use as many physical parameters as possible to determine the effect of the anesthesia (hoof testers, flexion, and so on). A patient may continue to show lameness in spite of the diseased area being anesthetized if other sources of lameness are contributing factors. However, there should still be partial improvement or a change in the gait. The lameness does not improve if it is due to a neurologic or mechanical problem. An improvement after local anesthesia should be followed by radiographic or ultrasound examination (or nuclear scintigraphy if available).

Complications

Infection due to improper skin preparation or concurrent cellulitis. Subcutaneous inflammation and skin sloughing may occur following **perineural anesthesia.** *Use sterile technique and a minimal amount of anesthetic to reduce risk. Rinse the distal limb with alcohol and wrap if multiple injections are performed.*

Joint or tendon sheath infection is a serious sequela to **intrasynovial anesthesia.** Monitor patient for pain or swelling for 2 weeks following a procedure. *Delay procedure if periarticular cellulitis is present. Do not place a needle through a contaminated wound.* If signs of severe inflammation are present, treat for possible iatrogenic infection and lavage joint.

Needle breakage is more likely in proximal joints with long, small-gauge needles. The needle is often difficult to retrieve in a standing horse. Use flexible needles (spinal needles) that bend rather than break. Adequate patient restraint minimizes this complication.

CAUTION: Anesthesia of the proximal limb may result in loss of motor function and stumbling. The distal limb should be wrapped to prevent abrasions and patients confined to a stall immediately following examination.

20 Arthrocentesis and Synovial Fluid Analysis

James A. Orsini and Christine Kreuder

Analysis of the synovial fluid from a joint or tendon sheath can be useful in differentiating among various diseases that affect these structures. Synovial fluid is an ultrafiltrate of plasma, and pathology of synovium-bathed structures is reflected in the fluid. Aspiration of synovial fluid from joints and tendon sheaths requires familiarity with the applied anatomy. Patient restraint and strict adherence to sterile technique are essential for safe arthrocentesis.

Equipment

- sedation (xylazine hydrochloride and butorphanol tartrate)
- twitch
- clippers
- material for sterile scrub
- sterile gloves
- needles (18–22-gauge) and 5–20-ml syringe (not Luer-Lok); see Figures 19–4 through 19–10 for needle size required for each joint. Needles and syringes should be kept sterile throughout the procedure.
- 25-gauge needle, 3-ml syringe, and 2% local anesthetic if anesthesia of skin is desired
- EDTA and plain Vacutainer tubes[1]
- culture material (Port-a-Cul,[2] blood culture bottles[3])

Procedure

- Clip or shave the site for arthrocentesis. Sites for arthrocentesis are identical to sites for intra-articular anesthesia in Figures 19–4 through 19–10.

  WARNING: Do not place the needle through an open or contaminated wound or an area of possible infection. Determination of joint involvement after trauma or infection often requires alternative needle placement if the usual site for joint access is contaminated in any way.
- Sedation is optional. Recommended dosage for adults: 0.3–0.4 mg/kg

---

[1]Vacutainer tubes. Becton-Dickinson Vacutainer Systems, Rutherford, NJ 07070.

[2]Port-a-Cul culture swab and transport system. Becton-Dickinson Microbiology Systems, Cockeysville, MD 21030.

[3]Septi-check, BB blood culture bottle. Roche Diagnostic Systems, Nutley, NJ 07110-1199.

xylazine with 0.01 mg/kg butorphanol IV. For neonatal foals: 0.1–0.2 mg/kg diazepam IV **slowly.**

- Place twitch.
- Perform a sterile scrub of the puncture site and any landmarks to be palpated.
- If the joint requires a 20-gauge or larger needle, place a bleb of 2% local anesthetic subcutaneously, using a 25-gauge needle.
- Using sterile gloves, detach the needle from the syringe and place the needle with a rapid thrust through the skin. Care must be taken not to damage the articular cartilage with the needle. Successful needle placement results in synovial fluid at the hub of the needle. Fluid may flow freely (particularly if the joint is distended), or it may need to be aspirated with a syringe. Digital pressure on other aspects of the joint usually increases the flow of fluid from the needle.

  Failure to obtain synovial fluid is often caused by placement of the needle opening within or adjacent to a ligament, cartilage, or synovial lining. Attempt to redirect or rotate the needle without exiting the skin. The needle may also become plugged with tissue during placement. If synovial fluid is not obtained after the needle is redirected, attempt arthrocentesis with a new needle.
- Collect the sample into a plain and EDTA (purple top) Vacutainer tube for culture and cytology respectively. Samples may be transported in the syringe used for collection—remove air and cap with a sterile needle. If the culture sample is not to be processed within 12 hours, place the sample in a blood culture bottle or Port-a-Cul transport system.

SYNOVIAL FLUID ANALYSIS

Color, clarity, volume, and viscosity of fluid collected are parameters immediately assessed. Normal synovial fluid is clear, slightly yellow, and completely free of particulate. Red streaks indicate trauma and bleeding caused by the needle during placement or aspiration; a uniform red or amber tinge may be due to chronic intra-articular injury. An increase in turbidity or a dark yellow color is caused by inflammation. The presence of particles or purulent material indicates serofibrinous inflammation, which is often associated with infection (septic arthritis or tenosynovitis).

Viscosity is directly related to the amount and quality of hyaluronic acid (HA) secreted by the synovial membrane. Depolymerization or dilution of hyaluronate from inflammation causes a decrease in viscosity. Viscosity is assessed subjectively by placing a drop of fluid between the thumb and a finger; the fluid should string out approximately 2–5 cm before breaking if the fluid is normal. Similarly, fluid expressed from a syringe should form a string about 5–7 cm in length.

Other important parameters are complete white cell count and differential. A slide prep is made with a drop of the synovial fluid and a drop of Wright stain. The quantity, type, and state of degeneration of the white cells is useful for characterizing the inflammation. Total protein quantifies the degree of inflammation. Normal synovial fluid does not clot as it lacks fibrinogen and other clotting factors present during inflammation. Glucose concentration in synovial fluid is compared with serum concentration and may be decreased due to

TABLE 20-1. Correlation of Synovial Fluid Parameters and Intra-articular Disorders

Condition	Appearance	Viscosity	Volume	Total Protein (gm/dl)	Nucleated Cells/L	Cytology Findings	Glucose (mg/dl)
Normal	Light yellow, clear	High	Low	<2.0	<0.4 × 10⁹/L	<20% neutrophils	Equal to blood
Nonseptic synovitis	Yellow, translucent	Low	Generally increased	<3.0	2–10 × 10⁹/L	>75% neutrophils (preserved)	25–50 mg/dl; lower than blood
Septic arthritis	Yellow-green, turbid	Low	Increased	3.0–6.0	30–100 × 10⁹/L	>90% neutrophils (degenerate) ± intracellular bacteria	<25 mg/dl
Degenerative joint disease (osteoarthritis)	Yellow, clear	Low (variable)	Low	<2.5	0.2–2 × 10⁹/L	10–30% neutrophils (preserved)	Equal to blood

1

consumption by inflammatory cells and bacteria. A Gram stain and culture are essential if a septic process is suspected. Negative culture results do not rule out infection, as bacteria are isolated in only 50% of the samples. PCR has not been shown to be of great benefit.

See Table 20–1 for correlation of synovial fluid with certain equine joint disorders.

Complications

See complications of intrasynovial anesthesia, p. 76.

21 Fluorescein Staining

James A. Orsini and Christine Kreuder

Fluorescein staining is an important diagnostic aid to identify diseases of the cornea and determine the patency of the nasolacrimal duct. The most common use of topical fluorescein is to localize corneal ulcers. Defects in the corneal epithelium selectively retain the dye and stain bright green by conversion of absorbed light to fluorescent light. This procedure is indicated whenever a corneal ulcer is suspected or there is a history of direct trauma to the eye.

Equipment

- fluorescein strip[1]
- 5-ml sterile saline in a syringe or collyrium (sterile eye wash)
- penlight or ophthalmoscope

Procedure

- Insert the fluorescein strip under the upper eyelid for 5 to 10 seconds, or the paper strip may be moistened with sterile saline and touched to the dorsal bulbar conjunctiva. When the patient blinks, the fluorescein distributes over the cornea. Direct contact of the impregnated fluorescein strip to the cornea causes excess staining and may be erroneously diagnosed as a corneal defect.
- Gentle flushing with saline or collyrium removes any excess stain.
- Use a direct light source to examine the entire eye for stain uptake. Very deep corneal ulcers may take up stain only along their outermost borders.
- Ultraviolet and cobalt blue light excite fluorescein, thereby facilitating detection of minute corneal epithelial defects.
- Patency of the nasolacrimal duct is verified if fluorescein staining appears at the nostril within 5 minutes.

---

[1]Fluor-i-strip (fluorescein sodium ophthalmic strip). Ayerst Laboratories, Inc., New York, NY 10017.

22 | Nasolacrimal Duct Cannulation

James A. Orsini and Christine Kreuder

Cannulation of the nasolacrimal duct is indicated whenever obstruction of lacrimal drainage is suspected. Clinical signs often seen with an obstruction include epiphora (tearing), staining beneath the eye, and discharge and swelling at the medial canthus. Cannulation is also a valuable method for delivering medications to the eye without having to manipulate the eye or eyelids. This is also a procedure required for dacryocystorhinography—used to define an acquired inflammatory lesion of the nasolacrimal duct. The duct is easily cannulated at its rostral opening where it emerges at the mucocutaneous junction on the ventrum of either nostril.

Equipment

- penlight
- 5–8-Fr. polypropylene catheter[1] (French conversion: each unit French = 0.33-mm diameter)
- 10- or 12-ml syringe filled with sterile saline
- gauze sponges
- sterile lubricant[2]

Procedure

- Reflect the alar fold of the nostril and locate the puncta of the nasolacrimal duct, utilizing a light source. The rostral duct opening is easily located on the ventral aspect of the nasal meatus. Some horses have two or more puncta in one nostril and only one is patent.
- Swab the inside of the nostril and place the minimally lubricated catheter in the duct. Slide the catheter at least 5 cm proximally.
- To flush the duct, place a finger over the puncta to hold the catheter in place and prevent the saline from exiting normograde. Attach the syringe and gently flush the duct retrograde. Patency has been achieved once the saline flows from the lacrimal puncta at the medial canthus of the eye.
- The catheter may be sutured in place for routine ophthalmic medication, using a butterfly taping technique.

---

[1]Polypropylene catheter. Monoject, Sherwood Medical, St. Louis, MO 63103.
[2]KY lubricating jelly. Johnson and Johnson Products, Inc., New Brunswick, NJ 08903.

23 Subpalpebral Catheter Placement

James A. Orsini and Christine Kreuder

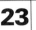

Horses requiring frequent or long-term topical administration of an eye medication are candidates for subpalpebral catheters. A catheter is placed through the eyelid, which allows one to deliver the medication while standing at the individual's withers. This system is ideal for difficult patients requiring frequent treatments. If complications do not occur, the catheter may remain in place for several weeks.

Equipment

- sedation (xylazine hydrochloride)
- 2% local anesthetic with 25-gauge, ⅝-inch needle, 5-ml syringe
- 12-gauge, 1.5-inch needle with hub removed
- Silastic tubing (0.03-inch ID × 0.065-inch OD)[1] polyethylene tubing (PE190)[2]
- feline indwelling catheter (20-gauge)[3]
- injection cap
- white tape
- 2-0 nonabsorbable suture on a straight needle
- suture scissors

Procedure

- Recommended dose for sedation: 0.4–0.6 mg/kg xylazine IV.
- Anesthetize the auriculopalpebral and supraorbital nerves innervating the upper eyelid (Fig. 23–1).
- Place the lavage system **deep** in the dorsal palpebral fornix to minimize tubing contact with the corneal surface.
- Lift the upper eyelid and insert the 12-gauge needle up through the conjunctiva and skin in the dorsolateral aspect of the lid.
- Insert the Silastic tubing into the lumen of the needle in the same upward direction. Once the tubing exits from the sharp end of the needle, pull

---

[1]Dow Corning Silastic tubing. Stortz Instrument Company, St. Louis, MO 63122.

[2]Intramedic nonradiopaque Polyethylene tubing. Clay Adams, Division of Becton-Dickinson and Co., Parsippany, NJ 07054

[3]Feline indwelling catheter (20-gauge). Sherwood Medical, 1915 Olive Street, St. Louis, MO 63103; (800) 428-4400.

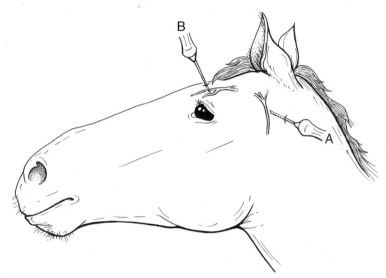

FIGURE 23–1. Needle placement for auriculopalpebral and supraorbital nerve blocks. *A*, Block the auriculopalpebral nerve as it runs along the zygomatic arch with 3–5 ml of local anesthetic. *B*, Block the supraorbital nerve at the ventral rim of the supraorbital fossa with 3–5 ml of local anesthetic.

the needle out and thread the tubing through the lid until 10 cm of tubing remains below the lid.

- Reinsert the needle up through the conjunctiva and skin in the dorsomedial aspect of the lid, 4 cm medial to the first insertion. Thread the tail end of the tubing through the blunt end of the needle.
- Remove the needle from the eyelid and tie several knots in the medial end of the tubing.
- Pull the knotted end of the tubing out of the lid and place six holes in the tubing with a 25-gauge needle. Place the holes 1 to 2 cm from the knot so that the eye medication distributes over the eye rather than leaks subcutaneously.
- Position the tubing and secure it dorsal to the eyelid in at least two areas on the forehead and near the poll. Place white tape around the tubing and suture the tape to the skin. Secure the tubing down the neck by taping it to a braided mane (Fig. 23–2).
- Insert a feline indwelling catheter (without the needle) into the tubing and attach an injection cap in order to have a portal for drug administration.
- Medication may be administered through the injection cap by standing at the withers of the patient. Fill the line with medication until drops are seen distributing over the cornea. Different medications may be mixed in the line. Continuous administration of ophthalmic solution may be delivered by a pressurized fluid bag attached to the mane or a surcingle.

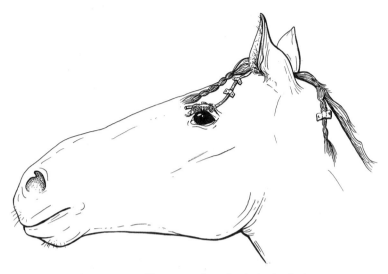

FIGURE 23–2. Placement of a subpalpebral catheter.

Complications

Corneal ulceration develops if the catheter scratches the cornea. Tubing should be soft and pliable and have no rough edges. *Lift the upper eyelid and check the position of the catheter several times daily to make sure it has not migrated over the cornea.*

A **swollen** and **irritated eyelid** occurs if the catheter migrates into the conjunctiva and medication goes into subcutaneous tissue. Some individuals rub their eyes because both the catheter and ocular disease are irritating. *Fly nets or hoods with eye cups prevent trauma to the catheter and the eye.* Use caution when manipulating sharp objects around the eye because sudden movement of even a properly restrained horse can cause puncture of the globe. *Guard the object's sharp end as much as possible.*

The holes in the Silastic tubing often become plugged with fibrin after several days. Retract the tubing from under the eyelid and flush medication through the holes by administering a new dose. If this is unsuccessful, make additional holes with a 25-gauge needle, taking care not to lacerate the tubing.

PART VII

Central Nervous System

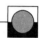

24 Cerebrospinal Fluid Collection

James A. Orsini and Christine Kreuder

Cerebrospinal fluid (CSF) analysis is indicated whenever disease of the central nervous system is suspected. Analysis helps rule in or out involvement of the central nervous system (CNS) (vs. a peripheral neuropathy), and specific changes in the CSF are well correlated to certain infectious diseases. CSF is assessed for a titer against *Sarcocystis neurona* if equine protozoal myelitis (EPM) is suspected.[1] Fluid may be aspirated from two sites, the lumbosacral space and the atlanto-occipital space. Collection from the atlanto-occipital space must be done under general anesthesia, which may be contraindicated in the severely neurologic adult.

Equipment

- twitch and/or sedation (detomidine and butorphanol tartrate)
- clippers
- material for sterile scrub
- sterile gloves
- 2% local anesthetic, 6-ml syringe and 22-gauge, 1.5-inch needle
- 15-cm (6-inch), 18-gauge spinal needle for lumbosacral aspirate or 9-cm (3.5-inch), 18-gauge needle for atlanto-occipital aspirate[2] (sterile)
- 12-ml syringe (sterile)
- EDTA and plain Vacutainer tubes[3]
- Culture[4] or Port-a-Cul[5] culture system
- stool to stand on to reach puncture site

---

[1]Sample required: two red-top tubes, one with serum and one with CSF fluid. Purple-top (EDTA) tube required for PCR.

[2]Spinal needles. Becton-Dickinson, Franklin Lakes, NJ 07417.

[3]Vacutainer tubes. Becton-Dickinson Vacutainer Systems, Rutherford, NJ 07070.

[4]Culturette collection and transport system. Becton-Dickinson Microbiology Systems, Cockeysville, MD 21030.

[5]Port-a-Cul tube. BBL Division of Becton-Dickinson and Company, Cockeysville, MD 21030.

- Styrofoam shipping container with ice packs and appropriate address labels for sample submission via 1 to 2 day delivery to:

EBI, A165 ASTeCC Building
University of Kentucky
Lexington, KY 40506-0286
Phone (606) 257-2300, ext. 226
Fax (606) 257-2489
or
Neogen Corporation
ELISA Technologies Division
628 Winchester Rd.
Lexington, KY 40505
Phone (606) 254-1221
Fax (606) 255-5532

Procedure

Collection from the Lumbosacral Space

- Restrain individual in stocks. Sedation is generally not necessary but is recommended. Recommended dosage: 0.01 mg/kg detomidine with 0.01 mg/kg butorphanol IV.
- See Figure 24–1 for landmarks for the lumbosacral tap.
- Wear sterile gloves and maintain sterility throughout procedure.
- Place a bleb of local anesthetic beneath the skin and 3 to 5 ml in the deeper muscle layers.
- With the patient standing squarely, insert a 6-inch spinal needle perpendicular to the midline. The subarachnoid space is approximately 11 to 15 cm deep to the skin in the adult. A loss of resistance is often felt as the needle passes into the subarachnoid space and there is often a sudden patient movement.
- Remove the trochar from the needle.
- Fluid frequently appears at the needle hub shortly after the subarachnoid space has been penetrated. Occlude both jugular veins with digital pressure to increase CNS pressure.
- If the initial sample appears blood contaminated, discard and use another syringe for additional sampling.
- Aspirate fluid with a syringe and place the sample into EDTA and plain Vacutainer tubes and onto a Culturette swab.

Collection from Atlanto-Occipital Space

- Place the patient under general anesthesia to maintain proper position of the head and neck. This spinal tap is performed over the cervical spinal cord close to the brain stem, and it is therefore possible to traumatize nervous tissue if the head or neck moves.
- Flex the patient's neck so that the head is at a right angle to the neck.
- See Figure 24–2 for landmarks for the atlanto-occipital aspirate.
- Clip area and perform a sterile scrub. Maintain sterility throughout the procedure.

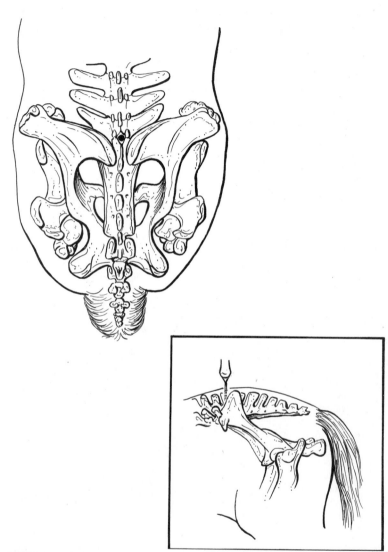

FIGURE 24–1. Needle placement for collection of CSF from the lumbosacral space. The LS space is generally palpable as a depression caudal to the sixth lumbar spinous process. Palpate the caudal edge of each tuber coxae and draw a line directly to midline to find the depression. This area (inset) is also immediately cranial to the prominence of each tuber sacrale. Angle the needle directly perpendicular to the vertebrae.

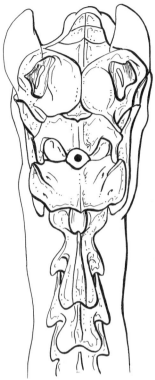
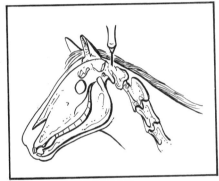

FIGURE 24–2. Needle placement for collection of CSF from the atlanto-occipital space. Palpate the cranial borders of the atlas and draw a line directly to midline. The site for puncture (inset) is 1 to 2 cm caudal to this line directly on midline. Angle the needle perpendicular to the cervical vertebrae.

- Using sterile gloves, insert the 3.5-inch spinal needle to a depth of 5–7 cm. Remove the trochar to determine placement in the subarachnoid space.
- Once CSF appears at the needle hub, aspirate the fluid with a syringe or allow the CSF to flow into collection tube.

CEREBROSPINAL FLUID ANALYSIS

CSF is examined grossly for color, clarity, and particulate matter. Normal CSF is clear and colorless. An increase in turbidity or particles occurs with inflammation and infectious processes. Red streaks in the fluid result from contamination during collection, whereas previous hemorrhage in the CNS creates a xanthochromic or yellow-colored sample. Total protein measurement and cytology (including total white cell and red cell counts) should be performed on every aspirate. Various changes in the cellular content are typical for specific disease processes. See Table 24–1 for correlation between abnormal parameters and

TABLE 24-1. Correlation of Cerebral Spinal Fluid Parameters and Central Nervous System Disorders

Condition	Appearance*	Total Protein* (mg/dl)	Total Nucleated Cells*/ml	Cytology Findings
Normal	Clear, colorless	40–90	0–10/ml	All mononuclear cells
Bacterial infection	White-amber to yellow, may be turbid	>200	>100/ml	↑ Neutrophils
Viral infection	Clear-turbid, colorless, amber	100–200	Low normal to increased	Predominantly lymphocytes
Hemorrhage or trauma	Uniformly red† or yellow‡	>100	0–variable	Macrophages, erythrophagia and neutrophils
Fungal infection	Clear to yellow	100–200	>100/ml	↑ Neutrophils
Protozoal infection§	Clear to yellow	40–200	0–40	Mixed macrophages, lymphocytes, and neutrophils

*Characteristic finding but may vary.
†Recent hemorrhage.
‡Past hemorrhage.
§<30% of horses with EPM have abnormal values.

CNS disease. Other parameters to assess are creatine phosphokinase level (normally less than 8 IU/dl) and glucose (normally between 55 and 70 mg/dl) level. The creatine phosphokinase (CPK) is found in fat and dura and, while the enzyme may be released with neuronal cell damage or degeneration, it is generally not a reliable monitor for CNS disease. Glucose levels are lower than normal with inflammation due to consumption of glucose by white blood cells and/or bacteria.

Complications

Trauma to the spinal cord or brain stem during needle placement, although rare, can cause serious neurologic impairment. *Minimize patient movement with stocks and/or sedation.*

Infection of the meninges, although rare, can be fatal; therefore maintain sterile technique.

Organ System Examination, Neonatology, Shock, and Temperature-Related Problems

PART I: Organ System Examination **94**
  25. Cardiovascular 94
  26. Gastrointestinal Emergencies and Other Causes of Colic 156
  27. Integumentary 238
  28. Liver Failure; Hemolytic Anemia 273
  29. Musculoskeletal 297
  30. Nervous System 337
  31. Ophthalmology 379
  32. Reproductive System 405
  33. Respiratory 434
  34. Urinary 462

PART II: Neonatology **473**
  35. Neonatology; Foal Cardiopulmonary Resuscitation 473

PART III: Shock and Temperature-Related Problems **538**
  36. Shock and Systemic Inflammatory Response Syndrome 538
  37. Temperature-Related Problems 543

Organ System Examination

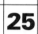

25 Cardiovascular

Virginia B. Reef

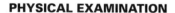

PHYSICAL EXAMINATION

A complete cardiovascular examination in the horse includes auscultation of the heart; auscultation of both lung fields; palpation of the precordium; palpation of the arterial pulses; evaluation of the venous system, mucous membranes, and capillary refill time; and an overall assessment of the horse's health. In the emergency setting, the horse is usually distressed, and only a resting examination is indicated. The patient's clinical condition should be assessed as quickly as possible so that the appropriate lifesaving treatment, if needed, can be instituted as soon as possible.

Auscultation of the Heart

This is performed from both sides of the individual's chest, evaluating heart rate, rhythm, and intensity of heart sounds and characterizing any murmurs or transient sounds detected that are associated with the cardiac cycle.

- The normal heart rate is 28–44 beats/minute in the adult at rest and may be up to 80 beats/minute in the foal (average in the equine neonate is 70 beats/minute).
- The most common normal rhythm in horses is sinus rhythm.
- Second-degree AV block is the most common vagally mediated arrhythmia detected in normal horses. It is detected in 15–18% of individuals on a resting electrocardiogram and in 44% of individuals during 24-hour continuous electrocardiographic monitoring.
- Sinus arrhythmia, sinus bradycardia, SA block, and SA arrest also occur in normal horses with high resting vagal tone.

Identify heart sounds and characterize their timing and intensity. Up to four heart sounds can be auscultated in normal horses (Table 25–1).

Auscultate the heart over all four valve areas (Fig. 25–1).

Characterize murmurs detected by their intensity, timing, duration, quality, point of maximal intensity, and radiation (Table 25–2).

- **Intensity**—the loudness of the murmur and the ability to detect the murmur upon palpation of the precordium. The murmur's intensity,

TABLE 25–1. **Equine Heart Sounds**

Sound	Genesis	PMI	Quality
S1	Early ventricular contraction, abrupt deceleration of blood associated with tensing of the AV valve leaflets and AV valve closure, opening of the semilunar valves, and vibrations associated with ejection of blood into the great vessels	L apex	Loud, high frequency Longer, louder Lower pitch than S2
S2	Closure of the semilunar valves, abrupt deceleration of blood in the great vessels, opening of the AV valves	L base	Loud, high frequency Sharper, shorter Higher pitch than S1
S3	Rapid deceleration of blood in the ventricles at the end of the rapid ventricular filling phase; transient AV valve closure may occur	L apex	Soft, low frequency Lower pitch than S2
S4	Vibrations associated with blood flow from atria to ventricle during atrial contraction; transient AV valve closure may occur	L base	Soft, low frequency Lower pitch than S1

PMI, point of maximal intensity; L, left.

1–6/6, is determined by the quantity and velocity of blood flow through the murmur's origin, its distance from the stethoscope, and the acoustic properties of the interposed tissue.
□ **Grade 1**—the softest audible murmur, detected only after minutes of intense listening
□ **Grade 2**—a soft murmur that is immediately detected at its point of maximal intensity
□ **Grade 3**—a louder, moderate-intensity murmur that is easily heard but lacks a precordial thrill
□ **Grade 4**—a loud murmur that has a faint precordial thrill palpable at the point of maximal intensity of the murmur
□ **Grade 5**—a louder murmur with a strong precordial thrill palpable at the point of maximal intensity of the murmur
□ **Grade 6**—the loudest possible murmur, with a strong precordial thrill that can be heard when the head of the stethoscope is removed from the chest
■ **Timing**—the phase of the cardiac cycle (systolic, diastolic, or both) that the murmur occupies
■ **Duration**—the length of time the murmur is detectable within each phase of the cardiac cycle
□ Early, mid, or late systolic—occurs in early (immediately following the first heart sound, S1), mid (midway between S1 and the second heart sound, S2), or late (immediately before S2) systole

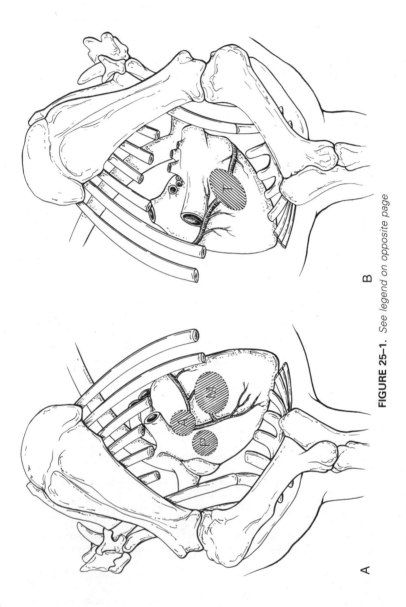

A

B

FIGURE 25-1. *See legend on opposite page*

TABLE 25–2. **Characterization of the Common Equine Cardiac Murmurs**

Murmur	Intensity (Grade)	Timing	Duration	Quality/Shape	PMI	Radiation
Physiologic	1–2	S	E, M, L, HS	low freq	A, P, Mi, T	
(flow)	1–3	D	E, M, L	decrescendo	A, P, Mi, T	
MR	2–6	S	HS, PS	mixed, plateau	Mi / A	DCa / DCr
MVP	2–6	S	M-L	crescendo	Mi	DCa
TR	2–6	S	HS, PS	mixed, plateau	T	DCr, DCa
TVP	2–6	S	M-L	crescendo	T	
AR	1–6	D	HD	low freq, musical, decrescendo	A	DCr apex (L)
PR	1–6	D	HD	low freq, musical, decrescendo	P	apex (R)
VSD	3–6	S	HS, PS	mixed, plateau	T	P

PMI, point of maximal intensity; S, systolic; D, diastolic; E, early; M, mid; L, late; HS, holosystolic; PS, pansystolic; HD, holodiastolic; A, aortic valve; P, pulmonic valve; Mi, mitral valve; T, tricuspid valve; DCa, dorsocaudal; DCr, dorsocranial; MR, mitral regurgitation; MVP, mitral valve prolapse; TR, tricuspid regurgitation; TVP, tricuspid valve prolapse; AR, aortic regurgitation; PR, pulmonic regurgitation; VSD, ventricular septal defect.

□ Holosystolic—occurs between S1 and S2 but does not encompass these heart sounds
□ Pansystolic—begins at the onset of S1 and ends at the completion of S2
□ Early, mid, or late diastolic—occurs in early (between S2 and the third heart sound, S3), mid (midway between S2 and S1), or late (between the fourth heart sound, S4 and S1) diastole
□ Holodiastolic—between S2 and S1
□ Continuous—throughout all phases of the cardiac cycle
■ **Quality**—the frequency (high, low, or mixed-pitch) and character (harsh, coarse, rumbling, scratchy, musical, honking, or blowing) of the murmur detected
■ **Shape**—determined by the phonocardiographic depiction of the intensity of the murmur over time (band- or plateau-shaped, crescendo-decrescendo or diamond-shaped, crescendo, decrescendo, or machinery)
■ **Point of maximal intensity**—the point of the thoracic wall (intercostal space or valve area) where the murmur is heard the loudest. This point should correspond to the area of the strongest precordial thrill if a precordial thrill is present.
■ **Radiation**—the direction in which the murmur intensity decreases most slowly. The radiation of the murmur is usually from the murmur's origin

FIGURE 25–1. Cardiac auscultation areas in the horse viewed from the left *(A)* and the right *(B)* side of the thorax. The shaded areas represent the respective valve areas. P, pulmonic valve, A, aortic valve, M, mitral valve, T, tricuspid valve.

in the direction of abnormal blood flow and is also determined by the murmur's intensity and physical characteristics of the chest.

Palpate the precordium over both sides of the chest to detect precordial thrills or abnormal apex beats (accentuated, faint, or displaced).

Rhythm disturbances are classified as bradyarrhythmias or tachyarrhythmias.

Evaluate the arterial pulses simultaneously with cardiac auscultation to determine that they are synchronous with every heart beat.

Assess the quality of the arterial pulses in the facial or transverse facial artery and in the extremities.

Evaluate the jugular vein, saphenous vein, and other peripheral veins for distention and pulsations.

Perform auscultation of both lung fields at rest and, if possible, with the patient breathing into a rebreathing bag. *The rebreathing bag should not be used at all, or should be used with care*, in individuals with severe respiratory distress.

Diagnosis of rhythm disturbances is made with an electrocardiogram.

Diagnosis and assessment of the severity of valvular, pericardial, myocardial, or great vessel disease are made with an echocardiogram.

THE ELECTROCARDIOGRAM

Obtain a complete 12-lead electrocardiogram (ECG) whenever possible (Table 25–3 and Fig. 25–2). In an emergency setting, the base-apex lead may be all that is needed to diagnose accurately the rhythm disturbance present in the equine patient. Occasionally, however, due to the extensive Purkinje fiber network present in the equine ventricle, it may be difficult to determine whether the rhythm disturbance detected is ventricular or supraventricular. In these situations at least two different leads are needed to determine the origin of the abnormal depolarization.

- The **base-apex lead** gives the clinician large, easy to read complexes, and the electrodes can usually be properly applied with minimal resistance from the horse.
- The base-apex lead can be easily obtained in the recumbent individual when obtaining a full 12-lead electrocardiogram may be difficult. The electrodes can be applied at the heart base and apex on the same side of the patient if necessary.
- The base-apex lead is the best **monitoring lead** for radiotelemetry ECG systems, continuous 24-hour Holter electrocardiographic monitoring, and monitoring cardiac rhythm in critical patients, during antiarrhythmic therapy or during pericardiocentesis.
- Heart rate can be quickly estimated at 25 mm/sec paper speed as "Bic pen" × 10.
- Transtelephonic ECG systems have one important disadvantage in an emergency setting. The clinician transmitting the ECG is usually not able to evaluate the electrocardiogram as it is being obtained because he or she does not see the ECG tracing. Instead, the clinician has to wait for the assessment of the person receiving the ECG to select an appropriate treatment.

2

TABLE 25–3. **Electrode Placement for Complete 12-Lead Electrocardiogram**

Lead I: LA—RA:	Left foreleg (left arm) electrode placed just below the point of the elbow on the back of the left forearm. Right foreleg (right arm) electrode placed just below the point of the elbow on the back of the right forearm.
Lead II: LL—LA:	Left hindleg (left leg) electrode placed on the loose skin at the left stifle in the region of the patella. Left foreleg (left arm) electrode placed just below the point of the elbow on the back of the left forearm.
Lead III: LL—RA:	Left hindleg (left leg) electrode placed on the loose skin at the left stifle in the region of the patella. Right foreleg (right arm) electrode placed just below the point of the elbow on the back of the right forearm.
aV$_R$: RA—CT:	Right foreleg (right arm) electrode placed just below the point of the elbow on the back of the right forearm. The electrical center of the heart or central terminal $\times$ $3/2$.
aV$_I$: LA—CT:	Left foreleg (left arm) electrode placed just below the point of the elbow on the back of the left forearm. The electrical center of the heart or central terminal $\times$ $3/2$.
aV$_F$: LL—CT:	Left hindleg (left leg) electrode placed on the loose skin at the left stifle in the region of the patella. The electrical center of the heart or central terminal $\times$ $3/2$.
CV6LL: V1—CT:	V1 electrode placed in the 6th intercostal space on the left side of the thorax along a line parallel to the level of the point of the elbow. The electrical center of the heart (central terminal).
CV6LU: V2—CT:	V2 electrode placed in the 6th intercostal space on the left side of the thorax along a line parallel to the level of the point of the shoulder. The electrical center of the heart (central terminal).
V10: V3—CT:	V3 electrode placed over the dorsal thoracic spine of T7 at the withers. Electrical center of the heart. The dorsal spine of T7 is located on a line encircling the chest in the 6th intercostal space (central terminal).
CV6RL: V4—CT:	V4 electrode placed in the 6th intercostal space on the right side of the thorax along a line parallel to the level of the point of the elbow. The electrical center of the heart (central terminal).
CV6RU: V5—CT:	V5 electrode placed in the 6th intercostal space on the right side of the thorax along a line parallel to the level of the point of the shoulder. The electrical center of the heart (central terminal).
Base-apex: LA—RA:	Left foreleg (left arm) electrode placed in the 6th intercostal space on the left side of the thorax along a line parallel to the level of the point of the elbow. Right foreleg (right arm) electrode placed on the top of the right scapular spine.

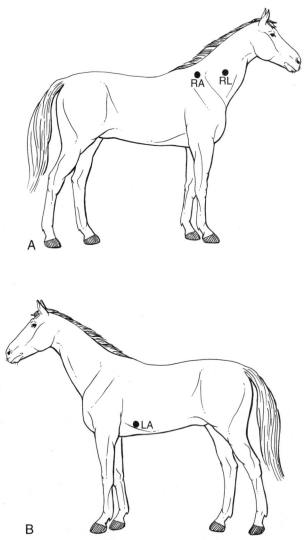

FIGURE 25–2. Sites for lead placement for obtaining a base-apex electrocardiogram *(A* and *B)* and a complete electrocardiogram *(C* and *D)* in a horse. The black circles represent the sites of attachment for the electrodes.

A, Position of the electrode placement on the right side of the patient for obtaining a base-apex electrocardiogram, using the electrodes from lead I. RA, right foreleg (right arm); RL, right hindleg (right leg).

B, Position of the electrode placement on the left side of the patient for obtaining a base-apex electrocardiogram, using the electrodes from lead I. LA, left foreleg (left arm).

2

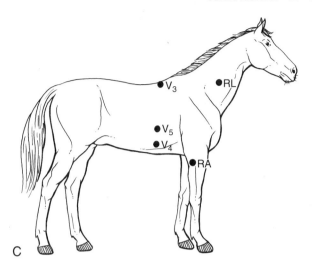

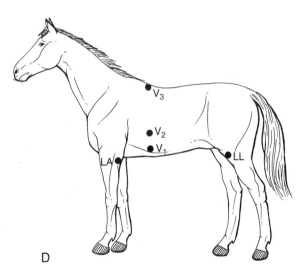

FIGURE 25–2 *Continued. C,* Position of the electrode placement on the right side of the patient for obtaining a complete electrocardiogram. RA, right foreleg (right arm); RL, right hindleg (right leg); V_3, third chest lead (V_{10}); V_4, fourth chest lead (CV_6RL); V_5, fifth chest lead (CV_6RU).

D, Position of the electrode placement on the left side of the patient for obtaining a complete electrocardiogram. LA, left foreleg (left arm); LL, left hindleg (left leg); V_1, first chest lead (CV_6LL); V_2, second chest lead (CV_6LU); V_3, third chest lead (V_{10}).

ARRHYTHMIAS

Cardiac arrhythmias occur commonly in horses and rarely require antiarrhythmic therapy. Certain cardiac arrhythmias, however, can be life-threatening and require emergency treatment. Rapid tachyarrhythmias and profound bradyarrhythmias are most likely to need immediate treatment to control the arrhythmia and relieve the signs of cardiovascular collapse.

An **electrocardiogram** is necessary to confirm the diagnosis of the rhythm disturbance auscultated and to choose the appropriate treatment.

Perform **continuous ECG monitoring** in all individuals with potentially life-threatening arrhythmias to monitor cardiac rhythm and response to treatment.

Bradyarrhythmias

Complete (Third-Degree) AV Block

- Rare
- Usually associated with inflammatory or degenerative changes in the AV node
- Severe exercise intolerance and frequent syncope are common
- Resting heart rate (ventricular rate) usually ≤ 20 beats/minute, with a more rapid, independent atrial rate

Auscultation

- Loud, regular first (S1) and second (S2) heart sounds
- Slow ventricular rate (≤ 20 beats/minute)
- Rapid, regular independent fourth (S4) heart sounds (usually ≥ 60/minute). Occasional "bruit de canon" sounds, caused by the summation of the fourth (S4) heart sound with another heart sound (S1, S2, or S3)

Electrocardiogram

- Rapid atrial rate (more P waves than QRS complexes)
- Regular P–P interval
- No evidence of AV conduction; no consistent relationship between P waves and QRS complexes (P–R intervals of different lengths)
- Abnormal QRS configuration (usually widened and bizarre) unassociated with the preceding P waves (Fig. 25–3)
- The dominant pacemaker is idionodal or idioventricular.

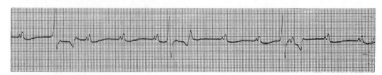

FIGURE 25–3. Base-apex electrocardiogram obtained from a horse with complete heart block. Notice the large, wide QRS complexes, which are not associated with the preceding P waves. There is complete A-V dissociation, with a rapid, regular atrial rate of 70/minute and a slow, regular ventricular rate of 20 beats/minute. The P–P interval is regular, and the R–R interval is regular. This electrocardiogram was recorded at a paper speed of 25 mm/sec with a sensitivity of 10 mm = 1 mV.

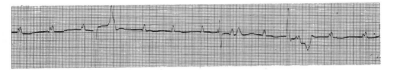

FIGURE 25–4. Lead II electrocardiogram obtained from a horse with complete heart block. Notice the large wide QRS complexes of differing configurations, which are not associated with the preceding P waves. There is complete A-V dissociation, with a rapid regular atrial rate of 70/minute and a slow, irregular ventricular rate of 30 beats/minute. The P–P interval is regular and the R–R interval is irregular. This electrocardiogram was recorded at a paper speed of 25 mm/sec with a sensitivity of 10 mm = 1 mV.

- R–R interval is usually regular but is irregular when more than one QRS configuration is present, associated with complexes arising from different areas in the ventricle (Fig. 25–4).

Treatment

Should be aggressive when diagnosed.

- **Vagolytic drugs**:
  - □ **Atropine** or **glycopyrrolate** should be administered **IV** at a dose of **0.005–0.01 mg/kg as a bolus.** Usually unsuccessful in restoring sinus rhythm; potential **side effects** include tachycardia, arrhythmias, decreased gastrointestinal motility, and mydriasis.
- **Corticosteroids**:
  - □ **Dexamethasone** is indicated in high doses **(0.05–0.22 mg/kg) IV (preferable), IM or PO,** in hopes that reversible inflammatory disease is present in the region of the AV node.
  - □ *Laminitis* is an undesirable side effect of corticosteroid usage in horses but occurs most frequently following prolonged use of large doses of corticosteroids. Immune suppression and iatrogenic adrenal insufficiency may also occur with prolonged use of corticosteroids. Exacerbation or recrudescence of viral and bacterial infections with corticosteroid usage is also a potential problem and should be considered in horses with suspected myocarditis.
- **Sympathomimetic drugs** to speed the idioventricular rhythm. These drugs should be used with care, or not at all, if other ventricular ectopy is present, because they may exacerbate ventricular arrhythmias.
  - □ **Isoproterenol** is indicated when syncope is present and if no ventricular ectopy is detected at a dose of **0.05–0.2 μg/kg/min.** Rapid tachyarrhythmias are an undesirable side effect. *If tachyarrhythmias occur, stop isoproterenol infusion and treat ventricular arrhythmias with lidocaine or propranolol.*
- **Implantation** of a **cardiac pacemaker**—definitive treatment for complete heart block, if no response is seen with corticosteroid therapy. A permanent transvenous pacemaker has been successfully implanted in a horse with complete heart block (Figs. 25–5 and 25–6). Temporary transvenous pacemakers may be tried in horses with advanced second-degree or complete AV block, until a permanent transvenous pacemaker can be inserted.

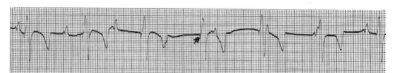

FIGURE 25–5. Base-apex electrocardiogram from a horse with complete heart block treated with a ventricular demand pacemaker (VVI) and a single pacing electrode in the right ventricle. Notice the pacing spike *(arrow)*, which initiates the ventricular depolarization at a rate of 50 beats/minute. There is a completely independent, slightly faster atrial rate of 60/minute and complete A-V dissociation. The QRS complexes appear widened and bizarre. The P–P interval is regular, and the R–R interval is regular. This electrocardiogram was recorded at a paper speed of 25 mm/sec with a sensitivity of 10 mm = 1 mV.

□ Temporary transvenous pacemakers are less successful in capturing the cardiac rhythm because these pacing wires are not anchored in the right ventricle but are, instead, free floating. The temporary pacing wires tend to float in the blood within the right ventricular chamber

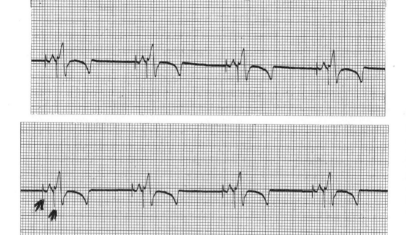

FIGURE 25–6. Continuous base-apex electrocardiogram obtained from a horse with complete heart block treated with a universal pacemaker (DDD) with an atrial pacing electrode in the right atrium and a ventricular pacing electrode in the right ventricle. Notice the pacing spike causing atrial depolarization *(first arrow)* and the pacing spike causing ventricular depolarization *(second arrow)*. Both the atrial and the ventricular rate are 50 beats/minute and are associated with one another. The P–P interval is regular, and the R–R interval is regular. These atrial electrodes have the ability to sense electrical depolarization of the atria and do not pace the atria if the sinus rate increases, thus allowing the patient to exercise. This electrocardiogram was recorded at a paper speed of 25 mm/sec with a sensitivity of 5 mm = 1 mV.

without making consistent contact with the right ventricular free wall. Contact between the pacing wire and the right ventricular free wall is necessary for the electrical impulse to result in ventricular depolarization.

Advanced Second-Degree AV Block

- May also be associated with severe exercise intolerance and collapse
- Can be seen with electrolyte imbalances, e.g. hypercalcemia, digitalis toxicity, and AV nodal disease
- Should be investigated thoroughly and treated aggressively (see above) in hopes of preventing progression of the conduction block to complete AV block

Auscultation

- Regular first (S1) and second (S2) heart sounds
- Slow to low-normal heart rate (usually 8–24 beats/minute)
- Fourth (S4) heart sounds preceding each S1 and regular S4 in pauses for each period of second-degree AV block

Electrocardiogram

- Rapid atrial rate
- Regular P–P interval
- Evidence of AV conduction (P–R intervals of similar lengths)
- Normal QRS configuration associated with the preceding P waves (Figs. 25–7 and 25–8)
- R–R interval is usually regular, but may be irregular in some individuals (Fig. 25–8).

Sinus Bradycardia, Sinoatrial Block

Sinus bradycardia, sinus arrhythmia, and **sinoatrial block** occur in fit horses but are less common than second-degree AV block.

Auscultation

- Regular first (S1) and second (S2) heart sounds with a pause in the rhythm (sinoatrial block) or rhythmic variation of diastolic intervals (sinus bradycardia and sinus arrhythmia)

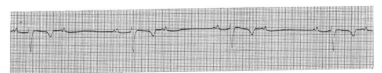

FIGURE 25–7. Base-apex electrocardiogram obtained from a horse with advanced second-degree A-V block with 2:1 conduction. Notice that every other P wave is not followed by a QRS complex, but every QRS complex present is preceded by a P wave at a normal P–R interval (440 msec). The P–P interval is regular, and the R–R interval is regular. The atrial rate is slightly increased at 50/minute with a slow ventricular rate of 30 beats/minute. This electrocardiogram was recorded at a paper speed of 25 mm/sec with a sensitivity of 5 mm = 1 mV.

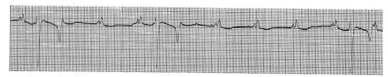

FIGURE 25–8. Base-apex electrocardiogram obtained from a horse with advanced second-degree AV block with variable conduction. Notice that every P wave is not followed by a QRS complex, but every QRS complex present is preceded by a P wave at a normal P–R interval (480 msec). The P–P interval is regular, and the R–R interval is regular. The atrial rate is slightly increased at 60/minute with a slower than normal ventricular rate of 20 beats/minute. This electrocardiogram was recorded at a paper speed of 25 mm/sec with a sensitivity of 5 mm = 1 mV.

- Slow to low-normal heart rate (usually 20–30 beats/minute)
- Fourth (S4) heart sound preceding each S1 usually auscultable
- No S4 in pauses for each period of sinoatrial block

Electrocardiogram

- Slow to low-normal atrial rate
- Irregular P–P interval
- Evidence of AV conduction
- Normal QRS complex associated with the preceding P waves
- R–R interval is rhythmically irregular (sinus bradycardia and sinus arrhythmia) or regularly irregular (sinoatrial block), with a diastolic pause equal to the number of beats blocked at the sinoatrial node.

Usually manifestations of high vagal tone

Disappear with exercise or the administration of a vagolytic (**atropine or glycopyrrolate at 0.005–0.01 mg/kg IV**) or sympathomimetic (**isoproterenol at 0.05–0.2 μg/kg/minute**) drug

Sinoatrial Arrest

An uncommon, vagally mediated arrhythmia in horses

Auscultation

- Regular first (S1) and second (S2) heart sounds with a prolonged pause in the rhythm (greater than two diastolic periods)
- Slow to low-normal heart rate (usually 20–30 beats/minute but may be lower if pathologic)
- Fourth (S4) heart sounds preceding each S1 usually auscultable
- No S4 in pauses for period of sinoatrial arrest

Electrocardiogram

- Slow to low-normal atrial rate
- Regularly irregular P–P interval
- Evidence of AV conduction
- Normal QRS complex associated with the preceding P waves
- R–R interval is regularly irregular, with a diastolic pause equal to more than two diastolic periods.

Should disappear with exercise and/or the administration of a vagolytic and/or sympathomimetic drug

Prolonged periods of sinoatrial arrest, profound sinus bradycardia, or high-grade sinoatrial block may indicate sinus node disease. *These individuals should be carefully evaluated with exercising electrocardiography and the response of the individual to vagolytic and sympathomimetic drugs determined.* Sinus node disease is rare in horses, but inflammatory and degenerative changes must be considered possible etiologies.

A course of high-dose corticosteroids (**dexamethasone** at **0.05–0.22 mg/ kg IV**) should be initiated for patients with life-threatening abnormalities of sinus rhythm in hopes that pacemaker implantation will not be necessary.

Sick Sinus Syndrome

Periods of profound sinus bradycardia and tachycardia—has not been reported in horses. Definitive treatment is pacemaker implantation.

Tachyarrhythmias

Atrial Fibrillation

- This occurs frequently in patients and rarely requires emergency therapy.
- Most horses have little or no underlying cardiac disease and present for exercise intolerance. Other presenting complaints include tachypnea, dyspnea, exercise-induced pulmonary hemorrhage, myopathy, colic, and congestive heart failure. Atrial fibrillation can also be an incidental finding during a routine examination.
- Resting heart rates are usually normal, although the rhythm is irregularly irregular and no fourth heart sound is auscultable.
- Intensity of peripheral pulses is irregularly irregular.
- Cardiac output in patients with atrial fibrillation and no significant underlying cardiac disease is normal at rest.

Auscultation

- Heart rate is usually normal (28–44 beats/minute), although atrial fibrillation can occur at any heart rate.
- Irregularly irregular diastolic periods
- Fourth (S4) heart sounds absent

Electrocardiogram (Fig. 25–9)

- Irregularly irregular R–R intervals
- No P waves
- Rapid baseline fibrillation "f" waves
- Normal QRS complexes

Patients with little or no underlying cardiac disease are candidates for conversion to sinus rhythm.

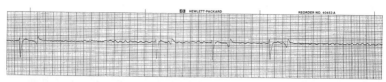

FIGURE 25–9. Base-apex electrocardiogram obtained from a horse with atrial fibrillation. Notice the irregularly irregular R–R intervals, the absence of P waves, and the presence of baseline "f" waves. The QRS configurations are normal, as is the ventricular rate (30 beats/minute). This electrocardiogram was recorded at a paper speed of 25 mm/sec with a sensitivity of 5 mm = 1 mV.

Treatment for Horses with Little or No Other Underlying Cardiovascular Disease

PATIENT PREPARATION

- An **IV catheter** should be placed before beginning the quinidine treatment for rapid venous access, in case arrhythmias develop.
- Prior to treatment, ensure an adequate whole body potassium status. This clinicopathologic evaluation should include determination of a plasma potassium level and fractional excretion of potassium in the urine.
  - □ To calculate the fractional excretion, urine and serum samples must be obtained simultaneously. Creatinine and potassium must be measured on both the urine and serum samples, and the fractional excretion of potassium is calculated using the following equation:

$$FE = \frac{urine\ (K^+)}{serum\ (K^+)} \times \frac{serum\ (Cr)}{urine\ (Cr)} \times 100$$

  - □ Normal fractional excretion of potassium is 23.3–48.1%.
  - □ A low fractional excretion of potassium indicates renal potassium conservation and a probable low total body potassium status.
    Red blood cell potassium determination has also been investigated by several researchers as a tool for assessing whole body potassium status, but reports of its reliability vary significantly.
- A **continuous electrocardiogram** (Fig. 25–10) should be obtained (easiest with radiotelemetry) throughout the entire treatment period to monitor cardiac rhythm and conduction times.

FIGURE 25–10. Contact electrodes in place under a surcingle for obtaining an electrocardiogram via radiotelemetry in a horse. *A*, Notice the withers pad and the surcingle in place in the girth area, with the telemetry box taped to the upper rings of the surcingle just below the withers. *B*, Notice the placement of the grounded electrodes on the left side of the patient underneath the moistened sponges and held in place by the surcingle. Care must be taken to ensure close contact between the patient's skin and the contact electrodes in the area near the withers as well as in the girth area. The upper grounded electrode (negative electrode) should be placed on the flat portion of the dorsal thorax while the lower grounded electrode (positive electrode) should be placed in the flat portion of the girth area or on the sternum, whichever area ensures better contact.

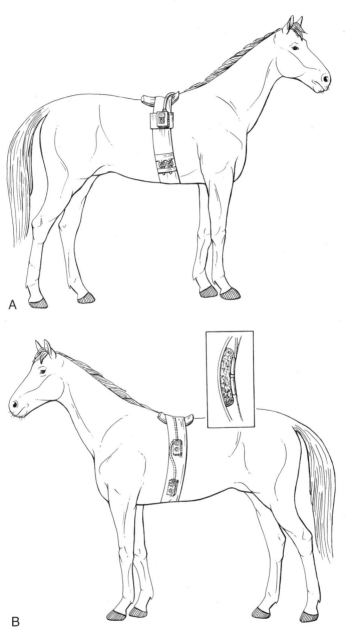

A

B

FIGURE 25–10. *See legend on opposite page*

If the **duration** of the arrhythmia is **recent**—ideally ≤ **2 weeks:**

- **Quinidine gluconate, 1–2.2 mg/kg,** should be administered **IV** as a bolus, every 10 minutes to effect, **not to exceed 12 mg/kg total dose.**
  - □ The average half-life of quinidine administered IV in horses is 6.5 hours, with a range of 4–12 hours.

If the atrial fibrillation is of more long-standing duration: > **2–4 weeks;** if there is **mild to moderate, but not severe, underlying cardiac disease** (mild to moderate tricuspid, mitral, or aortic regurgitation or mild myocardial dysfunction) and if **no signs of congestive heart failure:**

- **Quinidine sulfate** is administered **at 22 mg/kg via nasogastric intubation.**
- Quinidine sulfate should be administered via nasogastric intubation **every 2 hours until** the patient either **converts to sinus rhythm, shows adverse reactions or toxic side effects** to treatment with quinidine (Table 25–4) **or has received four to six treatments at 2-hour intervals** (most individuals with atrial fibrillation can tolerate only four treatments every 2 hours before exhibiting adverse or toxic side effects).
  - □ A **plasma quinidine concentration** should be determined **1 hour after the fourth treatment,** before continuing with the every-2-hour treatment interval, or when the patient exhibits adverse or toxic side effects of treatment.

> **Therapeutic concentration = 2–5 μg/ml**
> **Toxic concentration = > 5 μg/ml**

  - □ Treatment intervals should be prolonged to every 6 hours if plasma quinidine concentration is ≥ 4.0 μg/ml.
- **Treatment intervals** should then be **prolonged to every 6 hours until conversion** to sinus rhythm, **adverse reactions or toxic side effects develop** (rare on the every-6-hour treatment interval) **or** the owner elects to **discontinue treatment.**
- **Oral digoxin (0.011 mg/kg twice daily)** appears to be helpful in the conversion of some individuals that do not convert with quinidine alone, and it should be added on day 2 if conversion has not occurred.
  - □ Digoxin **should not be administered beyond day 2 without monitoring serum digoxin concentrations** (therapeutic concentration, 1–2 ng/ml).

The administration of digoxin and quinidine together results in rapid elevations of serum digoxin concentrations and the possible development of digoxin toxicity. Plasma digoxin concentrations nearly double with concurrent quinidine sulfate administration.

Digoxin toxicity may be manifested by anorexia, depression, colic and/or the development of other cardiac arrhythmias (Fig. 25–11).

- Patients being treated for atrial fibrillation with quinidine should be **monitored carefully** for **adverse reactions** and signs of **quinidine toxicity.**

TABLE 25–4. Adverse Reactions and Toxic Side Effects of Quinidine Sulfate/Gluconate Treatment

1. Depression
   Rx: Seen in all treated horses, no Rx indicated
2. Paraphimosis
   Rx: Seen in all treated stallions or geldings, no Rx indicated
3. Urticaria and/or wheals
   Rx: Discontinue quinidine; if severe, administer corticosteroids and/or antihistamines
4. Nasal mucosal swelling
   Snoring
   Rx: Monitor degree of air flow; discontinue quinidine if significant decrease in air flow through nares
   Upper respiratory tract obstruction
   Rx: Discontinue quinidine; if severe, administer corticosteroids and/or antihistamines, insert nasotracheal tube, preferably, or perform emergency tracheotomy
5. Laminitis
   Rx: Discontinue quinidine; administer analgesics and other treatment as needed
6. Neurologic
   Ataxia
   Rx: Discontinue quinidine; sign of quinidine toxicity
   Bizarre behavior—hallucinations?
   Rx: Discontinue quinidine; sign of quinidine toxicity
   Convulsions
   Rx: Discontinue quinidine; sign of quinidine toxicity; administer anticonvulsants as indicated
7. Gastrointestinal
   Flatulence
   Rx: Seen in many treated horses; Rx not indicated
   Diarrhea
   Rx: Usually resolves with discontinuation of Rx; discontinue Rx if diarrhea severe
   Colic
   Rx: Usually resolves with administration of dipyrone; use other analgesics as needed
8. Cardiovascular
   Tachycardia—supraventricular or ventricular—uniform, multiform, torsades de pointes
   Rx: See Table 25–5
   Prolongation of the QRS duration (>25% of pretreatment value)
   Rx: Discontinue quinidine; sign of quinidine toxicity
   Hypotension
   Rx: Discontinue quinidine; administer phenylephrine if needed (Table 25–5)
   Congestive heart failure
   Rx: Discontinue quinidine; administer digoxin if not already given
   Sudden death
   Rx: Cardiopulmonary resuscitation

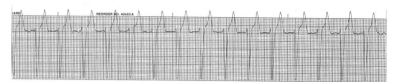

FIGURE 25–11. Base-apex electrocardiogram obtained from the horse in Figure 25–9 after treatment with quinidine sulfate and digoxin. This patient has atrial fibrillation with uniform ventricular tachycardia and digoxin toxicity. Notice the large wide QRS complexes that are ventricular in origin, the absence of P waves, and the presence of baseline "f" waves. This electrocardiogram was recorded at a paper speed of 25 mm/sec with a sensitivity of 5 mm = 1 mV.

- The detection of **any significant adverse reactions** or signs of **quinidine toxicity** (Table 25–4) should prompt **discontinuation of quinidine administration** and **may require additional treatment** if the induced problem is serious **(Tables 25–4 and 25–5).**
- Obtain a **plasma sample** for determination of plasma **quinidine concentration.** Plasma electrolyte concentrations and a creatinine level should also be determined if the adverse or toxic effects are cardiovascular.

ELECTROCARDIOGRAPHIC MONITORING FOR QUINIDINE TOXICITY AND ADVERSE REACTION

PROLONGATION OF QRS

Measure the duration of the QRS complex before each planned administration of quinidine and compare it with the pretreatment duration.

- **Prolongation of the QRS duration** to **greater than 25%** of the pretreatment QRS duration is an indication of **quinidine toxicity** (Fig. 25–12).
- Q–T interval prolongation also occurs.

RAPID SUPRAVENTRICULAR TACHYCARDIA

- Occurs in patients being treated for atrial fibrillation with quinidine associated with a sudden release of vagal tone at the AV node; is an idiosyncratic reaction and not associated with quinidine toxicity

> - Heart rates ≥ **200 beats/minute** occasionally occur and are potentially **life-threatening** (Fig. 25–13). **Immediate therapy (Table 25–5) is required** to slow the ventricular response rate and prevent deterioration of the patient's cardiovascular status.
>
> Administer **0.0022 mg/kg digoxin IV.**
> Administer **1 mEq/kg NaHCO₃ IV.**
> If **rate still high,** administer **propranolol at 0.03 mg/kg IV.**
> If **pressures still poor,** administer **phenylephrine at 0.1–0.2 μg/kg/min.**

- Associated with decreased cardiac output at rest and may deteriorate into other, more life-threatening ventricular arrhythmias (Fig. 25–14)

TABLE 25–5. **Treatment of Quinidine-Induced Arrhythmias**

1. **Determine whether arrhythmia is supraventricular or ventricular:**
   a. Obtain another ECG lead if unable to determine whether rhythm is supraventricular or ventricular. Look for change in QRS configuration from normal or preceding QRS configuration. **Record ECG during entire treatment** with radiotelemetry, if possible
   b. Obtain **blood pressure** if possible
   c. Don't panic!

2. **If arrhythmia is supraventricular:**
   a. If **rate is sustained in excess of 100 beats/minute:**
      Administer **digoxin at 0.0022 mg/kg IV (1 mg/1000#)** or **0.011 mg/kg PO (5 mg/1000#)**
   b. If **rate is sustained in excess of 150 beats/minute** and/or pressures are poor:
      (1) Administer **digoxin at 0.0022 mg/kg IV (1 mg/1000#);** can repeat dose once in relatively short period of time if necessary
      (2) Administer **NaHCO₃ IV at 1 mEq/kg (450 mEq/1000#)**
      If rate still high or pressures poor:
      (3) Administer **propranolol at 0.03 mg/kg IV (13.5 mg/1000#)** to slow heart rate
      (4) Administer **phenylephrine IV to effect at 0.1–0.2 μg/kg/min** up to 0.01 mg/kg total dose to improve blood pressure
      (5) Administer **verapamil at 0.025–0.05 mg/kg (11.25–22.5 mg/1000#) IV every 30 minutes,** can repeat up to 0.2 mg/kg (90 mg/.1000#) total dose

3. **If arrhythmia is ventricular:**
   a. If **wide QRS tachycardia** (torsades de pointes):
      Administer **magnesium sulfate IV at 1–2.5 gm/450 kg/min to effect up to 25 gm/1000#.** Administer in rapid IV drip over 10 minutes or bolus if necessary
   b. If **ventricular tachycardia is unstable:**
      (1) Administer **lidocaine HCl at 20–50 μg/kg/min or 0.25–0.5 mg/kg very slowly IV (225 mg/1000#);** can repeat in 5–10 minutes
      (2) Administer **magnesium sulfate IV at 1–2.5 gm/450 kg/min to effect up to 25 gm/1000#.** Administer in rapid IV drip over 10 minutes or bolus if necessary
      (3) Administer **procainamide IV at 1 mg/kg/min (450 mg/min/1000#)** to a maximum of 20 mg/kg (9 gm/1000#).
      (4) Administer **propafenone IV at 0.5–1 mg/kg (225–450 mg) in 5% dextrose slowly over 5–8 minutes.**
      (5) Administer **bretylium IV at 3–5 mg/kg (1.35–2.25 gm/1000#).** Can repeat up to 10 mg/kg total dose.

- Sustained ventricular response rates ≥ 100 beats/minute (Fig. 25–15) in patients being treated for atrial fibrillation with quinidine should also be treated and controlled, before continuing quinidine administration, to prevent further deterioration of the cardiac rhythm.

VENTRICULAR ARRHYTHMIAS ASSOCIATED WITH QUINIDINE

- If a large number of **ventricular premature depolarizations, ventricular tachycardia** (Fig. 25–16) or **multiform ventricular complexes** are detected, **quinidine administration** should also **cease.**

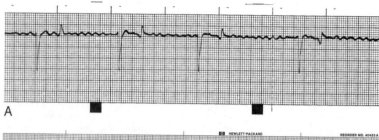

FIGURE 25–12. Base-apex electrocardiograms obtained from a horse with atrial fibrillation *(A)*, that was then treated with quinidine sulfate and developed prolongation of the QRS complex *(B)*. Notice the irregularly irregular rhythm with variable R–R intervals, no P waves, and baseline "f" waves in the pretreatment ECG *(A)* with a QRS duration of 100 msec. Following treatment with four doses of 22 mg/kg of quinidine sulfate, the QRS complexes prolonged to 140 msec *(B)*, and the ventricular rate increased to 60 beats/minute. Now large P waves are occurring regularly, buried in many of the QRS and T complexes associated with an atrial tachycardia (atrial rate of 150/minute) with block. A quinidine plasma concentration obtained at this time was elevated. These electrocardiograms were recorded at a paper speed of 25 mm/sec with a sensitivity of 5 mm = 1 mV.

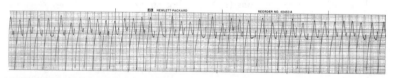

FIGURE 25–13. Base-apex electrocardiogram obtained from a horse with atrial fibrillation that developed a rapid supraventricular tachycardia with a heart rate of 210 beats/minute following the second dose of quinidine sulfate at 22 mg/kg. Notice the slightly irregular R–R intervals, the absence of P waves, and the normal orientation of the QRS complex for the base-apex lead. The "f" waves are not visible due to the rapid ventricular response rate. This electrocardiogram was recorded at a paper speed of 25 mm/sec with a sensitivity of 5 mm = 1 mV.

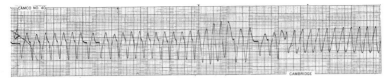

FIGURE 25–14. Base-apex electrocardiogram obtained from a horse with atrial fibrillation and rapid supraventricular tachycardia that developed after two doses of 22 mg/kg quinidine sulfate and then deteriorated into paroxysms of ventricular tachycardia. Notice the irregular R–R intervals, the absence of P waves, and the normal orientation of the QRS for a base-apex lead on the left side of the strip consistent with a rapid supraventricular tachycardia at a heart rate of 240 beats/minute in a horse with atrial fibrillation. This rhythm then deteriorates into a paroxysm of wide ventricular tachycardia, followed by a couple of normally conducted beats and then a period of more sustained ventricular tachycardia with a heart rate of 270 beats/minute. The "f" waves are not visible due to the rapid ventricular rate. This electrocardiogram was recorded at a paper speed of 25 mm/sec with a sensitivity of 2 mm = 1 mV.

□ If the ventricular arrhythmias do not disappear, IV administration of **antiarrhythmic drugs** should be instituted, usually beginning with **lidocaine at 20–50 μg/kg/min slowly IV (see Table 25–5).**

□ Ventricular arrhythmias induced by quinidine administration are usually idiosyncratic, associated with the proarrhythmic effect that all antiarrhythmic drugs possess, and not associated with quinidine toxicity (Fig. 25–16).

■ Quinidine-induced **torsades de pointes,** a wide ventricular tachycardia (Fig. 25–17), is more likely to occur in hypokalemic patients (Fig. 25–18). Therefore, every effort should be made before quinidine treatment to be sure that individuals have an adequate whole body potassium status.

□ **Intravenous magnesium sulfate** at an infusion rate of **1–2.5 gm/450 kg/minute** should be instituted immediately for quinidine-induced torsades de pointes.

SUDDEN DEATH

■ Probably associated with deterioration of rapid supraventricular or ventricular tachycardia to ventricular fibrillation or cardiac arrest

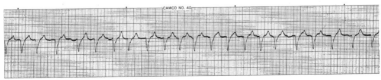

FIGURE 25–15. Base-apex electrocardiogram obtained from a horse with rapid atrial fibrillation and a heart rate of 130 beats/minute. Notice the irregular R–R intervals, the absence of P waves, and the small baseline "f" waves. This electrocardiogram was recorded at a paper speed of 25 mm/sec with a sensitivity of 2 mm = 1 mV.

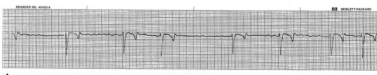

A

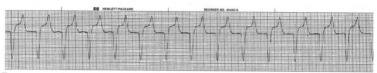

B

FIGURE 25–16. Base-apex electrocardiogram obtained from a horse with atrial fibrillation *(A)* that developed uniform ventricular tachycardia *(B)* 15 minutes after the first dose of quinidine sulfate was administered via nasogastric intubation at a dosage of 22 mg/kg. These electrocardiograms were recorded at a paper speed of 25 mm/sec with a sensitivity of 5 mm = 1 mV.

A, Notice the irregular R–R intervals, the absence of P waves, and the presence of baseline "f" waves characteristic of atrial fibrillation. The resting heart rate is 40 beats/minute.

B, Notice the wide and bizarre QRS complexes with the T wave oriented in the opposite direction to the QRS, consistent with complexes that are ventricular in origin. The ventricular complexes have a uniform configuration, and the heart rate is 90 beats/minute. The baseline "f" waves are barely visible on the electrocardiogram, and no P waves are present.

- Underscores the importance of continuous electrocardiographic monitoring (see Fig. 25–10) and rapid treatment of any arrhythmias that do occur

HYPOTENSION

Monitor pulse pressure or blood pressure for quinidine-induced **hypotension.** Discontinue quinidine administration; if hypotension is **severe,** administer **phenylephrine at 0.1–0.2 µg/kg/min to effect.**

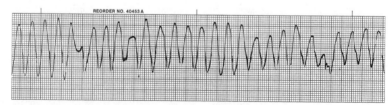

FIGURE 25–17. Base-apex electrocardiogram obtained from a horse with atrial fibrillation that had received two doses of quinidine sulfate (22 mg/kg each) and developed a wide ventricular tachycardia (torsades de pointes). Notice how the QRS complexes and T waves twist around the baseline and are difficult to distinguish from one another. The plasma potassium was normal at this time. This electrocardiogram was recorded at a paper speed of 25 mm/sec with a sensitivity of 2 mm = 1 mV.

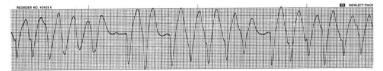

FIGURE 25–18. Base-apex electrocardiogram obtained from a horse with atrial fibrillation that had received six doses of quinidine sulfate (22 mg/kg each) and developed torsades de pointes, which was immediately treated with an intravenous infusion of magnesium sulfate. Notice the widened QRS complexes and T waves. Notice also the twisting of the QRS complexes and T waves around the baseline, which is still present although the torsades de pointes is resolving at this time. This horse was hypokalemic (2.4 mEq/L) and was receiving an infusion of intravenous magnesium sulfate at the time of this electrocardiogram. The ventricular rate is 110 beats/minute. An occasional "f" wave is seen. The fluids were subsequently spiked with KCl, and the wide QRS tachycardia resolved with magnesium and potassium replacement fluids. This electrocardiogram was recorded at a paper speed of 25 mm/sec with a sensitivity of 5 mm = 1 mV.

CONGESTIVE HEART FAILURE

- Occurs in individuals with severe underlying myocardial dysfunction or compensated congestive heart failure (inappropriate patients for conversion with quinidine)
- Negative inotropic effect of quinidine only manifested at higher drug doses
- Treat with **digoxin at 0.0022 mg/kg IV** and **furosemide at 1–2 mg/kg IV,** if needed.

UPPER RESPIRATORY TRACT OBSTRUCTION

Monitor nasal air flow for quinidine-induced **upper respiratory tract obstruction** secondary to nasal mucosal swelling.

- If air flow through the external nares decreases, discontinue quinidine administration.
  - □ **Insert a nasotracheal tube** if air flow through the external nares continues to decrease.
  - □ If severe, administer corticosteroids and/or antihistamines.
  - □ Emergency tracheotomy may be necessary in some patients if a nasotracheal is tube not inserted when a significant decrease in air flow is detected.

URTICARIA AND/OR WHEALS

- Discontinue quinidine administration.
- If severe, administer antihistamines and corticosteroids.

PARAPHIMOSIS

- Transient in all geldings and stallions
- Disappears with conclusion of treatment and return of plasma quinidine concentrations to negligible levels—not necessary to discontinue quinidine treatment

LAMINITIS

- Rare
- If digital pulses are increased, discontinue quinidine administration.
- If patient is uncomfortable, administer analgesics.

NEUROLOGIC SIGNS

- **Ataxia, bizarre behavior, seizures**
- Indicative of **quinidine toxicity**—discontinue quinidine treatment.
- Anticonvulsants may be indicated if seizures occur.

GASTROINTESTINAL SIGNS

- **Flatulence** is very common—quinidine administration need not be discontinued.
- **Oral ulcerations**—associated with oral administration of the drug, therefore **oral** administration of **quinidine sulfate** is **contraindicated.**
- **Diarrhea** usually is seen with higher doses of quinidine and usually resolves with discontinuation of quinidine treatment.
  - ☐ Only one reported case of quinidine-induced diarrhea culturing positive for *Salmonella* sp.
- **Colic** associated with **quinidine toxicity**—discontinue quinidine administration; analgesics as needed.

Treatment of Horses with Congestive Heart Failure and Atrial Fibrillation

- A small percentage of horses (10–15%), particularly draft breeds, with atrial fibrillation have severe underlying cardiac disease and present in congestive heart failure.
  - ☐ Resting heart rates in these individuals are elevated (> 60 beats/minute) and may exceed 100 beats/minute (Fig. 25–19).
  - ☐ Clinical signs of left-sided heart failure (pulmonary edema, coughing, tachypnea) and/or right-sided heart failure (generalized venous distention, jugular pulsations, and peripheral edema—pectoral, ventral, preputial, and limb) may be present.
  - ☐ Murmurs of tricuspid and/or mitral regurgitation are usually present, although patients with severe aortic regurgitation can also present in congestive heart failure.

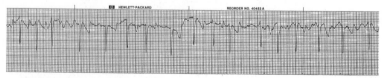

FIGURE 25–19. Base-apex electrocardiogram obtained from a horse with atrial fibrillation and congestive heart failure. Notice the rapid heart rate (110 beats/minute), the irregular R–R interval, the absence of P waves, and the presence of baseline "f" waves, consistent with atrial fibrillation. This electrocardiogram was recorded at a paper speed of 25 mm/sec with a sensitivity of 5 mm = 1 mV.

TABLE 25–6. **Drug Therapy for Horses with Myocardial and Valvular Heart Disease and Congestive Heart Failure**

Drug	Indications	Dose
Aspirin	Thrombophlebitis, endocarditis	5–20 mg/kg
Dexamethasone	Myocarditis, arrhythmias	0.05–0.22 mg/kg IV or IM
Digoxin	CHF, atrial tachyarrhythmias, control of rapid ventricular response in AF/atrial flutter	0.0022 mg/kg IV q12h (maintenance dose); 0.0044–0.0075 mg/kg IV q12h (loading dose administered for only two doses, rarely used); 0.0022–0.00375 mg/kg IV q12h to control ventricular response rate in AF; 0.011–0.0175 mg/kg PO q12h
Dobutamine	Cardiogenic shock, hypotension, complete AV block (emergency therapy)	1–5 μg/kg/min IV
Enalapril	Mitral and aortic regurgitation	0.25–0.5 mg/kg PO q12h or q24h
Furosemide	Edema	1–2 mg/kg as needed SQ, IM, or IV; 0.5–1 mg/kg PO q12h (maintenance)
Hydralazine	Mitral regurgitation	0.5–1.5 mg/kg PO q12h
Milrinone	CHF, low cardiac output	10 μg/kg/min IV; 0.5–1 mg/kg PO q12h

CHF, congestive heart failure; AF, atrial fibrillation; IV, intravenous; IM, intramuscular; SQ, subcutaneous; PO, per os.

- Treatment in these individuals is directed toward slowing the ventricular response rate (heart rate) and supporting the failing myocardium.
  □ **Digoxin (0.0022 mg/kg IV q12h or 0.011 mg/kg PO q12h)** is the drug of choice for both its vagal and positive inotropic effects (Table 25–6).
  □ If heart rate is not controlled adequately with digoxin alone, **propranolol** at **0.03 mg/kg IV** or **0.38–0.78 mg/kg PO q8h** may be added to further slow the ventricular response rate.

Ventricular Tachycardia

- The clinical signs of congestive heart failure become more severe the longer uniform ventricular tachycardia is present and the higher the heart rate.
- Clinical signs of congestive heart failure develop more rapidly in individuals with shorter cycle lengths and higher heart rates.
- Clinical signs of low output heart failure also develop more rapidly when the rhythm is multiform rather than uniform.

☐ Generalized venous distention, jugular pulsations, ventral edema, and pleural effusion develop in patients with sustained uniform ventricular tachycardia at a rate of ≥ 120 beats/minute.

☐ Occasionally, these patients also develop pericardial effusion, pulmonary edema, and ascites.

☐ Syncope has been detected in individuals with uniform ventricular tachycardia and a heart rate of ≥ 150 beats/minute.

Auscultation

- Rapid, regular rhythm if uniform; rapid, irregular rhythm if multiform
- Heart sounds often loud and varying in intensity

Electrocardiogram

- Elevated ventricular rate (usually > 60 beats/minute) with slower independent atrial rate
- Regular P–P interval
- P waves buried in QRS and T complexes (atrioventricular dissociation)
- Regular R–R interval (uniform) or irregular R–R (multiform) ventricular tachycardia
- Abnormal QRS and T wave configuration unrelated to the preceding P wave. All abnormal QRS complexes and T waves have same configuration (uniform) or several different QRS complex and T wave configurations are detected (multiform).
  ☐ **Uniform** ventricular tachycardia occurs when the ectopic focus originates from one place in the ventricle, creating only one abnormal QRS and T wave configuration (Fig. 25–20).
  ☐ **Multiform** ventricular tachycardia occurs when the ectopic ventricular complex originates from more than one focus in the ventricle, creating abnormal QRS and T complexes of different orientations (Fig. 25–21). Multiform ventricular complexes are associated with increased electrical inhomogeneity and instability and *an increased risk of a fatal ventricular rhythm developing.*
- **R on T,** a QRS complex occurring within the preceding T wave (Fig. 25–22), also indicates marked electrical inhomogeneity and instability and increases the chance for ventricular fibrillation to develop.
- Wide QRS tachycardia or **"torsades de pointes,"** in which the QRS and T complexes twist around the baseline (Fig. 25–23), is another ventricular rhythm that may rapidly deteriorate into ventricular fibrillation and result in sudden death.

Echocardiogram

- In most individuals the only abnormality is that associated with the rhythm disturbance.
- Severe concurrent myocardial dysfunction may be detected in horses with multiform ventricular tachycardia, indicating probable widespread myocardial necrosis (Fig. 25–24).

Treatment

Indicated if the patient is showing **clinical signs** at rest attributable to the dysrhythmia, the **rate** is **excessively high,** the rhythm is **multiform,** or **R on T** complexes are detected (Table 25–7).

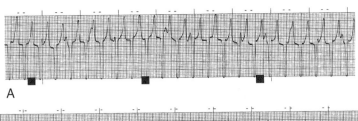

A

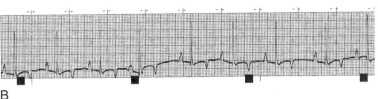

B

FIGURE 25–20. Lead II electrocardiogram obtained from a horse with uniform ventricular tachycardia before *(A)* and after *(B)* conversion.

A, Notice the large, negative QRS complexes with the T wave oriented in the opposite direction, which is an abnormal QRS configuration for lead II in the horse. Notice the rapid, regular ventricular rate of 150 beats/minute and the slower regular atrial rate of 90/minute. The R–R interval and P–P interval are regular. The P waves are buried in the QRS and T complexes and are unassociated with the QRS complexes. This electrocardiogram was recorded at a paper speed of 25 mm/sec with a sensitivity of 5 mm = 1 mV.

B, Notice the tall positive QRS complex with a negative T wave deflection following each P wave. Notice also that the P wave morphology changes some from beat to beat and that the P–P and R–R intervals are not perfectly regular. This electrocardiogram demonstrates a slight sinus arrhythmia with a wandering pacemaker at a heart rate of 50 beats/minute immediately following conversion from sustained uniform ventricular tachycardia. This electrocardiogram was recorded at a paper speed of 25 mm/sec with a sensitivity of 10 mm = 1 mV.

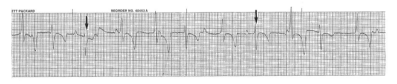

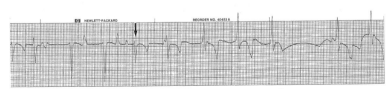

FIGURE 25–21. Continuous base-apex electrocardiogram obtained from a horse with multiform ventricular tachycardia. Notice the multiple different configurations of the QRS and T complexes, which appear widened and bizarre when compared with the few normal QRS and T complexes *(arrows).* The R–R intervals are irregular, but the P–P intervals are regular. The underlying atrial rate is 60/minute, with a heart rate of 70 beats/minute. This electrocardiogram was recorded at a paper speed of 25 mm/sec with a sensitivity of 5 mm = 1 mV.

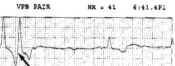

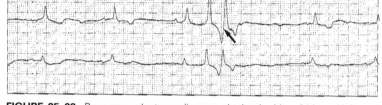

FIGURE 25–22. Base-apex electrocardiogram obtained with a 24-hour Holter recorder from a horse with multiple ventricular premature depolarizations, pairs of ventricular premature depolarizations, and paroxysms of ventricular tachycardia. Notice the R on T, which occurs with the pair of ventricular premature depolarizations *(arrow)*. The heart rate is 41 beats/minute. This electrocardiogram was recorded at a paper speed of 25 mm/sec.

TABLE 25–7. Indications for Urgent Treatment of Ventricular Tachycardia

Clinical signs of cardiovascular collapse
Rapid rate (>120 beats/min)
Multiform ventricular tachycardia
Detection of R on T

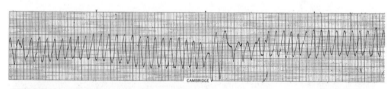

FIGURE 25–23. Base-apex electrocardiogram obtained from a horse with torsades de pointes ventricular tachycardia with a heart rate of 280 to 300 beats/minute. Notice the wide QRS tachycardia and the slurring of the distinction between the QRS complex and the T wave as the ECG appears to oscillate around the baseline. This electrocardiogram was recorded at a paper speed of 25 mm/sec with a sensitivity of 2 mm = 1 mV.

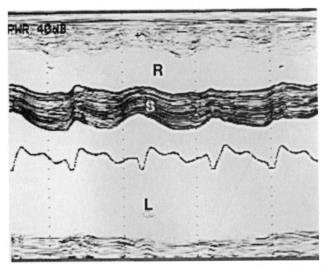

FIGURE 25–24. M-mode echocardiogram obtained from a horse with multiform ventricular tachycardia, severe left ventricular dysfunction, and left-sided congestive heart failure. Notice the lack of systolic thickening of the left ventricular free wall. This echocardiogram was obtained from the right parasternal window in the left ventricular position with a 2.5 MHz sector scanner transducer. An electrocardiogram is superimposed for timing. R, right ventricle; L, left ventricle; S, interventricular septum.

The selection of an **appropriate antiarrhythmic** for a patient with ventricular tachycardia depends upon the **severity of the arrhythmia,** the associated **clinical signs,** the **suspected etiology,** and the **availability** of appropriate antiarrhythmic **drugs** (Table 25–8).

- Lidocaine (without epinephrine) is readily available and is the most rapidly acting drug.
  - **Lidocaine** must be administered carefully and in small doses **(0.25–0.5 mg/kg slowly as a bolus)** due to the excitement and seizures associated with larger doses. *Diazepam (0.05 mg/kg IV) may be used to control the excitability or seizures that may result from lidocaine.*
  - Therapeutic plasma concentration is 1.5–5 μg/ml.
- **Quinidine gluconate (0.5–2.2 mg/kg IV as a bolus), procainamide (1 mg/kg/min IV),** and **propafenone (0.5–1 mg/kg in 5% dextrose IV)** are either administered more slowly or in graded doses (Table 25–8).
  - All have negative inotropic effects when administered at high doses but often are very effective in converting ventricular tachycardia in horses.
  - The principal metabolite of procainamide is *N*-acetylprocainamide (NAPA), which is also pharmacologically active. The half-life for procainamide administered intravenously is 3.5 ± 0.6 hours and for *N*-acetylprocainamide is 6.3 ± 1.5 hours. The therapeutic plasma concentration for procainamide is thought to be 4–10 μg/ml; for

TABLE 25-8. Antiarrhythmic Therapy

Drug	Indications	Dose
Atropine or glycopyrrolate	Sinus bradycardia, vagally induced arrhythmias	0.005–0.01 mg/kg IV
Breytylium tosylate	Life-threatening VT, ventricular fibrillation	3–5 mg/kg IV, can repeat up to 10 mg/kg total dose
Dexamethasone	VT, complete AV block	0.05–0.22 mg/kg IV or IM
Lidocaine[1]	VT, ventricular arrhythmias	20–50 µg/min; 0.25 mg/kg (bolus); 0.5 mg/kg very slowly IV to effect, can repeat in 5–10 min
Magnesium SO_4	VT	1–2.5 gm/450 kg/min to effect IV, not to exceed 25 gm total dose
Phenylephrine HCl	Quinidine toxicosis, arterial hypotension, excessive vasodilation	0.1–0.2 µg/kg/min; 0.01 mg/kg to effect
Phenytoin	Digoxin toxicity, atrial arrhythmias	5–10 mg/kg IV first 12 h, then 1–5 mg/kg IM q12h; 1.82 mg/kg PO q8h, may increase to 2.27 mg/kg PO q8h after 2–3 days if no drowsiness and to 2.73 mg/kg after 2–3 more days if no drowsiness
Procainamide	VT, AF, ventricular and atrial arrhythmias	1 mg/kg/min IV, not to exceed 20 mg/kg IV; 25–35 mg/kg q8h PO
Propafenone[2]	Refractory VT, AF, ventricular and atrial arrhythmias	0.5–1 mg/kg in 5% dextrose slowly IV to effect over 5–8 min; 2 mg/kg PO q8h
Propranolol	Unresponsive VT and SVT	0.03 mg/kg IV; 0.38–0.78 mg/kg PO q8h
Quinidine gluconate	VT, AF	0.5–2.2 mg/kg (bolus) q10min to effect; not to exceed 12[3] mg/kg IV total dose
Quinidine sulfate	AF, VT, atrial and ventricular arrhythmias	22 mg/kg via NG tube q2h until converted, toxic, or plasma [quinidine] = 3–5 µg/ml;[4] continue quinidine sulfate q6h until converted or toxic
Sodium bicarbonate	Quindine toxicosis, atrial standstill, hyperkalemia	1 mEq/kg IV; can be repeated
Verapamil	SVT	0.025–0.05 mg/kg IV, q30min; can repeat to 0.2 mg/kg total dose

[1]Lidocaine **without epinephrine** for intravenous injection.
[2]Not available for intravenous injection in North America.
[3]Most horses can tolerate only 12 mg/kg IV total dose if given as 1–2.2 mg/kg q10min.
[4]Not to exceed 6 doses q2h (most horses can tolerate only four doses q2h).

VT, ventricular tachycardia; atrial fibrillation; SVT, supraventricular tachycardia.

TABLE 25–9. **Adverse Effects of Antiarrhythmic Drugs**

Drug	Adverse Effects	CV Effects
Atropine	Ileus, mydriasis	Tachycardia, arrhythmias
Bretylium tosylate	GI	Hypotension, tachycardia, arrhythmias
Digoxin	Depression, anorexia, colic	SVPD, VPD, SVT, VT
Lidocaine	Excitement, seizures	VT, sudden death
Quinidine	Depression, paraphimosis, urticaria, wheals, nasal mucosal swelling, laminitis, neurologic, GI	Hypotension, SVT, VT, prolonged QRS and QT intervals, CHF, sudden death, negative inotrope
Phenytoin	Sedation, drowsiness, lip and facial twitching, gait deficits, seizures	Arrhythmias
Procainamide	GI, neurologic—similar to quinidrine	Hypotension, SVT, VT, prolonged QRS and QT intervals, sudden death, negative inotrope
Propafenone	GI, neurologic—similar to quinidine, bronchospasm	CHF, AV block, arrhythmias, negative inotrope
Propranolol	Lethargy, worsening of COPD	Bradycardia, 3° AV block, arrhythmias, CHF, negative inotrope
Verapamil		Hypotension, bradycardia, AV block, asystole, arrhythmias, negative inotrope

CV, cardiovascular; SVPD, supraventricular premature depolarizations; VPD, ventricular premature depolarizations; SVT, supraventricular tachycardia; VT, ventricular tachycardia; GI, gastrointestinal, CHF, congestive heart failure, COPD, chronic obstructive pulmonary disease.

N-acetylprocainamide, 7–15 μg/ml; and for procainamide and NAPA together, 10–30 μg/ml.

Intravenous propafenone, if available, should be reserved for patients with refractory ventricular tachycardia. Therapeutic plasma concentrations appear to be between 0.2 and 3.0 μg/ml in horses.

- **Propranolol (0.03 mg/kg IV)** also has negative inotropic effects and is rarely successful in converting horses with ventricular tachycardia.
  □ Propranolol should be tried, however, in patients that do not respond to other antiarrhythmics. Therapeutic plasma concentrations of propranolol may be 20–80 ng/ml in horses.
- **Magnesium sulfate (1–2.5 gm/450 kg/minute IV)** is often effective in refractory ventricular tachycardia in horses, is the drug of choice for quinidine-induced torsades de pointes, and has no negative inotropic effects.
  □ Magnesium sulfate is effective in individuals that are normomagnesemic or hypomagnesemic but is also usually administered slowly.

- **Bretylium tosylate (3–5 mg/kg IV)** should be reserved for individuals with severe, life-threatening ventricular tachycardia or ventricular fibrillation.

All antiarrhythmic drugs may have adverse effects and can also be proarrhythmic (Table 25–9).

CARDIOPULMONARY RESUSCITATION (CPR)

Cardiopulmonary resuscitation (CPR) in the horse should be approached utilizing the same systematic principles applied to CPR in humans and small animals; the major difference is the size of the patient with cardiac arrest. The "ABCD" of CPR reminds the clinician of the order in which cardiopulmonary resuscitation is approached. "A" stands for establishing an airway, "B" indicates to breathe for the patient, "C" indicates establishing circulation, and "D" represents drugs that should be administered.

Establish an Airway

- Easily established with the nasotracheal placement of a smaller endotracheal tube or the orotracheal placement of a larger endotracheal tube
  - ☐ If orotracheal or nasotracheal intubation is not possible, an emergency tracheotomy can be performed and the endotracheal tube inserted into the trachea through the tracheotomy site.
  - ☐ The cuff should be inflated and the endotracheal tube attached to a demand valve or anesthetic machine.
- If an endotracheal tube is not available, a 10-foot length of Tygon tubing with a 0.5-inch internal diameter should be inserted nasotracheally and attached to the flow regulator of an E oxygen cylinder.

Breathe for the Patient

- Four to six breaths/minute are reportedly adequate to maintain normal PaO_2 values in the horse.
- With a demand valve or large animal anesthetic machine, the rebreathing bag can be compressed to between 20 and 40 cm H_2O.
- The oxygen flow rate (100% O_2) should be adjusted so that there is moderate expansion of the thorax in 2–3 seconds.
- With Tygon tubing and intranasal oxygen, the horse's nose and mouth must be occluded and released alternately.

Establish Circulation in Cardiac Arrest

An **emergency** that **must be diagnosed and treated** as **quickly** as possible

- The peripheral arterial pulses should be checked and the heart auscultated to verify cardiac arrest.
- An electrocardiogram must be obtained to determine the type of cardiac arrhythmia present in the patient with cardiac arrest.

> - **Remember, an airway must be established and breathing initiated** for the individual **before** beginning to **re-establish circulation.**

- The horse should be in **lateral recumbency,** ideally in right lateral recumbency with the head level or lowered.
- An **electrocardiogram should be obtained** with external or internal cardiac massage to determine what rhythm is being generated or initiated during CPR.

2

External Cardiac Massage

- Forcefully and rapidly compress the horse's chest right behind the patient's elbow with the resuscitator's knee or hands (if the patient is small).
- Initiate at the rate of 60 to 80 compressions/minute.
- Difficult to perform in the adult and rarely successful
- Monitor the peripheral pulses to determine whether cardiac compressions are adequate.

Internal Cardiac Massage

- Only attempt if external cardiac compression is not successful.
- Associated with a large number of postoperative complications in the horse (pneumothorax, pleuropneumonia, and severe lameness)
- Successful intracardiac compression requires an incision in the 5th intercostal space with retraction of the fifth and sixth ribs or a 5th rib resection and manually compression of the left ventricle.
- Compress the heart 40–60 times/minute.
- Can be performed through an incision in the diaphragm in the patient undergoing exploratory celiotomy

Drugs That Are Administered

- **Determine the type of cardiac emergency** that is being experienced by the equine patient. Further therapeutic intervention depends upon whether **asystole** or **ventricular fibrillation** is present (Table 25–10).
- Administer drugs into a central vein (cranial vena cava), if possible, or otherwise into the jugular vein as close to the central vein as possible.

ASYSTOLE (Fig. 25–25)

- **Epinephrine** should be administered **IV (10–20 μg/kg/min)** (5–10 ml/ 500kg adult) or **intratracheally (20–40 μg/kg/min);** intracardiac as a last resort.
- Periods of asystole require immediate recognition and intervention to be treated successfully in horses.

VENTRICULAR FIBRILLATION (Fig. 25–26)

- Epinephrine is unlikely to be successful.
- Antiarrhythmic drugs with efficacy against ventricular fibrillation (preferable) or refractory sustained ventricular tachycardia should be administered.

TABLE 25–10. **Cardiopulmonary Resuscitation and Treatment in the Horse**

ESTABLISH AN AIRWAY

Nasotracheal placement of an endotracheal tube
Orotracheal placement of an endotracheal tube

ASYSTOLE

Initiate external cardiac massage
If no heart beat, inject epinephrine, 0.3–0.5 mg/kg, or 20–40 μg/kg/min, or 10–20 ml/
    500 kg in sterile saline intratracheally and ventilate vigorously for 4–5 breaths, or
    inject 0.03–0.05 mg/kg, or 10–20 μg/kg/min, or 5–10 ml/500 kg epinephrine IV
    Epinephrine is administered intracardiac (IC) as a last resort and is injected into the
    left ventricle cavity
Continue CPR, checking the peripheral pulse for effectiveness
Establish an IV line and administer lactated Ringer's solution rapidly
Re-evaluate CPR and ECG findings. If unable to establish a pulse within 2 minutes,
    open the chest at the 6th intercostal space and begin cardiac massage

VENTRICULAR FIBRILLATION

Initiate or continue CPR
Defibrillate:
    Administer bretylium tosylate intracardiac (IC)
    Use electrical defibrillator (DC or direct current) at appropriate watt-sec/kg. Use
        adequate amounts of electrode paste on the skin and no alcohol (flammable)
    Mix potassium chloride (1 mEq/kg) with acetylcholine (6 mg/kg) and inject IC

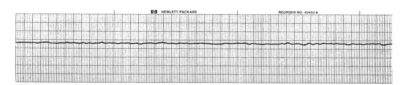

FIGURE 25–25. Base-apex electrocardiogram obtained from a horse with asystole. Notice the flat line with some baseline undulations and no evidence of atrial or ventricular electrical activity. This electrocardiogram was recorded at a paper speed of 25 mm/sec with a sensitivity of 5 mm = 1 mV.

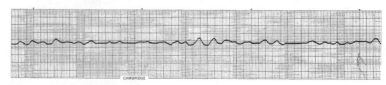

FIGURE 25–26. Base-apex electrocardiogram obtained from a horse with ventricular fibrillation. Notice the fine baseline fibrillation waves with no evidence of coordinated atrial or ventricular depolarization. This electrocardiogram was recorded at a paper speed of 25 mm/sec with a sensitivity of 5 mm = 1 mV.

□ Administer **bretylium tosylate at 3–5 mg/kg IV;** can repeat up to 10 mg/kg total dose.
■ Successful chemical defibrillation of an adult with antiarrhythmic drugs has not been performed.
■ Successful electrical defibrillation has been reported, however, in one 350-kg horse and in several foals.
■ Chemical or electrical defibrillation or both should be attempted, if the necessary drugs and/or defibrillator are available and the pre-existing condition of the patient is not terminal.

Intravenous fluids should be administered at the rate of 20 ml/kg/hr during resuscitation in the horse to maintain normal or elevated mean circulatory pressures. Maintaining normal or elevated mean circulatory pressure during CPR increases the probability of a favorable outcome in the dog and is likely also to do so in the equine patient.

Postresuscitation Treatment

■ **Calcium** in the form of calcium chloride or calcium gluconate **(0.1–0.2 mEq/kg slowly IV over 5–10 min),** *although highly controversial,* may be indicated to increase the force of myocardial contraction and counteracts the effects of hypocalcemia and hyperkalemia.
■ Once a **normal sinus rhythm** has been **restored, dobutamine (1–5 μg/ kg/min IV)** is the drug of choice for maintaining cardiac output and arterial blood pressure.
■ The use of sodium bicarbonate is controversial and is not indicated if circulation is rapidly restored, because large volumes of sodium bicarbonate can cause hyperosmolality, hypernatremia, hypocalcemia, hypokalemia, and decreases in the affinity of hemoglobin for oxygen.
  □ Small doses of sodium bicarbonate may be indicated to treat metabolic acidosis and hyperkalemia in horses that have experienced a prolonged period of cardiac arrest.

ELECTROLYTE DISTURBANCES CAUSING CARDIAC ARRHYTHMIAS

Hyperkalemia

■ Most frequently recognized in foals with uroperitoneum but is occasionally seen in adults, primarily those with acute renal failure
■ Also seen in Quarter Horses with hyperkalemic periodic paralysis (HPP)
  □ Clinical signs include stiffness, muscle weakness, muscle fasciculations, muscle spasm, respiratory stridor, recumbency, and death.
  □ Death occurs either secondary to paralysis of the pharyngeal and laryngeal muscles or from cardiac arrhythmias associated with hyperkalemia.
  □ Identify individuals predisposed to the development of HPP by testing for the HPP-type Na channel DNA. *Ventricular arrhythmias during exercise are more likely in individuals homozygous for HPP.*
■ Cardiac arrhythmias may or may not be detected, but an electrocardiogram should be obtained in adults or foals with a plasma potassium ≥ 6 mEq/L.

Electrocardiogram

- Tall, peaked T waves detected with plasma potassium values ≥ 6.2 mEq/L (Fig. 25–27)
- Progressive slowing of conduction and decreased excitability result in cardiac arrest or ventricular fibrillation.
  - □ Broadening and flattening of the P waves, prolonged P–R intervals, and bradycardia develop, with slowing of conduction and decreased excitability. *Atrial arrest or atrial standstill develops.*
  - □ Atrial and ventricular premature depolarizations and ventricular tachycardia have been reported.
  - □ Widened QRS complexes are further indications of severe (near lethal) hyperkalemia.
  - □ The Q–T interval is not a reliable indicator of hyperkalemia.

Treatment

- Uroperitoneum must be treated aggressively as soon as diagnosed, because these foals are at high risk for the development of cardiac arrhythmias, particularly under general anesthesia during surgical repair of the ruptured bladder, urachus, or ureter.
  - □ Ventricular premature beats, ventricular tachycardia, complete heart block, and atrial standstill have been reported in foals with uroperitoneum.
- **Sodium** deficit should be **replaced slowly** at the rate of **0.5 mEq/hr.**
  - □ **0.45–0.9% NaCl IV**
- **NaHCO₃** (1 mEq/kg) IV will help drive potassium intracellularly.
- Intravenous **5–50% dextrose** may also be needed to help drive the potassium intracellularly.
  - □ Administer **5% dextrose (0.5 ml/kg) and 0.9% NaCl IV.**
- If the foregoing measures are unsuccessful, administer **0.1 IU/kg regular insulin IV** with **0.5–1 gm/kg dextrose IV,** to help drive potassium into the cell. Add 5 ml of the foal's blood to the fluid to prevent the insulin from adhering to the fluid administration bag.
- If **severe cardiac arrhythmias** or atrial standstill is detected, **calcium gluconate** can be administered **slowly** (over a 10-minute period) **IV (4 mg/kg)** to effect.
  - □ Calcium gluconate should be discontinued if bradycardia occurs following calcium administration.

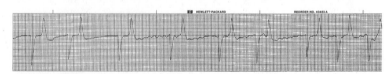

FIGURE 25–27. Base-apex electrocardiogram obtained from a horse with hyperkalemia (plasma K⁺ = 6.6 mEq/L) and a creatinine level of 24 mg/dl. Notice the tall tented T waves (2.5 mV) typical of hyperkalemia. This horse also had atrial fibrillation. Notice the irregular R–R intervals, absence of P waves, and presence of baseline "f" waves with a heart rate of 50 beats/minute. This electrocardiogram was recorded at a paper speed of 25 mm/sec with a sensitivity of 5 mm = 1 mV.

- Gradual drainage of the uroperitoneum should be performed in conjunction with intravenous fluid replacement therapy, as indicated earlier.
- Surgical correction of the uroperitoneum should occur following medical stabilization of the foal.

Hyperkalemic Periodic Paralysis

In adult **horses with HPP** experiencing an acute episode, e.g., recumbency, respiratory stridor, trembling:

- Serum K concentrations are often in excess of 6 mEq/L; draw blood to measure serum potassium concentration.
- Administer:
  □ **0.2–0.4 ml/kg of 23% calcium borogluconate solution IV**
  □ **6 ml/kg 5% dextrose solution IV** or **1 ml/kg 50% dextrose**
  □ **$NaHCO_3$ at 1–2 mEq/kg IV**
  □ Insulin may be used as indicated earlier but requires regular monitoring of the blood glucose concentration for the following 24 hours.

MANAGEMENT

- Feed diets low in potassium (timothy hay and Bermuda grass hay, no molasses).
- Keep horses in a regular exercise program.
- Kaliuretic diuretics such as acetazolamide (2–4 mg/kg PO q6h) or hydrochlorothiazide (250 mg IM or IV q6h) have been useful in reducing the frequency and severity of clinical signs and are expensive.
- Do not use affected individuals for breeding because the mode of inheritance is autosomal dominant.

Hypokalemia

- Commonly seen in individuals with heat exhaustion with hypochloremia, hypocalcemia, and metabolic alkalosis
- Also seen in patients with severe diarrhea

Electrocardiogram

- Prolongation of the Q–T interval is an indication of hypokalemia.
- Supraventricular and ventricular arrhythmias occur:
  □ Atrial tachycardia with block (Fig. 25–28) and junctional tachycardia are common supraventricular arrhythmias seen in patients with hypokalemia.
  □ Ventricular tachycardia, torsades de pointes, and ventricular fibrillation can occur with severe hypokalemia.

Treatment

- Replace calculated potassium deficit slowly IV, adding KCl at 20–40 mEq/L, not to exceed a rate of **0.5 mEq/kg/h.** Serum potassium concentrations should be monitored during treatment.
- Administer 0.1 gm KCl/kg PO if the GI tract is patent.

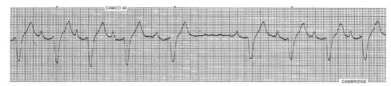

FIGURE 25–28. Base-apex electrocardiogram obtained from a horse with hypokalemia (plasma K^+ = 1.4 mEq/L), a sinus arrhythmia, and a heart rate of 50 beats/minute. Notice the markedly widened QRS and T complexes reflecting delayed conduction and abnormal ventricular repolarization. This electrocardiogram was recorded at a paper speed of 25 mm/sec with a sensitivity of 5 mm = 1 mV.

- Correct other electrolyte abnormalities, if present, and do not cause a diuresis with excessive IV fluids unless the patient is volume contracted.

Hypomagnesemia

Magnesium deficiency is usually associated with hypokalemia or hypocalcemia.

Electrocardiogram

- Serious ventricular arrhythmias are most likely in patients with significant hypomagnesemia, but supraventricular tachycardia (Fig. 25–29) and atrial fibrillation also occur in patients with severe hypomagnesemia.
- P–R interval prolonged, QRS complex widened, ST segment depressed, and T wave peaked

Treatment

Administer **Mg SO_4 IV** at a rate of **1–2.5 gm/450 kg/min** not to exceed 25 gm/450 kg followed by oral $MgSO_4$ supplementation (0.2–1 gm/kg).

Hypocalcemia

Hypocalcemic tetany, lactation tetany, transport tetany, and eclampsia are uncommon in horses.

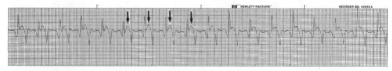

FIGURE 25–29. Lead II electrocardiogram obtained from a horse with severe hypomagnesemia (Mg^{++} = 0.7 mg/dl), hyperkalemia (K^+ = 6.2 mEq/L), and azotemia (creatinine = 6.0 mg/dl). Notice the rapid, regular rhythm with a ventricular rate of 100 beats/minute. The QRS complexes are normal for lead II, but the P waves are buried in the QT complex (arrows), consistent with a junctional tachycardia. The T waves are also large (≥ 1 mV and spiked in appearance). This electrocardiogram was recorded at a paper speed of 25 mm/sec with a sensitivity of 10 mm = 1 mV.

- When associated with lactation, often occurs following peak lactation, approximately 60–100 days postpartum
- Occasionally occurs following prolonged or strenuous exercise, especially in hot weather, in prolonged transport, or in individuals with diarrhea.
- Seen in patients fed a diet low or deficient in calcium. Magnesium may also be deficient in the diet, which can lead to multiple cases of hypocalcemia on a farm.
- Seen in individuals with cantharidin (blister beetle) toxicosis
- Hypoalbuminemia reduces the concentration of total serum calcium and protein-bound calcium *but not ionized calcium.*
  - □ To measure serum calcium more accurately in patients with hypoalbuminemia if ionized calcium cannot be measured:

corrected calcium = measured calcium (mg/dl) − albumin (gm/dl) + 3.5

Alkalosis reduces the concentration of ionized calcium in the blood. Two different clinical syndromes occur in horses with moderate to severe hypocalcemia:

- Individuals with a low serum calcium (5–8 mg/dl) and low serum magnesium:
  - □ Tachycardia, synchronous diaphragmatic flutter, laryngospasm with loud, labored breathing, trismus, protrusion of the nictitans, dysphagia, abdominal pain, goose-stepping or stiff hindlimb gait, and ataxia may be present.
  - □ Rhabdomyolysis, convulsions, coma, and death may ensue.
- Individuals with an even lower serum calcium (<5 mg/dl) and normal serum magnesium concentrations:
  - □ Flaccid paralysis, mydriasis, stupor, and recumbency are usually present.

Electrocardiogram

- Electrocardiographic abnormalities other than tachycardia are rarely seen.
- Atrial or ventricular premature beats or ventricular tachycardia is occasionally detected.
- Cardiac arrest or ventricular standstill may occur.
- $Q_{-o}T_c$ interval inversely correlated to ionized plasma calcium concentration

Treatment

- Intravenous infusion of **calcium gluconate** can be administered **slowly** (over a 10-minute period) **IV (4 mg/kg)** to effect.
- Analyze the horse's ration and ensure adequate calcium to phosphorus ratio (1.3–2 : 1) and adequate magnesium in the diet.

Hypercalcemia

- Seen in horses with chronic renal failure, lymphosarcoma, paraneoplastic syndromes, and hypervitaminosis D, and after ingestion of *Cestrum diurnum*
  - □ *Cestrum diurnum* contains 1,25-dihydroxycholecalciferol and may induce hypervitaminosis D.

□ Hyperphosphatemia also occurs and is an earlier and more reliable indicator of vitamin D intoxication.
- Results in soft tissue mineralization and mineralization of the heart and blood vessels (especially aorta, pulmonary artery, coronary arteries, and endocardium)

Electrocardiogram

- Initially heart rate slows, sinus arrhythmia and partial AV block are detected.
- Tachycardia and extrasystoles are a common finding.
- Atrial and ventricular tachycardia may occur.
- Q_o-T_c interval inversely correlates to ionized plasma calcium concentration.
- Terminally, cardiac arrest, ventricular fibrillation, or ventricular standstill occurs.

Treatment

- Search for the underlying cause of the hypercalcemia and remove or treat if possible.
  □ Discontinue all exogenous supplements containing calcium, phosphorus, and vitamin D and remove individuals from *Cestrum diurnum–*infected pasture.
- Emergency treatment is indicated in patients with cardiac disease, severe renal decompensation, and systemic disease with hypercalcemia in the 15–20 mg/dl range.
  □ Administer **0.9% NaCl IV** to expand the extracellular fluid volume and increase the glomerular filtration rate. Potassium (20 mEq/L), and magnesium (10 gm/L, not to exceed 25–30 gm over 30 minutes) supplementation of the intravenous fluids should be administered more slowly and/or be added to oral fluids.
  □ Begin diuretic therapy with a calciuretic diuretic such as **furosemide** at 1–2 mg/kg every 12 hours and keep intravenous fluid maintenance levels at 5 ml/kg/h (or at least equal to urine output).
  □ Administration of corticosteroids may reduce calcium concentrations and decrease the likelihood of soft tissue and cardiac mineralization by decreasing calcium loss from bone, decreasing intestinal calcium absorption, and increasing renal excretion of calcium. (Steroid-responsive hypercalcemias include lymphoma, lymphosarcoma, leukemia, multiple myeloma, thymoma, vitamin D toxicity, granulomatous disease, and hyperadrenocorticism.)
- Treatment with salmon calcitonin may be indicated if severe, prolonged hypercalcemia is present.

CONGESTIVE HEART FAILURE

Congestive heart failure has a multitude of causes in horses, both congenital and acquired. The majority of individuals presenting with congestive heart failure have acquired cardiac disease—either valvular heart disease, myocardial disease, or both. Severe cardiac arrhythmias, primarily ventricular tachycardia, also result in patients presenting with clinical signs of congestive heart failure.

Severe congenital cardiac disease is an uncommon cause of congestive heart failure in horses. Congestive heart failure in horses may develop slowly over a prolonged period of time or suddenly, requiring emergency intervention.

Individuals with **severe primary myocardial disease, acute onset of severe valvular heart disease** (mitral or aortic, Table 25–11) or **multifocal ventricular tachycardia** are most likely to present with clinical signs of **acute, left-sided heart failure** and require emergency treatment.

Clinical Signs of Acute, Left-Sided Heart Failure

- Anxiety, tachypnea, dyspnea, tachycardia, coughing, foamy nasal discharge, expectoration of a foamy fluid, lethargy, and exercise intolerance
  - □ Ruptured mitral valve chordae tendineae are the most likely cause of acute fulminant pulmonary edema in horses with primary valvular heart disease.
  - □ Patients with bacterial endocarditis may also present in acute left- or right-sided heart failure because of the rapid destruction of the valve apparatus by the vegetative lesion. The most common site of endocarditis in the horse is on the mitral valve and next, the aortic valve. The patients may also have fever, weight loss, and a shifting leg lameness. Systemic septic emboli frequently occur.
  - □ Acute severe myocarditis with severe left ventricular dysfunction is the most common cause of frank pulmonary edema in horses with primary myocardial disease. Many of these individuals have a history of fever (often a suspected viral, equine herpesvirus, or influenza infection) in the weeks or months preceding the signs of cardiac disease.
  - □ Most individuals with multifocal ventricular tachycardia and acute severe pulmonary edema also have severe myocardial disease.
- Weakness or syncope may occur, particularly with multifocal or rapid unifocal ventricular tachycardia.
  - □ Patients with ventricular tachycardia also have frequent jugular pulses.
- Arterial pulses are usually weak, and extremities may be cool.

TABLE 25–11. Clinical Signs and Physical Examination Findings in Horses with Acute Mitral or Aortic Regurgitation

Tachycardia—heart rate usually ≥ 60 beats/min
1. +/− Irregular rhythm—usually atrial fibrillation but may have atrial and/or ventricular premature contractions
2. Loud third heart sound
Tachypnea—respiratory rate usually ≥ 24 breaths/min with increased respiratory effort, flared nostrils, and prolonged recovery after exercise
Coughing—at rest, during or after exercise
+/− Expectoration of foamy fluid
Exercise intolerance or poor performance
Syncope—rare
Harsh inspiratory and expiratory vesicular sounds
Crackles or moist sounds—rare

- Cyanosis at rest is rarely detected but may occasionally be induced by exercise.

Auscultation

- Coarse breath sounds over the entire lung field in the majority of horses. Occasional individuals also have crackles or moist sounds detected in the perihilar or ventral lung field.
- The abnormal lung sounds are most frequently detected when the patient is taking deep breaths in a rebreathing bag.
    □ Horses easily become distressed when breathing in a rebreathing bag or with breath holding, often cough, may expectorate foamy fluid, and have a prolonged recovery time to resting respiratory rate.
- Cardiac murmurs are usually heard if severe valvular, congenital, or myocardial disease is the etiology of the congestive heart failure. Loud (grade 3/6–6/6), coarse, band-shaped, holosystolic, or pansystolic murmurs of mitral regurgitation are detected in the majority of patients with acute, left-sided heart failure.
    □ Murmurs associated with ruptured mitral chordae tendineae are usually loud and honking initially.
    □ Most individuals also have slightly quieter murmurs of tricuspid regurgitation.
    □ Some patients with bacterial endocarditis do not have a murmur.
    □ A small number of patients also have holodiastolic decrescendo murmurs of aortic regurgitation.
    □ Murmurs associated with a congenital defect, such as a ventricular septal defect, are infrequently detected.
- The cardiac rhythm is usually rapid and regular, unless multifocal ventricular tachycardia is the underlying cause of the congestive heart failure.
    □ Atrial fibrillation is more common in horses with chronic valvular regurgitation.
    □ Ventricular premature depolarizations or paroxysms of ventricular tachycardia may be present in individuals with bacterial endocarditis of the mitral or aortic leaflets.
- Loud third (S3) heart sounds may be heard associated with ventricular volume overload.

Treatment

> Emergency treatment for pulmonary edema should be instituted as soon as possible and should include **intravenous furosemide (1–2 mg/kg)** and **intranasal oxygen.** Drugs to reduce anxiety should be administered if needed. If the heart rate exceeds 120 beats/minute, ventricular tachycardia should be suspected.

ADDITIONAL DIAGNOSTICS

- An electrocardiogram to establish the underlying cardiac rhythm.
- An echocardiogram to evaluate myocardial function (Fig. 25–30), determine the severity of underlying congenital or valvular heart disease (Figs. 25–31 and 25–32), and look for evidence of pulmonary hypertension (Fig. 25–33).

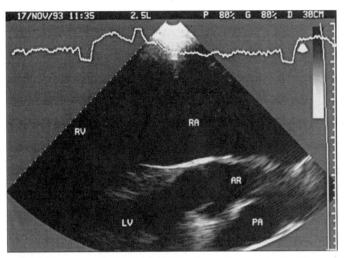

FIGURE 25–30. Long axis two-dimensional echocardiogram obtained from a horse with right ventricular cardiomyopathy, syncope, and congestive heart failure. Notice the markedly enlarged right atrium (RA) and right ventricle (RV) and the small pulmonary artery (PA) associated with severe pulmonary hypoperfusion. This echocardiogram was obtained from the right parasternal window in the left ventricular outflow tract position with a 2.5 MHz sector scanner transducer. The electrocardiogram is superimposed for timing. AR, aortic root; LV, left ventricle.

□ A dilated pulmonary artery is compatible with significant pulmonary hypertension and the possibility of impending pulmonary artery rupture (Fig. 25–33).

■ Cardiac isoenzyme levels of creatine kinase and lactate dehydrogenase should be obtained using protein electrophoresis to determine whether myocardial injury and necrosis have occurred. Elevated cardiac isoenzyme levels are a good indicator of myocardial cell damage; however, normal laboratory values do not rule out myocardial insult.

■ A chemistry profile, complete blood count, total protein content, and fibrinogen determination should also be obtained to ascertain whether there is an underlying disease process and to evaluate the severity of any renal compromise (usually prerenal azotemia).

If **ventricular tachycardia** is the **cause** of the acute congestive heart failure, **antiarrhythmic therapy** should be instituted as soon as possible. The selection of the appropriate antiarrhythmic drug depends upon the severity of the arrhythmia and the associated clinical signs (see earlier).

> If **sinus tachycardia, supraventricular tachycardia, or atrial fibrillation** is present, positive inotropic support should be instituted immediately and consist of either **intravenous digoxin (0.0022 mg/kg) or dobutamine (1–5 μg/kg/min).**

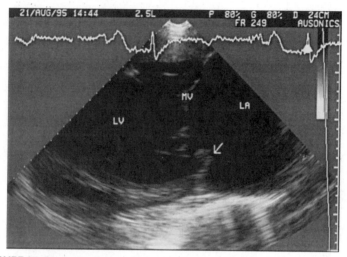

FIGURE 25–31. Long axis two-dimensional echocardiogram obtained from a horse with a ruptured chordae tendineae of the mitral valve *(arrow)* and acute left-sided congestive heart failure. This echocardiogram was obtained from the left parasternal window in the mitral valve position with a 2.5 MHz sector scanner transducer. An electrocardiogram is superimposed for timing. MV, mitral valve; LA, left atrium; LV, left ventricle.

- Modify the dose of digoxin (increase dosing intervals to once daily or decrease dose) if prerenal azotemia is present.
- After an initial clinical response, **oral digoxin (0.011 mg/kg) and furosemide (0.5–1 mg/kg)** can be instituted.
- Afterload reducers (vasodilators), such as **hydralazine (0.5–1.5 mg/kg PO q12h)** or angiotensin-converting enzyme (ACE) inhibitors (0.25–0.5 mg/kg enalapril PO q24h or q12h, if needed),** should be administered in horses with severe mitral and/or aortic regurgitation to improve cardiac output and reduce myocardial work.

If the horse has **bacterial endocarditis, broad-spectrum bactericidal intravenous antimicrobial therapy** (both gram-positive and gram-negative coverage) should be instituted after obtaining several blood cultures.

Right-Sided Congestive Failure

In contrast, patients with more **long-standing congenital, valvular, or myocardial disease** that gradually leads to the development of congestive heart failure frequently show little in the way of clinical signs referable to the respiratory system. These individuals usually present with clinical signs of **right-sided congestive heart failure** and rarely require emergency treatment.

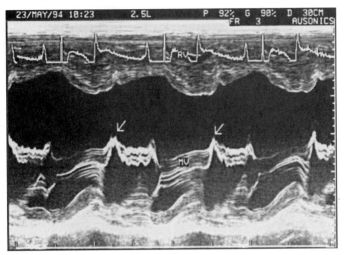

FIGURE 25–32. M-mode echocardiogram of a horse with acute, severe aortic regurgitation. Notice the marked separation between the mitral valve E point *(arrows)* and the interventricular septum; associated with marked left ventricular volume overload and dilatation of the left ventricular outflow tract. The septal leaflet of the mitral valve has high-frequency vibrations caused by turbulence in the left ventricular outflow tract associated with the regurgitant jet. This echocardiogram was obtained from the right parasternal window with a 2.5 MHz sector scanner transducer. An electrocardiogram is superimposed for timing. MV, mitral valve.

Clinical Signs

- May have tachypnea at rest, an occasional cough, prolonged recovery times to resting respiratory rate after exercise, with biventricular failure or a large pleural effusion associated with right-sided heart failure
- The veterinarian is usually consulted because the affected individual has developed preputial, pectoral, and/or ventral edema.
- Generalized venous distention and jugular pulsations are usually present.
- Syncope may be present in patients with severe right-sided congestive heart failure and decreased pulmonary blood flow.

Auscultation

- Coarse vesicular sounds at rest or with a rebreathing bag:
  - ☐ Crackles or moist sounds are rarely detected.
- Dullness may be detected in the cranioventral lung field on auscultation and/or percussion associated with a pleural effusion.
- Rarely, the heart may sound muffled because of a small pericardial effusion.
- Murmurs of mitral and tricuspid valvular regurgitation are frequently detected.
  - ☐ Occasionally affected individuals will also have murmurs of aortic

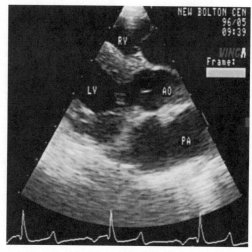

FIGURE 25–33. Long axis two-dimensional echocardiogram obtained from a horse with a ruptured chordae tendineae of the mitral valve and acute left-sided congestive heart failure. Notice the small diameter of the aortic root (AO) and the larger diameter of the pulmonary artery (PA), consistent with severe pulmonary hypertension. This echocardiogram was obtained from the right parasternal window in the left ventricular outflow tract position with a 2.5 MHz annular array transducer. An electrocardiogram is superimposed for timing. RV, right ventricle; LV, left ventricle.

regurgitation or a ventricular septal defect (or another, usually complex, congenital defect).
- The heart rate is usually elevated and irregularly irregular with atrial fibrillation.
- Patients with uniform ventricular tachycardia and congestive heart failure usually have a more rapid (> 120 beats/minute) and regular rhythm but present with similar clinical signs.
  □ These patients should be treated with antiarrhythmic drugs to correct the ventricular tachycardia (see earlier).
- Loud third (S3) heart sounds may be heard, associated with ventricular volume overload.

Treatment
Affected individuals should be started on **furosemide, positive inotropic drugs (usually digoxin), and vasodilators (hydralazine or ACE inhibitors)** as indicated earlier. **Intravenous** administration can be selected initially if the signs of congestive heart failure are severe, but most patients respond well to **oral** therapy, with clinical improvement noticed within 24 hours **(see Table 25–6).**

- Serum or plasma samples should be obtained for **digoxin concentrations** after several days of oral therapy to see whether adjustments in the dosage are necessary.
  □ **Peak** (sample obtained 1–2 hours after oral digoxin administration)

and **trough** digoxin concentrations should be obtained and should fall within the **therapeutic range of 1–2 ng/ml.**
  ☐ **Digoxin toxicity** has been reported in horses with digoxin concentrations > 2 ng/ml.
- Clinical improvement usually occurs with this treatment regimen within several days. However, due to the severity of the underlying cardiac disease in most horses with clinical signs of congestive heart failure, the improvement is usually of short duration (2–6 months).

Digoxin has a very narrow therapeutic to toxic range and therefore the patient should be monitored for any signs of **digoxin toxicity.**

- Anorexia, lethargy, colic, and the development of other cardiac arrhythmias have all been reported in horses with digoxin toxicity.
- **Hypokalemia potentiates the toxic effects** of digoxin, yet digoxin toxicity may cause extracellular hyperkalemia by interfering with Na-K pump, therefore **careful monitoring of the patient's potassium status is important.**
- Ectopic foci, usually atrial, develop with relatively small doses of digoxin in hypokalemic patients.
- The administration of **digoxin should be discontinued** in all individuals when digoxin toxicity is suspected and a blood sample obtained for serum or plasma digoxin, potassium, and creatinine concentrations.
  ☐ **Oral potassium** (40 gm/450 kg) supplementation if the patient is hypokalemic may be adequate if the clinical signs associated with digoxin toxicity are mild.
  ☐ **Intravenous potassium** (40 mEq/L) may be administered slowly in intravenous fluids to the hypokalemic patient if life-threatening arrhythmias are present.
  ☐ **Lidocaine (20–50 μg/kg/min)** is indicated for the treatment of ventricular arrhythmias associated with digoxin toxicity.
  ☐ **Phenytoin (5–10 mg/kg IV** first 12 hours, then 1–5 mg/kg IM q12h or switch to oral phenytoin, 1.82 mg/kg PO q12h) may be indicated in the treatment of supraventricular arrhythmias associated with digoxin toxicity. *Side effects of phenytoin* include a mild tranquilizing effect. Overdosing can lead to lip and facial twitching, gait deficits, and seizures. Do not use in conjunction with other medications, particularly trimethoprim-sulfa.
  ☐ Administer a cardiac glycoside–specific antibody or its Fab fragments **(Digibind),** which binds excess circulating digoxin and prevents further development of digoxin toxicity. This treatment should be reserved for patients with life-threatening digoxin toxicity and is very expensive. In humans with digoxin toxicity, this treatment results in a reversal of the digoxin-induced cardiac arrhythmias in nearly all patients and hyperkalemia, if present.
- Chronic administration of **high doses of furosemide** can lead to **hypokalemic metabolic alkalosis.**
  ☐ Plasma potassium should be regularly monitored (weekly).
  ☐ Feed individual a high-quality hay, such as alfalfa, that is rich in potassium.
  ☐ Oral potassium supplementation should be considered, in addition to

feeding a high-quality hay. KCl salt is not very palatable and must be gradually introduced into the horse's grain (1 tablespoon/feeding with gradual increases if the individual consumes up to 1 ounce q12h).

- Patients with bacterial endocarditis involving the pulmonic or tricuspid valve may have severe pneumonia or pulmonary thrombosis secondary to septic emboli. Tricuspid valve endocarditis has frequently been associated with septic jugular vein thrombophlebitis.

PERICARDITIS/PERICARDIAL EFFUSION

Pericarditis is uncommon in horses, but affected individuals usually present as an emergency with clinical signs of cardiovascular collapse. Concurrent or historical respiratory tract disease is present in approximately 50% of patients with pericarditis.

- Many patients with pericarditis exhibit signs of discomfort that are initially interpreted as abdominal pain and are, therefore, **usually referred for colic.**
- **Physical examination findings** at presentation include depression; tachycardia; generalized venous distention; pectoral, ventral, and preputial edema; and muffled heart sounds. Fever, lethargy, anorexia, jugular pulsations, weak arterial pulses, pericardial friction rubs, tachypnea, dullness in the cranioventral thorax, and weight loss may also be detected.
  □ Arrhythmias are infrequently detected, are usually atrial if present, and indicate the presence of concurrent myocarditis.
- Patients with pericarditis may also have a mild anemia, neutrophilic leukocytosis, hyperproteinemia, and hyperfibrinogenemia, particularly individuals with septic pericarditis.

Cardiac tamponade can occur when there is a rapid accumulation of fluid within the pericardial sac, impeding ventricular filling and resulting in a rapid decrease in cardiac output. The three determinants of the development of cardiac tamponade are the distensibility of the pericardial sac, the rate at which the fluid accumulation occurs within the pericardial sac, and the amount of fluid present within the pericardial sac.

- Cardiac tamponade should be suspected in any individuals with **rising venous pressure, tachycardia, muffled heart sounds, decreasing arterial blood pressure, and pulsus paradoxus.**
  □ Pulsus paradoxus is an inspiratory reduction in arterial blood pressure greater than 10 mm Hg.
- Central venous pressures of up to 43 cm of H_2O (normal CVP = 10–15 cm H_2O) have been reported in patients with cardiac tamponade, large pericardial effusions, or constrictive pericarditis.
- Right atrial, right ventricular, and pulmonary arterial end-diastolic pressures may be increased in individuals with cardiac tamponade.

Echocardiography is the **diagnostic modality of choice** for the assessment of the amount of pericardial fluid, its character, and the degree of cardiac compromise. Fibrinous effusive pericarditis is most common in horses, with the volumes of fluid associated with the pericarditis ranging from none visible to > 14 liters (Fig. 25–34). Fluid within the pericardial sac is usually anechoic to slightly hypoechoic in individuals with septic or idiopathic pericarditis. Sheets of fibrin with frondlike projections are usually imaged on the epicardial and

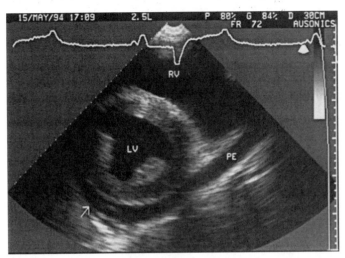

FIGURE 25–34. Short axis two-dimensional echocardiogram obtained from a horse with pericarditis. The arrow points to some fibrin within the pericardial sac. This echocardiogram was obtained from the right parasternal window in the left ventricular position with a 2.5 MHz sector scanner transducer. An electrocardiogram is superimposed for timing. LV, left ventricle; RV, right ventricle; PE, pericardial effusion.

pericardial surfaces. Occasionally, compartmentalization of this fluid can occur with walled-off areas developing in the pericardial sac. A concurrent pleural effusion is often present. Effusive pericarditis without fibrin is most common in patients with congestive heart failure, not in patients with primary pericardial disease. Hemopericardium has also been detected in several individuals associated with thoracic trauma and in one foal with penetration of the right ventricular free wall by a broken and dislodged intravenous catheter. Blood within the pericardial sac appears as echogenic swirling fluid.

- Excessive motion (swinging) of the right ventricular free wall is detected echocardiographically in patients with pericardial effusion (Fig. 25–35).
- Diastolic collapse of the right ventricular free wall occurs as the amount of pericardial fluid begins to increase and is first visualized in the right ventricular outflow tract as this area is easiest to compress.
- Early echocardiographic signs of cardiac tamponade include an inspiratory increase in the dimension of the right ventricle, an inspiratory decrease in the internal diameter of the left ventricle, and collapse of the right atrium during systole (right atrial inversion).
  - □ Right atrial inversion (Fig. 25–36) becomes more severe as the individual develops hemodynamically significant cardiac tamponade.
  - □ Doppler-detected increased tricuspid and decreased mitral inflow during exhalation are other indications of developing cardiac tamponade.
- Electrocardiography reveals small amplitude P, QRS, and T complexes caused by the damping of the electrical impulse by the surrounding pericardial fluid (Fig. 25–37).
- Electrical alternans, a cyclical variation in the size of the QRS complexes,

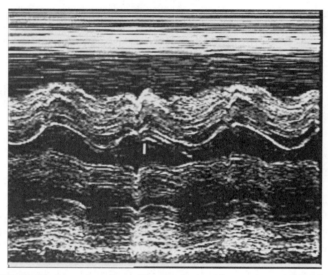

FIGURE 25–35. M-mode echocardiogram obtained from a horse with idiopathic pericarditis and a fibrinous pericardial effusion demonstrating the swinging pattern of right ventricular free wall motion. Notice the slight increase in right ventricular diameter associated with inspiration (I). This echocardiogram was obtained from the right parasternal window in the left ventricular position with a 2.5 MHz sector scanner transducer.

has also been reported in horses with pericardial effusion but is infrequently seen (Fig. 25–38). Electrical alternans is thought to be caused by the swinging motion of the heart in the pericardial fluid.

- A globoid cardiac silhouette is detected on thoracic radiography, usually with opacification of the ventral thorax due to a concurrent pleural effusion. However, this radiographic appearance cannot be definitively differentiated from other forms of cardiac enlargement, and good-quality lateral thoracic radiographs cannot be obtained with portable radiographic equipment, except in the foal.

Treatment

Pericardiocentesis is the diagnostic and therapeutic tool of choice for horses with pericarditis, as long as there is enough pericardial fluid to perform this procedure safely.

- **Echocardiography** should be **used to safely select a site** of pericardiocentesis and the placement of an indwelling tube, if significant volumes of pericardial fluid are imaged.
- In most horses with pericarditis, the **ideal site** is in the **left 5th intercostal space, above** the level of the **lateral thoracic vein** and **below** a line level with the **point of the shoulder** (over the left ventricular free wall and below the left atrium and atrioventricular groove).
  □ Lacerations of the left atrium coronary vessels or right ventricle are avoided if this site is chosen for pericardiocentesis.

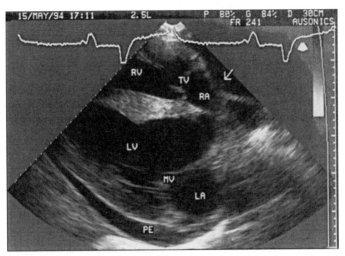

FIGURE 25–36. Two-dimensional echocardiogram obtained from a horse with pericarditis, demonstrating inversion of the right atrium *(arrow)*. This echocardiogram was obtained from the right parasternal window in the mitral valve position with a 2.5 MHz sector scanner transducer. An electrocardiogram is superimposed for timing. RA, right atrium; TV, tricuspid valve; RV, right ventricle; LV, left ventricle; MV, mitral valve; LA, left atrium; PE, pericardial effusion.

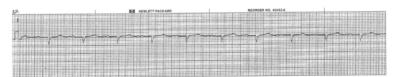

FIGURE 25–37. Base-apex electrocardiogram obtained from a horse with pericarditis, demonstrating damping of the P, QRS, and T waves from the pericardial effusion. Notice the tachycardia that is present (60 beats/minute), a common finding in horses with pericarditis. The P–P interval and R–R interval are regular. This electrocardiogram was recorded at a paper speed of 25 mm/sec with a sensitivity of 10 mm = 1 mV.

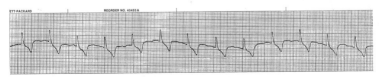

FIGURE 25–38. Base-apex electrocardiogram demonstrating electrical alternans in a horse with pericardial effusion. Notice the slight variation in the amplitude of the QRS complexes from 0.6 mV to 0.8 mV. The amplitude of the P, QRS, and T complexes is also damped. This electrocardiogram was recorded at a paper speed of 25 mm/sec with a sensitivity of 10 mm = 1 mV.

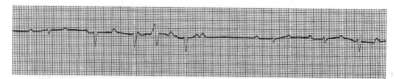

FIGURE 25–39. Lead II electrocardiogram obtained during pericardiocentesis in a horse with pericarditis. Notice the paroxysm of ventricular premature depolarizations. There are two different configurations of ventricular premature complexes in the paroxysm. The amplitude of the P, QRS, and T complexes is still very damped. This electrocardiogram was recorded at a paper speed of 25 mm/sec with a sensitivity of 10 mm = 1 mV.

- **Electrocardiographic monitoring** (base-apex as rhythm strip is preferable) should be performed during pericardiocentesis to monitor the patient for the development of arrhythmias induced by the procedure (Fig. 25–39).
- An **intravenous catheter** should be placed before beginning the pericardiocentesis for rapid venous access, in case arrhythmias do develop.
  - □ If a large number of ventricular premature depolarizations, ventricular tachycardia, or multiform ventricular complexes are detected, cease advancement of the pericardiocentesis catheter.
  - □ If the ventricular arrhythmias do not disappear, the intravenous administration of antiarrhythmic drugs should be instituted and/or the pericardiocentesis catheter withdrawn, depending on the severity of the arrhythmias detected. The catheter can then be repositioned once the arrhythmia has resolved.
- A large-bore (28–32 Fr) Argyle catheter containing a trocar should be inserted as an indwelling tube if there is a large volume of pericardial fluid and/or cardiac tamponade is present.
  - □ This tube can be used for both sample collection and pericardial drainage and lavage.
  - □ Smaller-bore (12–24 Fr) Argyle catheters containing a trocar can be used if the volume of fluid within the pericardial sac is small.
- The **sample** obtained should be submitted for **culture and sensitivity testing,** cytologic evaluation, and viral isolation, if possible (Table 25–12).
  - □ Streptococcal sp. have been **most frequently isolated** from horses with pericarditis, but *Actinobacillus equuli* has also been isolated from adults and foals with pericarditis.
  - □ A thoracocentesis should be also performed if a pleural effusion is present, and a transtracheal aspirate should be obtained if pulmonary disease is suspected. Culture and sensitivity testing of both these fluids should also be performed as this may yield the etiologic agent responsible for the concurrent pericarditis.

  Lavage of the pericardial sac, **following drainage** of the pericardial fluid, **markedly improves the prognosis** for patients with pericarditis.
- The pericardial sac should be lavaged with **2 or more liters of warm sterile 0.9% NaCl.**
  - □ The lavage fluid should be infused and **left in the pericardial sac for 0.5 to 1 hour,** followed by **drainage** of this fluid and the **instillation of**

TABLE 25–12. **Etiology of Pericardial Effusions in Horses**

Type of Effusion	Etiology	Cytologic Findings	Culture Results	Treatment
Blood	Neoplasia	Neoplastic cells (usually RBCs and lymphocytes)	No growth	Drainage and corticosteroid therapy (symptomatic only)
	Left atrial rupture (rare)	Blood	No growth	Intravenous fluids
	Aortic root rupture	Blood	No growth	Intravenous fluids
	Trauma	Blood	No growth unless penetrating wound to the pericardium	Drainage if cardiac tamponade; intravenous fluid support
	Iatrogenic injury (intravenous or cardiac catheterization or cardiac puncture)	Blood	No growth unless iatrogenic contamination	Drainage if cardiac tamponade; intravenous fluid support
Transudate	Congestive heart failure Hypoproteinemia		No growth No growth	
Exudate	Idiopathic pericarditis	Lymphocytes/plasma cells and red blood cells in large numbers	No growth, seroconversion to viral diseases possible	Drainage and lavage with sterile saline and instillation of broad-spectrum antibiotics, systemic broad-spectrum antibiotics until cytology and culture results negative for bacterial infection, then systemic corticosteroids
	Septic pericarditis	Neutrophils	+/– Positive culture (*Streptococcus* sp., *Pasteurella* sp.)	Drainage and lavage with sterile saline and instillation of broad-spectrum antibiotics, systemic broad-spectrum antibiotics until the results of culture and sensitivity testing available, minimum 4 weeks of antimicrobials

       1–2 liters of sterile 0.9% NaCl with 10–20 × 10⁶ IU Na penicillin/L or 1 gm gentamicin/L.

- □ This infusate should be **left** in the pericardial sac for the next **12 hours.**
- □ The **drainage, lavage, drainage,** and instillation of sterile fluid should **continue until ≤ 0.5 liter of pericardial fluid is obtained** at the time of the initial drainage or the pericardial catheter falls out and fluid does not reaccumulate.

- **Broad-spectrum systemic antibiotics should also be administered.**
  - □ The use of systemic and intrapericardial antimicrobials should continue until the cytologic examination and culture and sensitivity testing have ruled out a bacterial etiology of the pericarditis.
  - □ Although systemic concentrations of antibiotics are reached in the pericardial fluid with the administration of systemic antimicrobials alone, the use of intrapericardial antimicrobials increases by threefold the concentrations of antimicrobials in the pericardial fluid. This local increase in antimicrobial concentration appears to be helpful because of the fibrinous nature of pericarditis in horses and the rapid inactivation of many antimicrobial agents by the fibrin.
  - □ Long-term **(4–6 weeks)** of **systemic antimicrobial therapy** is indicated in individuals with **septic pericarditis.**

- Patients with pericarditis should **initially** be given a **guarded to cautiously optimistic prognosis,** until response to treatment with pericardial drainage and lavage is detected, at which time the prognosis can usually be changed to good for both life and performance.

- **Corticosteroids** (dexamethasone, 0.045–0.09 mg/kg IV q24h for 3 days followed by a tapering dose) are indicated in individuals with **idiopathic pericarditis** (often lymphacytic plasmocytic), once a bacterial etiology has been definitively ruled out.

- Therapy for septic or idiopathic pericarditis should continue for several weeks after the patient is afebrile and clinically normal, and the pericardial effusion has resolved. During this time the patient should be stall rested and hand walked, with subsequent turnout in a small paddock for an additional month.

- Echocardiographic re-evaluation is indicated at that time to determine whether the individual is ready to return to work.

- Intravenous fluids may be needed if the creatinine level is high, to prevent or treat renal failure.

IONOPHORE TOXICITY

Horses are uniquely sensitive to the cardiotoxic effects of several of the ionophores (monensin, salinomycin, and lasalocid). The LD_{50} for these ionophores in horses is much lower than that in other domestic species. The ionophores are primarily cardiotoxic, although other signs of systemic toxicity may also be detected in exposed individuals. Horses of any age or breed or either sex can be exposed to ionophore-contaminated feed. The contamination may come from feed accidentally contaminated at the feed mill or from accidental feeding of or exposure to ionophore-containing steer or poultry feed.

- Feed samples should be obtained for toxicologic analysis if ionophore exposure is suspected.

■ Gastrointestinal samples should be similarly analyzed in any individuals that have experienced sudden death.

Clinical Signs

■ Sudden death is often the first indication of exposure to high doses of ionophores.
■ Fever, depression, lethargy, restlessness, exercise intolerance, and profuse sweating are some of the signs first noticed by the owners and/or trainers of affected individuals.
■ Anorexia, poor appetite, and feed refusal are common because ionophore-contaminated feed is less palatable.
■ Muscle weakness, trembling, ataxia often occur.
■ Affected individuals may be polyuric and become oliguric or anuric.
■ Diarrhea, colic, and/or ileus has frequently been reported.
■ Muddy or injected mucous membranes with thready arterial pulses may be detected initially.
■ Cardiac arrhythmias may develop at any time after ionophore exposure but are most likely in the first few days to weeks after exposure.
■ Generalized venous distention, jugular pulses, ventral edema, and murmurs of mitral and/or tricuspid regurgitation may develop weeks to months following ionophore exposure.
■ Recumbency may occur without heart failure.

Diagnosis and Prognosis

■ **Echocardiography** is the **diagnostic modality of choice** in situations of suspected or known ionophore exposure, to determine the severity of the myocardial injury in exposed individuals.
  □ Patients with **normal left ventricular function** and a normal fractional shortening (normal fractional shortening = 30–40%) have an **excellent prognosis for life and performance.**
  □ Patients with slightly depressed fractional shortening have a good prognosis for life and a fair-to-good prognosis for performance.
  □ The detection of a **fractional shortening < 20%** in exposed individuals is a **grave** prognostic sign. Affected individuals with a fractional shortening of > 10 but < 20% may survive monensin exposure but have persistent left ventricular dysfunction and exercise intolerance.
  □ Individuals with a **fractional shortening of ≤ 10% do not survive monensin exposure** and are usually dead 24–48 hours following the echocardiographic examination (Fig. 25–40).
■ **Electrocardiographic abnormalities** may be detected in individuals recently exposed to ionophores but **are not good prognostic indicators** of the severity of the myocardial injury.
  □ Axis shifts, ST segment depression, T wave changes, atrial and ventricular premature beats, atrial fibrillation, ventricular tachycardia, and a variety of bradyarrhythmias have been reported in horses exposed to ionophores (Fig. 25–41).
  □ The majority of individuals exposed to ionophores in the field situation, however, do not have cardiac arrhythmias.

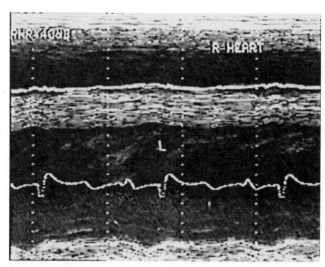

FIGURE 25–40. M-mode echocardiogram obtained from a horse with monensin toxicosis. Notice the minimal thickening of the left ventricular free wall and interventricular septum in systole. This echocardiogram was obtained from the right parasternal window in the left ventricular position with a 2.5 MHz sector scanner transducer. An electrocardiogram is superimposed for timing. L, left ventricle.

- **Elevations** in the **cardiac isoenzymes of CK and lactate dehydrogenase (LDH)** have been reported in some outbreaks of monensin toxicity but were detected only slightly or not at all in other field outbreaks.
  - □ The elevation of the cardiac isoenzymes of CK and/or LDH and the magnitude of their elevation were **not useful prognostic indicators** of survival or the severity of permanent myocardial injury.
- Other clinicopathologic abnormalities that have been reported include elevations of hematocrit, total plasma protein concentration, serum BUN, creatinine, osmolality, total bilirubin, serum glutamic oxaloacetic transaminase, serum aspartate aminotransferase, and serum alkaline phosphatase, as well as decreases in serum calcium and plasma potassium.

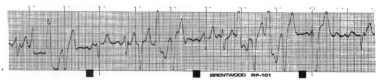

FIGURE 25–41. Lead II electrocardiogram obtained from a horse with monensin toxicosis and multifocal ventricular tachycardia. Notice the markedly different QRS complexes, some of which are occurring in rapid succession. The ventricular rate here is 110 beats/minute. This electrocardiogram was recorded at a paper speed of 25 mm/sec with a sensitivity of 5 mm = 1 mV.

□ None of these abnormal clinicopathologic abnormalities, however, is diagnostic of monensin or other ionophore exposure.

Treatment

- **Remove** the possibly **contaminated feed.**
- **Administer activated charcoal or mineral oil** to decrease further absorption of recently ingested feed.
- **Administer large doses of vitamin E** as soon as possible after exposure in an attempt to stabilize cell membranes and control peroxidation-mediated cell injury.
- Provide appropriate supportive care (Table 25–13).
- Exposed individuals should receive **stall rest** for a minimum of 2 months.
- **Digoxin is contraindicated in acute monensin exposure** because monensin and digoxin have an additive effect, causing calcium to flood into the myocardial cell. The use of digoxin in a patient recently exposed to monensin may result in the intracellular calcium sequestration mechanisms being further overloaded, increasing the amount and severity of myocardial cell injury and cell death.
  □ Monensin is a sodium-selective ionophore that makes the myocardial cell membrane more permeable to sodium. The sodium influx into the cell is followed by a calcium influx.
  □ Digoxin inhibits the $Na^+,K^+,ATPase$ pump, and this influx of sodium is also followed by an influx of calcium.

TABLE 25–13. **Approach to the Horse with Potential Ionophore Exposure**

Perform complete physical and cardiovascular examination.

Treat affected individuals with antiarrhythmics as needed to control life-threatening arrhythmias.

Pass nasogastric tube and administer activated charcoal or mineral oil in attempt to prevent further absorption of the ionophore.

Administer vitamin E or vitamin E and selenium as soon as possible.

Stall-rest exposed individuals and minimize stress.

Digoxin contraindicated if exposure recent.

Perform echocardiogram:
a. Evaluate myocardial function carefully, looking for myocardial hypokinesis, dyskinesis, or akinesis.
b. Evaluate myocardium for heterogeneity of muscle echogenicity (tissue characterization).

Obtain blood for determination of cardiac isoenzymes of CK (CK-MB) and LDH (LDH_1 and LDH_2 or HBDH).

Obtain electrocardiogram, including 24-hour continuous ECG, if possible.

CK, creatine kinase; CK-MB, isoenzyme of creatine kinase with muscle and brain subunits; LDH, lactate dehydrogenase; HBDH, hydroxybutyrate dehydrogenase.

AORTIC ROOT RUPTURE

Aortic root rupture in horses most frequently results in sudden death associated with massive hemorrhage into the thoracic cavity. If the aortic rupture is intracardiac rather than extrapericardial, the affected individual survives for a variable period of time. The longevity depends on the extent of the aortic rupture, the severity of the intracardiac shunt, the chamber(s) or structure into which the rupture occurred, the severity of the resultant cardiac (ventricular) arrhythmias, the patient's myocardial function, and the presence or absence of other cardiac disease. Several individuals with aortic rupture have lived for a year or more following the initial event.

- Affected individuals are usually **male,** primarily stallions, $\geq$ **10 years of age.**

Clinical Signs at Time of Rupture

- **Distress** (which is **usually interpreted initially as colic), tachycardia** (usually with rapid regular heart rates $\geq$ 120 beats/minute), jugular distention, and **jugular pulsations**
  - ☐ The rapid regular heart rate and jugular pulsations suggest a rhythm of **ventricular tachycardia.**

Physical Examination Findings

- Bounding arterial pulses, a loud continuous murmur with its point of maximal intensity in the right fourth intercostal space, and a loud third heart sound
  - ☐ Systolic murmurs of tricuspid regurgitation have also been reported in individuals with aortic root rupture.
- Auscultation of the abdomen usually reveals normal gastrointestinal sounds, and a rectal examination is also normal.

Diagnosis

- **Electrocardiography** usually reveals a **uniform ventricular tachycardia** (Fig. 25–42), with a heart rate ranging from 120–250 beats/minute (higher heart rates are possible but have not been recorded in horses with aortic root rupture).
- **Echocardiographic examination** reveals the **rupture in the aortic root** at the **right aortic sinus** or right sinus of Valsalva (Fig. 25–43).
  - ☐ Aneurysmal dilatation and rupture of the right sinus of Valsalva (Fig. 25–44) is detected in approximately half of affected individuals whereas in the other individuals, no pre-existing aortic root disease is detected.
  - ☐ The aortic root may dissect apically, down the interventricular septum (Fig. 25–45), with subsequent endocardial rupture into the right and/or left ventricle (most frequent), or rupture into the right atrium, tricuspid valve, and/or right ventricle.
  - ☐ Generalized cardiomegaly is common, and pulmonary artery dilatation is imaged in approximately half the patients with aortocardiac fistulas from aortic root rupture.

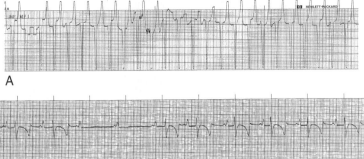

A

B

BRENTWOOD RP-100

FIGURE 25–42. Lead aVf electrocardiograms obtained from a horse with aortic root rupture and the presence of an aortic-cardiac fistula. Notice the presence of uniform ventricular tachycardia *(A)* at a ventricular rate of 160 beats/minute, which is successfully converted to sinus rhythm with 2° AV block *(B)* following treatment with quinidine gluconate, lidocaine, magnesium sulfate, and procainamide. The horse converted to sinus rhythm and a ventricular rate of 60 beats/minute with the procainamide infusion. This electrocardiogram was recorded at a paper speed of 25 mm/sec with a sensitivity of 5 mm = 1 mV.

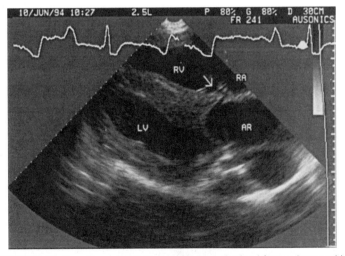

FIGURE 25–43. Two-dimensional echocardiogram obtained from a horse with an aortic root rupture and the presence of an aortic cardiac fistula (same horse as in Figure 25–42). Notice the defect in the right side of the aorta *(arrow)* just underneath the septal leaflet of the tricuspid valve. This echocardiogram was obtained from the right parasternal window just cranial to the left ventricular outflow tract view with a 2.5 MHz sector scanner transducer. RA, right atrium; RV, right ventricle; LV, left ventricle; AR, aortic root.

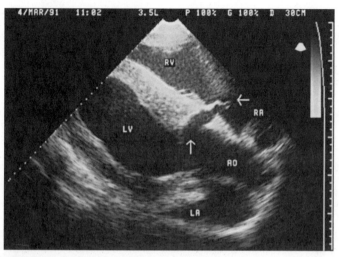

FIGURE 25–44. Two-dimensional echocardiogram obtained from a horse with a ruptured sinus of Valsalva aneurysm. Notice the communication *(vertical arrow)* between the aortic root (AO) and the right atrium (RA). Notice the torn aneurysmal tissue *(horizontal arrow)* floating in the right atrium. This echocardiogram was obtained with a 3.5 MHz sector scanner transducer from the right parasternal window slightly cranial to the left ventricular outflow tract view. RV, right ventricle; LV, left ventricle; LA, left atrium.

□ Aortic ruptures into the pericardial sac can occur but are uncommon and not localized to the right aortic sinus.

□ Pulsed wave, continuous wave, and color flow Doppler echocardiography and contrast echocardiography can be used to detect the intracardiac shunt flow and to attempt to semiquantify the severity of this shunt.

Treatment

■ **Correct the uniform ventricular tachycardia,** as indicated earlier, if the heart rate exceeds 120 beats per minute, the patient has clinical signs of cardiovascular collapse, the rhythm is multiform (not reported), or an R on T is detected in the electrocardiogram (not reported).

■ **Afterload reduction (enalapril, 0.25–0.5 mg/kg PO q24h or q12h or hydralazine, 0.5–1.5 mg/kg PO q12h)** is also indicated to help decrease the severity of the intracardiac shunt.

■ Diuretics and positive inotropic drugs may also be indicated if the individual presents with congestive heart failure.

Prognosis

■ Affected individuals must be given a **grave** prognosis for life and should not be used for performance, even if they improve clinically and/or

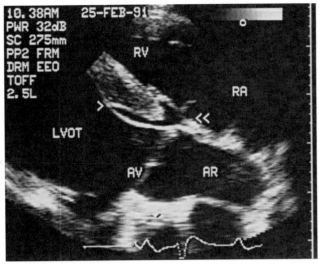

FIGURE 25–45. Two-dimensional echocardiogram obtained from a horse with a ruptured sinus of Valsalva aneurysm and subendocardial dissection of blood down the interventricular septum (same horse as in Figure 25–44). Notice the dissection of blood down the left (primarily) *(arrowhead)* and right side of the interventricular septum. The aortic cardiac fistula is between the right aortic sinus (depicted in Figure 25–44) and the right atrium *(double arrowheads)*. This echocardiogram was obtained with a 2.5 MHz sector scanner transducer from the right parasternal window in the left ventricular outflow tract view. RA, right atrium; RV, right ventricle; LVOT, left ventricular outflow tract; AV, aortic valves; AR, aortic root. An electrocardiogram is superimposed for timing purposes.

echocardiographically, as they will always be at increased risk for sudden death.

SUGGESTED REFERENCES

Baggot JD. The pharmacological basis of cardiac drug selection for use in horses. Equine Vet J 1995;Suppl 19:97–100.

Ellis EJ, Ravis WR, Malloy M, et al. Pharmacokinetics and pharmacodynamics of procainamide in horses after intravenous administration. J Vet Pharmacol Ther 1994;17:265–270.

McGuirk SM, Muir WW. Diagnosis and treatment of cardiac arrhythmias. Vet Clin North Am [Equine Pract] 1985;1:353–370.

Muir WW. Anesthetic complications and cardiopulmonary resuscitation in the horse. *In* Muir WW, Hubbell JAE: Equine Anesthesia. Monitoring and Emergency Therapy. St. Louis, Mosby–Year Book, 1991, pp 461–484.

Muir WW, Bednarski RM. Equine cardiopulmonary resuscitation—part II. Compend Contin Educ Pract Vet 1983;5:S287–S295.

Muir WW, McGuirk SM. Pharmacology and pharmacokinetics of drugs used to treat cardiac disease in horses. Vet Clin North Am [Equine Pract] 1985;1:335–352.

Muir WW, Reed SM, McGuirk SM. Treatment of atrial fibrillation in horses by intravenous administration of quinidine. J Am Vet Med Assoc 1990;197:1607–1610.

Reef VB. Echocardiographic examination in the horse: The basics. Compend Contin Educ
  Pract Vet 1990;12:1312–1320.
Reef VB. Echocardiographic findings in horses with congenital cardiac disease. Compend
  Contin Educ Pract Vet 1991;13:109–117.
Reef VB. Pericardial and myocardial diseases. *In* Koblick CN, Ames TR, Geor RJ, Trent
  AM: The Horse: Diseases and Clinical Management. New York, Churchill Living-
  stone, 1993, pp 185–197.
Reef VB. Echocardiographic evaluation of ventricular septal defects in horses. Equine Vet
  J 1995;Suppl 19:86–96.
Reef VB. Heart murmurs in horses: Determining their significance with echocardiography.
  Equine Vet J 1995;Suppl 19:71–80.
Reef VB, Bain FT, Spencer PA. Severe mitral insufficiency in horses: Clinical, echocardio-
  graphic, and pathologic findings. Equine Vet J, in press.
Reef VB, Reimer JM, Spencer PA. Treatment of equine atrial fibrillation: New perspec-
  tives. J Vet Intern Med 1995;9:57–67.

26 Gastrointestinal Emergencies and Other Causes of Colic

A. CLASSIFICATION AND PATHOPHYSIOLOGY OF COLIC

P. O. Eric Mueller and James N. Moore

A variety of enteric diseases may result in the manifestation of abdominal pain (**colic**) in horses. Abnormalities of the equine gastrointestinal tract are broadly classified as physical or functional obstructions. With a *nonstrangulating physical obstruction*, the mesenteric blood supply is intact but the bowel lumen is occluded. This may be caused by either intraluminal masses or reduction of the lumen by intramural thickening or extramural compression. *Strangulating obstruction* implies both luminal occlusion and a reduction or occlusion of the mesenteric blood supply. *Incarceration of intestine* through internal or external hernias, intussusception, or a greater than 180° twist of a segment of intestine on its mesentery may result in a strangulating obstruction. *Functional obstruction*, referred to as adynamic or paralytic ileus, may be idiopathic, result from inflammatory disease (e.g., duodenitis/proximal jejunitis and colitis), or be caused by serosal irritation due to surgical manipulation.

Intestinal obstruction prevents the aboral movement of gastrointestinal contents, resulting in distention of the intestine. As the distention increases, venous drainage from the intestinal wall is impaired and the mucosa becomes congested and edematous. **If the obstruction persists for a prolonged period** of time (>24 hours), **significant compromise of intestinal vascular integrity may result in mucosal ischemia.** With progressive distention, gastric, cecal, or colonic rupture may result. In strangulating obstructions, these events are combined with rapid tissue hypoxia and ischemia of the affected segment, leading to necrosis and transmural leakage of bacteria and endotoxin. Cardiovascular deterioration rapidly follows transperitoneal absorption of endotoxin, resulting in hypovolemia and endotoxic shock.

Diagnosis

Previous History. Previous colic episode, duration of colic, recent changes in management (feed, water, deworming, medication, exercise routine), breeding, pregnancy

Recent History. Degree and change in pain (looking at flank, pawing, kicking at abdomen, rolling), last defecation, sweating, treatment, and response to treatment

Physical Examination. Assess the following parameters immediately and completely during initial examination of the horse with a history of acute abdominal pain:

- **Attitude**
- **Observation of abdominal shape (distention)**
- **Body temperature, pulse, and respiratory rate—TPR**
- **Skin turgor, mucous membrane moisture and color, and capillary refill time (CRT)**
- **Abdominal auscultation and percussion**
- **Nasogastric intubation (quantity/characteristics of fluid)**
- **Rectal examination**

The *physical examination* starts with observation of the individual's external appearance and attitude. Abdominal distention is generally a sign of large intestinal disease, but it can occur with severe small intestinal distention. Multiple abrasions, particularly around the periorbital area, indicate that the patient recently experienced severe abdominal pain. Recent enlargement of an umbilical or abdominal hernia or the scrotum may indicate intestinal incarceration with obstruction or strangulation. Assess the degree of pain with the patient in a quiet environment.

Signs of abdominal pain in order of severity are:

- Lying down for excessive periods of time
- Inappetence
- Restlessness
- Quivering of the upper lip
- Turning of the head toward the flank
- Repeated stretching as if to urinate
- Kicking with the hind feet at the abdomen
- Crouching as if wanting to lie down
- Sweating
- Dropping to the ground and rolling

Severe, unrelenting pain may require analgesics before examination (Table 26–1).

TABLE 26–1. **Analgesics and Relative Efficacy for Control of Acute Abdominal Pain**

Analgesic	Trade Name	Dosage	Efficacy
Flunixin meglumine	Banamine	0.25–1.1 mg/kg IV or IM	Excellent
Detomidine hydrochloride	Dormosedan	5–40 µg/kg IV or IM[3]	Excellent
Xylazine hydrochloride	Rompun	0.2–1.1 mg/kg IV or IM[1, 3]	Good
Butorphanol tartrate	Torbugesic	0.02–0.08 mg/kg IV or IM[2, 5]	Good
Ketoprofen	Ketofen	1.1–2.2 mg/kg IV	Good
Meperidine hydrochloride	Demerol	1.1–2.2 mg/kg IV or IM[3, 5]	Good
Morphine sulfate		0.3–0.66 mg/kg IV[4, 5]	Good
Pentazocine	Talwin	0.3–0.6 mg/kg IV[5]	Poor
Chloral hydrate		30–60 mg/kg IV titrated	Poor
Dipyrone	Novin	10–22 mg/kg IV or IM	Poor
Phenylbutazone	Butazolidin	2.2–4.4 mg/kg IV	Poor

[1] Repeated administration may compromise cardiac output and colonic motility.
[2] Doses in upper range may cause ataxia.
[3] Intravenous administration may cause severe hypotension.
[4] *Use only with xylazine* (0.66–1.1 mg/kg IV) to avoid CNS excitement.
[5] Indicates a controlled substance.

Consider previous treatment by the owner or trainer when assessing the amount of abdominal pain present. Depression with mild to moderate abdominal pain and fever may indicate an inflammatory condition (enteritis or colitis). **In the absence of extreme muscle exertion, suspect inflammatory disease (enteritis, colitis, peritonitis) as the cause of abdominal pain accompanied by fever.** Loud "fluid and bubbling" sounds may be heard on abdominal auscultation in some patients with impending colitis. Ultrasound examination can be helpful in delineating enteritis (distended small intestine with increased motility) from strangulating obstruction (distended small intestine with no motility).

Tachycardia and tachypnea may serve as indicators of abdominal pain, cardiovascular shock, and endotoxemia.

Skin turgor, mucous membrane moisture and color, and CRT may aid in assessment of dehydration resulting from intestinal dysfunction. Mucous membrane moisture and color change from moist and pale pink to dry and red with a decrease in circulating blood volume. With the onset of shock and endotoxemia, mucous membrane color may progress to reddish-blue to purple (cyanosis).

Auscultate for *intestinal borborygmi* in all abdominal quadrants. Pain and inflammation related to the gastrointestinal tract results in decreased borborygmi. Increased borborygmi may be present early with enteritis or colitis, only to progress to ileus and cessation of the sounds as the bowel becomes progressively inflamed and distended. Increased borborygmi are present early in individuals with obstruction, but intestinal sounds decrease as the obstruction becomes complete. Simultaneous auscultation and percussion may reveal high-pitched sounds (pinging) due to cecal (right flank) or colonic (left flank) tympany. A sound similar to an ocean wave can be heard in some patients with sand impaction; if sand is suspected, perform auscultation of the ventral abdomen for 5 minutes.

Apply nasogastric intubation **immediately** in individuals demonstrating abdominal pain. Gastric decompression is essential to determine whether gastric distention is present and to provide relief to patients with primary or secondary gastric distention. Nasogastric reflux may be secondary to small intestinal obstruction or secondary ileus from large intestinal disease. Individuals with anterior enteritis characteristically have large volumes of reflux (10–20 L). Blood-tinged, foul-smelling reflux may indicate small intestinal strangulating obstruction or severe anterior enteritis. **If small intestinal obstruction or enteritis is suspected, it is essential to leave the tube in place to prevent spontaneous gastric rupture and subsequent death!**

A careful *rectal examination* is important when examining a horse demonstrating abdominal pain. Before beginning the examination, note the amount and consistency of fecal material in the rectum. Absence of fecal material, or the presence of dry, fibrin- and mucus-covered feces is abnormal and is consistent with delayed intestinal transit. Fetid, watery fecal material is often seen in horses with colitis. Examine in a consistent, systematic manner to minimize missing a lesion. Intra-abdominal structures palpable in the **normal horse**, starting in the left cranial abdominal quadrant and progressing in a clockwise direction, include:

- Caudal border of the spleen
- Nephrosplenic ligament
- Caudal pole of the left kidney
- Mesenteric root
- Ventral cecal band (no tension)
- Cecal base (empty)
- Small colon containing distinct fecal balls
- Pelvic flexure

The small intestine is not palpable unless an underlying abnormality exists. Determination of bowel distention of any form is important in formulating a tentative diagnosis.

Abnormal rectal examination findings include:

- Cecal distention
- Gas- or ingesta-distended small intestine, large intestine, or small colon
- Marked intramural or mesenteric edema
- Bowel malposition
- Herniation
- Impaction
- Intussusception
- Intra-abdominal mass, abscess, or hematoma formation
- Enterolithiasis
- Volvulus of the mesenteric root

Always examine the internal inguinal rings, urethra, and bladder (male) and reproductive tract and bladder (female). Sequential rectal examinations are often helpful in determining the rate and severity of disease and the need for surgical intervention.

Response to Analgesics. The amount of pain demonstrated by a horse with gastrointestinal disease is variable and depends on the individual pain threshold of the individual and the severity of disease present. In general, the greater the pain, the more severe the disease. In the later stages of disease, abdominal pain may be replaced by marked depression and cardiovascular deterioration as a result of bowel necrosis and systemic endotoxemia. Pain control is accomplished by gastric decompression via a nasogastric tube and administration of peripherally and centrally acting analgesics (see Table 26–1). Assessment of a patient's response to analgesics is helpful in determining the severity of disease and likelihood of successfully treating the patient with medical management. *Horses demonstrating unrelenting pain not responsive to analgesics require immediate surgical exploration or euthanasia.*

Clinicopathologic Evaluation

- Packed cell volume (PCV)
- Total plasma protein (TPP)
- Complete blood cell count (CBC)
- Blood gases (BG)
- Electrolyte determination

PCV AND TPP. Hypovolemia secondary to intestinal dysfunction results in dehydration. The PCV/TPP is the most accurate measurement to support a clinical assessment of dehydration in most individuals with abdominal pain.

	*PCV (%)**	*TPP (gm/dl)*
Mild dehydration	45–50	7.5–8.0
Moderate dehydration	50–60	8.0–9.0
Severe dehydration	≥ 60	≥ 9.0

Marked increases in PCV without corresponding increases or decreases in TPP, may indicate protein loss into the intestinal lumen or peritoneal cavity, or sympathetic and endotoxin-induced splenic contraction.

CBC. Most simple or strangulating obstructions do not cause a substantial change in the white blood cell count until the terminal stages of diseases. Acute inflammatory diseases (enteritis, colitis), however, often cause a leukopenia (< 4000 cells/μl). A marked leukopenia (< 1000 cells/μl) is seen with fulminant septic peritonitis secondary to acute bowel rupture. A mature neutrophilia and high TPP and fibrinogen may indicate chronic peritonitis secondary to abdominal abscessation.

BLOOD GASES. Acidemia with advanced hypovolemic shock may be noted. Evaluation of blood gases is essential for appropriate treatment of severe acid-base abnormalities, especially in those patients requiring general anesthesia and surgical treatment. Individuals with simple colon displacements may have a slight base excess, whereas patients with strangulating obstruction usually have a base deficit.

ELECTROLYTES. Determination of serum electrolytes is rarely helpful in making a diagnosis. A rare exception to this is acute abdominal pain caused by

---

*These values cannot be applied to nursing foals, which generally have lower PCV and protein.

hypocalcemia and ileus (synchronous diaphragmatic flutter may be present). Electrolyte determinations are essential for appropriate patient management before, during, and after surgical treatment. Hyponatremia and hypochloremia may suggest impending colitis.

Abdominocentesis (see p. 55). This useful diagnostic tool for assessment of intestinal compromise may be performed with an 18-gauge, sterile hypodermic needle or a blunt cannula (teat cannula or canine female urinary catheter). Collect fluid in a sterile tube containing EDTA for cytologic analysis of the fluid, and into a second sterile tube not containing additives for culture and sensitivity, if indicated. Fluid analysis includes specific gravity and protein determinations, and cell types, numbers, and morphology (see Table 16–1). Ultrasonography, using a 7.5 MHz transducer, may be useful in locating peritoneal fluid. *Be more cautious in performing abdominocentesis in foals because needle perforation of the bowel may lead to adhesions, and the teat cannula method may cause herniation of omentum unless performed in the most caudal aspect of the abdomen.*

Normal peritoneal fluid is odorless, nonturbid, and clear to pale yellow. The nucleated cell count should be less than 3000–5000 cells/μl, with a total protein concentration of less than 2.5 gm/dl. With early, simple obstruction of the small or large intestine, peritoneal fluid characteristically remains normal. With strangulating obstruction or severe intestinal inflammation, the peritoneal fluid may become serosanguineous, with increases in nucleated cell count and total protein concentration.

Dark, turbid fluid with the smell of ingesta, increased nucleated cell counts, and increased protein concentration indicate bowel necrosis and leakage. The presence of plant material and intracellular bacteria indicates bowel rupture (see Fig. 38–2) **(if this material has been collected by needle aspiration, it should be repeated with a teat cannula before diagnosing a ruptured viscus).**

Blood-tinged fluid indicates splenic puncture, intra-abdominal or iatrogenic hemorrhage, or intestinal necrosis.

With splenic puncture, the PCV of the fluid is greater than the peripheral PCV and contains high numbers of small lymphocytes. Fluid from intra-abdominal hemorrhage reveals a PCV less than that of peripheral blood, erythrocytophagia, and few to no platelets.

NOTE: The **absence of gross or cytologic abnormalities in the peritoneal fluid does not rule out compromised intestine.**

Some strangulating lesions, such as intussusceptions, external hernias, and epiploic foramen incarcerations may not demonstrate abnormalities in the peritoneal fluid owing to sequestration of the fluid in the omentum, intussuscipiens, or hernial sac.

If a sand impaction is suspected or marked cecal or colonic distention is present, an abdominocentesis should be performed only to confirm suspected bowel rupture.

If physical examination reveals other findings consistent with a surgical lesion and referral for surgery is contemplated, an abdominocentesis should not be performed in the field, due to the risk to the patient and examiner.

Medical Versus Surgical Management

Considerations in determining the need for exploratory surgery (see Table 26–2):

TABLE 26–2. **Indications for Exploratory Celiotomy in Horses Demonstrating Acute Abdominal Pain**

Severe, unrelenting abdominal pain[1]
Refractory to analgesics[1]
Increased heart rate[2]
Large quantities of gastric reflux[2]
Absence of borborygmi[2]
Abnormal rectal examination[2]
Serosanguineous abdominal fluid with increased total protein and nucleated cell count[2]

[1]These parameters alone are indications for emergency exploratory celiotomy.
[2]These parameters are not sole indications for emergency exploratory celiotomy but must be evaluated in view of other clinical findings.

- Pain
- Response to analgesic therapy
- Cardiovascular status
- Rectal examination findings
- Amount of gastric reflux
- Abdominocentesis results

A history of abdominal pain often requires reassessment of these parameters over time. A change in one or more clinical parameters may determine the need for surgical or medical management. Manifestation of **pain** and the response to analgesic therapy are the most valuable criteria in assessing the need for surgical intervention. **Individuals demonstrating unrelenting pain, or recurrent pain after administration of analgesics, are considered surgical candidates.**

Rectal examination is the next most valuable criterion for surgery. Demonstration of pain concurrent with abnormal rectal examination findings is a strong indicator. Failure of medical therapy, systemic cardiovascular deterioration, or changes in peritoneal fluid characteristics indicating intestinal degeneration are also indications for surgical intervention.

Treatment

Treatment for individuals demonstrating acute abdominal pain is directed at:

- Pain relief
- Stabilization of cardiovascular and metabolic status
- Minimizing the deleterious effects of endotoxemia
- Establishing a patent and functional intestine

This may be accomplished by one or more of the following therapeutic modalities:

- Analgesic therapy (see Table 26–1)
- Fluid therapy and cardiovascular support
- Laxatives and cathartics
- Antiendotoxin therapy
- Therapy for ischemia-reperfusion injury
- Antimicrobials

- Nutritional support
- Surgical intervention

Analgesic Therapy. Pain relief is accomplished by gastric decompression using a nasogastric tube and administration of peripherally and centrally acting analgesics (see Table 26–1). Perform gastric decompression (see p. 53) (approximately every 2 hours) through an indwelling nasogastric tube; it may be necessary to prevent distention, which can potentially lead to pain, gastric rupture, and death. Patients being referred for possible exploratory surgery should have an **indwelling nasogastric tube** in place during transport to the referral facility.

Fluid Therapy and Cardiovascular Support. IV administration of polyionic, balanced electrolyte solutions is necessary to maintain intravascular fluid volume. Hypertonic saline (5% or 7% NaCl, 1–2 L, IV) results in improved systemic blood pressure and cardiac output. *Hypertonic saline may be administered initially but **must** be followed by adequate fluid replacement with balanced crystalloid solutions (ideally within 1 hour after hypertonic saline).* Monitor hydration status with clinical assessment and PCV/TPP. Monitor blood gases and serum electrolytes and adjust the IV solutions to correct deficiencies.

If plasma protein concentration is less than 4.5 gm/dl and the patient is dehydrated, administer plasma (2–10 L, IV, slowly) or a synthetic colloid (Hetastarch) to maintain plasma oncotic pressure and avoid inducing pulmonary edema during rehydration with IV fluids.

Laxatives. Use to increase GI water content, soften ingesta, facilitate intestinal transit, and treat impactions of the cecum and large and small colons. *For maximal effect, oral and intravenous fluids should be administered concurrently.* Do not administer orally in patients with nasogastric reflux.

Commonly used laxatives:

- Mineral oil (6–8 L/500-kg body weight) can be administered to facilitate passage after the impaction begins to resolve; however, it is not useful to penetrate and hydrate the primary impaction.
- Magnesium sulfate (Epsom salt, 500 gm diluted in warm water/500-kg body weight, daily). Do not use longer than 3 days or in patients with decreased renal function to avoid enteritis and possible magnesium intoxication. *Preferred for large colon impactions.*
- Psyllium hydrophilic mucilloid (Metamucil, 400 gm/500-kg body weight every 6–12 h) until the impaction resolves. *Especially useful for sand impactions.*
- Dioctyl sodium sulfosuccinate (DSS, 10–20 mg/kg up to two doses, 48 hours apart). *May cause mild abdominal pain and diarrhea.*

Antiendotoxin Therapy. Antiserum (500–1000 ml) directed against the gram-negative core antigens of endotoxin (Endoserum, Immvac, Columbia, MO) can be administered IV diluted in a balanced electrolyte solution. Significant amounts of endotoxin have been reported in Endoserum. Endoserum should be warmed to room temperature and administered slowly to avoid undesired side effects, e.g., tachycardia, muscle fasciculations. Hyperimmune plasma directed against the J-5 mutant strain of *Escherichia coli* (Polymune-J, San Luis Obispo, CA, or Foalimmune, Lake Immunogenics Inc., Ontario, NY) or normal *equine plasma* (2–10 L), administered IV *slowly*, may be equally or more beneficial, supplying protein, fibronectin, complement, antithrombin III, and other inhibitors of hypercoagulability.

Therapy for Ischemia-Reperfusion Injury. If ischemia is suspected, dimethyl sulfoxide (DMSO), a hydroxyl radical scavenger, can be administered IV (100 mg/kg q8–12h) diluted to a 10% solution in a balanced electrolyte solution. Efficacy has not been proved. Kinetic studies support *q12h* use at the anti-inflammatory dose.

Antimicrobials. Not routinely administered to individuals that demonstrate acute abdominal pain unless an underlying infectious agent is suspected. Broad-spectrum antimicrobials are indicated in septic, neutropenic (< 2000 cells/μl) patients to minimize bacteremia and organ colonization by enteric organisms and in patients undergoing exploratory celiotomy.

Penicillin (22,000–44,000 IU/kg, IV q6h, or IM q12h) often is administered to individuals with duodenitis/proximal jejunitis (suspected agent: *Clostridium perfringens*, type A).

Nutritional Support. Individuals demonstrating abdominal pain should be withheld from hay and grain for 12–18 hours. If they do not have gastric reflux, they should be allowed free-choice water and have access to trace mineral salt. If the patient responds to initial treatment, it should be gradually returned to a normal diet over 24–48 hours (moist bran/alfalfa pellet mashes, grazing grass, hay, then grain). Individuals being referred for possible exploratory surgery **should not be fed** during transport to the referral facility.

Surgical Intervention. Candidates for exploratory celiotomy (Table 26–2):

- **Unrelenting pain**
- **Recurrent pain after administration of analgesics**
- **Systemic cardiovascular deterioration**
- **Changes in peritoneal fluid characteristics indicating intestinal degeneration**
- **Failure of medical therapy**

Ventral midline celiotomy is the surgical approach of choice, and specific treatments are discussed under each gastrointestinal disorder.

B. DISORDERS OF THE MOUTH AND SALIVATION (PTYALISM)

Michael Ball and Thomas J. Divers

Acute salivation (ptyalism) may be caused by the inability to swallow normally produced saliva—e.g., choke (see pp. 166–168) by neurologic disturbances (see Section 30, p. 337), or from excessive production of saliva. A thorough physical examination and history are necessary to differentiate between local causes and a focal manifestation of a generalized disease to arrive at an accurate diagnosis. **The most common causes of excessive salivation are red clover poisoning and choke in adults. In foals the cause is usually gastric ulceration (see pp. 173–175).**

The cause may be found in the mouth and diagnosed on oral examination in some cases. Evaluate the entire oral cavity, looking for a laceration, ulcerations, vesicular disease, foreign body, abscess of tooth root or soft tissue, a fractured tooth, injury to the palate, or evidence of chemical injury. Sedation (detomidine with butorphanol) and the *careful* use of an equine mouth speculum may be needed to improve examination of the mouth. *Without proper sedation, the mouth speculum becomes a dangerous weapon to the examiner if the patient "throws" its head*; excessive biting on it by the individual may cause a fractured tooth.

Localized Causes

- The most common equine foreign body is a wooden stick large enough to become lodged between the upper arcade of teeth or a smaller stick penetrating the soft tissue of the pharyngeal cavity or soft palate.
- Evaluate the tongue for blisters, ulceration, or cellulitis.
- Burrs or grass awns may be stuck in the mouth and cause salivation. This may be a farm problem.
- Patients that have licked mercury blister compounds are prone to severe oral erosions.
- Most vesicles are idiopathic, but consider vesicular stomatitis, which appears most commonly in New Mexico and Colorado, occurring every 3 to 7 years. Immune-mediated pemphigus vesicular formation in the oral cavity occurs but is rare.
- *Actinobacillus lignieresii* can cause wooden tongue in the horse.
- Consider also sialadenitis, fractured teeth, or fractured bones of the mouth.
- Primary pharyngitis or epiglottiditis, retropharyngeal lymphadenopathy, guttural pouch empyema, pharyngeal edema, and choke are other frequent causes of ptyalism.

Diagnosis

Ancillary diagnostics include radiography, ultrasonography, and endoscopy of the mouth and/or pharyngeal area. Ultrasonography may elucidate an area that can be aspirated for cytology and culture. Observe carefully from a distance to note whether the ability to prehend, masticate, and swallow is retained. In some cases, a complete oral examination under anesthesia may be necessary before a cause can be determined.

Treatment

Treatments may include:

- Removal of foreign bodies
- Tooth extraction
- Antibiotic therapy for infectious causes
- Intravenous fluids
- Nonsteroidal anti-inflammatory drugs (NSAIDs)
- Other symptomatic treatment:
  - 2% potassium per manganate as a mouth disinfectant
  - Furacin/prednisolone spray for pharyngeal edema and inflammation

Penicillin is often the initial choice for an antibiotic since many commensal oral organisms are sensitive to it. Some cases may require a tracheotomy if laryngeal/pharyngeal swelling is compromising the airway. Regarding fluid therapy, it is important to remember that, in the horse, the anion of highest concentration in saliva is chloride, with a relatively low concentration of bicarbonate. When an individual develops an acid-base disturbance primarily from salivary loss, it is usually a hypochloremic metabolic alkalosis, and therefore fluid therapy consisting of 0.9% sodium chloride with 20 mEq/L KCl is used.

Systemic Causes

Slaframine toxicity (see Chapter 40) (slobber syndrome), caused by the ingestion of red clover (hay or more commonly pasture) that has been infected with the fungus Rhizoctonia leguminicola, can cause excessive salivation. The clinical signs usually resolve within 48–96 hours after withdrawal from the affected forage; mortality is rare.

Other toxicities include organophosphates/carbamates, monensin, NSAID toxicity, acorn, oleander, potato, and cantharidin (blister beetle). An index of suspicion regarding potential exposure to toxins or chemical irritants that may have been ingested is necessary.

Other systemic diseases that may cause salivation include **botulism, equine protozoal myelitis,** leukoencephalomalacia, and renal and liver disease.

C. DISORDERS OF THE ESOPHAGUS

P. O. Eric Mueller and James N. Moore

The most common clinical problem affecting the horse's esophagus is obstruction of the lumen (choke), which may occur either as a single acute episode or as a chronic, intermittent problem. In either case, these conditions are treated as emergencies. If the condition recurs, then a diverticulum or stricture should be considered as a possible cause.

ESOPHAGEAL OBSTRUCTION

Most often acute esophageal obstruction results from obstruction of the esophageal lumen with food, wood chips, or bedding. These problems arise in individuals with ravenous eating habits, especially older horses being fed pelleted feeds. **The most common clinical signs are excessive salivation, retching, coughing with saliva, and food dripping from the nostrils.** In most instances, an enlargement may be palpated over the trachea if the obstruction is in the cervical region and is of recent origin. Over time, the swelling and muscle spasm in this region make it difficult to delineate the mass. The likelihood that the obstruction is in the cervical portion of the esophagus increases if the patient retches immediately after attempting to swallow. There is a 10- to 12-second delay between the swallow and the onset of retching if the obstruction occurs in the distal esophagus.

Diagnosis and Medical Treatment of Choke

Confirm the diagnosis by endoscopy, or by passing a nasogastric tube and meeting an obstruction in the esophagus. Initial aim of treatment: to reduce the patient's level of anxiety and allow the esophageal musculature to relax.

Tranquilize the affected individual with acepromazine and provide further sedation with *xylazine* or *detomidine*. Withhold *water and feed until esophageal obstruction can be safely ruled out*. **If choke is suspected, advise owners to remove hay and water immediately.** Frequently, these conservative treatments are sufficient to relax the esophagus and allow the obstruction to pass on its own within 4–6 hours.

To reduce the likelihood of aspiration pneumonia, administer one dose (0.02 mg/kg IV) of atropine to decrease salivation; *do not repeat owing to its side effects on the gastrointestinal tract!*

If this treatment is unsuccessful in relieving the choke in 4–6 hours, administer further treatment, including gentle lavage. *With the patient sedated with xylazine or detomidine, causing the patient to lower its head, pass a stomach tube to the proximal extent of the obstruction*; gently push a small volume of water through the tube and against the obstructing mass. Gently massage the obstructed area while the mass is advanced with the end of the stomach tube. This process may need to be repeated several times to aid breakup of the blockage. Careful manipulation is essential to avoid esophageal injury and secondary stricture or esophageal perforation.

IV fluids are an important supportive treatment in more prolonged choke cases to prevent dehydration and worsening of the esophageal obstruction.

If more aggressive lavage is required, a warmed, cuffed endotracheal tube passed intranasally *into the esophagus* provides the security of an inflatable cuff and can prevent aspiration of water during lavage of the esophagus. Warming the tube before passage facilitates passage by making it more pliable. Fluid can then be pumped through the endotracheal tube or through a small-diameter stomach tube that has been passed inside the larger endotracheal tube. The lavage solution is commonly warm water and/or a mixture of glycerin and DSS.

An alternative procedure is to pass the endotracheal tube into the trachea and inflate the cuff before flushing the esophagus. If the obstruction cannot be resolved or if the patient becomes unmanageable under sedation, general anesthesia, with the head positioned down, is required for more aggressive lavage.

Prophylactic antimicrobials are indicated for all choke cases because of the potential for aspiration pneumonia. Generally a broad-spectrum combination of antibiotics is administered for 5–7 days (e.g., procaine penicillin G, 22,000 IU/kg IM q12h initially and/or trimethoprim-sulfa, 20–30 mg/kg PO q12h after the obstruction is relieved). If aspiration is known to have occurred, copious lavage is performed. If respiratory signs develop or crackles are present on auscultation or thoracic ultrasound, indicating abnormalities of the pleura, add metronidazole (15–25 mg/kg PO q8h).

Once the obstruction is resolved, initially offer the patient only water, because esophageal dilation postobstruction increases the likelihood of reimpaction for 48 hours. Advise the owner to withhold feed for 48 hours, or if impractical, to allow small amounts of a soft diet to prevent recurrence of the obstruction. Endoscopic examination after the obstruction is relieved allows evaluation of the esophageal mucosa and provides information concerning the likelihood of secondary complications (e.g., reobstruction, stricture, perforation).

Surgical Treatment

If all attempts to dislodge the obstruction are unsuccessful, surgical intervention is indicated. Although several procedures are used to treat strictures, diverticula, tumors, and other rare causes for obstruction, cervical esophagotomy is the only emergency procedure.

Cervical esophagotomy is performed under local or general anesthesia. The decision depends on the temperament of the individual, the type of obstruction, cost, and the surgeon's preference. Make an incision either on the midline or ventral to the left jugular vein over the obstruction. Once the obstructed portion of the esophagus can be identified, attempt extraluminal massage and manual breakdown of the mass before entering the esophagus. If these are unsuccessful, make a longitudinal incision distal to the obstruction on the ventral or ventrolateral aspect of the esophagus. These sites are used to aid in ventral drainage if the incision is left open to heal by second intention or if dehiscence of the primary incision occurs. A 2–3-cm incision is made in the muscular layer of the esophagus, and the mucosa is grasped with forceps and incised. A sponge forceps is used to remove the obstructing mass.

A stomach tube is then passed normograde and retrograde to ensure a patent lumen. To suture the esophagus, a simple continuous 3–0 monofilament polydioxanone or polypropylene suture is placed in the mucosa and submucosa, with the knots in the lumen of the esophagus. Close the muscular layer of the esophagus, using an interrupted pattern of absorbable material; place a suction drain adjacent to the esophagus and close the subcutaneous tissues. The suction drain remains in place for 48 hours, all food is withheld, and fluids administered IV. Feed the patient a slurry of pelleted feed for 8–10 days, beginning on postoperative day 5.

Alternatively, use a second esophagotomy distal to the site of the obstruction to feed the patient a gruel and water mixture through an indwelling stomach tube sutured in place. This tube can be used for 10 days, allowing the sutured proximal esophagotomy time to heal by first intention. If dehiscence occurs, a traction diverticulum may develop but is usually associated with few complications.

If necrotic tissue is debrided at the obstruction site, a stomach tube is recommended. Suture the tube in place and feed the patient a gruel and water mixture through it for 10 days. The stoma is left to heal by second intention after tube removal.

Prognosis and Complications

The prognosis for survival with simple esophageal obstruction is excellent. The prognosis is favorable for individuals with pulsion diverticula but poor if strictures occur requiring resection and anastomosis of the esophagus. Aspiration pneumonia is a serious sequela, to be recognized early and treated aggressively. Use ultrasonography to determine the severity of the aspiration pneumonia. The incidence of these complications is directly related to the time for resolution of the primary obstruction. Therefore, treat aggressively, with particular care given to potential iatrogenic complications. Choke in the miniature horse foal is not unusual and has a guarded prognosis.

ESOPHAGEAL PERFORATION

Causes for esophageal perforation (rupture) include:

- Chronic obstruction
- Swallowed perforating foreign body
- Penetrating external wounds
- Repeated, traumatic nasogastric intubation
- Extension of an infection from surrounding tissues

Clinical signs vary from a fistula draining saliva and feed material with open perforation to severe cervical swelling, cellulitis, abscessation, and subcutaneous emphysema with closed esophageal perforation. Dyspnea may develop and require emergency tracheotomy.

Confirm the diagnosis by endoscopy, radiography, or contrast radiography. Small perforations may be difficult to detect using endoscopy. Survey radiographs may reveal subcutaneous emphysema, and positive contrast studies may demonstrate leakage of the aqueous media into the surrounding tissues.

Treatment

- Acute (6–12 h) perforations may be debrided and closed primarily if sufficient viable esophageal tissue is present.
- Maintain affected individuals NPO for 48–72 hours following surgery to allow time for mucosal healing and minimize postoperative fistula formation.
- Administer broad-spectrum antimicrobial therapy. Antimicrobial combinations commonly used include
  □ Na^+/K^+ penicillin, 22,000–44,000 IU/kg IV q6h, and aminoglycosides: gentamicin, 2.2 mg/kg IV q8h/6.6 mg/kg IV q24h or amikacin, 6.6 mg/kg q8h/19.8 mg/kg IV q24h
  □ Metronidazole, 15–25 mg/kg PO q6h, for anaerobes
- IV-balanced, polyionic fluids to correct electrolyte and acid-base abnormalities *and/or if aminoglycosides are being given*
- NSAIDs
- Tetanus prophylaxis

If primary closure is not possible, adequate ventral drainage is established to minimize extension of the cellulitis along fascial planes, which could result in septic mediastinitis and pleuritis.

Nutritional supplementation via an esophagostomy and indwelling nasogastric tube placement distal to the site of perforation, or total parenteral nutrition (TPN), may be required during the convalescent period.

Prognosis and Complications

Prognosis for acute esophageal perforation is fair if rapid, aggressive therapy is instituted and primary closure of the defect is possible. In chronic cases, the prognosis is guarded because of the high probability of secondary complication such as esophageal stricture, reobstruction, and septic mediastinitis and/or pleuritis.

D. DISORDERS OF THE STOMACH

P. O. Eric Mueller, James N. Moore,
and Thomas J. Divers

ACUTE GASTRIC DILATION

Primary gastric dilation is believed to be associated with the ingestion of highly fermentable feed, such as grass clippings and/or excessive amounts of corn or other grain. Secondary gastric dilation occurs when fluid from the small intestine accumulates in the stomach because of ileus, obstruction of the small intestinal lumen, strangulation obstruction involving the small intestine, or severe inflammation of the small intestine. In one study of 50 horses with gastric rupture, individuals drinking water from a bucket, stream, or pond were at greater risk of gastric rupture than individuals having access to an automatic waterer.

- Horses exhibit signs of severe pain and increased heart and respiratory rates due to pain and diaphragmatic pressure.
- If the dilation is primary, the patients' mucous membranes are pale, and on rectal examination the spleen may be palpated displaced caudally by the enlarged stomach. If the dilation is secondary to a problem involving the small intestine, the patient may exhibit signs of toxicity, the peritoneal fluid may reflect intra-abdominal ischemia (discoloration with erythrocytes, increased WBC count and protein concentration), and several loops of distended small intestine may be palpable on rectal examination.
- In some cases spontaneous regurgitation may occur immediately before the stomach ruptures along its greater curvature.

Treatment

For acute abdominal pain, the primary goal is to relieve intragastric pressure by passing a medium- or large-bore stomach tube. *Lidocaine may be needed to relax the cardiac sphincter, and it may be necessary to create a "siphon" effect to ensure that all excess fluid is removed from the stomach.* Once emergency care is given, perform a complete physical examination to determine the cause. In primary dilation, the individual should remain pain-free once the pressure is relieved. If the dilation is secondary to a small intestinal problem, relief is transient. If the stomach ruptures, the patient immediately appears comfortable, followed by rapid deterioration caused by endotoxic and cardiovascular shock. Ingesta is evident in the peritoneal fluid, and the serosa of the intestines are roughened on rectal examination; euthanasia is recommended.

Prognosis

The prognosis for primary dilation is excellent, provided the intragastric pressure is rapidly relieved. Prognosis for secondary gastric dilation depends on the underlying disease and duration of the condition before beginning treatment.

GASTRIC IMPACTION

Occurs infrequently. The most common causes:

- Grain overload
- Dry, impacted ingesta
- Gastric squamous cell carcinoma

If the impaction is associated with causes other than squamous cell carcinoma, the patient may show signs of moderate to severe pain. Most often these patients do not show evidence of systemic toxicity unless the grain overload has progressed, resulting in signs of acute laminitis. Individuals with impacted ingesta in the stomach may be in uncontrollable pain, necessitating immediate exploratory surgery. The diagnosis in these cases is made at surgery.

Treatment

At surgery, intragastric administration of 2–3 liters of water through a 3-inch needle is placed through the stomach wall intra-abdominally. Redirect the end of the needle, infiltrating different areas of the mass, followed by gentle massage. Postoperative care: lavage of the stomach and drainage through a large-bore stomach tube.

Prognosis

Guarded.

EMERGENCY GRAIN OVERLOAD

Clinicians are often called on emergency to examine and treat a horse that has accidentally ingested an excessive amount of grain (either commercially prepared concentrate or a cereal grain hay such as barley). If the individual has no clinical signs on examination, the following treatment is recommended:

- Pass a stomach tube and check for gastric reflux; if there is no reflux, administer 1 lb Epsom salt ($MgSO_4$) or 1 lb activated charcoal mixed in 1 gallon warm water (per 500-kg adult) via *gravity* (funnel) *flow.*
- 0.3 mg/kg flunixin meglumine IV or IM q8h for 48h
- 0.5 mg/kg doxylamine succinate SQ q6h for 24h (other favorite antihistamines may be substituted)
- Remove all feed for 24 hours.

Prognosis

Should be excellent if the treatment is given before any clinical signs.

SYMPTOMATIC GRAIN OVERLOAD

The clinical signs most frequently noted are colic, marked abdominal distention, severe lameness (laminitis), trembling, sweating, polypnea, and, less frequently, diarrhea. Clinical findings include bright red to purple membranes, tachycardia, absence of intestinal sounds (some pings may be found on simultaneous auscultation and percussion of the abdomen), gastric reflux, and colonic distention with tight bands palpated on rectal examination.

CBC usually reveals severe polycythemia, neutropenia with a left shift, and vacuolization of neutrophils (toxic changes).

Treatment

- IV fluid therapy. Hypertonic saline initially, but this must be followed within 1–2 hours by administration of a polyionic fluid at 2–4 L/hr for the adult; 23% calcium borogluconate, 500 ml, can be administered but must be diluted with several liters of polyionic fluids. Add KCl, 20–40 mEg, to each liter of fluids after urination is noted.

- Administer plasma if possible (2–4 L/adult). Hyperimmune plasma containing antibodies against endotoxin is preferred but not essential.
- Flunixin meglumine IV (1 mg/kg IV initially and 0.3 mg/kg q8h after signs of colic are no longer evident).
- Pass a nasogastric tube and leave in place to relieve gastric distention. If there is no gastric reflux, 0.5 lb of charcoal should be administered in 0.5 gallon warm water (per 500-kg adult) via *gravity flow*.
- Pentoxifylline (8.4 mg/kg PO q8h) may also be administered if there is no gastric reflux. Pentoxifylline may inhibit cytokine production.
- Remove feed, bed heavily, and/or apply frog pads to the feet.
- Aggressive and early treatment for laminitis if signs of founder are noted

Prognosis

The prognosis with marked clinical signs is poor. **If severe abdominal pain and marked abdominal distention are present, a very poor prognosis should be given, and affected individuals generally die within 24 to 48 hours with even the most aggressive therapy.** If the abdominal distention is becoming severe but the cardiovascular system seems stable and you are certain of the diagnosis, two additional treatments may be attempted:

- Trocarize the cecum; if that fails to relieve the distention,
- 0.005–0.01 mg/kg of neostigmine SQ during heavy sedation, to evacuate the fermented gas.

If signs of laminitis occur before the intestinal signs diminish, a very grave prognosis is warranted.

GASTRIC ULCERS (ADULTS)

Gastroduodenal ulcers were first identified as a cause of abdominal pain in foals, and more recently gastric ulcers have been documented in adults. Although affected individuals are often asymptomatic, ulcers may be a cause of colic in both young and older horses. The etiology is unknown but is thought to be related to physiologic stress, high grain:low pasture diets and/or the administration of NSAIDs.

In adults, ulcers cause signs ranging from severe acute pain to chronic intermittent low-grade colic, poor appetite, and poor body condition. Most commonly gastric ulcers in adults involve the squamous epithelial mucosa adjacent to the margo plicatus. Ulcers may be implicated as the cause if signs of colic develop after eating. Affected individuals may roll or may remain standing and continually paw. The diagnosis is confirmed on the finding of ulcers on gastroendoscopy (after feed is withheld for 18 hours) and lack of other abnormalities affecting the gastrointestinal tract, response to treatment with histamine type 2 (H_2)-receptor antagonists, and healing of ulcers with treatment.

Treatment

Clinical disease believed to be caused by ulcers responds to ranitidine (6.6 mg/kg PO q8h) or other H_2 or proton pump blockers within 24–72 hours, with an improvement in ulcer appearance in 75% of cases. *If there is no clinical response within 72 hours after H_2-receptor antagonist treatment at the recommended dose, suspect another cause for the pain.* Remove the individual from training and feed a safe feed most conducive to more persistent consumption (e.g., grass).

Prognosis

The prognosis for adults is good to excellent with treatment and removal from training.

GASTRIC ULCERS IN FOALS

Gastric ulcers are common in foals and may lead to pain, interference with nursing, and general loss of condition. Gastric ulceration is caused by disequilibrium between ulcerogenic and protective factors in the stomachs of foals. Many physiologic stress factors can lead to this imbalance, including a recent episode of diarrhea, (the highest risk factor), and the use of NSAIDs in the foal.

Diagnosis

Common Clinical Signs

- Grinding of teeth (bruxism)
- Excessive salivation (ptyalism)
- Rolling on the back, particularly after nursing

Ancillary Tests

The signs are so commonly characteristic of gastric ulceration that ancillary tests usually are not indicated. However, gastroscopy may be used to confirm a diagnosis of gastric ulceration. Older foals (>60 days) commonly have severe lesions on the lesser curvature (nonglandular portion) of the stomach. In younger foals or in those associated with NSAID administration, lesions can be more severe in the glandular area. **Occult fecal blood tests are not indicated, as a negative result does not rule out gastric ulceration.**

Treatment

- Administer either H_2-antagonists *or* proton-pump blockers, in combination with sucralfate, as follows. *In severe cases, it is best to administer initial therapy IV.*
  - □ **H_2-Antagonists**
    Famotidine: 0.5–1.0 mg/kg IV q24h, or 3–4 mg/kg PO q24h
    Ranitidine: 1.5 mg/kg IV q8h, or 6.6 mg/kg PO q8h
    Cimetidine: 6.6 mg/kg IV or 12–20 mg/kg PO q8h

☐ There should be a response to H$_2$-antagonist therapy in 3–5 days. If not, other possibilities include duodenal stricture (especially in older foals) and inadequate therapy.

☐ **Proton-pump blocker**

Omeprazole: 0.5 mg/kg IV q24h, followed by 1–4 mg/kg PO q24h. (Its granular nature can make it more difficult to administer; a gel formulation may soon be available.)

☐ **Sucralfate**

1–2 gm (or 2–4 gm in large foals) PO q6h. **This may not be effective for nonglandular ulcers.** NOTE: Because sucralfate is in gel form and decreases absorption of concurrently administered drugs, do not administer at the same time as oral H$_2$-antagonists. Administer simultaneously with IV H$_2$-blockers.

- Pain may be managed with xylazine, detomidine, or butorphanol. Do not use NSAIDs as they may promote gastric ulceration. If repeated doses of xylazine, detomidine, or butorphanol fail to diminish pain, an antacid "cocktail" (approximately 0.5 liters of Pepto-Bismol/Mylanta mixed with 0.5 liters of warm water, 100 ml of Maalox-TC liquid, and 1 cup activated charcoal) may provide immediate relief from pain. This should be administered via a soft nasogastric tube after sedation.

- Supportive therapy must be initiated to correct/diminish (as much as possible) the predisposing factors. For example, if the foal has diarrhea, fluid therapy would likely be indicated. If there is clinical evidence of severe gastroesophageal reflux (marked salivation and/or obvious distention of the esophagus) or the esophagus is noted on gastroscopic examination to be severely eroded, bethanechol, 0.03 mg/kg SC q8h, should be administered until the signs improve.

- Misoprostol: 4 μg/kg PO q12h should be administered if gastric ulcers are believed caused by NSAIDs.

Prognosis

If the predisposing cause can be corrected and the foal responds to treatment within 3–5 days, the prognosis is good for a return to full function. Duodenal stricture is a serious complication that would prevent a favorable prognosis. **Perforations may occur, although most are seen without noticeable characteristic signs of gastric ulceration.**

Prevention

Minimize the risk factors. Treat diarrhea promptly and minimize the use of NSAIDs (especially if the foal is dehydrated). Administer prophylactic treatment to moderately or severely ill foals or stressed foals (those receiving frequent treatments) with oral sucralfate and/or an acid inhibitor drug. There is a general impression among equine neonatologists that sucralfate is effective in preventing ulcers in stressed foals, although this has not been documented.

NOTE: If the history or condition of the foal suggests that the problem may not be acute, pass a nasogastric tube after sedation. If there is a large amount of gastric reflux, the foal should undergo further diagnostic testing (barium radiographs) to rule out duodenal stricture.

DUODENAL OR GASTRIC PERFORATION

Usually occurs in foals younger than 8 weeks old. Risk factors include the use of NSAIDs and stresses on the foal, including diarrhea. Many cases occur with minimal warning signs of gastric ulceration.

Diagnosis

Common Clinical Signs

Foals are often found acutely depressed and/or colicky with a tight abdomen, increased heart and respiratory rates, and a high fever but may continue to nurse. Often diarrhea accompanies duodenal perforations, either present before the perforation or as a consequence of the endotoxemia.

Ancillary Tests

- Ultrasound—large amounts of flocculent fluid are seen.
- Abdominocentesis—to confirm septic peritonitis

Treatment

Euthanasia except for those cases with a small leak that may upon exploratory surgery be found to be sealed by the omentum.

Prevention

NSAIDs generally should not be administered to young foals, **especially foals with diarrhea**. If a NSAID has been administered to a foal, initiate treatment with H_2-antagonists. Do not rely on sucralfate alone to prevent ulcers if NSAIDs are being used.

E. DISORDERS OF THE SMALL INTESTINE CAUSING COLIC

P. O. Eric Mueller and James Moore

INTUSSUSCEPTION

Small intestinal intussusception usually occurs in younger horses and involves an invagination of a segment of bowel (**intussusceptum**) and mesentery into the lumen of an adjacent distal segment of bowel (**intussuscipiens**). Continued peristalsis draws more bowel and its mesentery into the intussuscipiens, causing venous congestion, edema, infarction and necrosis of the involved segment; small intestinal obstruction and strangulation result.

Intussusception results from alterations in intestinal motility. Predisposing factors:

- Enteritis
- Maladjustment of septic foals in intensive care units
- Abrupt dietary changes
- Heavy ascarid *(Parascaris equorum)* or tapeworm *(Anoplocephala perfoliata)* infestation
- Anthelmintic treatment
- Intestinal anastomosis

In most cases, no specific factor is identified. Jejunojejunal and jejunoileal intussusceptions are more common in foals, whereas ileocecal intussusceptions are more common in adults.

Diagnosis

- Clinical signs of jejunojejunal and ileocecal intussusception vary with the degree and duration of the condition.
- Most commonly, intussusception leads to complete intestinal obstruction and strangulation of the intussusceptum, causing an acute onset of unrelenting abdominal pain.
- Nasogastric reflux develops, and progressive dehydration and hypovolemia rapidly follow.
- Rectal examination reveals loops of distended small intestine, and occasionally the intussusception may be palpated. With an ileocecal intussusception, a turgid segment of bowel may be palpable within the cecum.
- Increased peritoneal protein concentration and nucleated cell count reflect devitalization of the affected bowel. Changes in the peritoneal fluid, however, may not accurately reflect the degree of intestinal compromise owing to isolation of the devitalized intussusceptum within the intussuscipiens.
- In foals, the intussusception is usually identified using ultrasound.

Chronic ileocecal intussusception with partial obstruction causes intermittent or continual abdominal pain, weight loss, poor general physical condition and varying degrees of anorexia and depression. This may continue for weeks to months, but eventually leads to an acute episode of severe abdominal pain corresponding to a complete obstruction of the intestine.

Treatment

Initial therapy is supportive:

- Gastric decompression
- Balanced polyionic IV fluids (e.g., lactated Ringer's solution)
- Analgesics (e.g., xylazine ± butorphanol tartrate or flunixin meglumine)
- Monitoring of physiologic and clinical parameters (pain, nasogastric reflux, heart rate (HR), mucous membranes, hematocrit (HCT), PCV/TPP, borborygmi)
- Surgical exploration is indicated if an intussusception is suspected.

Exploratory surgery includes:

- Ventral midline exploratory celiotomy
- Manual reduction of the intussusception
- Resection and anastomosis of the affected intestine

Some intussusceptions cannot be reduced due to length of bowel involved, venous congestion, and edema; these require en bloc resection and anastomosis. Even if the intestinal segment appears viable, consider resection and anastomosis because of the possibility of mucosal necrosis, serosal inflammation, and postoperative adhesion formation.

Prognosis

With early diagnosis and surgical repair, prognosis is good. If the intussusception is advanced and irreducible, prognosis is poor due to the likelihood of ileus, peritonitis, and postoperative adhesion formation.

VOLVULUS

A volvulus is the rotation of a segment of intestine around the long axis of its mesentery. Although most cases are not accompanied by a predisposing lesion, adhesions, infarctions, intestinal incarcerations, pedunculated lipomas, and meso-diverticular bands can predispose to volvulus. Abrupt dietary changes and verminous arteritis have also been implicated. The length and segment of the intestine involved are variable; the ileum is frequently involved because of its fixed attachment at the ileocecal junction.

Diagnosis

- Acute onset of progressive, moderate to severe, continuous pain that may initially respond to analgesics. Analgesic effectiveness rapidly decreases as the disease progresses.
- Rapid, progressive cardiovascular deterioration occurs as evidenced by poor peripheral perfusion (rapid, weak pulse, hyperemic or cyanotic mucous membranes, and a prolonged CRT).
- Hypovolemia and hemoconcentration develop rapidly.
- **Nasogastric reflux is often present, but in contrast to simple obstructions, decompression may not provide pain relief.**
- Rectal examination usually reveals moderate to severe small intestinal distention, and occasionally a tight mesenteric root. Mild tension on the mesentery may elicit a pain response.
- Lack of palpable small intestinal distention *does not rule out* the possibility of a strangulating lesion, because the distended intestine may be beyond the reach of the examiner.
- Abdominocentesis may yield normal or serosanguineous fluid with increased peritoneal protein concentration (> 3.0 gm/dl) and nucleated cell count ($>10,000$ cells/μl). The devitalized portion of intestine may be isolated from the peritoneal cavity (e.g., within the omental bursa), and the peritoneal fluid analysis, therefore, may not accurately reflect the degree of intestinal change.
- Abdominal ultrasound reveals dilated nonmotile small intestine.

Treatment

Initial therapy is supportive:

- Gastric decompression
- Balanced polyionic IV fluids (e.g., lactated Ringer's solution) with plasma
- Analgesics (e.g., xylazine ± butorphanol tartrate or flunixin meglumine)
- Monitoring of physiologic and clinical parameters (pain, nasogastric reflux, HR, mucous membranes, HCT, PCV/TPP, borborygmi)
- Surgical exploration is indicated if a volvulus is suspected.

Exploratory surgery includes:

- Ventral midline exploratory celiotomy
- Identification of the strangulated portion of intestine
- Determining the direction of rotation of the affected segment by palpation of the mesentery
- After correction, evaluate intestinal viability and perform resection and anastomosis if needed

Prognosis

Prognosis depends on the duration of illness and amount of intestine involved in the volvulus—good with early detection and rapid treatment. In patients with long-standing strangulation, postoperative peritonitis, ileus, and adhesion formation are common sequelae. When resection of greater than 50% of the small intestine is needed, there is a high incidence of postoperative complications (malabsorption, weight loss, and liver damage).

HERNIATION

Herniation of the small intestine is classified as internal or external. **Internal hernias** occur within the abdominal cavity and do not involve a hernial sac. Examples are displacement of the small intestine through the epiploic foramen, mesenteric defects, and rents in the gastrosplenic and broad ligaments. **External** hernias extend outside the limits of the abdominal cavity and include inguinal, umbilical, ventral abdominal, and diaphragmatic hernias.

Epiploic Foramen Herniation

The epiploic foramen is a potential opening, approximately 4 to 6 cm in length, that separates the omental bursa from the peritoneal cavity. It is bounded dorsally by the caudate lobe of the liver and caudal vena cava, and ventrally by the right lobe of the pancreas and portal vein. Cranially, it is limited by the hepatoduodenal ligament and caudally by the junction of the pancreas and mesoduodenum. Adults (> 8 years) are predisposed to epiploic foramen entrapment due to enlargement of this space by atrophy of the right caudate lobe of the liver. Herniation through the foramen may occur as a right to left (from the lateral side) or as a left to right (from the medial side) displacement.

Diagnosis

- An acute onset of moderate to severe pain that may initially be responsive to analgesics. The effectiveness of analgesics decreases as the disease progresses.
- Rapid cardiovascular deterioration occurs, with hypovolemia and hemoconcentration developing rapidly.
- Nasogastric reflux is present, but decompression may not provide pain relief.
- Rectal examination reveals moderate to severe small intestinal distention.
- Some individuals may exhibit mild signs of pain with no nasogastric reflux or palpable intestinal distension. The lack of palpable small intestinal distention does not rule out a strangulating lesion, because the distended intestine may be beyond the reach of the examiner. Ultrasound generally reveals distended nonmotile bowel.
- In these patients, abdominocentesis is useful in determining the severity of the lesion and the need for surgical intervention. Peritoneal fluid analysis may reveal normal or serosanguineous fluid with increased protein concentration (>3.0 gm/dl) and nucleated cell count ($>10,000$ cells/μl). The devitalized portion of intestine within the omental bursa may be isolated from the rest of the peritoneal cavity, and, therefore, fluid obtained via abdominocentesis may not accurately reflect the severity of intestinal compromise.

Treatment

Initial therapy is supportive:

- Gastric decompression
- Balanced polyionic IV fluids (e.g., lactated Ringer's solution)
- Analgesics (e.g., xylazine $\pm$ butorphanol tartrate or flunixin meglumine)
- Monitoring of physiologic and clinical parameters (pain, nasogastric reflux, HR, mucous membranes, HCT, PCV/TPP, borborygmi)
- Surgical intervention if epiploic entrapment is suspected

Exploratory surgery is frequently needed to confirm the diagnosis and includes:

- Ventral midline exploratory celiotomy
- Decompression of the bowel, careful manual dilation of the foramen, and reduction of the hernia
- Trauma during dilation of the foramen can result in life-threatening rupture of the caudal vena cava or portal vein.
- Evaluate intestinal viability and perform resection and anastomosis if necessary.

Prognosis

Depends on the duration of illness, the length of intestine requiring resection, and difficulty encountered reducing the hernia.

Gastrosplenic Ligament Incarceration

Incarceration of the small intestine through the gastrosplenic ligament is uncommon. Anatomically, the ligament attaches the greater curvature of the stomach to the hilus of the spleen and continues ventrally with the greater omentum. Defects in the ligament are generally acquired secondary to trauma. The distal jejunum and ileum are most commonly involved, with herniation occurring in a caudal to cranial direction.

Diagnosis

Clinical signs are similar to those for patients with epiploic foramen herniation:

- Acute onset of severe abdominal pain, positive nasogastric reflux, small intestinal distention on rectal examination, and rapid systemic deterioration
- Distended small intestine may not be palpable early in the disease due to the cranial location in the abdomen.
- Abdominocentesis may yield normal to serosanguineous fluid, with an increased total protein and nucleated cell count. Severity of the signs depends on the location, duration, and extent of the lesion.
- Exploratory celiotomy is frequently needed for a definitive diagnosis.

Treatment

Initial therapy is supportive:

- Gastric decompression
- Balanced polyionic IV fluids (e.g., lactated Ringer's solution)
- Analgesics (e.g., xylazine ± butorphanol tartrate or flunixin meglumine)
- Monitoring of physiologic and clinical parameters (pain, nasogastric reflux, HR, mucous membranes, HCT, PCV/TPP, borborygmi)
- Surgical intervention if a strangulating obstruction is suspected

Exploratory surgery:

- Ventral midline exploratory celiotomy
- Reduction of the hernia
- The ligament is relatively avascular and digital enlargement of the rent facilitates reduction of the incarceration with minimal risk of life-threatening hemorrhage.
- Resection and anastomosis of devitalized bowel
- The defect in the ligament is not closed.

Prognosis

Depends on the duration of illness and length of intestine resected (see Epiploic foramen herniation).

Mesenteric Defects

Defects or rents in the mesentery, broad ligaments, or greater omentum provide a potential space for intestinal incarceration or strangulation. Mesenteric defects most often occur in the small intestinal mesentery and less commonly in the large and small colon mesentery. Defects commonly are acquired as a result of blunt abdominal trauma or surgical manipulation of bowel and mesentery. A segment of intestine may pass through the defect, becoming incarcerated or strangulated. A mesodiverticular band, a congenital remnant of a vitelline artery and its associated mesentery, extends from one side of the mesentery to the antimesenteric border of the jejunum or ileum and is a common site for incarceration. This tissue normally atrophies during the first trimester; failure to atrophy results in formation of a triangulated mesenteric sac. A loop of intestine may become incarcerated in the sac, leading to mesenteric rupture and resulting herniation and strangulation.

Diagnosis

Clinical signs are similar to those for patients with a volvulus:

- Acute onset of abdominal pain
- Nasogastric reflux with small intestinal distention on rectal examination
- Systemic cardiovascular deterioration
- Abdominocentesis reveals normal to serosanguineous fluid with increased protein concentration and nucleated cell count. Severity of the signs depends on the location, duration, and severity of the lesion.

Treatment

Initial therapy is supportive:

- Gastric decompression
- Balanced polyionic IV fluids (e.g., lactated Ringer's solution)
- Analgesics (e.g., xylazine ± butorphanol tartrate or flunixin meglumine)
- Monitoring of physiologic and clinical parameters (pain, nasogastric reflux, HR, mucous membranes, HCT, PCV/TPP, borborygmi)
- Surgical intervention if a strangulating obstruction is suspected

Exploratory surgery is needed for definitive diagnosis and includes:

- Ventral midline exploratory celiotomy
- Reduction of the hernia
- The hernial ring may require manual dilation to reduce the hernia.
- Closure of the mesenteric defect
- Resection and anastomosis of devitalized bowel
- Defects near the root of the mesentery are difficult to close due to limited exposure.

Prognosis

Depends on the duration of illness and the length of intestine needing resection. The prognosis is poor if difficulty is encountered reducing the hernia and closing the defect.

Inguinal Hernia

Acquired inguinal hernias in stallions are associated with breeding or strenuous exercise and cause acute onset of abdominal pain. A sudden increase in intra-abdominal pressure or an enlarged internal inguinal ring may predispose to an inguinal hernia. Inguinal hernias are commonly unilateral and occur frequently in Standardbred, Saddlebred and Tennessee Walking horses. Inguinal herniation and evisceration occur as a sequela to castration.

Congenital inguinal hernias in foals usually close spontaneously as the foal matures and only occasionally cause intestinal problems, e.g., if the hernia cannot be reduced or if it is very large. A scrotal herniation may require surgical correction when the bowel ruptures through the parietal tunic.

Diagnosis

Acquired inguinal and scrotal herniations in the stallion can produce acute intestinal obstruction requiring emergency surgical intervention. Incarcerated bowel is strangulated with hypovolemic and endotoxic shock following, causing systemic cardiovascular deterioration. The hernia is usually indirect and unilateral, with the incarcerated intestinal segment descending through the vaginal ring and contained within the tunica vaginalis.

Affected individuals demonstrate a rapid onset of moderate to severe abdominal pain. Palpation of the scrotum may reveal a firm, swollen, cold testicle on the affected side, but early scrotal swelling may be absent. A swollen and slightly turgid tail of the epididymis may be palpated in early cases owing to passive congestion. The loop of herniated small bowel may be palpable per rectum passing through the internal inguinal ring.

The signs of strangulating obstruction, tachycardia, dehydration, endotoxemia, and cardiovascular deterioration, develop with time. Abdominocentesis reveals fluid with an increased total protein and nucleated cell count. Peritoneal fluid analysis may not accurately reflect the severity of intestinal compromise owing to sequestration of fluid within the scrotum.

Herniation and rupture of the vaginal tunic in newborn foals may cause mild pain and depression, local edema, and subsequent abscessation.

Treatment

Initial therapy is supportive:

- Gastric decompression
- Balanced polyionic IV fluids (e.g., lactated Ringer's solution)
- Analgesics (e.g., xylazine ± butorphanol tartrate or flunixin meglumine)
- Monitoring of physiologic and clinical parameters (pain, nasogastric reflux, HR, mucous membranes, HCT, PCV/TPP, borborygmi)
- Surgical intervention is inguinal or scrotal herniation is suspected

Exploratory surgery:

- Ventral midline exploratory celiotomy
- An inguinal incision to achieve adequate surgical exposure and reduction
- Reduction and resection and anastomosis of the affected bowel
- Unilateral castration and inguinal herniorrhaphy usually required

Inguinal herniation in newborn colts may be contained in the vaginal tunic or may rupture through the tunic and lie subcutaneously; those within the vaginal tunic may be manually reduced and generally correct spontaneously. Those that rupture through the tunic or those that are very large and cannot be reduced require surgical repair through inguinal and scrotal incisions.

Prognosis

Good if reduction and repair are performed within hours of herniation, before strangulation ensues. The prognosis worsens with increasing duration before correction. The prognosis for breeding soundness is good if only one testicle is involved.

Diaphragmatic Hernia

Diaphragmatic hernia may be congenital or acquired and is an unusual cause of abdominal pain in horses. Most often it results from strenuous exercise, a hard fall, hitting something while running, or being hit by a car. Pregnant or periparturient mares are also at risk.

Diagnosis

Clinical signs seen with diaphragmatic hernia include abdominal pain, tachypnea, and dyspnea. The severity of signs depends on the size of the hernia opening and degree of visceral herniation. The presence of viscera within the thoracic cavity may reduce the intensity of lung sounds and cause dullness on percussion. Radiography or ultrasonography (Fig. 26–1) is helpful in diagnosing fluid or ingesta-filled loops of intestine in the thoracic cavity. Blood gases may indicate respiratory compromise and hypoxemia. *Thoracocentesis* and *abdominocentesis* may reveal blood-tinged fluid with an increased total protein and

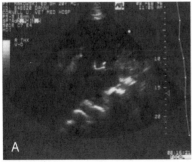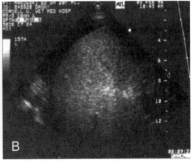

FIGURE 26–1. *A,* Ultrasound of the thorax of a 20-year-old gelding with mild pain, sternal edema, and thoracic effusion. The 5-mHz scan shows multiple loops of small intestine (white reflections) in the thoracic cavity and an unusually well-defined posterior vena cava. To the left of the screen is fluid and fibrin. *B,* Ultrasound from the same horse showing the liver in the thoracic cavity.

nucleated cell count, supporting the presence of devitalized bowel. An exploratory celiotomy is often necessary for a definitive diagnosis.

Treatment

Initial therapy is supportive:

- Gastric decompression
- Balanced polyionic IV fluids (e.g., lactated Ringer's solution)
- Analgesics (e.g., xylazine ± butorphanol tartrate or flunixin meglumine)
- Supplemental oxygen therapy (if necessary)
- Monitoring of physiologic and clinical parameters (pain, nasogastric reflux, HR, mucous membranes, HCT, PCV/TPP, borborygmi)

Exploratory surgery:

- Ventral midline exploratory celiotomy
- Reduction, resection, and anastomosis of the affected bowel
- Closure of the diaphragmatic defect by suturing or use of a synthetic mesh (Marlex, Proxplast)

Prognosis

Prognosis for surgical repair is guarded to poor because of difficult surgical exposure and a high incidence of postoperative complications, septic pleuritis, implant failure, and hernia recurrence. The prognosis is better in young individuals as a result of the improved surgical exposure.

PEDUNCULATED LIPOMA

A common cause of small intestinal strangulation or obstruction in horses > 10 years of age. Lipomas attach to the mesentery by a fibrovascular stalk of variable length. They are frequently incidental findings on exploratory surgery or necropsy; these masses have the potential to incarcerate a segment of small intestine and produce strangulating obstruction.

Diagnosis

Pedunculated lipomas should be considered in the differential diagnosis in individuals > 10 years of age demonstrating signs of small intestinal obstruction. Clinical signs:

- Acute abdominal pain
- Hemoconcentration
- Decreased borborygmi
- Nasogastric reflux usually present but may be absent early in the disease.
- Multiple loops of small intestine are palpable on rectal examination, and increases in peritoneal total protein concentration and nucleated cell count reflect the degree of intestinal compromise.

Treatment

Initial therapy is supportive:

- Gastric decompression
- Balanced polyionic IV fluids (e.g., lactated Ringer's solution)
- Analgesics (e.g., xylazine ± butorphanol tartrate or flunixin meglumine)
- Monitoring of physiologic and clinical parameters (pain, nasogastric reflux, HR, mucous membranes, HCT, PCV/TPP, borborygmi)
- Surgical intervention if a strangulating obstruction is suspected

Exploratory surgery:

- Ventral midline exploratory celiotomy
- Ligation and transection of lipoma
- Resection and anastomosis of the affected bowel
- Remove any lipomas found at surgery to minimize recurrence

Prognosis

Favorable with early diagnosis and prompt treatment. If devitalized bowel cannot be resected or if peritonitis is severe, the prognosis is guarded to poor.

ILEAL IMPACTION

The ileum is the most common site for small intestinal intraluminal impactions. Incidence varies with geographic location—more common in Europe and the southeastern United States. The etiology is unknown; an association with fine, high-roughage forage and coastal Bermuda hay has been implicated. Ingesta accumulates in the ileum, causing an obstruction. Spasmodic contraction and absorption of water from the ileal lumen worsen the impaction. Mesenteric vascular thrombotic disease, tapeworm infestation *(Anoplocephala perfoliata)*, and ascarid impaction *(Parascaris equorum)* are less common causes. Ileal hypertrophy should be considered in older horses with histories of chronic colic.

Diagnosis

Clinical signs are variable and depend on the duration of the impaction:

- Moderate to severe abdominal pain due to focal intestinal distention and spasmodic contraction around the impaction. Affected individuals usually respond transiently to analgesics.
- Rectal palpation reveals multiple loops of moderate to severely distended small intestine; early examination may reveal a 5–8-cm-diameter, firm, smooth-surfaced ileum originating at the cecal base and coursing from the right of the midline obliquely downward and to the left side.
- Nasogastric reflux may be absent in the early stages; during the 8–10 hours following the initial episode of colic, small intestinal and gastric distention develops, resulting in recurrence of signs of pain and progressive dehydration.
- Gastric decompression often provides temporary pain relief. Borborygmi become diminished or absent, and intestinal distention without motility is seen on ultrasound examination.

- CBC, electrolytes, blood gases, and abdominocentesis are frequently within normal limits.
- Hemoconcentration and increased total peritoneal protein and nucleated cell count may occur with long-standing impaction.

Treatment

Initial therapy is supportive:

- Gastric decompression
- Balanced polyionic IV fluids (e.g., lactated Ringer's solution)
- Analgesics (e.g., xylazine ± butorphanol tartrate or flunixin meglumine)
- Monitoring of physiologic and clinical parameters (pain, nasogastric reflux, HR, mucous membranes, PCV/TPP borborygmi)
- The impaction may resolve with medical therapy; more commonly surgical intervention is needed.

Exploratory surgery:

- Ventral midline exploratory celiotomy
- Reduction of the obstruction by extraluminal massage
- Mixing of the impaction with jejunal fluid or infusion of the impaction with sterile saline or sodium carboxymethylcellulose to facilitate reduction
- With marked mural edema and congestion, a jejunal enterotomy facilitates emptying of the ileal contents without excessive manipulation of the bowel.
- Resection and anastomosis (ileocecostomy or jejunocecostomy) may be needed if additional problems exist, e.g., ileal hypertrophy, mesenteric vascular thrombotic disease.

Prognosis

Good if no additional problems exist, e.g., ileal hypertrophy, and guarded if ileocecostomy or jejunocecostomy is needed because of postoperative ileus and the high incidence of intra-abdominal adhesions.

ASCARID IMPACTION

Heavy ascarid *(Parascaris equorum)* infestation can lead to intraluminal obstruction in foals, weanlings, and yearlings. Affected individuals have a history of a poor parasite control program leading to heavy infestation with ascarids. *Impaction commonly follows use of one of the highly effective anthelmintics, piperazine, pyrantel, or organophosphates*, or tranquilizers and/or general anesthetics. Ivermectin, although highly effective, has a relatively slow onset of action and therefore is not commonly implicated in the development of ascarid impactions. Intestinal rupture, peritonitis, and intussusception are potential sequelae. Foals develop an immunity to the parasite by 6 months to 1 year of age. Consequently, this condition is uncommon in adults.

Diagnosis

Clinical signs depend on the duration and degree of small intestinal obstruction and include unthriftiness, poor hair coat, and mild to severe abdominal pain. Nasogastric reflux is usually present and may contain ascarids. Rectal examination reveals multiple loops of distended small bowel. The diagnosis is based on signalment, history, and signs consistent with small intestinal obstruction.

Treatment

Partial obstruction of the intestine with ascarids may be treated medically with:

- Intestinal lubricants, e.g., mineral oil
- Balanced polyionic IV fluids (e.g., lactated Ringer's solution)
- Analgesics (e.g., xylazine ± butorphanol tartrate or flunixin meglumine)
- Low-efficacy or slow-onset anthelmintics (fenbendazole, ivermectin) are preferred to prevent further recurrence.

Ventral midline exploratory surgery is needed to relieve the obstruction:

- With complete obstruction, or if medical therapy is unsuccessful.
- Multiple enterotomies may be needed to remove the ascarids.

Prognosis

Good if medical treatment is successful, and guarded if surgery and multiple enterotomies are performed because of the high incidence of intra-abdominal adhesions.

DUODENITIS/PROXIMAL JEJUNITIS

Characterized by transmural inflammation, edema, and hemorrhage in the duodenum and proximal jejunum. The stomach and proximal small intestine are moderately distended with fluid, whereas the distal jejunum and ileum are usually flaccid. Histologic lesions include hyperemia and edema of the mucosa and submucosa, villous epithelial degeneration and sloughing, neutrophil infiltration, hemorrhage in the muscular layer, and fibrinopurulent exudation on the serosa. The cause of this extensive intestinal damage is unknown; *Clostridium perfringens* is a presumed etiologic agent and frequently can be cultured from the gastric reflux.

Proximal small intestinal distention, gastric reflux, dehydration, and hypovolemic and endotoxic shock result from the intestinal damage. The inflammation and damage may alter intestinal motility, causing adynamic ileus.

Diagnosis

Clinical signs:

- Acute abdominal pain
- *Large volumes of nasogastric reflux fluid* (red to greenish-brown)
- Absent borborygmi
- Tachycardia

- Dehydration
- Slight increase in body temperature (38.6° to 39.1°C)
- Hyperemic mucous membranes
- Increased HCT
- Moderate to severe small intestinal distention on rectal examination. However, early in the disease, small intestinal distension may be absent.
- Distended proximal small intestine with thickened wall and mild to moderate motility on ultrasound examination

Clinical laboratory findings:

- Increased PCV and total plasma protein (hemoconcentration)
- Increased creatinine concentration indicating prerenal or renal azotemia
- Increased peritoneal total protein concentration
- Mild to moderate increase in nucleated cell count (5000 to 25,000 cells/μl)
- Hypokalemia
- Sometimes metabolic acidosis
- CBC may reveal a normal, increased (neutrophilia due to inflammation), or decreased (neutropenia and left shift due to endotoxemia and consumption) WBC count.
- Gram stain of the gastric reflux shows a large number of large gram-positive rods (Fig. 26–2).

The clinical findings can be confused with strangulating or nonstrangulating obstruction. **After nasogastric decompression, the abdominal pain usually decreases, being replaced by depression in patients with duodenitis/proximal jejunitis.** Abdominal pain with serosanguineous abdominal fluid is supportive of a strangulating obstruction, but serosanguineous abdominal fluid may be seen with proximal enteritis.

Treatment

- Voluminous gastrointestinal reflux is produced for 1–7 days, requiring gastric decompression through an indwelling nasogastric tube every 2 hours to prevent distention, pain, and gastric rupture.
- Food and oral medication are withheld until small intestinal borborygmi return.
- IV administration of a balanced crystalloid solution to maintain intravascular fluid volume

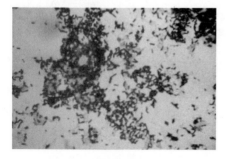

FIGURE 26–2. Gram stain of gastric fluid from a horse with proximal duodenitis-jejunitis that demonstrates many large gram-positive rods (compatible with *Clostridium perfringens*).

- Monitor blood gases and serum electrolytes (Na^+, K^+, CL^-, HCO_3^-, Ca^{+2}) daily and adjust the IV solution to correct any deficiencies.
- Low-dose flunixin meglumine, 0.25 mg/kg IV q8h, to reduce the adverse effects of arachidonic acid metabolites (thromboxane A_2 and prostaglandins)
- Antiserum (Endoserum) directed against gram-negative core antigens (endotoxin) administered IV diluted in a balanced electrolyte solution; hyperimmune plasma directed against the J-5 mutant strain of *E. coli* (Polymune-J or Foalimmune), or normal *equine plasma* (2–10 L) administered IV *slowly* may be equally beneficial, supplying protein, fibronectin, complement, antithrombin III, and other inhibitors of hypercoagulability.
- Heparin 100 u/kg SQ q12h may decrease the incidence of laminitis.
- A 10% dimethyl sulfoxide (DMSO) solution can be administered IV (100 mg/kg q8h or q12h).
- Na^+ or K^+ penicillin (22,000–44,000 IU/kg IV q6h) or procaine penicillin (22,000–44,000 IU/kg IM q12h) for *Clostridium perfringens*, as the proposed etiologic pathogen
- Motility modifiers may be useful in reducing gastric reflux and may decrease the cost of treatment and complications associated with frequent passage of the nasogastric tube.
- Recommendations: lidocaine 2%, slow IV bolus, 1.3 mg/kg (approximately 20 ml/450-kg adult) followed by 0.05 mg/kg/min infusion
- And/or cisapride, 0.1–0.2 mg/kg IV q8h; 0.3 mg/kg PO q8h
- Monitor serum creatinine concentration and urine output after fluid therapy because secondary renal failure is common.
- Laminitis is a common complication. The feet should be monitored and treatment incorporated in the medical therapy, including:
  - □ Heavily bedded stall with shavings or sand
  - □ Remove shoes, trim and balance feet, apply frog supports (lily pads).
  - □ Lower limb support bandages
  - □ Phenylbutazone (2.2–4.4 mg/kg PO or IV q12h)
  - □ Acepromazine (0.02 mg/kg IM q8h) (for its vasodilatory properties)
  - □ Nitroglycerin cream, 1″ strip q24h over palmar (posterior) digital arteries
- With prolonged (>7 days) nasogastric reflux, bowel decompression or intestinal bypass via a standing right flank laparotomy or ventral midline celiotomy may be used to augment medical therapy.

Prognosis

With aggressive medical management, the disease resolves in most cases. Sequelae that adversely affect the prognosis include laminitis, renal failure, intraabdominal adhesion formation, pharyngeal or esophogeal injury, and gastric rupture. Individuals with a red gastric reflux appear to be more prone to complications.

NONSTRANGULATING INFARCTION

The disease involves infarction (necrosis due to loss of blood supply) of the intestine without a strangulating lesion. Commonly, postmortem examination reveals the cause to be thrombus formation at the cranial mesenteric artery from damage by migration of fourth and fifth stages of *Strongylus vulgaris* larvae. It is hypothesized that infarction is the result of hypoxia induced by vasospasm.

Diagnosis

A poor parasite control program may predispose individuals to nonstrangulating ischemia and/or infarction. The disease also occurs in individuals regularly treated with anthelmintics. Clinical signs of variable severity range from depression to moderately severe abdominal pain:

- Heart rate, respiratory rate, and body temperature may be normal or increased, with hyperemic mucous membranes suggesting endotoxemia or inflammation due to migrating parasites.
- Rectal examination findings may be normal or include distended small intestine.
- Pain, fremitus, or thickening is commonly evident on palpation of the mesenteric root.
- Auscultation of the abdomen may reveal normal, increased, or decreased borborygmi.
- Gastric reflux may be present due to functional obstruction of the intestinal segment.
- PCV, total plasma protein, and creatinine may be increased secondary to dehydration.
- Peripheral blood examination may reveal a normal, decreased (neutropenia with a left shift due to endotoxemia), or increased (neutrophilia due to inflammation) WBC count.
- Total plasma protein may be increased owing to the chronic inflammation caused by parasites or decreased as a result of protein loss through damaged intestinal mucosa.
- Abdominal fluid is normal or contains increased total protein (>3.0 mg/dl) and WBC count up to 200,000 cells/μl.

Treatment

- Balanced crystalloid IV fluids to correct dehydration and enhance reperfusion of the affected intestinal segments
- Maintain gastric decompression.
- Broad-spectrum antimicrobial drugs (K^+ penicillin, 22,000 IU/kg IV q6h and gentamicin, 2.2 mg/kg IV q8h or 6.6 mg/kg IV q24h, if peritonitis present)
- Flunixin meglumine, 0.25 mg/kg IV q8h, to reduce thromboxane production and increase mesenteric perfusion
- 10% dimethyl sulfoxide solution, 100 mg/kg IV q8–12h to decrease superoxide radical injury during reperfusion
- Aspirin (20 mg/kg PO every other day) and heparin (40–100 IU/kg IV or SQ q6–12h) for thrombosis. Monitor the HCT closely for RBC agglutination and decreasing HCT secondary to heparin administration.
- Exploratory surgery in patients nonresponsive to medical therapy

Prognosis

The prognosis is poor in patients requiring surgery for intestinal resection. Ischemia not obvious at the time of exploratory surgery may progress to infarction. Ileus and adhesions are common postoperative complications. Large segments of intestinal involvement may be too extensive for resection. Identification and resection of affected small or large intestinal segments is sometimes successful using fluorescein dye, Doppler ultrasound, or surface oximetry to determine intestinal viability.

F. DISORDERS OF THE LARGE INTESTINE CAUSING COLIC

P. O. Eric Mueller and James N. Moore

CECAL IMPACTION

Frequently, inflammatory bowel conditions also predispose the colon (especially the small colon) to impactions and may be associated with positive *Salmonella* sp. fecal cultures. In many cases, a predisposing factor is never identified.

Cecal impaction occurs secondary to other diseases, especially those associated with endotoxemia, surgery, or chronic pain, due to septic metritis, infectious arthritis, fractures, and corneal disease.

Diagnosis

Clinical findings:

- Anorexia
- Reduced fecal output
- Mild to severe abdominal pain
- **NOTE: Occasionally there are few prodromal signs, e.g., only slight depression.**
- Abdominal distention may be present but is often absent. With severe impaction, abdominal auscultation reveals a right-sided "cecal ping."
- Heart rate varies with the severity of pain, and mucous membranes are usually pink and tacky.
- Nasogastric reflux is unusual unless cecal dysfunction results in ileus of the small intestine.
- PCV, plasma protein, and creatinine levels are increased secondary to dehydration. In cases of cecal perforation, peritoneal total protein concentration and nucleated cell count are increased.

Diagnosis is confirmed on rectal examination; the ventral cecal taenia is tight and displaced ventral and medial. Dry ingesta is palpable in the body and base of the cecum, with moderate amounts of gas filling the base. The cecal distention may make the dorsal and medial cecal taenia readily palpable and the left colon and small colon empty.

Treatment

Medical management for individuals with mild to moderate cecal impaction:

- Nothing PO except water if negative gastric reflux
- Administer three times the daily maintenance requirement of fluid (balanced crystalloid solutions with 20 mEq/L KCl) IV and oral water to rehydrate the impaction: 6–8 L of water/500 kg q2h through an indwelling nasogastric tube.
- Laxatives to facilitate rehydration of impacted material (see Disorders of the Large and Small Intestine, Treatment)
- Reintroduce feed, slowly to avoid recurrence.
- Feed grass, water-soaked pellets, and bran mashes for the first 24–48 hours.

Surgical management is recommended for:

- Uncontrollable pain
- Very severe impactions (extremely tight medial cecal band)
- Unsuccessful medical therapy
- Characteristics of peritoneal fluid suggesting cecal compromise
- The surgical options via ventral midline celiotomy include:
    - ☐ Extraluminal massage
    - ☐ Typhlotomy and evacuation
    - ☐ Partial or complete typhlectomy
    - ☐ Cecocolic anastomosis
    - ☐ Ileocolic anastomosis
    - ☐ Jejunocolic anastomosis
- Jejunocolic or ileocolic anastomosis is considered superior to cecocolic anastomosis because it has fewer long-term sequelae. Complete typhlectomy through a right paralumbar laparotomy is difficult, and fecal contamination of the abdomen a problem.

Prognosis

For patients with mild to moderate cecal impaction without underlying cecal dysfunction, good. Severe cecal impactions requiring surgical treatment are complicated by peritonitis, adhesions, perforation, and death; prognosis with severe impaction is guarded.

CECAL PERFORATION

Site is generally the medial or caudal surface of the base due to excessive tension on the cecal wall as a result of severe impaction. Perforation is also associated with late gestation and parturition; the pathogenesis remains unknown, with tapeworm *(A. perfoliata)* infestation being implicated.

Diagnosis

Signs of cardiovascular shock secondary to septic peritonitis. The rate of deterioration is directly related to the degree of peritoneal contamination. Rectal examination reveals enlargement of the cecum with emphysema and roughening of the serosa of the cecal base. The peritoneal fluid, obtained via teat cannula, has an increased or decreased nucleated cell count and increased total protein concentration, with degenerative white cells and intracellular and extracellular bacteria, and plant material.

Treatment

Treatment is symptomatic only:

- Balanced, polyionic, IV fluids
- Broad-spectrum antimicrobials
- Flunixin meglumine

Prognosis

Poor; grave if fecal contamination occurs, due to septic peritonitis and endotoxic shock.

LARGE COLON IMPACTION

Occurs at two sites of narrowing, the pelvic flexure and transverse colon, where retropulsive contractions (propagation in an oral direction) retain ingesta for microbial digestion. These contractile patterns may contribute to impactions. Predisposing factors:

- Poor dentition
- Ingestion of coarse roughage
- Inadequate fluid intake
- Stress associated with transportation
- Intense exercise resulting in hypomotility
- Inadequate water intake
- Excessive fluid loss through sweating

Diagnosis

Clinical findings:

- Anorexia
- Abdominal distention
- Decreased fecal output
- Mild, initially intermittent to severe abdominal pain
- Heart rate varies with the degree of pain, and mucous membranes are pink and tacky.
- Nasogastric reflux uncommon unless ileus of the small intestine or compression of loops of small intestine occurs
- Packed cell volume, total plasma protein, and creatinine increased when clinical dehydration present
- With complete luminal obstruction, marked abdominal distention
- Rectal examination reveals impacted ingesta with varying degrees of distention of the pelvic flexure and ventral colon, and in severe cases, the colon is palpable in the pelvic canal.
- Impactions in the transverse colon are not palpable.

In chronic, severe cases, distention of the colonic wall may cause pressure necrosis of the bowel wall and peritonitis. The peritoneal fluid total protein and nucleated cell count reflect intestinal compromise. Abdominal pain is usually severe and unrelenting, and signs of toxemia (hyperemic and/or cyanotic mucous membranes), tachycardia, and tachypnea are apparent.

Treatment

- Withhold food to prevent continued accumulation of ingesta.
- Allow access to water if there is no nasogastric reflux.
- Medical management:
  - □ Patients with mild impactions respond to administration of water and mineral oil or magnesium sulfate (preferred) and electrolytes via nasogastric tube.
  - □ IV fluids (4–5 L/hr/450 kg) and laxative therapy are needed for moderate to severe colon impactions.
  - □ Analgesics as needed
- Surgical decision based on:
  - □ Unsuccessful medical management
  - □ Unrelenting abdominal pain
  - □ Rectal examination reveals large colon displacement.
  - □ Endotoxemia, cardiovascular deterioration
  - □ Changes in peritoneal fluid indicating intestinal compromise
- Ventral midline exploratory celiotomy:
  - □ Extent of impaction
  - □ Other abnormalities: colon displacement, enterolith(s)
  - □ Pelvic flexure enterotomy
  - □ Lavage lumen of colon to evacuate ingesta.

Prognosis

For medical management of mild to moderately severe large colon impactions, good. For surgical correction of severe impaction, fair to good unless necrosis of the intestinal wall or colonic devitalization results in intestinal perforation.

SAND IMPACTION

Ingestion of sand while grazing or eating hay on closely grazed pastures in areas with sandy soil may result in sand impaction. The ingested sand settles in the large colon where it accumulates and eventually results in a nonstrangulating obstruction.

Diagnosis

Clinical signs:

- Similar to those for large colon impaction; the signs of pain are frequently acute.
- Auscultation of the cranial ventral abdomen, when performed for 4–5 minutes, may reveal a sound similar to an ocean wave.

- Sand may be palpated on rectal examination and found in feces placed in water; the ingesta floats in water and the sand settles to the bottom of the container.
- The impaction is commonly palpable on rectal examination in the pelvic flexure or cecum, whereas impactions in the right dorsal (most common) or transverse colon are not palpable.
- Abdominocentesis, if performed, should be done with **extreme caution** to avoid enterocentesis due to the location of the sand-filled colon on the ventral abdominal floor.
- The sand's irritating effect on the colonic mucosa can cause diarrhea.
- Under the weight of the sand, degeneration and necrosis of the bowel wall may result in endotoxemia and peritonitis.

Treatment

- Medical management:
  - Frequently responds to early administration of fluids and laxatives (mineral oil)
  - Psyllium hydrophilic mucilloid (Metamucil) is the most effective laxative: 400 gm/500 kg q6h until the impaction resolves. Once in contact with cold water, the mucilloid forms a gel that can be difficult to pump through a nasogastric tube; therefore, the tube must be in place and the mixture administered immediately. The gel lubricates and binds with the sand, moving it distally and relieving the obstruction.
  - Continue psyllium treatment at 400 gm/500 kg once a day for 7 days to remove residual sand. Alternating psyllium and mineral oil may prevent obstruction associated with retrograde movement of sand and psyllium.
- Surgical management:
  - Ventral midline exploratory celiotomy in patients that fail to respond to medical treatment or have other abnormalities, e.g., colon displacement
  - Remove sand through a pelvic flexure enterotomy.
  - Sand can cause extensive damage to the colon wall: postoperative ileus, bowel wall degeneration, peritonitis
- Preventive management:
  - Do not overgraze pastures.
  - Hay supplement when needed and do not feed on the ground
  - Add psyllium treatment prophylactically to feed to remove sand from the colon.
  - Psyllium, 400 gm/500 kg, once a day for 7 days, is recommended for preventive treatment every 4–12 months, depending on sand exposure.
  - Flavored or soluble psyllium may be more palatable than nonflavored forms.

Prognosis

Medical prognosis for patients with mild to moderately severe sand impaction is good. Surgical prognosis for a severe sand impaction is good unless necrosis or devitalization of the intestinal wall results in rupture of the colon.

CECOCOLIC INTUSSUSCEPTION

An unusual cause of intestinal obstruction, resulting from invagination of the apex of the cecum through the cecocolic orifice into the right ventral colon. The entire cecum may invaginate into the colon and become strangulated. Etiology is unknown, although conditions causing aberrant intestinal motility, such as parasites, diet changes, impaction, mural lesions, and motility-altering drugs, have been implicated. Cecocolic intussusception is more common in individuals < 3 years of age.

Diagnosis

Patients with strangulating intussusception may present with signs of acute, severe abdominal pain. In contrast, affected individuals with chronic nonstrangulating intussusception may have mild to moderate abdominal pain, depression, weight loss, and scant, soft feces. The intussusception is frequently palpable per rectum as a large mass in the right caudal abdomen; if the ileum is involved, distended small intestine is palpable. A firm mass palpable in the cecal base and/ or the right ventral colon is confirmatory. Abdominocentesis reveals increases in peritoneal total protein and nucleated cell count; these changes may not be evident until late in the disease because the cecum is sequestered within the ventral colon. Failure to respond to medical therapy leads to exploratory surgery and a definitive diagnosis.

Treatment

- Ventral midline exploratory celiotomy
- Reducing the intussusception is difficult because of mural edema and adhesions between the serosal surfaces.
- If extraluminal reduction is successful, cecal viability is assessed, and if required, complete or partial typhlectomy performed.
- Reduction and resection of the devitalized portion of cecum, may be performed through an enterotomy in the right ventral colon if extraluminal reduction is impossible.

Prognosis

If the apex of the cecum is involved and extraluminal reduction is possible, prognosis is fair. If reduction requires an enterotomy or the entire cecum is involved, prognosis is poor because of the risk of septic peritonitis.

LARGE COLON DISPLACEMENTS

The left ventral and dorsal colons are freely movable, allowing for intestinal displacement and volvulus. The cause is unknown; alterations in colonic motility, excessive gas production, rolling secondary to abdominal pain, dietary changes, excessive concentrate intake, grazing lush pastures, and parasites have been implicated. Generally, no etiologic factor is identified.

Right dorsal displacement of the colon is a displacement of the left colon lateral to the cecum, lying between the cecum and the right body wall. Commonly, the pelvic flexure moves lateral to the cecum, in a cranial to caudal direction, and rests at the sternum. Displacement may be accompanied by a variable degree of volvulus.

Left dorsal displacement of the colon is a displacement of the left colon to a position between the dorsal body wall and the nephrosplenic (renosplenic) ligament. It is unknown whether the colon passes through the nephrosplenic space from a cranial to caudal direction or migrates dorsally, lateral to the spleen.

Diagnosis

Clinical signs:

- Abdominal pain and abdominal distention, the severity of which depend on the duration and amount of colonic tympany. The signs generally develop rapidly and are more severe than with impaction because of tension on the mesentery and greater colonic tympany.
- The displacement may place pressure on the duodenum, causing nasogastric reflux.
- Peritoneal fluid is usually normal in the early stages of displacement, with increases in peritoneal total protein and nucleated cell count in chronic displacements.

A **right dorsal displacement,** on rectal palpation, is characterized by mild to severe gas distention of the cecum and/or colon with large colon taeniae palpable lateral to the cecum or horizontally crossing the pelvic inlet.

A **left dorsal displacement,** on rectal palpation, is characterized by mild to severe gas distention of the cecum and/or colon, with large colon taeniae palpable coursing cranial and to the left, dorsal to the nephrosplenic ligament; signs of pain are elicited when the nephrosplenic area is palpated; and the spleen is rotated caudally, away from the left body wall due to tension on the ligament. Several loops of moderately distended small intestine may be palpable if it is secondarily involved. Decompression of the stomach and cecum provides temporary pain relief.

Treatment

Right dorsal displacement is corrected by:

- Ventral midline exploratory celiotomy
- Examining the colon for volvulus and correcting the displacement

Enterotomy is unnecessary unless the colon is secondarily impacted.

Left dorsal displacement—nonsurgical correction (Figure 26–3):

- General anesthesia with the patient positioned in right lateral recumbency; hobbles are placed on the hindlimbs, and the patient is positioned in dorsal recumbency.
- The hindlimbs are lifted to raise the hind end of the patient off the ground; the abdomen is vigorously balloted.
- The large colon falls cranially and to the right.
- The patient is then rolled 360 degrees back to right lateral recumbency and allowed to recover.

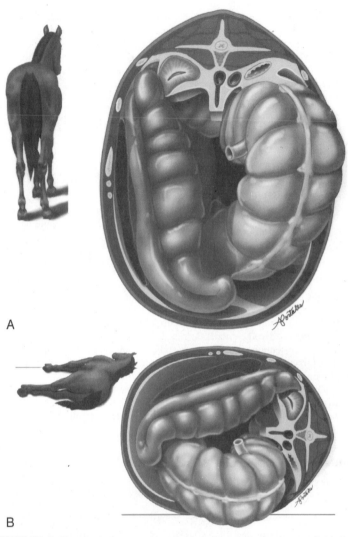

FIGURE 26–3. Nonsurgical correction of a left dorsal displacement of the large colon. *A,* Caudal view of the standing horse with the left ventral and dorsal colons entrapped over the nephrosplenic ligament. *B,* The horse is anesthetized and placed in right lateral recumbency.

- Rectal palpation is performed to assess the position of the colon with the patient in lateral recumbency or after recovery.
- If unsuccessful, the procedure may be repeated several times; it is reported to be 70% to 90% successful in patients with a stable cardiovascular system and without severe colonic distention or devitalization.

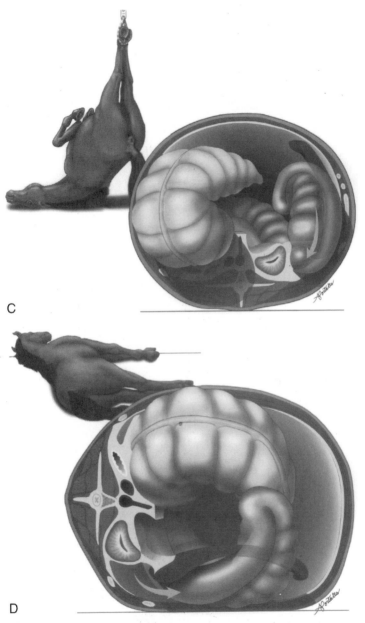

C

D

FIGURE 26–3 *Continued. C,* Hobbles are placed on the hind limbs and the patient is positioned in dorsal recumbency; the hind limbs are lifted to raise the hind end off the ground; the large colon falls cranially, lateral, and to the right *(arrow). D,* The patient is then positioned in left lateral recumbency; this allows the colon to continue to fall ventral and lateral to the spleen *(arrow).*

Illustration continued on following page

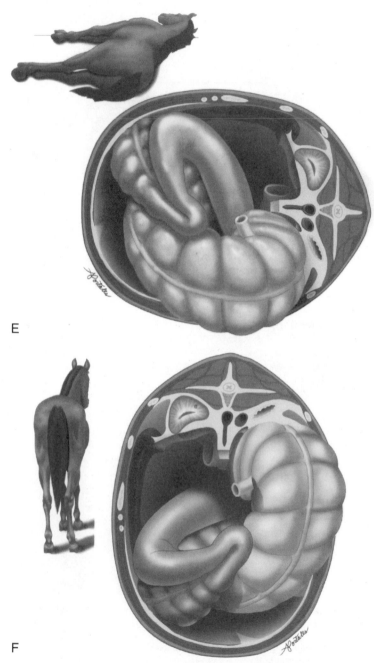

E

F

FIGURE 26–3 *Continued. See legend on opposite page*

■ An additional nonsurgical method is to administer phenylephrine, 4–8 mg/450–kg adult slowly IV to contract the spleen, followed by light exercise for 5–10 minutes; re-examine rectally. NOTE: Do not use in severely volume-depleted or cardiovascularly unstable patient.

Potential complications of nonsurgical correction (rolling) include:

■ Worsening or recurrence of the displacement
■ Iatrogenic colonic or cecal volvulus
■ Cecal or colonic rupture

Left dorsal displacement—surgical correction is performed when:

■ Colonic distention is severe.
■ Evidence of intestinal devitalization on peritoneal fluid analysis
■ Increased risk of colonic or cecal rupture and resulting fatal peritonitis

2

Prognosis

For complete recovery, good to excellent. Incidence of adhesions and laminitis with large colon displacements is low.

LARGE COLON VOLVULUS

This is a rotation of the ventral and dorsal colons on their long axes and frequently includes the cecum. Viewing the horse in dorsal recumbency, the colon usually twists in a counterclockwise direction (Figure 26–4). The large colon and cecum can rotate on the vertical axis of the mesentery (volvulus). Rotations of 360° cause the colon to lie in an apparently normal position with the mesenteric root occluded. Large colon volvulus is one of the **most severe** and **fatal** acute abdominal emergencies in horses. The etiology is unknown, but hypomotility secondary to dietary changes, electrolyte imbalances, and stress may predispose the colon to excessive gas accumulation and volvulus. There is a **higher incidence of colon volvulus** in **periparturient mares.** Large colon volvulus recurs in 20% to 30% of colic cases.

Diagnosis

■ Colonic volvulus (>180°) causes an acute onset of *severe* abdominal distention and continuous abdominal pain only mildly responsive or refractory to analgesic therapy. Xylazine or detomidine alone or in combination with butorphanol provides transient pain relief.
■ Tachycardia, tachypnea, and blanched or congested mucous membranes are usually present.

FIGURE 26–3 *Continued. E*, The 360° rotation is then completed by rolling the patient into sternal recumbency (not shown) and then back to right lateral recumbency, with the colon coming to rest in a position medial to the spleen. *F*, The patient is allowed to recover; if the procedure is successful, the colon assumes a position ventral and medial to the spleen. Rectal palpation is performed to assess the position of the colon.

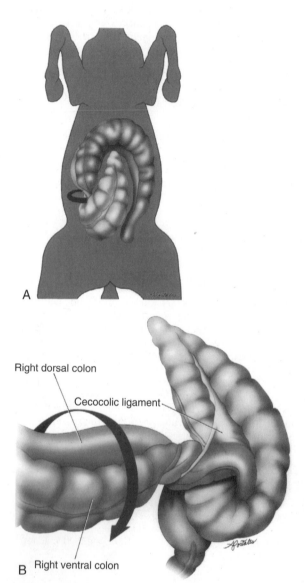

FIGURE 26–4. Large colon volvulus. *A*, ventral view of a horse in dorsal recumbency with a 360° counterclockwise (arrow) volvulus of the large colon. *B*, Right lateral view of a horse in dorsal recumbency with an 180° counterclockwise *(arrow)* volvulus of the large colon.

- Respiratory acidosis may develop if colonic distention impairs normal respiratory function.
- Serosanguineous peritoneal fluid with an increased total protein concentration and nucleated cell count reflect intestinal ischemia and necrosis.
- Rectal palpation reveals severe colonic distention, frequently accompanied by mural and mesenteric edema secondary to venous congestion. Taeniae may be palpable traversing the abdomen, **but a complete rectal examination is frequently impossible because of the marked colonic distention.**
- Rotations (twists) ≤180° may present with moderate pain only and a slow deterioration.

Treatment

Successful treatment requires an **early diagnosis** and **emergency surgical correction.**

- Ventral midline exploratory celiotomy
- Decompression and enterotomy often necessary to facilitate correction
- Affected bowel typically appears blue-gray initially and becomes red to black after reperfusion.
- Nonviable colon requires resection or humane destruction of the individual.
- 95% of the ascending colon may be resected without adversely affecting colonic function.
- Plasma, DMSO, and heparin may be useful in attenuating "reperfusion injury."

Prevention of Recurrence

Colopexy, or suturing the lateral taenia of the left colon to the abdominal wall, is performed by some surgeons to reduce the incidence of recurrence. Tearing of the adhesion, suture failure, and colon rupture are reported complications. Elective colon resection is also performed to minimize recurrence; this procedure is preferred for performance athletes.

Prognosis

Depends on early diagnosis and surgical intervention. Intestinal ischemia and necrosis rapidly progress to hypovolemia, endotoxemia, peritonitis, and irreversible shock. Therefore, the prognosis is poor unless surgery is performed within a few hours of onset of clinical signs. In some patients, postoperative absorptive dysfunction, diarrhea, and protein-losing enteropathy occur, which may be short lived or permanent.

ATRESIA COLI

This congenital absence or closure of a portion of the intestine presents in three forms:

1. Membrane atresia—a tissue diaphragm occludes the bowel lumen
2. Cord atresia—a fibrous cord connects the noncommunicating ends of the bowel
3. Blind-end atresia—the *most common type*, in which there is no connection or mesentery between the noncommunicating ends of bowel.

Atresia coli results from ischemia of the affected segment during development; the condition is believed to be a hereditary condition. **Lethal white foal disease** is an autosomal recessive pigmentary disorder in which newborn paint foals demonstrate albinism coupled with congenital defects of the intestinal tract, most commonly atresia coli. These defects are not compatible with life.

Diagnosis

Abdominal pain in the newborn during the first 12 to 24 hours of life and lack of meconium stool are the first signs. Digital palpation of the rectum reveals mucus and no meconium. Abdominal radiography may reveal an enlarged segment of colon with no obvious obstruction; contrast radiography is needed to confirm the diagnosis. Abdominal distention and pain are indications for surgical exploration. A meconium impaction is the primary rule out (see Disorders of the Small Colon and Rectum).

Treatment

Surgical correction is the only treatment:

- Ventral midline exploratory celiotomy
- The distance and size disparity between the affected bowel segments make anastomosis difficult.
- The aboral segment is often too small for an end-to-end anastomosis; a side-to-side anastomosis may be required but is often not possible due to the excessive distance between the proximal and distal intestinal segments, thereby necessitating euthanasia.

Prognosis

Guarded owing to the difficult technical aspects of performing the anastomosis in this part of the intestine.

NONSTRANGULATING INFARCTION

See this topic under Disorders of the Small Intestine.

ULCERATIVE COLITIS (NSAID Toxicity)

See Chapter 39.

G. DISORDERS OF THE SMALL COLON AND RECTUM

P. O. Eric Mueller and James N. Moore

SMALL COLON IMPACTION AND FOREIGN BODY OBSTRUCTION

Caused by dehydration of fecal matter, or by a foreign body or enterolith (see Enterolithiasis). If complete, abdominal pain is severe. Tympany and secondary ileus of the proximal small and large colons occur secondarily to the obstruction. The diagnosis is confirmed by palpating the impaction or gas-distended loops of small colon on rectal examination. The small colon is identified by its characteristic single wide band on its antimesenteric side.

Foreign body impactions occur more commonly in younger horses (< 4 years old), because they are curious, e.g., eat portions of hay nets, rubber fencing, bits of rope, and string. **Small colon impactions are very common in miniature horses.** They are frequently accompanied by inflammatory bowel diseases, e.g., salmonellosis.

Treatment

Medical treatment:

- Analgesics
- Large volumes of balanced, polyionic intravenous fluids
- 6–8 L of water q2h through an indwelling nasogastric tube if no gastric reflux
- Warm water enemas to soften the fecal material. **CAUTION:** *Use extreme care to prevent rectal perforation.*

Surgical treatment:

- Needed with unrelenting pain, severe gas distention, or failure of medical treatment
- Ventral midline exploratory celiotomy
- Enemas and extraluminal massage of the small colon to break down the impaction
- Enterotomy to remove a foreign body or enterolith(s)
- Pelvic flexure enterotomy and evacuation of large colon ingesta
- Patients with small colon impactions frequently culture positive for *Salmonella* sp.; these individuals may become toxic with secondary laminitis, peritonitis, and adhesions. Role of *Salmonella* sp. in development of the impaction is unknown.

Prognosis

Fair to good for individuals with foreign body obstructions or simple impactions of the small colon, and guarded if a positive culture for *Salmonella* sp. is identified. **Rectal examination of horses with small colon impactions presents a greater risk of perforation.**

ENTEROLITHIASIS

Enteroliths are concretions of magnesium and ammonium phosphate crystals deposited around a nidus, frequently a piece of wire, stone, or nail. May be single or multiple and do not cause a clinical problem until they become lodged in the transverse or small colon. The *specific geographic distribution* of the condition (California, Florida, Indiana) has led to speculation that undetermined constituents of the soil and water in these areas may be inciting causes. Enterolithiasis is most commonly seen in middle-aged individuals (5–10 years of age), with the condition being over-represented in Arabians and miniature horses.

Diagnosis

- Affected individuals may have a history of *chronic weight loss* and recurring acute bouts of mild to moderate abdominal pain *or* acute, severe abdominal distention and pain with no previous history of colic.
- The obstruction most commonly is at the proximal small colon or transverse colon; smaller enteroliths are located distally in the small colon. When the obstruction is complete, pain is severe and distention of the colon is marked.
- Heart and respiratory rates are increased, with pink mucous membranes.
- Rectal examination reveals colonic and cecal distention.
- Peritoneal fluid is generally normal unless the wall of the colon is compromised.
- *Abdominal radiography* may confirm the diagnosis of enterolithiasis, but in the field this can be performed only in miniature horses.
- Patients with chronic enterolithiasis often have gastric ulcers, which may confound the diagnosis.

Treatment

- Central midline exploratory celiotomy
- Decompression of the distended colon and cecum
- Small, freely movable enteroliths are removed through a pelvic flexure enterotomy.
- Large enteroliths in the transverse colon and proximal small colon are removed through a large colon enterotomy at the diaphragmatic flexure.
- If an enterolith has a *polyhedral* shape, multiple enteroliths are present.

Prognosis

Good, with survival rates of 65% to 90%.

MECONIUM IMPACTION

A common cause of acute pain in newborn foals is retention of meconium in the small colon and rectum. It occurs more frequently in males, weak newborns after a dystocia, and foals >340 days of gestation.

Clinical signs:

- Acute abdominal pain during the first 24 hours after foaling
- Tachycardia
- Repeated attempts to defecate
- Rolling
- Abnormal stance
- Swishing the tail
- Abdominal tympany if obstruction of the small colon is complete (Fig. 26–5).

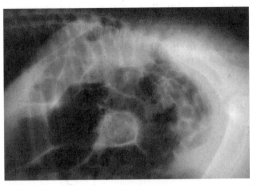

FIGURE 26–5. Radiograph of the abdomen of a 2-day-old foal with meconium impaction of the colon causing severe gaseous distention. Surgery was required to correct the problem.

The foal appears transiently normal for short periods and nurses. The diagnosis is often confirmed by digital palpation of meconium impaction in the distal small colon and rectum.

Treatment

- Soapy warm water enemas delivered by gravity flow through a soft rubber tube
- Intravenous, balanced polyionic fluids
- Mineral oil
- Sedatives as needed
- Ventral midline exploratory celiotomy in refractory individuals and for those with proximal impactions (see Fig. 26–5), using enemas and extra-luminal massage of the affected colon
- Small colon enterotomy rarely necessary

NOTE: *Repeated enemas and/or enemas with caustic solutions results in rectal edema and irritation* and a syndrome that mimics meconium impaction. Foals receiving several enemas often become very toxic.

Prognosis

Excellent.

MESOCOLIC RUPTURE

A condition affecting mares during parturition, resulting in tearing of the mesentery of the small colon and complicated by prolapse of the rectum, bladder, uterus, vagina, and/or small intestine. Multiparous mares > 11 years old are at greatest risk.

Clinical signs of abdominal pain develop during the first 24 hours postpartum and are complicated by intra-abdominal hemorrhage and peritonitis. The mare's clinical condition deteriorates rapidly if the blood supply to the small colon is compromised or the intestine is entrapped in the mesocolic rent. Rectal examination reveals impaction or tympany of the small colon.

Treatment

- Ventral midline exploratory celiotomy
- Resection and anastomosis of the affected small colon
- Colostomy if the tear involves the mesorectum

Prognosis

Poor due to ischemia of the small colon, difficult surgical exposure, and complications associated with the colostomy, e.g., prolapse of the proximal small colon through the colostomy stoma and adhesions.

RECTAL TEARS

A complication of performing a rectal examination is the risk of a rectal tear, and the incidence is highest in young, nervous, anxious individuals; older horses with a weakened rectal wall, e.g., small colon impactions; and patients that strain during rectal examination. There is a higher incidence in Arabians, presumably due to their size; stallions and geldings are at greater risk than mares. The tears occur at the 10–12 o'clock position, 25–30 cm from the anus. The tear is longitudinal and hypothesized to occur where blood vessels penetrate the intestinal wall.

Rectal tears are classified as:

Grade I: mucosa or submucosa
Grade II: muscular layer only
Grade III: mucosa, submucosa, and muscular layers without serosal penetration, including mesorectum
Grade IV: tears involving all layers and extending into the peritoneal cavity

NOTE: Grades III and IV are life-threatening, with cellulitis, abscessation, and acute septic peritonitis as sequelae. The diagnosis is confirmed by careful examination of the tear after the patient is sedated and the rectum evacuated. Intraluminal lidocaine gel or epidural anesthesia facilitates rectal examination.

Treatment

- Immediately begin broad-spectrum antimicrobials.
- IV, balanced polyionic fluids
- NSAIDs
- **Grade I** tears are treated conservatively unless the tear can be easily sutured using 2–0 or 0 polydioxanone (PDS, Ethilcon, Somerville, NJ) in a simple continuous pattern. These tears heal with minimal to no complications.
- **Grade II** tears, because of the lack of frank blood in the lumen of the rectum, frequently are not diagnosed at the time of injury; they are identified weeks later when a perirectal fistula or abscess develops.

- **Grade 3 or 4 tears** require
  □ Atropine to reduce peristalsis
  □ Packing of the rectal lumen from the anus to cranial to the tear
  □ A colostomy to divert feces from the site and prevent peritoneal contamination. NOTE: Grade 4 tears necessitate a colostomy; in grade 3 tears a colostomy is recommended (Fig. 26–6).
  □ A loop colostomy is performed under general anesthesia or sedation and local anesthesia, with the colostomy exiting through the left flank.
  □ Alternatively, the proximal end of the distal small colon is oversewn and the distal end of the proximal small colon exits from the flank as a diverting colostomy.
  □ If the patient is placed under general anesthesia, a large colon enterotomy is performed to reduce fecal bulk exiting from the colostomy.
  □ A rectal liner (Rectal Ring, Regal Plastic Co., Detroit Lakes, MN) is used in grade III tears to bypass the tear and obviate the need for a colostomy.
  □ Grades III and IV tears heal by second intention; the loop colostomy is reversed after the tear heals.

Prognosis

Excellent for grades I and II rectal tears, guarded for grade III tears, and guarded to poor for grade IV tears.

RECTAL PROLAPSE

Caused by straining secondary to constipation, obstipation, dystocia, colitis, urethral obstruction, or foreign body impaction of the distal small colon and/or rectum. In some cases no known predisposing cause can be identified. The condition occurs more commonly in mares and is classified based on severity:

- **Type I** prolapse involves only the rectal mucosal and submucosa and appears as a large circular anal swelling.
- **Type II** involves the entire rectal wall and is called a "complete" prolapse; the ventral portion of prolapsed tissue is thicker than the dorsal portion.
- **Type III** includes invaginated peritoneal rectum and/or small colon and is difficult to distinguish from a type II prolapse.
- **Type IV** involves intussuscepted peritoneal rectum or small colon beyond the anus, with a palpable invagination adjacent to the intussuscepted intestine, distinguishing it from a type III prolapse.

Treatment

Type I or type II prolapse:

- Reduce the edema in the tissues with topical application of glycerin or dextrose and apply Vasoline.
- Reduce the prolapse under epidural anesthesia.
- Tranquilize unless contraindicated
- Place a purse-string suture in the anus.

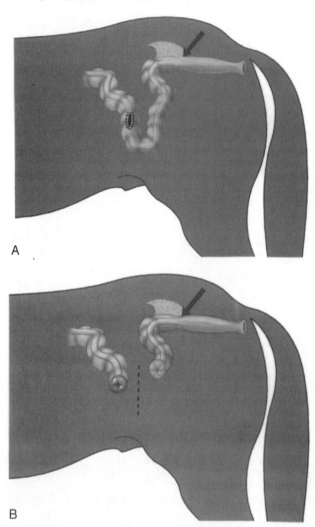

FIGURE 26–6. Colostomy techniques. *A*, Diagram of a loop colostomy and *B*, a diverting colostomy positioned in the left flank. The location of the rectal tear is depicted by the arrows. The loop colostomy is performed at the initial flank incision. The diverting colostomy is performed in a separate incision, cranial to the initial flank incision *(dotted line)*.

- Stool softeners, e.g., mineral oil
- Submucosal resection if medical treatment is unsuccessful
- Type III or IV requires a celiotomy to reduce the intussusception.
- A colostomy is necessary for Type IV due to compromise of the blood supply to the affected bowel.

Prognosis

Types I and II prolapse, good; guarded to poor for types III and IV.

H. Colic in the Late-Term Pregnant Mare

P. O. Eric Mueller and James N. Moore

Colic in the mare during the last trimester of pregnancy is often a diagnostic challenge. GI disorders must be ruled out by careful clinical examination, but the large, gravid uterus often precludes a complete rectal examination. The effect of the colic episode on the fetus is always of concern, because abortions can result in substantial emotional and financial loss. The overall postcolic abortion rate of mares is between 16% and 18%. Endotoxemia and intraoperative hypoxia or hypotension during colic surgery in the last 60 days of gestation has been associated with a higher incidence of abortion. Causes of colic in late-term pregnant mares not associated with the gastrointestinal tract include:

- Abortion/premature parturition
- Uterine torsion
- Hydroallantois
- Ruptured prepubic tendon

Pregnant mares with colic and endotoxemia during the first 2 months of pregnancy may benefit from treatment with progestin supplementation, Alternogest 22–44 mg PO q24h for 450 kg adult or injectable progesterone 150–300 mg/450 kg adult IM q24h for 100–200 days of pregnancy. The adverse effects of chronic endotoxemia in late pregnancy may be inhibited by administering NSAIDs.

ABORTION/PREMATURE PARTURITION

Mares may present with signs of mild to moderate abdominal pain, with minimal udder development. Vaginal examination reveals loss of the cervical plug and relaxation of the cervix. This finding alone does not indicate impending abortion as similar findings occur in many normal mares days or weeks before delivery. Rectal examination often reveals the fetus to be positioned within the birth canal.

Treatment

Treatment is supportive and directed at an uncomplicated delivery and postpartum care of the mare. Postmortem examination of the aborted fetuses and placenta may determine the cause of the abortion, e.g., equine herpesvirus 1; isolate the mare until the examination results are available.

UTERINE TORSION

Consider uterine torsion a possible cause of colic in late-term pregnant mares. It usually occurs from 8 months of gestation to term. Unlike cows, in which the torsion is most often diagnosed at term, mares affected near term are usually not in labor when clinical signs are first evident. Also unlike the cow, torsion usually occurs cranial to the cervix and vagina, thereby minimizing the benefit of a vaginal examination in making the diagnosis. The degree of torsion ranges from 180° to 540° and occurs in either direction with equal frequency. Uterine rupture can occur secondary to torsion and is an uncommon complication.

Diagnosis

Mild to moderate intermittent abdominal pain is the most consistent sign; however, some mares may demonstrate severe, unrelenting pain. A mild increase in heart and respiratory rates may also be present. Diagnosis is made by signalment, history, and rectal examination findings. Rectal palpation of the broad ligaments reveals them to be tight as they cross the caudal abdomen, below and above the cervix. Palpation of the dorsal most ligament, and occasionally the body of the uterus, indicates the direction of the torsion. In a *clockwise torsion*, as viewed from behind, the *left broad ligament is pulled tight over the uterus, coursing to the right, in a horizontal to oblique direction.* For a counterclockwise torsion, the opposite is true.

Treatment

Early recognition and intervention are essential for a successful outcome for both the mare and foal. The optimal method of correction depends on the condition of the mare and fetus and the stage of gestation.

Nonsurgical Correction—Rolling

See Fig. 32–2, p. 417.

Surgical Correction—Preferred

FLANK CELIOTOMY

Provides the *least stress* for the foal and mare; can be performed during any stage of gestation.

- Performed in the standing mare under sedation (xylazine or detomidine ± butorphanol) and local anesthetic infiltration along the proposed incision site
- Controversy exists as to the preferred side of entry relative to the direction of the torsion. Many prefer to enter the abdomen from the side to which the torsion is directed (e.g., right flank for a clockwise torsion).
- If the abdomen is entered from the side to which the torsion is directed, the surgeon's hand is passed ventrally to the uterus, and the uterus is lifted and rotated upward to correct the torsion.
- If the abdomen is entered on the side opposite that to which the torsion is directed (e.g., right flank for a counterclockwise torsion), the surgeon's hand is passed dorsally to the uterus, and the uterus is pulled toward the surgeon to correct the torsion.
- Correction may be facilitated by grasping the limbs of the fetus through

the wall of the uterus and *gently* "rocking" the uterus to gain sufficient momentum for complete rotation and final correction.

VENTRAL MIDLINE CELIOTOMY

This approach provides the best exposure for assessment and manipulation of the gravid uterus. Indications for ventral midline celiotomy include *uterine rupture, uterine tearing, and uterine devitalization.* This approach also allows for identification and correction of concurrent intestinal disorders. It can be performed during any stage of gestation.

- A standard ventral midline celiotomy
- If hysterotomy is indicated, the ventral midline approach provides the best surgical exposure.
- Ventral midline celiotomy *should be reserved for cases not amenable to nonsurgical correction or flank celiotomy* because of the associated risks of general anesthesia to the mare and foal.

Prognosis

Good to excellent for complete recovery and future breeding soundness of the mare with uterine torsion. Fetal viability depends on the duration and degree of torsion. Abortion rates following uterine torsion have been reported between 30% and 40%.

UTERINE RUPTURE (also see p. 418)

May result as a complication of manipulation during dystocia or during an apparently normal foaling; may also be a sequela to *uterine torsion* or *hydroallantois.* The tear usually occurs at the dorsal aspect of the uterus.

Diagnosis and Treatment

Suspect uterine rupture in any mare demonstrating postpartum abdominal pain. Large ruptures may result in significant blood loss and produce signs of hemorrhagic shock. Diagnosis is confirmed on vaginal and uterine examination. **If a uterine tear is suspected, irrigating solutions should not be infused into the uterus.**

- Broad-spectrum antimicrobials
- Balanced, polyionic intravenous fluids
- Plasma and/or synthetic colloids
- NSAIDs
- Peritoneal drainage
- Allow small tears to heal by second intention; close larger tears primarily, which requires general anesthesia and ventral midline celiotomy.

Prognosis

Depends on the size of the tear, duration before recognition and treatment, degree of peritoneal contamination, and nature of the intrauterine contents. Good for small tears recognized early and poor for large tears with an emphysematous fetus and gross peritoneal contamination.

HYDROALLANTOIS

See p. 419.

RUPTURED PREPUBIC TENDON

The prepubic tendon is a strong, thick, fibrous structure that attaches to the cranial border of the pelvis and provides attachment for the rectus abdominis, oblique abdominis, gracilis, and pectineus muscles. It forms the medial borders of the external inguinal rings. Hydroallantois, twins, or fetal giants may predispose to prepubic tendon rupture.

Diagnosis

Must be differentiated from a ventral hernia, both of which occur most frequently in late-term pregnant mares. Ventral hernias may respond favorably to surgical repair, in contrast to prepubic tendon rupture for which the prognosis is poor.

Clinical signs:

- Severe, progressive, ventral abdominal swelling and edema, with the *pelvis tilted cranially and ventrally. The mammary gland also assumes a more cranioventral position.*
- Mild to moderate abdominal pain is usually evident, and the *mare is reluctant to walk.* In contrast, mares with a *ventral hernia are not reluctant to walk, and the pelvis and mammary gland are in a normal position.*
- Identification of the defect by external palpation may be difficult due to the excessive edema formation.
- *Rectal examination and ultrasonography* are helpful in differentiating prepubic tendon rupture from ventral herniation.

Treatment

- In mares near term, early induction of parturition and *assisted foaling* may be required.
- An *exploratory celiotomy* ± a cesarean section should be performed immediately in mares that demonstrate intractable pain or systemic deterioration, or in which a concurrent incarcerating intestinal lesion is suspected.
- Stabilized mares should be confined to stall rest, placed in abdominal support bandages, and administered NSAIDs.
- A *low bulk, pelleted feed* should be fed to decrease the volume of ingesta.
- These mares may foal normally; however, they should be *observed closely* and assisted with foaling if necessary.

Prognosis

Stabilized mares not in pain may successfully raise a foal but should not be used for breeding. Prognosis for long-term survival is poor.

I. PERITONITIS

P. O. Eric Mueller and James N. Moore

Peritonitis, an inflammation of the peritoneal cavity, is classified according to origin, primary versus secondary; onset, peracute, acute, or chronic; extent of involvement, diffuse versus localized; and presence of bacteria, septic versus nonseptic. It is generally acute, diffuse, and secondary to gastrointestinal compromise or infectious disease. Severity depends on the etiologic agent, virulence of the organisms, host defenses, extent and site of involvement, recognition of problems, and treatment. Generally the aboral sites, cecum to small colon, contain more bacteria and anaerobes and therefore are associated with more severe disease. The organisms frequently cultured are enteric aerobes *(Escherichia coli, Actinobacillus* sp., *Streptococcus equi* or *S. zooepidemicus, Rhodococcus),* and anaerobes *(Bacteroides, Peptostreptococcus, Clostridium,* and rarely *Fusobacterium).*

Causes

- Idiopathic
- Perforation of the gastrointestinal or genitourinary tract
- Infectious disease
- Trauma
- Iatrogenic after abdominal surgery

Diagnosis

Clinical signs depend on the etiology, extent, and duration of disease. *Local* peritonitis has minimal systemic signs; *diffuse* peritonitis has signs of endotoxemia and septicemia, abdominal pain, pyrexia, anorexia, weight loss, and diarrhea.

Peracute peritonitis due to intestinal rupture causes severe signs of endotoxemia, depression, and rapid cardiovascular deterioration; severe abdominal pain, sweating, muscle fasciculations, tachycardia, red to purple mucous membranes with increased capillary refill time; dehydration; and depression.

In acute diffuse peritonitis, death occurs in 4–24 hours after the primary insult. Fever and abdominal pain may not be seen and depend on the stage of endotoxic shock. Ileus and gastric reflux may develop secondary to peritoneal and serosal inflammation. The rectal examination may be normal or reveal dry, emphysematous, "gritty" serosa and peritoneum and distended large and small intestine secondary to ileus.

Affected individuals with localized, subacute to chronic peritonitis present with signs of depression, anorexia, weight loss, intermittent fever, ventral edema, intermittent abdominal pain, and mild dehydration.

Clinical laboratory findings:

- Increased PCV
- Increased (hemoconcentration) or decreased (protein loss into the peritoneal cavity) total plasma protein concentration
- Hyperfibrinogenemia
- Increased creatinine concentration—prerenal or renal azotemia
- Metabolic acidosis

With severe endotoxemia, CBC reveals:

- Marked leukopenia—neutropenia and left shift due to endotoxemia and consumption in peracute and acute peritonitis
- Leukocytosis—neutrophilia due to inflammation and hyperfibrinogenemia in chronic peritonitis

Collect peritoneal fluid in an EDTA tube for cytology, total protein, and WBC determination. Collect samples for bacterial culture in a sterile tube. Peritoneal fluid analysis reveals:

- Increased total protein concentration and nucleated cell count—20,000–400,000 cells/μl
- Cytology—free or phagocytized bacteria in leukocytes
- Gram stain for initial evaluation and selection of antimicrobial agents while awaiting culture and susceptibility results

Treatment

Prompt and aggressive treatment is needed:

- Treatment of the primary disease
- Pain relief
- Reversal of endotoxic and hypovolemic shock
- Correction of metabolic and electrolyte abnormalities
- Correction of dehydration
- Correction of hypoproteinemia
- Broad-spectrum antimicrobial therapy
- Intravenous administration of a balanced electrolyte solution to maintain intravascular fluid volume
- Hypertonic saline (7% NaCl, 1 to 2 L IV) improves systemic blood pressure and cardiac output. Hypertonic saline administered initially must be followed by adequate fluid replacement with a balanced crystalloid solution.
- A total plasma protein concentration of ≤4.5 gm/dl requires administration of plasma, 2 to 10 L IV slowly, to maintain plasma oncotic pressure and minimize pulmonary edema during rehydration with IV fluids.
- Antiserum (Endoserum) against gram-negative core antigens (endotoxin) IV, diluted in a balanced electrolyte solution. Hyperimmune plasma directed against the J-5 mutant strain of *E. coli* (Polymune-J, Foalimmune) or normal *equine plasma* (2–10 L) administered IV, *slowly*, may be equally beneficial, supplying protein, fibronectin, complement, antithrombin III, and other inhibitors of hypercoagulability.
- Flunixin meglumine, 0.66–1.1 mg/kg IV q12h, or low-dose, 0.25 mg/kg IV q8h, to reduce the adverse effects of arachidonic acid metabolites.

These drugs should be used with *caution* in hypovolemic, hypoproteinemic patients to avoid gastrointestinal and renal toxicities.
- Monitor blood gas and serum electrolytes and correct deficiencies.
- Start antimicrobial therapy immediately after a peritoneal fluid sample has been obtained for culture and susceptibility. Antimicrobial combinations commonly used include:
  □ Na^+/K^+ penicillin, 22,000–44,000 IU/kg IV q6h, and/or
  □ Aminoglycosides: gentamicin, 2.2 mg/kg IV q8h/6.6 mg/kg IV q24h or amikacin, 6.6 mg/kg q8h/19.8 mg/kg IV q24h
  □ Metronidazole, 15–25 mg/kg PO, or suppository q6h for anaerobes
- Duration of antimicrobial therapy depends on:
  □ Severity of the peritonitis
  □ Etiologic agents
  □ Response to treatment
  □ Complications—thrombophlebitis, abdominal abscessation
- Use clinical signs and sequential evaluation of clinicopathologic parameters and peritoneal fluid to assess response to treatment. Generalized septic peritonitis may require from 1–6 months of antimicrobial therapy.
- After stabilization, surgical intervention to correct the primary problem and reduce peritoneal contamination by abdominal drainage, peritoneal lavage, and peritoneal dialysis

Prognosis

Prognosis depends on the severity and duration of the disease, primary etiologic agent, and complications—intra-abdominal adhesion formation, laminitis, endotoxic shock. Fair to good in mild, acute, diffuse peritonitis if prompt, aggressive treatment of the underlying problem is successful or if it is unknown. Prognosis is poor for severe abdominal contamination or intestinal perforation.

J. DIARRHEAL DISEASES—ADULTS

Thomas J. Divers

ACUTE DIARRHEA

Fever, colic, and diarrhea are the clinical signs caused by enteritis in horses. In many cases, the colic precedes the diarrhea and may be severe. This is especially true in young foals. Adult diarrhea is virtually always a result of colonic dysfunction, hence the terms "colitis" and "diarrhea" are often used synonymously. In foals, diarrhea is most severe with small intestinal dysfunction. Division in this section into adults, weanlings-yearlings, and foals is made because of age differences, although some of the etiologic agents, e.g., *Salmonella* spp., can affect all age groups.

Acute colitis is almost always an emergency in adults. Salmonellosis, Potomac horse fever (PHF), and drug-induced colitis (antibiotics, NSAID toxicity) are the most common causes. Approximately 50% of the cases go undiagnosed (idiopathic). Affected individuals may present with *colic* and/or *fever before the onset of diarrhea*. Take the rectal temperature in patients with abdominal pain! Make a presumptive diagnosis of acute colitis in the presence of fever with fluidy gut sounds (the sound of fluid rushing through pipes).

Causes

Salmonella *and Potomac Horse Fever (PHF)*

Many cases of PHF show fever, depression, and anorexia without diarrhea. **PHF is a common reason for fever in endemic areas during the summer months**. Bloody diarrhea may be more common with *Salmonella* but can be seen with other causes also. Although the clinical signs of salmonellosis and Potomac horse fever *(Ehrlichia risticia)* are indistinguishable, their epidemiology has some important differences such as presence or absence of stress factors (e.g., *Salmonella*) and seasonal (PHF most common in Northeast, North Central and Mid-Atlantic states from June to November) and geographic incidence.

Antibiotic-Induced Diarrhea

The history is important in assessing this possibility. It generally occurs 2–6 days after initiation of antibiotic treatment (although cases occur 1–2 days after discontinuing treatment). It is believed to result from pathogenic *Clostridium difficile* or *C. perfringens* overgrowth and/or the inflammatory and secretory impact on the colon; this is rarely proved. A decrease in roughage consumption may predispose the individual to enteric clostridiosis. All antimicrobial drugs, especially those given orally, have the potential for causing diarrhea. The most commonly implicated drugs are:

- Oral trimethoprim-sulfa—mostly in stressed, transported, or postoperative cases
- **Erythromycin in individuals > 6 months of age**—rarely occurs in mares with foals being treated with erythromycin
- Tetracycline—IV tetracycline **rarely** causes diarrhea in horses and has received an undeserved bad reputation. Nevertheless it should be considered as a possible cause, especially in stressed individuals.
- Penicillin V administered orally in doses > 66,000 IU/kg
- Ceftiofur, occasionally

NSAID Toxicity

Can occur from excessive administration of either oral or parenterally administered phenylbutazone, flunixin meglumine, or ketoprofen. Phenylbutazone is believed to be more damaging to the GI tract than the other two. **Affected individuals generally develop hypoproteinemia early in the disease and usually have plasma protein levels < 4.5 gm/dl (adults) before the diarrhea.** The protein is lower in foals. *The very low protein at the onset or before the diarrhea is not diagnostic for NSAID toxicity but highly suggestive.* Colic may also be more common with NSAID toxicity than other colitis cases.

Cyathostomiasis

Acute diarrhea associated with encysted cyathostomes may occur in yearlings or adults. Affected individuals are generally thin prior to the onset of diarrhea and have a questionable history regarding proper parasite control. Onset of clinical signs is most common in October through April. The history is important in making a tentative diagnosis of cyathostomiasis diarrhea. Fever may be absent, as may leukopenia. The fecal examination for parasites may not be helpful since the encysted larvae are the problem. A rectal biopsy should be taken; eosinophils or finding the cause of an encysted larva is supportive of the disease. Small adult strongyles may be observed in the manure or on the rectal sleeve after examination in a small percentage of cases.

Colitis X

This is a "catch-all" term for acute colitis, endotoxemia, and anaphylaxis. *There are multiple causes!* Segmental edema of the colon is characteristic. Stress and/or a change in feed may precede the acute disease. The syndrome is seen on a few occasions in horses recently (2–5 days) introduced to winter grazing.

Acute collapse and signs of shock are characteristic, although some individuals have a more prolonged course. Severe pain, mild abdominal distention, and fever are common. There may be severe diarrhea, mild "cow flop" manure, or no manure passed. The colon may palpate to be edematous on rectal examination, and in a few cases blood is observed in the manure. Sometimes, the affected individuals may improve initially with therapy but within a few days have a sudden demise. Necropsy reveals severe edema (sometimes hemorrhage) of the colon and/or cecum. The lesions may be segmental.

Fecal specimens should be submitted for *Salmonella* spp. and *Clostridium* spp. culture and *Clostridium* toxin assay. They are usually negative. Clinical pathology data are typical of those observed in many patients with endotoxemia and colitis (leukopenia, left shift, toxic-appearing neutrophils, thrombocytopenia, hyponatremia, hypochloremia, hypocalcemia, and acidosis).

General Diagnostic Tests for Acute Adult Colitis

- Routine hematology, including CBC, chemistry panel (hypochloremia and hyponatremia with azotemia are the most common findings early in all colitis diseases).
- PHF titer ($> 1{:}640$ on most individual fluorescent antibody tests is diagnostic in an unvaccinated individual; $> 1{:}2560$ *often* diagnostic in a vaccinated individual, although some vaccinated individuals may have higher titers and not be infected). A few infected individuals have lower than expected titers initially but seroconvert later.
- Polymerase chain reaction (PCR) (EDTA blood sample on ice—ship express mail) for PHF—(Cornell Diagnostic Laboratory) should be used in addition to IFA to confirm the diagnosis. Fecal culture is used to help diagnose *Salmonella*. Repeated samples (5–10 gm) are required. If the sample cannot be submitted immediately to a reference laboratory, place fecal material in a cup (not refrigerated) or place feces (10%) in a whirl pack of selenite or Ames transport media for storage. If you do your own culturing, it is best to perform direct culture on selective media. Place some feces in enrichment (Selenite F) media for later plating. *Salmonella* cultures are most often positive as the manure firms. Fecal cultures may also be tested for *Salmonella* using PCR. (Cornell Diagnostic Laboratory, Ithaca, NY 14853, (607)253-3900; or Diagnostic and Biologic Technologies, Inc., San Antonio, Texas 78258, 800-336-3060 Fax 210-496-2517.)

- *Clostridium* overgrowth is suspected to be the cause of antibiotic-induced colitis, although the specific relationship has not been identified. Feces should be submitted for *Clostridium* spp. culture and toxin assay. (Cary-Blair Transport Media, Meridian Diagnostics, Cincinnati, OH 45244 should be used for *Clostridium* culture.) Frozen feces shipped overnight is recommended for toxin assay. Send samples to Diagnostic Laboratory, New York State College of Veterinary Medicine, Cornell University, Box 786, Upper Tower Road, Ithaca, NY 14851; (607) 253–3333. For anaerobic culture and toxin assay when specific media are not available, at least 50 ml should be transported overnight to an appropriate laboratory. If more than 24 hours are required for laboratory submission, the sample should be sent on dry ice. A Gram stain on the feces is often helpful and with clostridiosis there are a majority of uniformly large gram-positive organisms. If *C. difficile* is the etiologic agent, many of the organisms may have spores.
- It is not routinely recommend performing an abdominocentesis unless peritonitis is suspected (see Peritonitis, Table 16–1). The peritoneal fluid in patients with severe colitis often has an increase in protein. This finding rarely affects therapy, but the procedure increases the subcutaneous abdominal edema associated with hypoproteinemia. *Stallions, with ventral edema, may develop severe cellulitis of the scrotum.*
- It is also not routine to perform rectal examinations on individuals with acute colitis unless the patient is colicky or has abdominal distention.

Treatment

Specific Treatment for Abdominal Pain Associated with Acute Colitis

Pass a nasogastric tube; perform a rectal examination and abdominocentesis to help rule out obstructive disease in those individuals *with persistent pain.* If, in addition to the history and laboratory findings, the information suggests colitis, assume the abdominal pain is a result of ileus, fluid distention of the bowel, edema of the bowel, stretching of the mesentery, mucosal ulcerations, and/or infarction of the bowel.

Intravenous calcium therapy may be useful in relieving the ileus in some cases. Lidocaine (2%) can be given IV, 1.3 mg/kg as a slow bolus, followed by 0.05 mg/kg/min as a continual infusion. If there is no gastric reflux, cisapride, 0.3 mg/kg PO, can be administered. In patients with colitis that are very painful and have a large ping over the base of the cecum, decompress the cecum (p. 59). If no other treatment is effective in relieving the pain or improving motility and fecal output, and you believe the pain is associated with colonic edema and pooling of fluid in the bowel and ileus, a single treatment with dexamethasone (0.5 mg/kg) may reduce the colonic edema and relieve the abdominal pain. Two to 4 liters per adult of hydroxyethyl starch (hetastarch) or plasma with or without DMSO (1 gm/kg) IV can be administered to reduce colonic edema.

Administer flunixin meglumine, 0.3 mg/kg IV q8h for endotoxemia; a larger dose, 1.0 mg/kg IV, can be administered once or twice for severe abdominal pain. Flunixin should not be used at the higher dose if NSAID toxicity is a possible diagnosis. Xylazine, detomidine, butorphanol, or ketoprofen can be used on a short-term basis to control pain. If a long-term effect is required, chloral hydrate may be administered, as a sedative, to effect.

General Treatment for Colitis, Regardless of the Cause

- Fluid therapy, with KCl (20 to 40 mEq/L) added and/or HCO_3^- as needed
  - □ Bicarbonate is rarely indicated initially unless the venous pH is extremely low (< 7.1). Always add potassium to the fluids (20–40 mEq/L) as soon as it becomes apparent that the patient is urinating.
  - □ Lactated Ringer's and Plasmalyte are preferred in most cases. In patients with severe colitis, replace *at least* half the plasma volume in the first 6–8 hours.
  - □ Administer hypertonic saline, 4 ml/kg IV, if severe hypotensive shock is suspected or as a means of cardiovascular support until continually administered IV fluids can be started.
  - □ Plasma: 2 liters minimum, has many advantages beyond its specific antiendotoxic antibodies. It contains fibronectin, antithrombin III, and other beneficial proteins. NOTE: plasma with antibodies against lipopolysaccharide is recommended. It is preferred not to use the commercially available hyperimmune serum because of the adverse effects associated with endotoxin found in the product.
- Low-dose flunixin meglumine: 0.25 mg/kg q8h initially; continue until signs of toxemia, fever, leukopenia, and so forth have resolved.
- Activated charcoal (commercial grade): 0.5 kg/500-kg horse PO—check for gastric reflux first.
- Pentoxifylline, 8.4 mg/kg PO q12h (for the more critically ill patients). This has been shown to decrease cytokine production in vitro following endotoxin challenge and may make red blood cells more deformable. The effect in vivo is unknown.
- One study found that polymyxin B, when administered at 600 u/kg IV slowly just prior to endotoxin challenge in foals, diminished the detrimental effects of the endotoxin. A noticeable clinical response in patients has not been frequently seen and therefore routine use is not recommended.

Specific Treatment for Adult Colitis

Antibiotic therapy has not been shown to be of any benefit for *Salmonella* in *adults*; however, most prefer to administer antibiotics, IM or IV, for adult salmonellosis. Ceftiofur, 1.5 mg/kg IV q12h is recommended.

Risks associated with antibiotic use include:

- Fungal colitis and pneumonia, seen occasionally with broad-spectrum antibiotics, including ceftiofur,
- Nephrotoxicity if aminoglycosides are used *(do not use aminoglycosides in patients with diarrhea unless they are on IV fluids and creatinine is being monitored).*

POTOMAC HORSE FEVER

- Tetracycline: 6.6 mg/kg IV diluted 1 part tetracycline and 3 parts saline q12h for 3–5 days. *The earlier in the course of the disease it is administered, the better the response.*

NSAID TOXICITY

- Plasma: 4–8 liters
- Sucralfate: 6–8 gm/adult q6–12h
- Misoprostol (Cytotec) 4 μg/kg PO q12h. Mild diarrhea and increase in rectal temperature have been seen after administration.
- Many individuals with NSAID toxicity have colic without diarrhea. The history, clinical examination, and finding of low total serum protein supports a tentative diagnosis. Treatment is plasma and polyionic fluids, sucralfate, Cytotec, and feeding a low-residue diet (no hay) with slow introduction of up to 0.5 cup dietary linseed oil added twice daily.

ANTIBIOTIC-INDUCED DIARRHEA

- Metronidazole: 15 mg/kg q6h PO. Expect improvement within 3 days or discontinue treatment.
- Use analgesics only if the preceding treatments are ineffective in controlling pain.
- Dipyrone or xylazine can be used.

CYATHOSTOMIASIS

- Moxidectin (American Cyanamid), 400–500 μg/kg PO once, or fenbendazole, 10 mg/kg daily for 5 days

Additional Treatment for All Causes of Colitis

- Unless the patient is in pain, offer free-choice water with and without electrolytes, including NaCl (15 gm); dextrose (15 gm), either anhydrous dextrose or 30 ml 50% dextrose, baking soda (12 gm); and KCl (10 gm), per gallon of water.
- Feed grass hay either without grain, or in small amounts.
- A wrap should be placed on the tail and the perineal-scrotal area protected with petroleum jelly from the effects of diarrhea. **Caution: If tail wraps are applied, be sure they are not too tight; do not use Vetwrap**.
- Monitor closely for signs of laminitis. Some clinicians routinely use frog pads as a prophylactic treatment. Topical nitroglycerin cream over palmar (posterior) digital arteries can be used.
- Take measures to prevent exposure of other individuals (via contact with feces or feces-contaminated equipment or personnel) until a diagnosis is confirmed.
- Use care in placing the jugular catheter since patients with colitis are prone to thrombophlebitis. Use a Mila catheter (Mila International, Inc., Covington, KY 41011) for patients with colitis and other conditions that are likely to receive large volumes of IV fluids for several days and/ or are at high risk of thrombosis—e.g., rapid drop in protein, severe hemoconcentration, and/or marked leukopenia with toxic changes.

□ Obtain samples from the transverse facial sinus (p. 3) and save the jugular veins for catheter placement.

Prognosis

Variable. The most difficult cases to manage are those that remain painful or are very toxic and produce scant, watery manure in the first 24 hours; *the prognosis is poor*. The prognosis for individuals with diarrhea caused by NSAIDs is poor to grave. Prognosis is associated with appetite; those that continue to eat have a better prognosis.

Degree of hemoconcentration: patients with a PCV of 60–65 or more have a poor prognosis, as do those with purple mucous membranes. These patients may recover from the colitis but seem to have a higher incidence of failure to gain weight, laminitis, and renal failure.

Laminitis: guarded to poor prognosis with ongoing colitis. If the patient is to be a performance individual and it develops laminitis associated with the colitis, **a *marked* improvement in the laminitis within 3 days of treatment must be seen or the prognosis for returning to performance is poor**.

Renal failure: fair prognosis if polyuria occurs with fluid therapy; otherwise grave. Most horses with acute colitis are azotemic, often having serum creatinine concentrations of 5.0–7.0 mg/dl. Most show a rapid decline in serum creatinine to normal range within 24–36 hours, suggesting that the azotemia is mostly prerenal. Suspect acute renal failure if the patient does not urinate after several liters of polyionic fluids or 2 liters of hypertonic saline and if the plasma potassium is >5.5 mg/dl. NOTE: that plasma and serum potassium may be falsely elevated if the plasma or serum remain with the red cells for several hours.

CANTHARIDIN INTOXICATION (BLISTER BEETLE POISONING)

Cantharidin is the toxic principle found in the male and inseminated female blister beetles (*Epicauta* spp.). The "three-striped" blister beetles (Fig. 26–7) are most often associated with the toxicity. The beetles feed on alfalfa in mid to late summer and can be incorporated into **alfalfa hay** during processing,

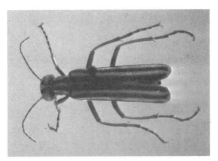

FIGURE 26–7. "Three-striped" blister beetle. (Courtesy of Dave Schmidt, Texas A&M University.)

especially when cutting and crimping occur simultaneously. Ingestion of the beetles or the toxin (released when the beetles are crushed) causes direct damage to the *oral mucous membranes and the GI mucosa*. Once absorbed from the GI tract, the toxin is rapidly excreted by the kidneys, damaging the *renal parenchyma* as well as the mucosa of the lower urinary tract in the process. Direct *myocardial* damage can occur with cantharidin intoxication. *As few as 5–10 beetles are lethal.*

Diagnosis

Clinical manifestations are not specific and vary with the amount of toxin ingested. The signs seen are associated with shock, gastrointestinal and urinary tract irritation, renal insufficiency, myocardial failure, and **hypocalcemia** within hours to days following ingestion of contaminated alfalfa hay (rarely pellets).

Clinical Signs and Findings

- Increased heart and respiratory rates
- Elevated temperature
- Abdominal pain—most common
- Anorexia
- Depression
- Sweating
- Oral irritation—salivation, playing in water
- Frequent attempts to urinate
- Diarrhea ± blood—uncommon
- Cold extremities
- Increased HCT and capillary refill time (CRT)
- Muddy, congested mucous membranes
- *Synchronous diaphragmatic flutter (thumps)**
- Erosions of the oral mucosa
- Stiff gait*
- Hematuria and/or hemoglobinuria
- Sudden death
- Neurologic signs

Isolation of cantharidin can be made from urine or stomach contents. However, levels fall dramatically within 3 days of ingestion and may require several hundred milliliters be submitted to detect it. One or more pints of urine can be submitted to the Diagnostic Laboratory at Texas A&M University, College Station, Texas 77843. Gastric contents and kidney should be submitted from postmortem samples.

Treatment

Remove the toxin.

- Evacuate the GI tract.

---

*Indicative of hypocalcemia.

□ Mineral oil in repeated doses serves as a laxative and binds the lipid-soluble toxin. **Mineral oil should be administered prophylactically to all potentially poisoned individuals**.

■ Diuresis: Begin as early as possible to increase toxin excretion. Administer furosemide, 0.25–1.0 mg/kg IV *ONLY* after adequate rehydration.

Supportive care:

■ Fluid therapy—as indicated by serum electrolyte determination, urine production, and serum creatinine
   □ If synchronous diaphragmatic flutter exists, to the first day's replacement fluids add calcium borogluconate—24 mg calcium/kg body weight (~ 500 ml Ca borogluconate per adult diluted in several liters of fluids with magnesium sulfate—6 mg/kg body weight).
   □ ADMINISTER IV SLOWLY—not subcutaneously.
   □ Monitor cardiac rhythm—discontinue if cardiac irregularities develop or worsen.
■ Analgesics: flunixin meglumine, 1.1 mg/kg IM or IV
■ Corticosteroids: dexamethasone, 0.25 mg/kg IV bolus, occasionally used
■ Broad-spectrum antibiotics: Ceftiofur—NOT aminoglycosides or sulfonamides
■ If renal failure is present, determine whether the failure is oliguric (see p. 462).

Prognosis

Guarded in most cases. If a lethal dose has been ingested, no treatment reverses the effects. Heart rate, respiratory rate, and serum creatinine should be monitored in patients that survive several days—increases indicate deterioration. An increase in the cardiac and GI enzyme CK-MB is an unfavorable finding.

Prevention

The beetles feed in mid to late summer, therefore alfalfa harvested before June is less likely to be contaminated. NOTE: Know where the alfalfa is harvested. Instruct owners who grow their own alfalfa to inspect their fields before cultivation and avoid harvesting in areas with insect swarms. Alternatively, fields may be treated with malathion before cutting, but appropriate withdrawal times should be observed. The toxicity of cantharidin does not decrease with storage, and the pelleting process does not denature it.

K. DIARRHEA IN NURSING FOALS

Thomas J. Divers

NECROTIZING ENTEROCOLITIS

This is a common cause of *colic* and *diarrhea* (sometimes hemorrhagic) in young foals, usually within the first week and sometimes within the first day of life. It is thought to be caused by the anaerobic organisms *Clostridium perfingens* (most commonly type A or C), *C. difficile*, or *Bacteroides fragilis*. It may affect only one foal on a farm, often with no recognizable predisposing factors. Orphan foals fed milk replacers and maladjusted foals seem to be at increased risk. Diarrhea caused by *C. perfringens* type A or *C. difficile* may be a farm problem.

Clinical Signs

- Colic often precedes the diarrhea by a few hours and can be severe.
- Mild to moderate abdominal distention generally precedes the diarrhea.
- There may be some reflux after passage of a soft nasogastric tube but more commonly reflux is absent or minimal.
- *Fever* is usually present!
- The diarrhea is bloody in some cases of *C. perfringens*.

Diagnosis

Diagnosis is based on clinical findings, history of fever, leukopenia, low serum sodium and chloride, and fluidy bowel sounds. Rule out other causes of colic. **The most common causes of colic in young foals are enteritis and meconium impaction.** Radiographic examination of the foal can be performed using 85 kVp and 20 mA with rare earth screen cassettes; this is useful in distinguishing colic/enteritis from surgical conditions, e.g., intussusceptions. Diffuse gas distention of the small intestine is supportive of enteritis (Fig. 26–8). With small intestinal surgical conditions gas distention generally is less diffuse; instead, a few distinct inverted U loops of bowel are seen (Fig. 26–9).

Ultrasound examination of the ventral abdomen is helpful in differentiating strangulating lesions from enteritis as a cause of the abdominal pain; 7.5-MHz probe (with standoff) is ideal. With enteritis, the small intestinal wall is more hypoechoic and thickened than normal (Fig. 26–10), and motility may be increased. With strangulating lesions, motility is usually absent. The ultrasound examination should be performed with the foal standing if possible.

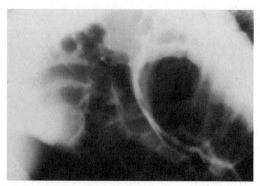

FIGURE 26–8. Radiograph of the abdomen of a 1-week-old foal with gaseous distention of the intestinal tract. The foal developed diarrhea within 4 hours after the radiograph was taken.

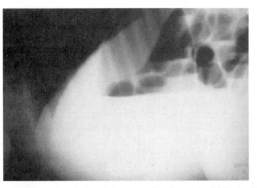

FIGURE 26–9. Radiograph of the abdomen of a 2-week-old foal with abdominal pain. Intussusception was found on exploratory celiotomy.

Perform abdominocentesis only if a strangulating lesion is suspected and only after ultrasound examination has identified a discrete fluid pocket. **Indiscriminate abdominocentesis in foals is fraught with complications: hypodermic needles frequently puncture the bowel lumen in foals, which may cause peritonitis and adhesions. Teat cannulas may cause herniation of omentum at the site of the centesis, but this can be reduced by performing the aspirate in the more caudal abdomen.**

Fecal cultures should be submitted for *Clostridium* spp. identification (Port-a-Cul anaerobic tube, Becton-Dickinson, Cockeysville, MD 21030) and toxin assay (place feces in fecal cup) and *taken to the laboratory directly or shipped overnight on ice. A Gram stain of the feces is helpful in the diagnosis if there are an abundant number of large gram-positive rods.* Blood cultures should be performed since many of the foals are blood culture–positive for *Clostridium perfringens.*

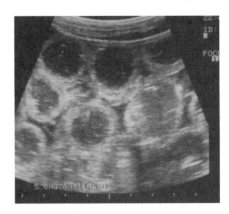

FIGURE 26–10. Ultrasound of the abdomen of a 1-day-old foal with *Clostridium perfringens* diarrhea. Note the thickened bowel wall.

Treatment

- Control pain in colicky foals to minimize injury. **Begin with dipyrone, 5 ml IV, or butorphanol, 4–6 mg IM/IV. If the pain is not controlled, administer xylazine, detomidine, carprofen, or ketoprofen, but limit repeated administrations. Avoid flunixin meglumine if possible**. Foals with colic, ileus, and severe/progressive "gaseous" abdominal distention that are unresponsive to appropriate medical treatment (see later), and are believed *not* to have an obstructive disorder, can be administered neostigmine, 0.2–0.4 mg SQ, with a short-acting anesthetic in an attempt to evacuate the gas.
- Intravenous fluids—lactated Ringer's solution. Add KCl (20 mEq/L) if the foal is hypokalemic or if sodium bicarbonate and dextrose have been administered and the foal is urinating. Additional potassium is generally needed in foals with diarrhea for more than 2 days or foals receiving large volumes of IV fluids. If the foal appears weak, add 100 gm of dextrose/L unless the Dextrostix indicates normal blood glucose. If the blood glucose is normal, add 50 gm/L. **Continual administration of intravenous fluids is seldom practical since the mare is often in the way and the foal may be colicky. Alternatively, foals can be administered 1 to 2 liters of fluids by bolus over 20 to 30 minutes two to six times daily, depending on the clinical condition of the foal.**
- Plasma: 2 liters administered IV. Preferably the plasma should have antibodies against endotoxin, although the lipopolysaccharide antibodies may not be as important as some naturally occurring factors in plasma—e.g., antithrombin III.
- If the foal is in hypotensive shock and the plasma and polyionic fluids do not improve the condition (as determined by blood pressure monitoring or clinical impressions—e.g., poor capillary refill, severe and persistent tachycardia, and cold extremities), administer dopamine (5–10 μg/kg/min) or dobutamine (10–20 μg/kg/min) in a slow IV drip. If this does not improve the blood pressure, methylene blue, 5–8.8 mg/kg, can be administered IV slowly.
- Antibiotics: intravenous penicillin, 44,000 IU/kg IV q6h; amikacin,* 6.6 mg/kg q8h (loading dose: 7.5 mg/kg); and metronidazole, 15 mg/kg PO q12h (for 3–5 days)
- Gastric ulcer prophylaxis:
  - ☐ Sucralfate, 2 gm PO q6h
  - ☐ Ranitidine, 1.5 mg/kg IV q8h, or cimetidine, 6.6 mg/kg IV q8h or famotidine, 0.7 mg/kg IV q24h. Once the pain subsides, these drugs can be given PO (see pp. 173–174).
  - ☐ Allow the foal to nurse.

Prognosis

Initially guarded, as intestinal necrosis may rapidly progress, but if the foal survives the first 2 days of the enteritis, the prognosis usually improves dramati-

---

*Administer amikacin only after urine production has been noted. Administer metronidazole only if the feces have a large number of gram-positive rods on Gram stain. There are other contagious causes of diarrhea in young foals, generally viral, that do not benefit from metronidazole therapy.

cally. Cachexia may become a problem if the foal does not improve within 3 days, and parenteral nutrition may be required.

FOAL SALMONELLOSIS

Clinical Findings

- Fever (usually $> 103°F$), depression, tachycardia, tachypnea, and variable diarrhea.
- The diarrhea may be scant, profuse, or bloody; tenesmus may be noted.
- Clinical findings more often result from the bacteremia/endotoxemia rather than from intestinal fluid and electrolyte loss.
- The sclera is often injected, and a green discoloration of the iris may be noted (presumably a result of septicemia-induced uveitis).
- Lameness may be caused by septic arthritis or physitis.
- Rales, resulting from hematogenous pneumonia, may be heard on thoracic auscultation.
- Stupor or seizure may be a result of meningitis or severe electrolyte abnormalities, e.g., hyponatremia.

Horses are susceptible to salmonellosis at any age, and outbreaks are not uncommon in nursing to weanling foals. In many cases of salmonellosis in nursing foals, it is presumed that the mare is the source of the infection. **It is unusual to find clinical signs in both the mare and the foal, although both are usually feces-positive for the *Salmonella* species**.

Diagnosis

Blood can be collected in a BBL Vacutainer (Becton-Dickinson, Cockeysville, MD 21030) for blood culture. *To reduce the cost of submitting every blood culture tube to the laboratory, it can be incubated or left at room temperature for 24–48 hours; if the broth becomes turbid it should be submitted for culture.* Feces can be obtained by digital examination (be careful not to initiate severe tenesmus); the feces sample should be placed in Ames transport medium for aerobic culture* (10% feces). Aerobic organisms that may be significant in foals with diarrhea include all *Salmonella* spp., some *Escherichia coli, Aeromonas hydrophila, Yersinia, Enterocolitica, Campylobacter* spp.,* *Streptococcus*, and *Pseudomonas* spp. *Salmonella*-selective media and selenite enrichment media should both be used for fecal cultures. Complete blood count usually reveals neutropenia with a left shift, toxic changes in the neutrophils, and high-normal to increased fibrinogen. A low platelet count suggests disseminated intravascular coagulation (DIC).

Electrolytes and Chemistries

Acidosis, hypochloremia, hyponatremia, and azotemia are the most common findings. If the azotemia is caused in part by intrinsic renal failure, the potassium level may be high. If the diarrhea has been present for more than 24 hours and

---

*Use Campy Thio transport medium for *Campylobacter*.

renal function is normal, especially if bicarbonate-dextrose has been administered, *life-threatening hypokalemia could be present.*

Treatment

The emphasis is on fluid therapy, antibiotics, and good nursing care.

Fluid Therapy

- Any balanced electrolyte product is acceptable, but a polyionic fluid is preferred over normal saline (which is an acidifying fluid). Use hypertonic saline only if the polyionic fluids are unsuccessful in correcting clinically apparent or measurable hypotension. NOTE: If hyponatremia is severe (<115 mEq/L), administer 1–2 ml/kg hypertonic saline as a bolus at 30-minute intervals until serum Na is 125–130 mEq/L but **NO HIGHER.**
- Potassium chloride (20 mEq/L) should be added to the fluids once urination is seen or if the plasma K is <3.5 mEq/L!
- If the foal remains severely depressed and acidotic in spite of the polyionic fluid therapy, administer isotonic sodium bicarbonate (1.25% solution or 12.5 gm baking soda/gallon sterile water). If sodium bicarbonate therapy is used, add additional KCL (20–40 mEq/L).
- One or preferably more liters of equine plasma with antibodies against LPS should be administered. The plasma is helpful not only in combating endotoxemia and DIC but also in improving the cardiodynamic effect gained from the administration of polyionic fluids.

Antibiotic Therapy

- Ticarcillin/clavulanic acid, 44 mg/kg IV q6h; amikacin,* 6.6 mg/kg IV or IM q8h or 19.8 mg/kg IV q24h; or ceftiofur, 5 mg/kg IV q8h, and amikacin provide appropriate antimicrobial treatment for salmonellosis in foals. *The use of effective antibiotics, administered at high doses early in the disease, is extremely important.*

Antiulcer Prophylaxis/Therapy

- Ranitidine, 1.5 mg/kg IV or 6.6 mg/kg PO q8h; famotidine, 0.7 mg/kg IV q24h or 2.8 mg/kg PO q24h; or omeprazole, 0.5 mg/kg IV q24h
- Sucralfate, 2 gm PO q6h, preferably 30–60 minutes before the administration of the preceding antiulcer medications. Carprofen, 1.5 mg/kg PO q24h or 0.7 mg/kg IV q24h, is believed to be less ulcerogenic than flunixin meglumine.

Additional Therapy

- *If, and only if,* the foal has clinical or laboratory findings that suggest life-threatening endotoxemia, administer 0.25 mg/kg of flunixin meglumine (Banamine) after fluid therapy has been initiated.

---

*Do not administer the amikacin until the foal has been observed to urinate a normal amount.

Nursing Care

- **Examine joints to detect early evidence of septic arthritis/physitis and monitor for lameness**.
- Place a plastic bag on the base of the tail using Elasticon, **wrapped loosely**, with a separate strip extending dorsally over the midsacral area. **Do not use Vetwrap or apply the Elasticon too tightly**. Clean the perineal area and apply petroleum jelly.
- If the foal is colicky, administer dipyrone (5–10 ml IV), butorphanol (4–6 mg IM/IV), xylazine (0.6–1.0 mg/kg IV or IM), detomidine, or ketoprofen. Limit the number of times they are administered!
- Apply a topical ophthalmic corticosteroid and atropine (1%) to the eye four to six times daily if uveitis is apparent and *if there is no corneal ulcer.*
- Do not separate the mare and foal. It is probable that the mare is already feces culture-positive for *Salmonella*, and the stress of separation could be detrimental to both.

ROTAVIRUS DIARRHEA

Rotavirus (group A) is the most common infectious cause of diarrhea. As a rule, several foals in a barn are affected over several days. **The diarrhea is watery, yellow to yellow-green, and has a characteristic nonfetid smell**. Onset of infection and clinical disease varies from a couple of days to several weeks. Affected foals are frequently seen to be depressed and not nursing normally before observing diarrhea. After the diarrhea begins, the foal's attitude may become more alert and nurse more vigorously. If dehydration or severe acidosis (bicarbonate <18 mEq/L) develops, the foal becomes more depressed. Mild abdominal pain may be noted early in the disease; signs of pain (odontoprisis/bruxism, rolling, and ptyalism) later in the course of the diarrhea are suggestive of gastric ulcers.

Diagnosis

The history, age and clinical findings as described are important in making a clinical diagnosis.

Collect feces in a cup and submit to a laboratory for enzyme-linked immunosorbent assay (ELISA) for the viral antigen. (Foals that have had the disease for several days may be negative.)

Monitor CBC and electrolytes if the foal becomes depressed or if the diarrhea has been present for several days. Immature neutrophils and toxic changes within the neutrophils are not characteristic of rotavirus infection and suggest a more severe disease process (e.g., necrotizing enterocolitis or salmonellosis). Hypochloremia, hyponatremia, hypokalemia, and acidosis may develop, and these indicate a need for fluid therapy.

Foal heat diarrhea is common in 7–12-day-old foals and should be considered as a differential for diarrhea in a bright and alert foal of this age.

Treatment

Generally, treatment may not be needed if the foal is bright and alert and has normal electrolytes and IgG >800 mg/dl (in foals <10 days of age).

- Two oz bismuth subsalicylate via dose syringe q6h may be of some medical value.
- If the foal is depressed and not nursing, administer 500–750 ml of warm electrolyte solution via nasogastric tube. Examine the tube for gastric reflux and administer the electrolyte solution only by gravity flow (funnel). Commercial electrolyte replacers with only glucose, glycine, Na, K, and Cl, e.g., Resorb, Ion-aid, are preferred. These should be mixed so they are nearly isotonic (300 mM/L).
- If the foal is still colicky, markedly depressed, and/or has significant electrolyte abnormalities, administer IV fluid therapy, 20 ml/kg of lactated Ringer's with 20 mEq/L KCl or another balanced electrolyte solution two to four times daily, depending on the severity of the diarrhea and the clinical condition of the foal.
- Administer antiulcer medication (see pp. 173–174) to all foals requiring IV therapy or repeated administration of oral fluids. Provide electrolyte fluids and free water.

Measures to prevent spread of the disease:

- Isolate all affected foals.
- Personnel should enter the stall last during daily treatment or cleaning.
- Place a foot bath with a newer generation of quaternary ammonium or hypochlorite outside the stall and wear boots and coveralls when entering the stall.
- Wash hands with disinfectant soaps.
- Keep pets and birds away from the stall.
- NOTE: Other unidentified infectious viral diarrheal diseases in foals are likely.

CRYPTOSPORIDIA

Cryptosporidium parvum–associated diarrhea occurs in catabolic foals being treated for other illnesses. *C. parvum* also may cause diarrhea in older nursing foals and sometimes appears without identifiable stress factors. In severe cases, electrolyte abnormalities and volume depletion may cause death. Diagnosis can be made by fecal flotation with a saturated sugar solution and identifying several 4.5–5.5-μm-diameter oocysts. Submit a fresh sample and a sample in 10% formalin to a parasitology laboratory for confirmation since experience is helpful in the microscopic identification of the oocyst.*

Treatment

Generally supportive, with fluid and electrolyte replacement therapy and ulcer prophylaxis as discussed for rotavirus diarrhea. Paromomycin, 100 mg/kg, administered PO q24h for 5 days, can be administered, but efficacy is unproven in foals. A concentrated hypochlorite solution is reported to be the disinfectant of choice. It can be killed by steam heat. Cleaning of the stall is very important

---

Eimeria and *Giardia* spp. may be found in the feces of foals and adults, but there is no proof that they are pathogenic to horses.

since reinfection may occur. Most transmission is from foal to foal and not from the mare. *Hand washing should be adhered to strictly since zoonotic potential is a real possibility.*

ENTEROTOXIGENIC *ESCHERICHIA COLI*

E. coli (both pili- and enterotoxin-positive) can cause diarrhea in young foals (usually 2 to 3 weeks of age). It commonly affects one foal on a farm.

Clinical Signs

- Watery diarrhea
- Moderate to severe depression
- Acidosis
- Fever is usually absent.
- Signs of gastric ulceration are common.

Diagnosis

Submit feces for rotavirus detection (ELISA), electron microscopy, aerobic cultures, and parasite examination for *Cryptosporidia*. A heavy growth of mucoid *E. coli* should be submitted to a laboratory that can test the organism for adhesion and enterotoxin.

Treatment

Similar to treatment for other causes of foal diarrhea.

- Intravenous fluids (lactated Ringer supplemented with KCl and plasma in early stages)
- If the foal becomes severely acidotic, depressed, and stops nursing, administer isotonic bicarbonate (1.25% solution or 12 gm mixed in a liter of sterile water) with 20–40 mEq/L of KCl IV.
- Administer prophylactic antiulcer medication (see pp. 173–174).
- Give affected foals a broad-spectrum antibiotic (e.g., ceftiofur, 1.5–2.0 mg/kg IV q12h).

FETAL DIARRHEA

Diarrhea in the newborn foal with obvious staining of the amnionic fluid at birth is not unusual. Affected foals are depressed, may have signs of sepsis, and are at high risk of aspiration pneumonia from the meconium-stained amnionic fluid.

Treatment

- Suction the trachea to remove the meconium fluid.
- Broad-spectrum antibiotics (as for *Salmonella*, see p. 230)
- Polyionic fluids and plasma
- If respiratory signs develop or worsen 24–48 hours after birth and aspiration of meconium amnionic fluid has occurred, dexamethasone,

0.1–0.25 mg/kg, can be administered to reduce the chemical pneumonitis. A lower-dose therapy should be continued for 2–3 days if there is improvement from the initial treatment.

L. DIARRHEA IN WEANLINGS AND YEARLINGS

Thomas J. Divers

RHODOCOCCUS EQUI

R. equi may cause diarrhea in foals 3 weeks of age up to yearlings. The diarrheal syndrome may or may not be associated with *R. equi* pneumonia in the younger foals (<4 months of age). Septic physitis and/or arthritis may accompany the diarrhea, and abdominal abscessation also occurs in affected foals.

Diagnosis

This can be difficult! If there are a large number, e.g., more than 10^5 of *R. equi* organisms/gm of feces, or over 100 colonies per plate from a swab of feces taken from the affected foal—and other known causes are ruled out—a tentative diagnosis of *R. equi* diarrhea can be made. Additional documentation of the organism as the pathogen can be done based on the presence of specific antigens associated with virulence (85-kbp plasmid and associated 15–17-kDa antigens). Serology is probably of little or no positive predictive value in diagnosing *R. equi* diarrhea. A negative result may help rule out the disease.

Treatment

- Administer erythromycin stearate, phosphate, or estolate, 25 mg/kg q8h PO, and rifampin, 5 mg/kg q12h PO. If there is evidence of systemic involvement, e.g., septic physitis, vancomycin, 4.3–7.5 mg/kg administered IV slowly (diluted with 1 liter of fluid), may improve treatment success and adds to the cost of treatment.
- Administer intravenous fluids, e.g., lactated Ringer's, with 20 mEq/L KCl to replace the fluid and electrolyte loss.
- Administer plasma (2–4 liters), with antibody directed against endotoxin, to valuable foals and/or those foals with severe hypoalbuminemia. This therapy improves the efficacy of the polyionic fluids and may provide some additional protection against endotoxemia.
- Medication to prevent or treat gastric ulceration (see pp. 173–174).
- Apply a topical corticosteroid ophthalmic ointment and 1% atropine ointment to the eyes if a **nonulcerative** uveitis is apparent. This is most commonly detected by a green discoloration of the iris.

Prognosis

Variable, and is guarded to poor if arthritis, physitis, or abdominal abscessation is present. Otherwise, fair to good with appropriate treatment. Foals that have weight loss preceding the diarrhea have a more guarded and often grave prognosis if mesenteric abscessation is present.

ANTIBIOTIC-INDUCED DIARRHEA

This is most commonly associated with the oral administration of trimethoprim-sulfa products or **erythromycin**. Nursing foals generally tolerate erythromycin well, but weanlings and older horses occasionally have severe "gaseous" colic, diarrhea, and toxemia associated with its administration. **Most antibiotic-induced diarrheas occur 2–6 days after beginning the drugs**. It does not seem to be related to the brand/preparation of erythromycin or trimethoprim-sulfa used.

Clinical Signs

- Colic usually precedes the diarrhea, with moderate to severe gaseous distention of the bowel and abdomen.
- Signs and findings of toxemia (scleral injection, tachycardia, cold extremities) may be severe!
- The diarrhea is often fetid but may not be different from that of salmonellosis.

Laboratory Findings

- Clinical pathology findings are nonspecific and often include elevations of PCV, BUN, and creatinine.
- Serum sodium and chloride levels are decreased, and the bicarbonate level may be low depending on the severity of the disease.
- The neutrophil count may be decreased or increased, but toxic changes can be seen in the neutrophils.
- Submit fecal samples for *Salmonella* spp. and *Rhodococcus* culture and for *C. difficile* and *perfringens* culture and toxin assay (see p. 220). In spite of the suspicion that *C. difficile* or *perfringens* is often involved in antibiotic-induced diarrhea, the organism or toxin in the feces of affected individuals is found only sporadically.

Treatment

- Control abdominal pain with dipyrone, 22 mg/kg IV, butorphanol, 0.05 mg/kg IM or IV, administered after xylazine, 0.5–1.0 mg/kg. Limit the number of times these drugs are used.
- IV fluids: *Any polyionic fluid suffices. Volume is the most important consideration*; add KCl at 20 mEq/L unless:
  - □ Oliguria is noted
  - □ Creatinine is >5 mg/dl
  - □ Potassium is >5.0 mEq/L

Bicarbonate is generally not needed and is administered if the foal is very depressed and/or the bicarbonate concentration is < 16 mEq/L. Isotonic sodium bicarbonate can be prepared by mixing 12.5 gm of baking soda in 1 liter of sterile water; 20–40 mEq KCl is usually added to each liter of bicarbonate. If 0.9% NaCl is used, this may cause acidosis. Hypertonic NaCl (4 ml/kg) can be administered as a single dose treatment if severe hypotension is present.

- Plasma: 1–2 L IV to improve hemodynamics and alleviate the effect of endotoxin-derived mediators of septic shock. More than 2 liters may be required for severe hypoalbuminemia and edema.
- Flunixin meglumine: Administer 0.25 mg/kg in cases with clinical signs or laboratory findings suggestive of severe endotoxemia; carprofen, 0.7 mg/kg IV q24h or 1.5 mg/kg PO q24h, in other cases.
- Sucralfate: 2–4 gm q6h to foals receiving NSAIDs and weanling foals with severe diarrhea
- Antiulcer medication (see pp. 173–174)
- Metronidazole: 15 mg/kg PO q8h. Recommended only for antibiotic-induced colitis. If no improvement within 3 days, discontinue the treatment.

SALMONELLOSIS

In *weanlings*, treat same as salmonellosis in foals (see pp. 229–230). In *yearlings*, same as treatment in adults (see pp. 220–223).

SUGGESTED REFERENCES

Colic

Baxter G. The steps in assessing a colicky horse. Vet Med 1992;87(10):1012–1018.

Spurlock S, Ward M. Fluid therapy for acute abdominal disease. *In* White N (ed): The Equine Acute Abdomen. Philadelphia, Lea & Febiger, 1990, pp 160–172.

Steckel R. Diagnosis and management of acute abdominal pain (Colic). *In* Auer J (ed): Equine Surgery. Philadelphia, WB Saunders, 1992, pp 348–360.

White N. Examination and diagnosis of the acute abdomen. *In* White N (ed): The Equine Acute Abdomen. Philadelphia, Lea & Febiger, 1990, pp 102–147.

White N, Moore J. Treatment of endotoxemia. *In* White N (ed): The Equine Acute Abdomen. Philadelphia, Lea & Febiger, 1990, pp 173–177.

Mouth and Salivation

Hintz HF. Mold, mycotoxins and mycotoxicosis. Vet Clin North Am Equine Pract 1990;6:419–431.

Esophagus

Whitehair KJ, Coyne CP, Cox JH, DeBowes RM. Esophageal obstruction in horses. Compend Cont Educ Pract Vet 1990;12(1):91–96.

Stomach

Dowling PM. Therapy of gastric ulcers. Can Vet J 1995;36:276–277.

Murray MJ. Endoscopic appearance of gastric lesions in foals: 94 cases (1987–1988). J Am Vet Med Assoc 1989;195(8):1135–1141.

Murray MJ. Gastric ulceration in horses: 91 cases (1987–1990). J Am Vet Med Assoc 1992;201(1):117–120.

Small Intestine

Doran R, Allen D, Orsini J. Small intestine. *In* Auer J (ed): Equine Surgery. Philadelphia, WB Saunders, 1992, pp 360–378.

Hance S, Clem M, DeBowes R, Welch R. Intra-abdominal hernias in horses. Compend Cont Educ 1991;13(2):293–298.
Mueller P, Parks A, Baxter G. Small intestinal diseases of horses: Diagnosis and surgical intervention. Vet Med 1992;87(10):1030–1036.

Large Intestine
Gaughan E, Hackett R. Cecocolic intussusception in horses: 11 cases (1979–1989). J Am Vet Med Assoc 1990;197(10):1373.
Harrison I. Equine large intestinal volvulus: A review of 124 cases. Vet Surg 1988;17(2):77–81.
Kalsbeek H. Further experiences with non-surgical correction of nephrosplenic entrapment of the left colon in the horse. Equine Vet J 1989;21(6):442–443.
Ross M, Hanson R. Large intestine. *In* Auer J (ed): Equine Surgery. Philadelphia, WB Saunders, 1992, pp 379–407.

Small Colon and Rectum
Murray R, Green E, Constantinescu G. Equine enterolithiasis. Compend Contin Educ 1992;14(8):1104–1112.
Ruggles A, Ross MW. Medical and surgical management of small colon impaction in horses: 28 cases (1984–1989). J Am Vet Med Assoc 1991;199(12):1762–1766.

Colic in the Late-Term Pregnant Mare
Boening KJ, Leendertse IP. Review of 115 cases of colic in the pregnant mare. Equine Vet J 1993;25(6):518–521.
Santschi EM, Slone DE, Gronwall R, Juzwiak JS, Moll D. Types of colic and frequency of postcolic abortion in pregnant mares: 105 cases (1984–1988). J Am Vet Med Assoc 1991;199(3):374–377.

Peritonitis
Hawkins J, Bowman K, Roberts M, Cowen P. Peritonitis in horses: 67 cases (1985–1990). J Am Vet Med Assoc 1993;203(2):284–288.

Diarrheal Diseases
Durando MM, Mackay RJ, Stalley LA. Effects of polymyxin B and *Salmonella typhimurium* antiserum on horses given endotoxin intravenously. Am J Vet Res 1994;55(7):921–927.
Mair TS. Outbreak of larval cyathostomiasis among a group of yearlings and 2-year-old horses. Vet Rec 1994;135:598–600.

Cantharadin Intoxication
Schmitz DG. Cantharidin toxicosis in horses. J Vet Intern Med 1989;3(4):208–215 (color pictures included).

Diarrhea in Nursing Foals
Byars TD. Approach to foal diarrheas. Proceedings AAEP 1992;38:177–182.
Cohen ND. Cryptosporidial diarrhea in foals. Proceedings 13th Annual Veterinary Medical Forum 1955;735–738.

Diarrhea in Weanlings and Yearlings
Nordman P, Kersledjian JJ, Ronco L. Therapy of *Rhodococcus equi* disseminated infections. Antimicrob Agents Chemother 1992;36(6):1244–1248.

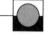

27 Integumentary

A. WOUND HEALING AND WOUND MANAGEMENT

Ted S. Stashak

Anatomy

- Skin is one of the largest and most important organ systems.
- Derived from two embryonic germ layers:
  - □ Epidermis from ectoderm, which has the ability to regenerate
  - □ Dermis (corium) from mesoderm, which cannot completely regenerate
- Skin thickness varies in the horse from 1.0–5.0 mm.
- Primary function is to protect and maintain homeostasis of the underlying structures.

Epidermis

- Epidermis is made up of five stratified squamous cell layers (Fig. 27–1).
- Nourishment is by diffusion of fluids from the capillary beds in the dermis.
- Stratum basale (base layer) has two nucleated cell types:
  - □ Keratinocytes constantly reproduce and push upward toward the surface to replace cells that have sloughed off the surface.
  - □ Melanocytes are responsible for producing the melanin that gives hair and skin its color.
- Stratum spinosum (prickle-cell layer)—cells in this layer are nucleated and become activated to reproduce when the outer epidermal layers are stripped off.
- Stratum granulosum (granular cell layer)—composed of cells that are in the process of dying, with nuclei that are shrinking and undergoing chromatolysis
- Stratum lucidum (clear cell layer)—made up of non-nucleated keratinized cells and is present only in hairless areas of the body
- Stratum corneum (horny cell layer)—composed of fully keratinized dead cells that are constantly being shed from the surface as scales. This layer forms a barrier that protects the underlying tissue from irritation, invasion of bacteria and noxious substances, and fluid and electrolyte losses.

Dermis

- Papillary layer, lies below the epidermis
- Reticular layer, extends from the papillary layer down to the subcutaneous tissue

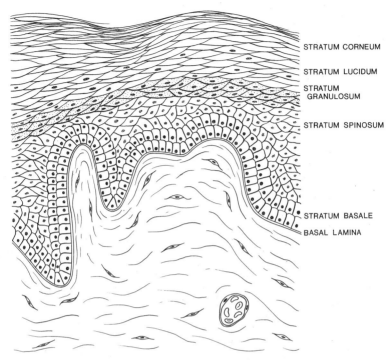

FIGURE 27–1. The layers of the epidermis. The stratum spinosum and stratum basale are collectively referred to as the stratum germinativum. (From Stashak TS: Wound Healing. *In* Jenning PB, ed: The Practice of Large Animal Surgery. Philadelphia, WB Saunders, 1984.)

- Contains a rich supply of blood vessels, lymphatics, hair follicles, sebaceous and apocrine sweat glands, and sensory nerve endings (Fig. 27–2)
- Fiber types:
  - Collagenous
  - Reticular
  - Elastic
- Cell types:
  - Fibroblasts
  - Histiocytes
  - Mast cells

WOUND HEALING

Phases

- Inflammatory
- Debridement
- Repair
- Maturation

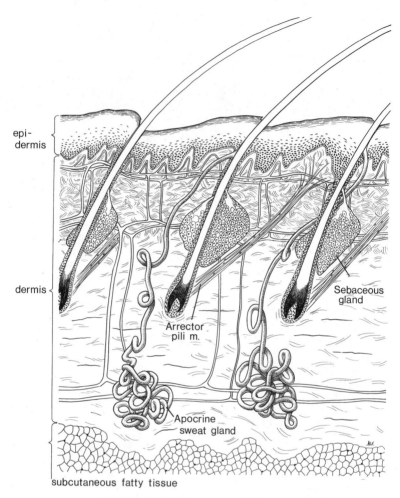

epi-
dermis

dermis

Sebaceous
gland

Arrector
pili m.

Apocrine
sweat gland

subcutaneous fatty tissue

FIGURE 27–2. The anatomy of the skin.

Inflammatory Phase

- Acute response affected by the severity of the injury
- Characterized by a vascular and cellular response protecting the body against excessive blood loss and invasion of foreign substances
- Fibrocellular clot that develops and maintains internal hemostasis and forms a scaffold for repair. Dehydrates superficially to form a scab, which acts like a bandage, protecting the wound from external contamination
- Factors affecting duration:
  - □ Degree of trauma
  - □ Nature of injury

□ Foreign substances (foreign bodies)
□ Infection
- NOTE: *Treatment with nonsteroidal anti-inflammatory drugs (NSAIDs), proper cleansing and debridement of the wound, and selection of appropriate antibiotics can influence the duration.*

Debridement Phase

- Neutrophils and monocytes, chemotactically stimulated by leukotaxine and lymph nodes–promoting factor, migrate into the wound and begin the clean-up process.
- Primary function of neutrophils:
  □ Ingestion of microorganisms by phagocytosis
  □ Lysosomal enzymes contribute to the inflammatory response.
  □ Aid the mononuclear cells in further breakdown of dead tissues
- Monocytes:
  □ Become macrophages on entering the wound
  □ Phagocytize dead tissues and debris
- Important function of monocytes:
  □ Produce many growth factors
  □ *Attract fibroblasts into the wound* and may stimulate them to undergo maturation for collagen synthesis
- Duration depends on amount of devitalized tissue, the degree of contamination, and whether infection develops; consequently, the value of *surgical debridement, effective lavage, good hemostasis, and adequate drainage of a wound is paramount.*

Repair Phase

EPITHELIALIZATION

- Basal cells of the epidermis begin to separate, duplicate, and migrate toward areas of cell deficit.
- Epithelial cells migrate underneath the scab and detach it by secreting proteolytic enzymes.
- Epithelial cells continue to migrate on the surface of a wound until like cells are contacted.
- The scab falls off when epithelialization is complete.
- Basal cells begin to reproduce to restore the normal thickness of the epidermis.
- Important *factors* that inhibit epithelialization include:
  □ Infection
  □ Excessive production of granulation tissue
  □ Repeated dressing changes
  □ Extreme hypothermia
  □ Desiccation of the wound surface
  □ Reduction in oxygen tension
- Epithelialization can be accelerated by the application of certain growth factors, topical antimicrobials (e.g., triple antibiotic ointment), and the use of semiocclusive dressings (e.g., Telfa).

FIBROPLASIA

- Fibroblasts advance along the previously formed fibrin lattice within the clot and begin secreting the ground substance.
- Collagen is synthesized by the fibroblasts predominantly from hydroxyproline and hydroxylysine.
- Immature tropocollagen fibrils bind together to form a mature collagen fiber.
- As collagen increases, the ground substance decreases, and wound strength improves with maturity.

GRANULATION TISSUE

- Result of proliferating capillaries that form vascular loops
- Vascular loops grow behind the fibroblasts and form multiple anastomoses.
- Lymphatics develop at a slower rate.
- *Granulation tissue* formation in an open wound is beneficial:
  □ Provides a surface for epithelial cells to migrate over
  □ Is resistant to infection
  □ The process of wound contraction is centered around its development.
  □ Carries the fibroblast responsible for collagen formation
- NOTE: *Healing of wounds in the distal extremities in horses is prompt and excessive, tending toward abnormal repair, which can result in exuberant granulation tissue formation.*

WOUND CONTRACTION

- A process in which an open skin wound reduces in size by centripetal movement of full thickness skin toward the wound's center
- Independent of epithelialization
- Modified fibroblasts called *myofibroblasts cause contractile properties of skin*—found in granulation tissue adjacent to the wound.
- Works best where the skin is relatively loose. In these areas, wound contraction is usually sufficient to bring about complete closure of the wound, with minimal scar formation.
- *Where skin is under tension, a wider scar is formed.*
- Contraction stops when
  □ Contact inhibition of like cells occurs.
  □ Tension of surrounding skin equilibrates with pulling forces of contraction.
  □ Exuberant granulation tissue impedes the wound's ability to contract.
  □ Full-thickness skin grafts are applied to the wound before the fifth day of healing.

Maturation Phase

- Characterized by a reduction in fibroblast numbers with an equilibration of collagen production and collagen lysis. Functionally oriented collagen fibers begin to predominate as nonfunctional ones are dissolved. Despite the reduction in fibroblasts, blood vessels, and collagen fibrils, the tensile strength of the wound increases.

- Wound tensile strength results from
  - □ Alignment of collagen along lines of tension, collagen cross-linking
  - □ Formation of more collagen contact bundles

SELECTED FACTORS THAT AFFECT WOUND HEALING

Anemia and Blood Loss

- Normovolemic anemia unrelated to malnutrition or chronic disease does not appear to affect wound healing until the packed cell volume (PCV) goes below 12.
- Hypovolemic anemia due to blood loss with vasoconstriction can impair wound healing. Reduced oxygen tension renders the wound more susceptible to infection by altering phagocytic mechanisms.
- Wound healing should progress normally if you correct
  - □ Anemia, with PCV < 12%
  - □ Chronic infection
  - □ Malnutrition
  - □ Hypovolemia

Malnutrition and Protein Deficiency

Wound Healing

- Impaired with mild to moderate short- or long-term protein energy malnutrition
- Direction the patient is moving metabolically (positive or negative) at the time of injury or surgery is most important.
- Hypoproteinemia adversely affects wound healing by impairing
  - □ Fibroplasia
  - □ Neoangiogenesis
  - □ Wound remodeling
  - □ Wound tensile strength gain
- *Plasma protein < 6 gm/dl results in markedly retarded healing.*
- Impairment in wound healing is easily reversed by providing adequate nutrition.

Recommendations

- Offer balanced nutrition in adequate amounts before elective surgery and/or after wounding and emergency surgery.
- Feeding D-L-methionine to protein-deficient patients reverses the retardation in wound healing. D-L-Methionine converts to cysteine, which serves as an important cofactor in collagen synthesis and disulfide cross-linking as collagen matures.
- Generally, vitamin deficiencies are not a problem. *Exception*: When individuals are chronically debilitated and undernourished, consider vitamin supplementation.

Nonsteroidal Anti-Inflammatory Drugs

- Because inflammation is a part of the wound-healing process, it is logical that anti-inflammatory drugs such as phenylbutazone, aspirin, indomethacin, and flunixin meglumine would affect wound healing.
- These drugs are useful because they
  □ Diminish pain from inflammation
  □ Improve overall well-being
  □ Encourage ambulation, resulting in improved circulation
  □ Reduce the adverse effect of endotoxins on wound healing
- *Recommendation: Administer the least amount to obtain the desired effect.*

Corticosteroids

- Administered in moderate to large amounts within the first 5 days after injury, they significantly retard wound healing.
- Retard healing by stabilizing the lysosomal membrane, preventing release of enzymes responsible for initiating the inflammatory response.
- Also suppress:
  □ Fibroplasia
  □ Ground substance formation
  □ Collagen formation
  □ Capillary proliferation
  □ Granulation tissue formation
- Also retard:
  □ Wound contraction
  □ The gain in tensile strength
  □ Epithelialization
- NOTE: *Have little effect when given 5 days after wounding*

Trauma

- Excessive trauma, within the wound or from other sites (e.g., multiple lacerations or fractures):
  □ Prolongs the early phase of healing
  □ Decreases the gain in tensile strength
  □ Makes the wound more susceptible to infection
  □ Results in excessive scar production
- Delay in wound tensile strength is observed as long as 15 days post-trauma.
- Delay in gain of wound tensile strength is proportional to the degree of trauma.
- *Tissue trauma can be reduced by*:
  □ Debriding the wound completely
  □ Reducing surgery time
  □ Using isotonic/iso-osmolar lavage solutions
  □ Maintaining hemostasis
  □ Reducing fluid accumulation in tissues

□ Apposing tissues with the proper tension with nonreactive suture material
□ Systemic antibiotics and NSAIDs are also important.
□ If excessive blood loss, intravenous fluids improve capillary perfusion.

Infection

■ Wound infection results when the number of organisms reaches a concentration of 10^6 organisms/gram of tissue or 10^6 organisms/milliliter of fluid.
■ Contaminated wounds with lesser concentrations of organisms may become infected when
□ Foreign bodies are present.
□ Excessive necrotic tissue is left in the wound.
□ Hematoma develops.
□ Local tissue defenses are impaired (burn patients or immunosuppressed patients).
□ The vascular supply is altered.
■ Wounds contaminated with dirt have a higher risk of infection owing to specific infection-potentiating fractions (IPFs) found in the organic components, and inorganic fractions.
■ Infection delays healing by
□ Mechanically separating the wound edges with exudate
□ Releasing endotoxins, which inhibit growth factors and collagen production
□ Reducing the vascular supply (a result of mechanical pressure and a tendency to form microthrombi in small vessels adjacent to the wound)
□ Increasing cellular responses, with prolongation of the inflammatory and debridement phases of wound healing
□ Bacteria also produce proteolytic enzymes that digest collagen.

Methods to Reduce Infection in Elective Surgery

■ *The best way to prevent infection in a surgical wound is*
□ Reduce surgery time
□ Aseptic technique
□ Meticulous hemostasis
□ Elimination of dead space and use of suction drains if necessary
□ Selection of nonreactive sutures
□ Proper suturing techniques and appropriate antimicrobials

Methods to Reduce Infection in a Traumatic Wound

■ *The best way to prevent infection in the traumatic wound is*
□ Proper wound preparation
□ Ample lavage
□ Thorough debridement
□ Systemic antimicrobial administration with broad-spectrum coverage
□ Culture and sensitivity to direct your selection when applicable

- Topical antibiotics
  - ☐ Can retard wound healing, especially some ointments or creams (e.g., nitrofurazone [Furacin] and gentamicin creams).
  - ☐ Solutions are most useful when applied to wounds before closure or in lavage solutions.
  - ☐ Creams and ointments remain in contact with the wound longer, prevent desiccation of the wound surface, and are best used under bandages and on exposed wounds.
  - ☐ Topical antimicrobials are most effective when applied within 3 hours of the injury.

Antiseptics for Skin Preparation

- The two most commonly used surgical scrubs for skin preparation are povidone-iodine (Betadine) and chlorhexidine (Hibiclens).
- Rinsing with saline or 70% isopropanol does not make a difference in antimicrobial effect.
- A disadvantage to povidone-iodine is skin reactions, particularly in small animals.
  - ☐ Occasionally an acute skin reaction in horses with povidone-iodine occurs but is rare.
  - ☐ More common in the horse after clipping, scrubbing and rinsing with 70% alcohol, spraying with povidone-iodine solution, and bandaging
  - ☐ Skin reactions include subcutaneous edema and skin wheal formation.
- The mechanical effect of scrubbing the wound with these antiseptic soaps can be helpful in removing debris and reducing bacterial concentration on the wound's surface. However, if the soap is not thoroughly rinsed from the wound, there is a marked delay in wound healing

Antiseptics for Wound Lavage

- *Bacteria adhere to the wound surface by an electrostatic charge.*
- Lavage solutions are most effective when delivered by a fluid jet of at least 7 psi on the wound.
- This pulsatile pressure can be achieved by
  - ☐ Forcefully expressing lavage solutions from a 35–60-ml syringe through an 18-gauge needle
  - ☐ Using a spray bottle
  - ☐ A "Water Pik"
  - ☐ Pressure equal to or above 7 psi *cannot* be achieved by gravity flow or lavage with a bulb syringe.
- Pressures of 10–15 psi have been shown to be approximately 80% effective in removing soil-potentiating factors and adherent bacteria from a wound.
- The Water Pik delivers 40–50 ml/min at 10–15 psi at the low-intermediate setting and is the most effective for heavily contaminated wounds. Pressures of 10–15 psi can also be achieved with a spray bottle.
- **CAUTION**: *Care must be taken so contaminants are not driven deeper within the wound and loose fascial planes are not inadvertently separated.*

Povidone-Iodine Solution

- Commonly used to lavage wounds because of its broad antimicrobial spectrum
- The free iodine gives the solution its antimicrobial activity and is complexed with polyvinylpyrrolidone to increase its stability; reduces irritation and staining.
- The complexing tightly binds the iodine and reduces the free iodine for antimicrobial activity.
- Diluting the solution uncouples the bond, making more free iodine available for antimicrobial activity.
- NOTE: *Povidone-iodine solutions diluted to 0.1% and 0.2% (1–2 ml/ 1000 ml) concentrations are best for wound lavage.*

Chlorhexidine Diacetate Solution

- Has a wide antimicrobial spectrum
- Commonly used as lavage solution
- When applied to the intact skin, its antimicrobial effect is immediate, and it has a lasting residual effect due to binding to protein in the stratum corneum.
- Chlorhexidine diacetate 0.05% has more bactericidal activity than povidone-iodine.
- NOTE: *Currently, 0.05% chlorhexidine (1:40 dilution of the 2% concentrate) solution is recommended for wound lavage. Greater concentrations can be deleterious to wound healing.*
- NOTE: Avoid contact with eyes; ocular toxicity has been documented.

Hydrogen Peroxide

- Common wound irrigant
  □ Narrow antimicrobial spectrum
  □ Has little value as an antiseptic
  □ Is an effective sporicide
- 3% hydrogen peroxide is damaging to tissues and cytotoxic to fibroblasts.
- Can cause thrombosis in the microvasculature adjacent to wound margins
- NOTE: *Hydrogen peroxide is not recommended for wound lavage.*

Wound Debridement

- Debridement reduces the number of bacteria and removes the contaminants (dead tissue, foreign bodies), which alters the local defense mechanisms.
- The standard approach is sharp debridement, converting a contaminated wound to a clean one.
- Chemical debriding agents are available; however, their effect on wound healing and reduction in the incidence of infection has not been elucidated.
- Debridement dressing includes
  □ Adherent open mesh gauze (e.g., 4 × 4 gauze sponges)

□ Wet-to-dry packing—using 4 × 4 mesh gauze or sheet cotton soaked in sterile 0.9% saline

Suturing Techniques and Suture Material

- Suturing and the material chosen influence wound healing.
- Simple interrupted sutured skin wounds, when compared with simple continuous sutured skin wounds, have
  □ Less edema
  □ Increased microcirculation
  □ 30%–50% greater tensile strength after 10 days
- NOTE: *Use interrupted sutures when impaired healing is anticipated and excessive tension is present.*
- Simple interrupted sutures cause less inflammation than vertical mattress and far-near–near-far patterns.
- Loosely approximated wounds are stronger at 7, 10, and 21 days postoperatively than wounds tightly secured with sutures.
- Recommendation
  □ Just appose wound edges.
  □ Avoid overreduction of tissues.
  □ Use tension-suturing techniques when excessive tension present (Fig. 27–3).
- Synthetic absorbable and nonabsorbable sutures cause less reaction than surgical gut, cotton and silk.
- Monofilament sutures are less reactive than twisted and braided materials.

Hematoma and Seroma

- Collection of blood or serum in tissues delays healing by mechanically separating the wound.
- If expanding fluid pressure is sufficient, it can alter the blood supply.
- Blood/serum provide excellent media for bacterial growth.
- Hemoglobin inhibits local tissue defenses and iron is necessary for bacterial replication; the ferric ion plays a role in increasing bacterial virulence.

Bandaging and Dressing

- Bandaging is considered beneficial for the following reasons:
  □ The wound is protected from further contamination.
  □ The pressure reduces edema.
  □ Exudate is absorbed.
  □ Bandages increase temperature and reduce CO_2 loss from the wound surface, thus reducing pH.
  □ Bandages immobilize a part and reduce additional trauma (e.g., a wound on the dorsal surface of the hock).
- Adherent dressings (open mesh gauze):
  □ Beneficial when applied during the debridement phase
  □ Deleterious when used during the repair phase of wound healing

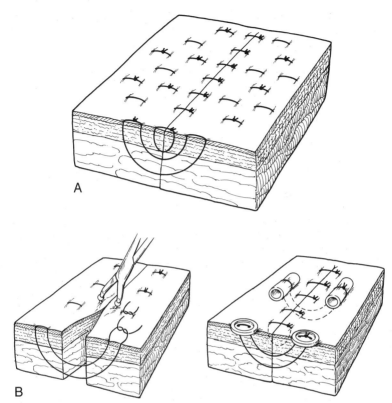

FIGURE 27–3. Tension suture patterns. A, Plain tension suturing technique, using vertical mattress sutures. B, Quill tension suturing technique, using vertical mattress sutures with supports. (From Stashak TS: Equine Wound Management. Philadelphia, Lea & Febiger, 1991.)

□ Aid the debridement of wounds by removing the absorbed exudate and necrotic tissue fragments
- Nonadherent semiocclusive dressings (e.g., Telfa, petroleum-impregnated gauze, and Dermaheal):
  □ Most beneficial when applied to the wound during the repair phase
  □ Wounds dressed with Telfa heal more rapidly than wounds dressed with amnion, mitriflex, and Biodres.
  □ Complete occlusion of wounds of the distal extremity promotes exuberant granulation tissue and mixed infections, which delay wound healing.
- Calcium alginate–dressed wounds heal at same rate as wounds dressed with Telfa.
- NOTE: *Telfa appears to be the dressing of choice during the repair phase of wound healing.*

- Hydrophilic dressings, such as copolymer flakes and dextranomer beads, stimulate the diffusion of wound fluids through the tissue, from inside to outside, and bathe the tissue and the fluids absorbed into the dressing.
  - □ By this process, tenacious coagulums and debris on the wound surface are diluted and drawn into the dressings.
  - □ They have not met wide acceptance.
- NOTE: *Clinically, the adherent dressings should be used only in the very early phases of wound healing when debridement is needed. After a healthy granulation tissue bed is formed, the use of nonadherent semiocclusive dressings such as Telfa is recommended.*

Dehydration and Edema

- Dehydration of the wound surface delays epithelialization by desiccation of the marginal epithelial cells, scab development.
- Poor perfusion of peripheral tissues in the dehydrated patient is believed the reason wound healing is delayed.
- The cause, extent, and location of the edema determine its effect on healing
  - □ Mild to moderate dependent edema unassociated with chronic disease processes or infection has little detrimental effect on wound healing.
  - □ Severe edema alters the vascular dynamics within the wound, which affects wound healing.
- *Treatments with NSAIDs, pressure bandaging, sweats under a bandage, and hydrotherapy are most beneficial in the treatment of edema associated with the limbs. Hand-walking exercise may be beneficial in the reduction of edema in regions of the upper body that cannot be bandaged.*

Blood Supply and Oxygen Tension

- Healing wounds depend on adequate microcirculation to supply nutrients and oxygen for healing.
- Alteration in the microcirculation can occur from
  - □ Applications of bandages or casts too tightly
  - □ Seroma formation
  - □ Tying sutures too tightly
  - □ Local trauma
  - □ The use of local anesthetics with vasoconstrictive agents
- Oxygen is required for cell migration, multiplication and synthesis of collagen, and protein in healing wounds.
- The migration and synthetic capabilities of the wound fibroblast depend on the rate at which revascularization occurs.
- Anything that impairs blood flow and subsequent delivery of oxygen retards wound healing.

Temperature and pH

- Wounds heal faster at higher temperatures and lower pH.
- Healing is accelerated at ambient temperatures of 30°C compared with 18–20°C.

- Lower temperatures, 12–20°C, reduce tensile strength in wounds by 20%, and alternating warm and cold temperatures delay wound healing.
  - □ The inhibitory effect on wound healing of lowering temperatures is a result of reflexive vasoconstriction and reduction of local blood flow.
- The use of warm hydrotherapy accelerates healing of sutured wounds and is beneficial during the inflammatory and debridement phase of healing of open wounds. *(It delays healing of open wounds if applied during the repair phase.)*
  - □ Moist heat above 60°C causes thermal injury to cells.
  - □ Moist heat at 49°C is optimum for acceleration of hemostasis in a newly incised wound.
  - □ Warm water hydrotherapy accelerates wound healing by increasing the blood flow.
- Acidification of a wound promotes healing by increasing the release of oxygen from hemoglobin.
- Alkalinity results from loss of CO_2 from the wound and/or from urease-producing bacteria in the wound.
- Bandaging is beneficial in increasing the wound surface temperature and decreasing the loss of carbon dioxide.

PRINCIPLES OF WOUND MANAGEMENT

- A rapid assessment of the wound should be followed by a physical examination, including the vital signs.
- A minor wound should not divert attention from more serious problems, such as
  - □ Hemorrhagic shock
  - □ Exhaustion
  - □ Cerebral contusion associated with head injuries
- The goal is to return the patient to a functional and cosmetic status as soon as possible.

History

- Historical features of the injury can be helpful in determining the approach to wound care.
- How long since the injury? Initially it was accepted that wounds treated within 6–8 hours after injury could be sutured with little risk of infection—the "golden period." Although this can be used as a rough guideline, other factors must be considered.
- Factors that contribute to a wound's susceptibility to infection:
  - □ Mechanism of injury
  - □ How the wound was managed
  - □ Degree and type of contamination
  - □ Location and type of wound
  - □ Virulence of the organism
  - □ Patient's immune status

Mechanism of Injury

- What caused the injury influences the patient's susceptibility to infection.
  - □ Lacerations caused by sharp objects such as metal, glass, and knives generally are resistant to infection.
  - □ Shear wounds from barbed wire, sticks, nails, and bites are more susceptible to infection because of the degree of soft tissue damage.
  - □ Soft tissue trauma from entanglement/entrapment or impact with a solid object or a kick is more susceptible to infection because of the degree of the soft tissue injury.
- *The greater the magnitude of the energy on impact, the more severe the soft tissue damage and the greater the alteration in blood supply.*

How the Wound Was Managed

- Substances such as lye, kerosene, gasoline, gentian violet, and pine tar are still used in wound care by some horse owners. Wounds treated with these substances *should not* be sutured by primary closure because the tissue damage is more extensive than can be seen, making the wound more susceptible to infection.

Degree and Type of Contamination

- Wounds contaminated with feces and dirt are at a high risk of infection despite treatment.
  - □ Feces have up to 10^{11} microorganisms/gram.
  - □ Infection-potentiating factors (IPFs) found in soil have organic components and inorganic clay fractions. These highly charged particles react directly with white cells and antibodies to alter their normal function and reduce bactericidal effectiveness. As few as 100 microorganisms cause infections in wounds contaminated with these factors.

Location and Type of Wound

- Generally, wounds involving the head region are more resistant to infection than those involving the distal extremities. Reason: the blood supply is better.
- Wounds with flaps that lack a good blood supply are more susceptible to infection.
- Degloving wounds that encircle the limb and damage the periosteum and paratendon are also more susceptible to infection due to lack of blood supply. Osteomyelitis and septic tendinitis can be sequelae.

Virulence of the Microorganism

- Generally, the more virulent the organisms, the greater the chances of infection.
- Fewer than 10^6 organisms can cause infection.

Immune Status of the Patient

- Poor health from chronic disease or insufficient nutrition can result in an altered immune status, making the patient more susceptible to infection.

Initial Wound Examination

- *The most important criteria in the decision on treatment of a wound are based on the physical examination of the wound and the patient.*
- Tissues adjacent to the wound edges are palpated for swelling and tissue temperature. Swollen, cool, discolored tissues indicate vascular compromise.
- The edges of the wound are separated to assess the extent of the wound and degree of contamination.
- *Avoid direct digital palpation of the wound until the wound is clipped, scrubbed, and lavaged.*
- Replace a skin flap into its normal position to identify tissue deficits.
- Using this approach provides insight into choice of treatment and prognosis.
- Factors affecting selection of the treatment:
  - ☐ Duration since injury
  - ☐ Wound location and depth
  - ☐ Has a synovial structure been penetrated?
  - ☐ Configuration of the wound
  - ☐ Degree of contamination
  - ☐ Severity and nature of the trauma
  - ☐ Economics
  - ☐ Patient temperament
  - ☐ Physical status
  - ☐ Intended use of horse

Wound Preparation

- Preparation of the wound for further examination is important.
- Some patients require sedation before wound preparation.
- Avoid using phenothiazine tranquilizers in hypovolemic shock.
- Regional perineural anesthesia is useful for wounds of the distal extremities, and regional infiltration of a local anesthetic is used elsewhere.
- Direct infiltration of the wound with a local anesthetic is acceptable after the wound is cleaned.
- Protect the wound with sterile moist gauze sponges, clip a wide area of hair around the wound, and shave the wound edges with a recessed head razor to prevent damage to the infundibulum of the hair follicle. *Dampen the hair with water or coat lightly with K-Y water-soluble jelly to prevent hair from falling into the wound.*
- Sponges used to pack the wound are discarded and replaced by new ones.
- Scrub the clipped area at least three times with antiseptic soap and rinse between scrubs with sterile 0.9% saline solution.
- The wound bed is gently cleaned with antiseptic soap and sterile gauze sponges, followed by lavage.
- The detergent base in antiseptics is neutralized with lavage.

Wound Lavage

- The mechanical effect of lavaging the wound with solutions under pressure is important for the removal of adherent contaminants and bacteria.
- Deliver lavage solutions by fluid jet and impact the wound with at least 7 psi (10–15 psi has been shown to be most effective). These pressures can be achieved using a spray bottle or Water Pik set at a low-intermediate setting.
- The addition of antiseptics and antibiotics to the lavage solution is effective in preventing wound infection. Povidone-iodine (0.1%–0.2%; 1–2 ml of PI/1000 ml of sterile solution) or chlorhexidine diacetate (0.05%) (1:40 dilution of the 2% concentrate) is effective and preferred.
- Lavage is discontinued before the tissues take on a "waterlogged" appearance and become discolored by a gray hue.

Wound Exploration

- After the wound is cleaned and free of devitalized tissue and debris, it is explored digitally using sterile gloves.
- A sterile probe is helpful in identifying the depth of the wound, a foreign body, or if bone is contacted, and can be used in conjunction with plain radiography.
- Synovial fluid is identified by stringing it between the thumb and forefinger; if questions remain, submit a sample for cytologic examination and culture/sensitivity.
- If you suspect that a synovial structure has been penetrated, place a needle in the synovial cavity at a site remote to the wound. If synovial fluid can be retrieved, it is submitted for cytology and culture/sensitivity. Following this, sterile saline solution is injected into the synovial structure; if the joint capsule has been violated, fluid is seen at the wound. If a synovial structure is involved, it is lavaged with 3–5 liters of sterile saline or crystalloid solution, followed by lavage with 1 liter of a 10% DMSO solution. Intrasynovial instillation of antibiotics is recommended.
- Ultrasound examination can document tendon and ligament injury and help in locating and identifying foreign bodies.

WOUND CLOSURE

- **Primary closure** is used for
  - Fresh, minimally contaminated wounds, with a good blood supply, not involving vital structures
  - Wounds of the head region
  - Flap wounds with a good blood supply
  - Wounds of the upper body when a good cosmetic result is required
- **Delayed primary closure** is used for
  - Severely contaminated, contused, or swollen wounds (and for wounds that involve a synovial structure)
- **Secondary closure** is used for
  - Chronic wounds with a compromised blood supply. When a healthy bed of granulation tissue develops, the wound is closed.

- **Second intention healing** is used for
  - □ Large wounds over moveable areas, such as the pectoral and gluteal regions
- Skin grafting is used when tissue deficits exceed the capability of wound contraction and epithelialization.
- Reconstructive surgery is used for a better cosmetic and functional end-result in a healed wound.

Primary Closure

Wound Preparation

- The wound is cleaned, lavaged, explored, and debrided.
- The skin and wound are scrubbed with antiseptic soap, after which the skin is rinsed with sterile saline and the wound is lavaged.
- The wound is then explored digitally, or with a probe.
- Excisional debridement is most effective in removing contaminants and bacteria in the superficial layers of the wound.
- After debridement is complete, the wound and surrounding skin are lavaged with a 0.1% povidone-iodine/sterile saline solution.
- Change surgical gloves, redrape if applicable, and use a new set of instruments for closure.
- Instill water-soluble, nonirritating antimicrobials in wounds if blood supply is questionable.

Suturing

- Sutures should just appose the tissues with minimal tension.
- Use the fewest number of sutures to close the wound effectively.
- Sutures should be used in deeper tissue to appose fascial layers, retinacula and joint capsules, and transected flexor tendons or ligaments.
- *Using a large number of sutures increases the chances of infection.*
- Synthetic monofilament absorbable and nonabsorbable sutures cause minimal inflammatory response and are preferred.

Tension Sutures

- Tension-suturing patterns are employed to reduce the tension on the primary suture line.
- Widely placed vertical mattress sutures with or without support, using buttons, gauze, or rubber tubing, are effective in reducing tension on the primary suture line (see Fig. 27–3).
  - □ Tension sutures with supports are used in regions that cannot be effectively bandaged (e.g., upper body and neck regions).
  - □ Tension sutures without supports are used in regions that are bandaged, or where a cast is applied.
- Tension sutures are removed in 4–10 days, depending on the appearance of the wound; staggered removal is preferred: removing half the sutures initially and the remaining half later.

Drains

- Drains are used when a large dead space remains after suture closure.
- Drains must be maintained in a sterile environment.
  - ☐ Use a sterile bandage for the extremities.
  - ☐ Use a sterile stent bandage for the upper body.
- *Drains should be sutured proximally, traverse the wound adjacent to but not directly underlying the sutured skin edges, and exit adjacent to the distal extremity of the wound. They should also be sutured at the point of exit.*
- The drain should exit from a separate incision adjacent to the wound edges. This placement of the drain reduces the chances of retrograde infection directly involving the suture line.
- Drains are usually left in place for 24–48 hours but may remain longer if drainage persists.

Delayed Primary Closure

- Delayed primary closure is closure of a wound before granulation tissue forms, usually within 4–5 days after injury.
- Healing and tensile strength gain are not appreciably affected by delayed closure.
- Before suture closure, the wound is maintained in a sterile environment under pressure bandage and assessed at bandage changes, daily or every other day. Antibiotics and NSAIDs are usually administered during this period.
- *Clean wounds with reduced swelling and a clear, serous, nonodoriferous surface fluid are candidates for closure.*
- The wound is clipped, shaved, cleaned, and debrided as needed, following the same principles described for primary closure.
- "Degloving" injuries require special consideration because they generally involve the cannon bone region, and the periosteum and paratendon are often compromised.
  - ☐ Bone devoid of periosteum and tendon without paratendon lack sufficient blood supply to support the development of granulation tissue, and they are more prone to infection.
  - ☐ There is an increased risk of bone sequestrum or tendon degeneration with continued infection if the blood supply is not able to support healing.
  - ☐ If delayed primary closure is used, the loose skin is held in place by a few sutures to provide a soft tissue covering for the exposed tendon and bone, which should provide sufficient blood supply to prevent bone infection and tendon degeneration until wound reconstruction.

Secondary Closure

- Secondary closure is used for chronic, severely contaminated, or infected wounds after granulation tissue formation. Heel bulb lacerations are frequently treated this way.
- The wound is cleaned, lavaged, cultured if necessary, debrided, and

placed in a bandage. Appropriate antimicrobials and NSAIDs are administered. Bandage changes are done daily until the exudative response is diminished and signs of infection are gone.

- Generally it takes 4–6 days before a healthy bed of granulation tissue appears that is free of infection.
- Reconstruction involves removal of the exuberant granulation tissue and apposition of the wound edges.
- If a large dead space exists, a drain is used to prevent the accumulation of serum within the wound.

Second Intention Healing

- Second intention healing depends on wound contraction and epithelialization to close the wound. It is used in cases of large tissue loss and wounds of the upper limbs, body, and neck.
- Wounds are prepared as for primary and delayed primary closure, except that wounds above the extremities are left uncovered. Appropriate antimicrobials and NSAIDs are administered. Bandage changes are done daily until the exudative response is diminished and signs of infection are gone.
- The uncovered wounds are cleaned daily to remove the exudate and tissue debris.
- The exposed skin below the wound is cleaned and covered with petroleum jelly to prevent serum burns. The distal limb is supported with bandages.
- When a healthy bed of granulation tissue forms, the frequency of cleaning is reduced and antimicrobials discontinued unless skin grafting is planned.
- If a skin flap is present or the wound is gaping, use a few well-placed sutures to support the wound.

Exuberant Granulation Tissue

- Wounds of the distal limb, below the carpus and tarsus, with large tissue deficits present a special problem with the development of exuberant granulation tissue.
- Factors believed involved in the formation of exuberant granulation tissue include
  □ Increased movement
  □ Lack of soft tissue covering
  □ Excessive contamination
  □ Reduced blood supply to the distal extremities
- Treatment is directed at preventing the formation of exuberant granulation tissue, using pressure bandages and casts.
- Excessive granulation tissue is managed in the following ways:
  □ Application of a steroid-antibiotic ointment and pressure bandage
  □ *Steroids applied to newly formed granulation tissue have very little effect on delaying wound healing when applied after 5 days.*
  □ Granulation tissue protruding above the skin surface, forming a fibrogranuloma, is excised, followed by a pressure bandage or cast.
- Caustics and astringents effectively remove and prevent the formation of

granulation tissue by chemical destruction. Chemicals are not selective and destroy migrating epithelial cells, resulting in prolonged healing, increased inflammation, and excessive scarring.

SELECTION OF WOUND SUPPORTS

Bandages

- Bandages are applied over wounds of the extremities to protect the wound from additional contamination, prevent edema, absorb secretions, and prevent movement.
- Wounds are generally covered with a nonadherent dressing, followed by application of a conforming gauze.
- For pressure, elastic adhesive bandage is applied over the conforming gauze, followed by a cotton bandage.
- If further immobilization is important, additional layers of cotton are used, or a polyvinyl chloride splint is incorporated into the bandage and/ or a cast applied.

Casts

- A cast is generally recommended with lacerations of the coronary band, heel bulbs, dorsal surface of the fetlock, degloving injuries, and injuries to tendons and ligaments.
- Additionally, casts are used after repair of deep lacerations perpendicular to the long axis of the wound to minimize movement of the fetlock, carpus and/or hock, and tension on the wound.
- If these wounds are not immobilized with a cast, dehiscence can occur.
- NOTE: *Wounds of the distal extremities that are sutured under tension are generally managed with a cast.*

B. BURNS AND ACUTE SWELLINGS

Thomas J. Divers

THERMAL INJURY (BURNS)

Thermal injury to the horse is typically rare. Most cases involve barn fires, lightning, electricity, caustic chemicals, or friction. The majority of burns are superficial, easily managed, and inexpensive to treat, and heal in a short period of time. More serious burns, on the other hand, may result in rapid, severe "burn shock" or hypovolemia with associated cardiovascular changes (smoke inhalation and corneal ulceration are also of considerable concern). Treatment of these severe and extensive burns is difficult, expensive, and time consuming. Before treatment, it is recommended that the patient be carefully examined with regard to cardiovascular status, pulmonary function, ocular damage, and extent/ severity of the burns, and that prognosis be discussed with the owner.

History and Physical Examination

- A good history helps determine the cause and severity of burns. Skin typically takes a long time to absorb heat and also a long time to dissipate the absorbed heat. Therefore, the longer the individual is exposed, the worse the situation and prognosis.

- It is **imperative** that the entire patient be examined, not just the burns. Horses frequently become severely hypovolemic and shocky as well as have respiratory difficulty. Thermal injuries may cause significant immune system suppression.

Clinical Signs/Findings

- Skin burns are most common on the back and face. Erythema, pain, vesicles, and singed hair are common findings.
- An increase in heart and respiratory rates
- Abnormal discoloration of mucous membranes is common.
- Blepharospasms and/or epiphora may indicate corneal damage.
- Coughing may indicate smoke inhalation.
- Fever

Laboratory Findings

- Shock (decreased cardiac output, low total solids and blood volume, increased vascular permeability)
  □ Anemia may be severe and steadily progressive.
- Hemoglobinuria
- Hyperkalemia—may occur early but later the patient becomes hypokalemic with blood volume expansion.

Classification of Burns

Superficial

- Thickened, erythematous epidermis
- Typically painful
- Heal readily by epithelialization
- Prognosis excellent*

Partial Thickness

- Severe subcutaneous edema
- Inflammation
- Typically very painful
- Heal by epithelialization from deeper skin appendages
- Prognosis good*

Full Thickness

- No dermis remaining
- Damage to underlying tissue structures
- No cutaneous sensation

---

*Assuming there is minimal ocular and respiratory involvement.

- Healing requires time and epithelialization from the wound edges. Skin grafting may be required.
- Prognosis can be poor, depending on extent.

Management and Treatment
Superficial Burns

- Typically not life-threatening
- Immediately cool affected area (ice or cold water) to draw heat out of tissues and decrease continued dermal necrosis.
- Topical water-soluble antibacterial creams: aloe vera or silver sulfadiazine creams are good.
  - ☐ Prevents infection
  - ☐ Decreases thromboxane activity
- Pain control—nonsteroidal administration of flunixin meglumine (Banamine), phenylbutazone (Butazolidin), ketoprofen (Ketofen)

Partial Thickness Burns

- Typically not life-threatening
- Treatment is same as for superficial burns.
- Typically cause vesicle/blister formation. Leave intact for 36 hours, then open by removing the top and applying copious antibacterial cream.
- A bandage, if possible, is a good idea as long as it is not tight, allows drainage, and does not stick to the wound. Change daily.

Full Thickness Burns

- Potentially life-threatening—*Treat shock first.*
- Treat as for superficial and partial thickness burns.
- Clip surrounding hair and debride all devitalized tissue.
- Copious lavage with sterile polyionic fluid with or without chlorhexidine (0.05% solution) is beneficial.
- Apply moist bandage with antibacterial cream. A shroud (sheet) soaked in antiseptic solution (e.g., povidone-iodine, chlorhexidine diacetate) and draped over the topline of the patient works well for dorsal burns.
  - ☐ Change bandage frequently and debride devitalized tissue as it appears.
  - ☐ Leave eschar intact.

Burn Shock—Life-Threatening

- Large volumes of lactated Ringer's solution (LRS) may be required. Alternatively, use hypertonic saline, 4 ml/kg, with plasma, followed by more isotonic fluids.
- Use LRS until electrolytes dictate otherwise.
- Carefully monitor hydration status, lung sounds, and cardiovascular status.
- Administer plasma. (NOTE: As a general rule in a 450-kg adult, 1 liter of plasma increases the total solids 0.2 gm/L.)

- Gradually increase grain availability, add 4–8 oz vegetable oil, and feed free-choice alfalfa hay.
  - □ Individuals with significant burns have a negative nitrogen balance and an increased metabolic rate with high energy demand. Gradually increasing the grain, adding fat, and offering free-choice alfalfa hay increases caloric intake and helps restore nitrogen balance.
  - □ If smoke inhalation is a concern or there is evidence of burns around the face, hay should be water soaked and fed on the ground, paper used as bedding, and good ventilation provided.
- Anabolic steroids, boldenone undecylenate (Equipoise), may be used to help restore nitrogen balance.
- Dimethyl sulfoxide (DMSO) administered IV, 1 gm/kg for the first 24 hours, may decrease inflammation and pulmonary edema.
  - □ If pulmonary edema is present and is unresponsive to DMSO and furosemide treatment, administer dexamethasone, 0.5 mg/kg IV once only.
- If there are respiratory signs or smoke inhalation is suspected, begin systemic antimicrobial therapy. Use penicillin IM to protect against oral contaminants colonizing the airway. Broad-spectrum antimicrobial therapy may encourage fungal growth. If respiratory signs worsen, a transtracheal aspirate should be performed, and additional broad-spectrum antimicrobial therapy administered based on Gram stain, culture, and sensitivity.

Complications

Wound Infection

Severe burns become infected. Most infections are caused by normal skin flora.
- *Pseudomonas aeruginosa, Staphylococcus aureus, Escherichia coli*, beta-hemolytic streptococcus, *Streptococcus* spp., *Klebsiella pneumoniae, Proteus, Clostridium*, and *Candida* are commonly isolated.
- It is appropriate to change antibacterial creams as needed to control infection.
  - □ Silver sulfadiazine is effective against gram-negative organisms such as *Pseudomonas*.
  - □ Aloe vera is reported to have antiprostaglandin and antithromboxane properties as well as providing pain relief, decreased inflammation, stimulation of cell growth, and antibacterial/antifungal activity.

Smoke Inhalation

See p. 447.

Corneal Ulceration/Eyelid Burns

- If the lids are swollen, apply ophthalmic antibiotic ointment to the cornea q 6 h.
- Examine the cornea for ulceration initially and twice daily. If damaged,

debride the necrotic cornea after tranquilization and topical anesthetic application.

- Apply antibiotics and cycloplegics (atropine) topically. Do **not** use corticosteriods.
- A third eyelid flap may be needed to protect the cornea from a necrotic eyelid.
- Silver sulfadiazine can be used around the eyes but not chlorhexidine.

Laminitis

See p. 323.

Kidney Damage

See Acute Renal Failure, p. 462.

Pruritus

- Frequently seen in healing burns and may require sedation throughout most of the healing process
- Acepromazine (injectable or granules) works well.
- Antihistamines may also be effective.

ACUTE SWELLINGS—EDEMA

Acute edematous conditions in the horse most commonly result from increased hydrostatic pressure, septic inflammation, or local or general immune response. Acutely occurring hypoproteinemia is a less common cause. Inflammatory conditions, both septic and immunologic, are usually painful to the touch. Edema resulting from increased hydrostatic pressure is less painful and in many cases nonpainful.

Purpura Hemorrhagica

- Consider this with any unexplained vasculitis and edema.
- Edema most commonly seen in the limbs and ventral abdomen and often moderately painful to the touch. May form elsewhere in the body, causing *respiratory distress* (*laryngeal swelling* and *pulmonary edema*), *colic, heart failure* (*distress* and *trembling*), or *myositis* (*stiffness*).
- **Fever and petechiae of mucous membranes are seen in approximately 50% of cases**.
- There is often a history of respiratory infection or exposure to *Streptococcus equi* (most frequent) or *S. zooepidemicus* in the preceding 2–4 weeks.

Diagnosis

- Made by CBC, creatine kinase (CK), aspartate aminotransferase (AST), platelet count, serum IgA, and serology for serum streptococcal M protein antibody and immune complexes (performed by Dr. John Timoney, Gluck Equine Research Center, University of Kentucky; (606) 257 1531).

- A skin specimen from an edematous area using a 6-mm Baker biopsy punch (Baker Cummins Pharmaceuticals Inc., Miami, FL 33178; (800) 347 4774) can be submitted in formalin to look for vasculitis. Detection of immunoglobulin deposition is rare, and submission in special media (Michel's) or snap freezing is recommended. The biopsy should not be taken in an area over an important structure (e.g., tendon).
- There is often a mature neutrophilia with CK and AST frequently elevated, with or without signs of myositis.
- A normal platelet count > 90,000 cells/μl is expected.
- An elevation in plasma protein is common, with an elevated IgA and a high antibody response to streptococcal M protein. However, high antibody response to streptococcal M protein can also be found in some normal horses.
- Severe proteinuria and even *hematuria* occur in some patients.

Differentials

Equine viral arteritis (EVA), infectious anemia, *Ehrlichia equi,* and Lyme disease. Be careful interpreting positive Lyme and EVA titers. Many normal horses in endemic areas have a titer to *Borrelia.* IFA antibody titer greater than 1:1280 is considered suspect for Lyme disease and additional testing with kinetic ELISA (<1:400) immunoblots and PCR (performed at Cornell University Diagnostic Laboratory [607] 253 3900) might be indicated. Most Standardbreds are serologically positive for EVA.

Treatment

- Corticosteroids: Dexamethasone, 0.04–0.16 mg/kg IV or IM q24h. Begin therapy at 0.08 mg/kg. If no response in 24–48 hours, the dosage needs to be increased or the diagnosis reconsidered. Continue at the clinical response dose for 2–3 days after signs resolve, and reduce the dosage over 7–14 days. Recurrence of clinical signs may occur as the steroid dosage is decreased or withdrawn.
  □ If corticosteroids are contraindicated, a plasma exchange can be attempted. Remove 8 ml/kg of the affected patient's blood and replace with 8 ml/kg compatible plasma.
  □ In mild cases, corticosteroids may not be needed.
- Antibiotics: Aqueous penicillin, 22,000 IU/kg q6h IV, or procaine penicillin, 22,000 IU/kg q12h IM during steroid therapy
- Furosemide, 0.5–1.0 mg/kg IV or IM q12–24h for 1–2 days for severe edema
- Leg wraps and hydrotherapy for limb edema
- Tracheotomy for life-threatening laryngeal edema (see p. 44).

> This is a serious disease with potential life-threatening complications in some cases. There is no single diagnostic test; purpura hemorrhagica is a clinical diagnosis. Clients should be informed of the risks of corticosteroid associated laminitis, generally low, and that laminitis may result from purpura-induced vasculitis.

Acute Onset of Edema in All Four Limbs

- This common occurrence may affect more than one individual on a farm.
- Fever is often present. Edema and fever affecting several individuals is often due to *equine herpes virus I, influenza, unidentified viruses*, or, less commonly, *viral arteritis*.
- Viral arteritis presents with ventral edema and focal areas of painful edema elsewhere on the body. Vasculitis caused by viral arteritis (EVA) may result in sloughing of the skin. Other viral infections usually do not cause as severe a vasculitis.

Diagnosis

- Made by history, clinical signs, virus isolation, and serology

> ***Hoary alyssum* poisoning is a toxic cause of limb edema, fever, and occasionally mild diarrhea affecting groups of horses in the northeastern/northcentral United States.** A member of the mustard family, the plant is evidently palatable to horses. Clinical signs usually occur 18–36 hours after consuming hay or pasture with large amounts of *Hoary alyssum* and resolve within 2–4 days of removal of contaminated hay.

Treatment

- NSAIDs: Dipyrone, 22 mg/kg, IV or IM, or phenylbutazone, 4.4 mg/kg PO q24h, as supportive therapy for viral infections.
- Corticosteroids: Prednisone, 1 mg/kg PO q24h, or dexamethasone, 0.04 mg/kg PO, IV, or IM q24h, **if the edema is progressive or persists more than 7 days.** Precaution: Auscultate the lungs and initiate prophylactic antibiotic therapy.
- Antibiotic: Ceftiofur, 1–5 mg/kg IV or IM q12h
- Cold hydrotherapy and leg wraps to decrease the swelling

Acute Edema Affecting Only One Horse in Group

Acute edema of all four limbs and/or ventral abdomen, generally accompanied by fever, may affect only one individual. Differential includes

- *Equine infectious anemia* (EIA)
- *Ehrlichiosis*
- *Borreliosis* (Lyme disease, which is probably rare)
- *Onchocerca*
- Pre- or *postfoaling ventral edema*
- *Purpura hemorrhagica* (see pp. 262–263)
- *Autoimmune hemolytic anemia* (see p. 284)
- *Autoimmune thrombocytopenia*
- *Right-sided heart failure* (see p. 138)
- *Ventral abdominal hernia*

- *Acute septic cellulitis* (see p. 267)
- *Idiopathic causes*

Equine Infectious Anemia (EIA)

The acute clinical syndrome caused by equine infectious anemia is rare but may cause *fever, edema, hemoglobinuria, jaundice, depression*, and *petechial or ecchymotic hemorrhages*. A Coggins test should be performed, although sero-conversion may not be present at the onset of the disease, requiring retesting 10–14 days later. If the individual survives and/or pending the diagnosis, it should be kept in a screened stall at least 200 yards from other horses.

Equine Ehrlichiosis (EE)/Equine Granulocytic Ehrlichiosis (EGE)

- *Ehrlichia equi* is a common cause of edema and fever in horses in certain areas of the western United States, e.g., northern California, as well as eastern New York and other northeastern states.
- The organism is spread by ticks (incubation period may be 1–9 days), which can frequently be found on the horse.
- Signs: *Depression, anorexia, ataxia, limb edema, fever*, and *petechial hemorrhages*
- Laboratory findings: *Thrombocytopenia, leukopenia*, and *mild anemia*. The organism (morula) is usually seen in the neutrophils with a Giemsa stain.
- Serology (sent to the University of California–Davis, Texas A&M University, or Louisiana State University) can be useful to confirm the diagnosis, if the disease has been present for several days.

Treatment

Tetracycline, 6.6 mg/kg IV q12h for 5–7 days, is effective.

Lyme Disease

Frequently cited as a cause of fever, lethargy, stiffness, edema, and malaise in horses in the northeastern United States.

> Lyme disease most commonly causes chronic lameness and rarely requires emergency treatment. Serologic results are quite variable, with some laboratories having IFA titers of 1:1200 and others reporting negative results on an identical sample.

A high IFA or enzyme-linked immunosorbent assay (ELISA) result (>1:1200) and strong reaction on immunoblot support the diagnosis. PCR on synovial membrane biopsy (send to Cornell Diagnostic Laboratory) may be required to confirm the diagnosis.

Treatment

If a horse exhibits the aforementioned clinical signs and has a high (> 1:1200) or changing titer to *Borrelia* with a strong positive immunoblot reaction, and if other diseases have been ruled out, then treat with intravenous tetracycline, 6.6 mg/kg IV q12–24h. A response should be seen in 3–5 days if the diagnosis is correct. Ceftiofur and doxycycline are used for longer term treatment of Lyme arthritis.

Onchocerca

Reaction to *Onchocerca cervicalis* larvae following anthelmintic therapy does not require treatment unless the ventral edema is very painful or the individual is febrile. In these cases, use dexamethasone, 0.05 mg/kg q24h, and antibiotics, ceftiofur, penicillin, or TMP-S.

Pre- or Postfoaling Ventral Edema

Rule out hernia, ruptured prepubic tendon (see p. 214), mastitis (see p. 429), cellulitis. If the mare is in good health and the edema is progressive, administer two dexamethasone (5 mg)/trichlormethiazide (200 mg) boluses PO q24h (ground-up, mixed in molasses). *This dose of dexamethasone is unlikely to produce abortion in late pregnant mares. Nevertheless, it should be used only when infectious causes have been ruled out and the edema is progressive.*

Idiopathic

Most individual cases are responsive to corticosteroids. May occasionally be seen as a herd outbreak in weanlings, yearlings, or adults, often with a respiratory and/or ocular component. If no septic cellulitis or abnormal lung sounds but progressive edema with severe pain, treat with steroids.

Anaphylactoid Reactions Causing Edema

Prior sensitization to an antigen is not always required for an anaphylactoid reaction. The most common drugs causing a reaction are vaccines, vitamin E and selenium, anthelmintics, penicillin, trimethoprim/sulfa, anesthetics, and NSAIDs. Many of the reactions to parenterally administered penicillin, TMP/S, and anesthetics that cause collapse are not immunologic in origin and are covered under *Adverse Drug Reactions* (see Chapter 39). **Anaphylactic reactions generally occur within minutes to 12 hours and may persist for several days. The clinical signs are *urticaria, dyspnea, sweating, collapse*, and occasionally *laminitis*.** Diagnosis is based on history of exposure.

Treatment

- Urticaria only—Antihistamine: Doxylamine succinate, 0.5 mg/kg IV or IM slowly, if cardiovascular status stable. Urticaria persists in many cases and may need to be treated with oral prednisolone, 0.4–1.6 mg/kg q24h or every other day for several days.

- Respiratory distress: Epinephrine 1:1000 (as packaged), 3–6 ml/450 kg given *slowly* IV, or 3–10 ml/450 kg IM in less severe cases. Tracheotomy (see p. 44) if laryngeal edema present. Furosemide, 1 mg/kg IV.
- Cardiovascular collapse and hypotension (poor pulse, pale membranes): epinephrine or 2 liters hypertonic saline or dobutamine, 50 mg/500 ml in dextrose solution administered over 10–20 minutes to a 450-kg horse (5–10 μg/kg/min).
- Corticosteroids: Dexamethasone, 0.25 mg/kg IV, may be used in addition to the previous therapies listed if the edema is rapidly progressive.

Idiopathic Urticaria

Occurs in either a generalized or local form. The generalized form is often a persistent problem, although immediate response to corticosteroids or antihistamines is often good. Local edema (ocular, nasal, laryngeal) may occasionally occur, without known cause. Conjunctival edema of one or both eyes is the most common.

Treatment

- Ocular: Ophthalmic corticosteroids after a *careful* and *complete* examination of the eye and fluorescein stain *reveals no corneal erosion.*
- Skin urticaria—Antihistamine or corticosteroids: Hydroxyzine hydrochloride, 1.0–1.5 mg/kg q8–12h, or prednisone, 0.5 mg/kg PO q24h. This form may recur for weeks or months.

Cellulitis

Septic cellulitis is the most common cause of painful inflammatory edema in horses. Usually associated with a wound or a local reaction to an injection. Pain and progressive swelling are the characteristic findings. Diagnosis is based on Gram stain and culture of a sample of the fluid. Anaerobic culture tubes (Port-A-Cul, Becton-Dickinson Microbiology Systems, Cockeysville, MD 21030) are recommended. Probe the wound to establish drainage and to search for a foreign body. Ultrasound with a 7.5 MHz probe to localize and evaluate the fluid and to look for hyperechoic foreign bodies.

> *Staphylococcus aureus* and *Clostridium* spp. infections are very common etiologic agents of severe and often rapidly spreading cellulitis in the horse.

Staphylococcal infections may result from blunt trauma, e.g., starting gate, bruise to the hock, without a noticeable break in the skin. *Staphylococcal and clostridial infections are considered the most pathogenic causes of cellulitis in the horse.*

Treatment

- Antibiotics:
  - □ Penicillin, 40,000 IU/kg IV q6h, and gentamicin,* 6.6 mg/kg q24h IV, if severe and rapidly progressive and if there is the probability of a mixed bacterial infection.
  - □ *If an anaerobic infection is suspected based on smell of the exudate and/or subcutaneous gas, add metronidazole, 15–25 mg/kg PO q6-8h, to the treatment.*
  - □ In less severe cases or when **only gram-positive cocci (Staph.) are seen on Gram stain, ceftiofur and/or trimethoprim/sulfa may be used.** Rarely, vancomycin is required.
- Hydrotherapy: Septic and aseptic (injection site) cellulitis, cold water therapy for the first 24 hours, followed by warm water therapy
- Support-wrap if on an extremity
- NSAID: Phenylbutazone, 4.4 mg/kg q12h for 2–3 days
- NOTE: Should tetanus toxoid or antitoxin or both be given to horses with a wound?
  - □ Tetanus toxoid is administered to **all** patients. If on routine vaccination prophylaxis, antitoxin is not given.
  - □ If the wound has occurred in an individual less than 2 years of age with questionable tetanus vaccination, use antitoxin (preferably a product with low incidence of serum hepatitis associated with administration of TAT).

> **Antitoxin should be administered to adults only if there is no history of previous tetanus toxoid vaccination.**

- Surgical drainage

Malignant Edema — Clostridial Myositis

Most commonly occurs on the chest from a wound, at the site of a nonantibiotic intramuscular injection, or from perivascular injections. The most common IM-administered drug associated with malignant edema is flunixin meglumine, probably because it is the nonantibiotic drug most frequently administered IM.

- Clinical signs: Acute painful swelling, which is warm and soft and becomes cool and firm, subcutaneous crepitus, a stiff neck after a cervical injection, inability to lower the head, and, rarely, ataxia.
- **Subcutaneous crepitus is absent in many cases of clostridial myositis**.
- Diagnosis: Made by needle aspirate and Gram stain to look for large, gram-positive bacilli. Place the fluid sample in anaerobic culture media (Port-A-Cult) and send a slide for fluorescent antibody examination.

---

*If using gentamicin, check serum creatinine every 2–3 days and be sure the patient is producing urine.

Treatment

- Antibiotics: **Penicillin**, 40,000 IU/kg IV q4–6h, and metronidazole, 15–25 mg/kg PO q6h, or per rectum, 25–30 mg/kg q6h
- **Surgical incision and drainage** or a radical incision may be needed if the disease appears rapidly progressive or no improvement seen after 24 hours of antimicrobial treatment
- Oral anti-inflammatory therapy: Phenylbutazone, 4.4 mg/kg PO q12–24h
- Hydrotherapy
- Tetanus prophylaxis

Lymphangitis

This is a serious emergency. Two important points:

- **The longer the leg remains swollen, the more severe the anatomic disruption of the lymphatics.**
- **The greatest chance of obtaining a positive bacterial culture is the untreated acute case**.

There is often an *acute progressive swelling of one hindlimb.* **Acute bacterial lymphangitis may cause limb swelling, with serum oozing through the skin**. Fungal infections are usually nodular and slower to develop. Acutely affected individuals are febrile and frequently very lame. Diagnosis is based on ultrasound examination using a 7.5-MHz probe revealing numerous dilated vessels (lymphatics). The gross and ultrasound appearance of the limb is fairly uniform compared with cellulitis. A wound may or may not be present on the leg. Culture of the fluid should be attempted using a 22-gauge needle to minimize damage to the limb and avoid vessels. **An etiologic agent generally is not identified**.

Treatment

- Antibiotics: Trimethoprim/sulfa, 20–25 mg/kg PO q12h, or tetracycline, 6.6 mg/kg IV q12h, or others that are effective against *Staphylococcus aureus*
- Anti-inflammatory: Phenylbutazone, 4.4 mg/kg IV or PO q12h
- Aggressive hydrotherapy with cold water. Use a Jacuzzi, hydrotherapy, or cold boot if available (P. I. Medical, Athens, TN (800) 963 9632). If the patient can get its leg in the boot, the constant pressure of the water decreases the size. Prompt reduction in the swelling may minimize damage to the leg.
- Pentoxifylline, 8.4 mg/kg PO q8–12h to improve circulation in the severely swollen leg
- Support-wrap on the opposite leg, and monitor closely for laminitis
- Moderate walking
- Furosemide, 1 mg/kg IV or IM q12–24h for two treatments, or trichlormethiazide/dexamethasone (Naquasone) for *recurrent* cases *without* fever
- Support-wrap with furacin-sweat applied to affected leg.

The owners should be advised that this is a serious disease, the etiologic agent is rarely identified, the prognosis is guarded unless there is a rapid response to therapy, and recurrence is common.

Corynebacterium pseudotuberculosis

An acute and progressive swelling in the pectoral area, mammary gland, ventral abdomen, inguinal area (causing swelling of one limb), or sporadically elsewhere on the body. It can cause nodular lymphangitis and affects horses in the western United States. Ultrasound examination reveals deep abscesses proximal to the swelling.

Treatment

- Drainage and systemic procaine penicillin, 20,000–44,000 IU/kg q12h IM

Hematoma

Acute swelling due to vessel rupture and blood collection. A common cause is a kick. If the swelling is not progressive, the hematoma is allowed to organize and surgical drainage considered at a later date. If the skin is injured, administer antimicrobials, e.g., penicillin. NOTE! Rule out thrombocytopenia as the cause of the hematoma, before administering intramuscular injections, by examining the mucous membranes for petechial hemorrhages. If the hematoma is rapidly progressive, an artery may have been ruptured, or rarely a large vein. **Most rapidly progressive hematomas of the limbs are associated with a fracture, e.g., fractured pelvis and laceration of the iliac artery**. Severe lameness also suggests a fracture. If no cause for the hematoma is found and it is progressive in spite of medical treatment, consider surgery to locate and ligate the vessel.

Treatment

- Phenylbutazone, 4.4 mg/kg PO q12–24h, because it has little effect on platelet function. Butorphanol, 0.01–0.02 mg/kg IV, 2–5 minutes after a low doseage of xylazine, 0.2–0.4 mg/kg IV, for sedation
- Polyionic fluids: no hypertonic saline when first examined.
- Pressure wrap if possible.
- Whole blood transfusion if hemorrhage is progressive, patient is deteriorating, and/or if PCV drops to <18% within 12 hours after the start of bleeding.

> NOTE: Caution is advised in using the PCV as a guide for transfusion because it can be quite variable between patients during the first 12–18 hours. If thrombocytopenia is present, the blood should be freshly collected in a plastic container for transfusion.

- Aminocaproic acid, 20 mg/kg, mixed in 3 liters of saline may be used for prolonged bleeding.

Nutritional Myopathy

Acute muscle swelling caused by selenium deficiency is rare but may occur. Swelling of the masseter and pterygoid muscles (masseter myopathy) results in a severe swelling of the facial muscles and protrusion of the conjunctiva. Affected individuals appear stiff and reluctant to chew but can eat. The urine is frequently dark colored and strongly positive for occult blood (myoglobin) on urine dipstick examination. This is usually a disease of poorly fed horses. Blood (whole blood, plasma, or serum) is collected for measurement of selenium (normal, 15–25 mg/dl) and serum creatine kinase.

Treatment

- Selenium, 0.05 mg/kg/adult **IM**, repeat in 3 days if the diagnosis is confirmed.
- DMSO, 1 gm/kg diluted IV, once as ancillary therapy
- Warm compresses on the affected area
- Nursing care for any tissue compromised by the swelling, e.g., conjunctiva
- Phenylbutazone, 4.4 mg/kg PO q12h

Snake Bite, Spider Bite, and Bee Sting

Occasionally these result in severe swellings in horses. Snake bites are more common on the noses of horses, causing airway obstruction and hemolysis (see *Nasal Obstruction*, p. 44). Black widow spiders can cause hot, painful swellings. The diagnosis is supported by finding the spider in the stall. Fire ants can cause an acute swelling, particularly of the distal extremities, and are common in the southeastern United States where they build large mounds (nests). Bee stings cause acute, painful swellings and are occasionally fatal if in large numbers. Bee stings are identified by circular areas of edema with a stinger in the center of the swelling.

Treatment

- Antihistamine: Doxylamine succinate, 0.5 mg/kg; hydroxyzine hydrochloride, 1.0–1.5 mg/kg
- Corticosteroids: Dexamethasone, 0.04 mg/kg IM **if severe**
- Epinephrine, 3–7 ml (1:1000 solution)/450 kg adult slowly IV or SQ, only in cases with systemic (anaphylactic) involvement and respiratory distress
- **Airway maintenance: Place a short endotracheal tube in the nasal passages before the swelling becomes severe, to prevent the need for tracheotomy. This is especially important in individuals bitten on the nose by a snake**.
- Broad-spectrum antibiotics for snake bites, e.g., penicillin, 44,000 IU/kg IV q6h, and gentamicin,* 6.6 mg/kg q24h and metronidazole, 15 mg/kg PO q6–8h, or 25–30 mg/kg per rectum q8h
- Tetanus toxoid
- NSAID therapy for snake bites: flunixin meglumine, 0.8 mg/kg q12h IV for 3 days. **Because of the size of the patient, the frequent time delay**

---

*Monitor serum creatine, hydration status, and urine production.

between the bite and clinical recognition of the problem, and the possibility of an adverse reaction, antivenin is rarely indicated.

Fly Bites

Rarely require emergency treatment. Occasionally severe reactions seen to horse flies (core of necrotic tissue in the center of the swellings), stable flies, horn flies, or black flies (characteristic hemorrhagic center in the urticarial swelling). Rarely, large numbers of black fly bites may cause death.

Other Causes of Acute Dermatitis

Contact dermatitis, photosensitivity, and drug eruptions can require emergency treatment. Photosensitivity is caused by liver disease, most commonly from toxic plants or less commonly from mycotoxins on the plants. Drug eruptions in the form of multifocal dermatitis bizarre in appearance or distribution may occur at any time during treatment or within a couple of days of discontinuing treatment.

Treatment

- Corticosteroids, topical or systemic (in severe cases only), for contact dermatitis or photosensitivity
- Removal of the causative agent

Acute and Severe Pruritus

Most common in the summer months due to acute *Culicoides* hypersensitivity. Drug eruptions (see above), stinging nettle, fire ants, and other insect bites can cause intense pruritus. Also consider neurologic disorders such as rabies or self-mutilation syndrome in stallions.

Treatment

- Corticosteroids: Prednisone, 2 mg/kg, to control itching in severe cases.

SUGGESTED REFERENCES

Wound Healing and Management

Baxter GM, Doran RE, Moore JN. Management of lower leg wounds with delayed closure in horses. Proc 32nd Annual Meeting Am Assoc Equine Pract 1986;341–347.

Booth LC. Wound Management. Vet Clin North Am 1989; 5(3).

Fogdestam I. A biomechanical study of healing rat skin incisions after delayed primary closure. Surg Gynecol Obstet 153(2):191–199, 1981.

Fretz PB, Martin GS, Jacobs KA. Treatment of exuberant granulation tissue in the horse. Evaluation of four methods. Vet Surg 1983;12:137–140.

Lindsay WA. Reconstructive Surgery. Prob Vet Med 1990;2(3):397–550.

Peacock EE, Jr. Wound Repair. 3rd ed. Philadelphia, WB Saunders, 1984.

Rodeheaver GT, Petty D, Thacker JG, et al. Wound cleaning by high pressure irrigation. Surg Gynecol Obstet 1975;141:357.

Stashak TS. Suture patterns used for wound closure in veterinary surgery. Proc 24th Annual Meeting Am Assoc Equine Pract 1978;383–394.

Stashak TS. Equine Wound Management. Philadelphia, Lea & Febiger, 1991.

Swain SF. Wound healing. *In* Surgery of Traumatized Skin. Philadelphia, WB Saunders, 1980, pp 70–115.

Burns and Acute Swellings

PURPURA HEMORRHAGICA
Divers TJ, Timoney JF. Group C streptococcal antigen-antibody immune complex disease in horses. Proc Am Coll Vet Intern Med, San Diego, 1992, pp 304–305.

EQUINE INFECTIOUS ANEMIA
Lucas MH, Davies THR. Equine infectious anemia. Eq Vet Educ 1995;7(2):89–92.

IDIOPATHIC URTICARIA
Fadok VA. Overview of equine papular and nodular dermatoses. Vet Clin North Am 1995;11(1):61–63.

MALIGNANT EDEMA
Rebhun WC, Shin SJ, King JM, Baum KH, Patten V. Malignant edema in horses. JAVMA J Am Vet Med Assoc 1985;187(7):732–736.

NUTRITIONAL MYOPATHY
Step DL, Divers TJ, Cooper B, Kallfelz FA, Karcher FL, Rebhun WC. Severe masseter myonecrosis in a horse. J Am Vet Med Assoc 1991;198(1):117–119.

28 Liver Failure; Hemolytic Anemia

Thomas J. Divers

ICTERUS (JAUNDICE)

Icterus usually indicates *hemolytic disease, liver failure*, or a *physiologic* cause (Fig. 28–1). These can usually be separated with a good history, clinical examination, and a few laboratory tests. If a significant problem is found in another organ system, e.g., pleuritis, then the icterus is probably a physiologic icterus associated with anorexia. Physiologic icterus in adults is believed to result from anorexia, increased plasma free fatty acids (FFA), and competition between FFA and bilirubin for hepatic uptake. *Icterus in young, septic foals is very common and may be a result of multiple physiologic mechanisms.* The best way to detect clinical icterus is by examining the membranes of the sclera, mouth, and vagina.

History

- If physiologic, history indicates inappetence for more than 2 days.
- If neurologic signs or photosensitivity are present, suspect liver failure.

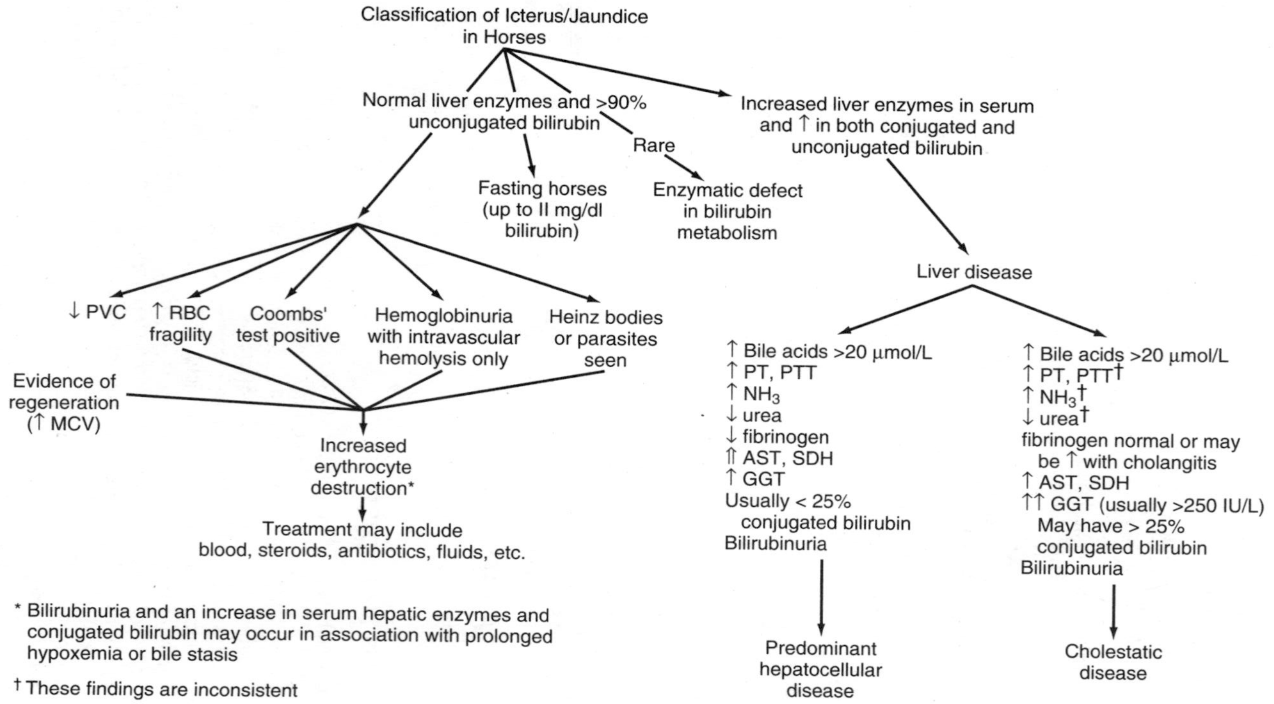

FIGURE 28–1 *See legend on opposite page*

Classification of Icterus/Jaundice in Horses

Normal liver enzymes and >90% unconjugated bilirubin

Increased liver enzymes in serum and ↑ in both conjugated and unconjugated bilirubin

Rare

Enzymatic defect in bilirubin metabolism

Fasting horses (up to II mg/dl bilirubin)

Liver disease

↓ PVC

↑ RBC fragility

Coombs' test positive

Hemoglobinuria with intravascular hemolysis only

Heinz bodies or parasites seen

Evidence of regeneration (↑ MCV)

Increased erythrocyte destruction*

Treatment may include blood, steroids, antibiotics, fluids, etc.

↑ Bile acids >20 µmol/L
↑ PT, PTT
↑ NH₃
↓ urea
↓ fibrinogen
⇑ AST, SDH
↑ GGT
Usually < 25% conjugated bilirubin
Bilirubinuria

Predominant hepatocellular disease

↑ Bile acids >20 µmol/L
↑ PT, PTT†
↑ NH₃†
↓ urea†
fibrinogen normal or may be ↑ with cholangitis
⇑ AST, SDH
↑↑ GGT (usually >250 IU/L)
May have > 25% conjugated bilirubin
Bilirubinuria

Cholestatic disease

* Bilirubinuria and an increase in serum hepatic enzymes and conjugated bilirubin may occur in association with prolonged hypoxemia or bile stasis

† These findings are inconsistent

274

- During late summer and fall in Eastern United States, incidence of both liver failure and hemolysis is increased since both red maple poisoning and Theiler's disease are more prevalent during this time.
- With either liver failure or hemolysis, urine color is dark red, bright red, black, or orange.

Diagnostic Tests

- □ If a urine sample is collected, dipstick examination is helpful.
- □ *Physiologic icterus*: Usually no abnormalities on urinalysis.
- □ *Liver failure*: Usually bilirubinuria (shaking may produce a green foam)
- □ *Hemolysis*: Strong reaction to occult blood and occasionally reaction to bilirubin if the hemolytic disease is of several days' duration.
- Best tests for determining the cause of icterus:
  - □ Packed cell volume (PCV) and total protein: Low PCV and normal to high total protein are most compatible with hemolysis. Pink plasma confirms intravascular hemolysis.
  - □ Gamma glutamyl transaminopeptidase (GGT): Elevations in the serum confirm liver disease.
  - □ Bilirubin: Increases in direct and indirect bilirubin with an elevation in GGT and a normal to high PCV indicate liver failure. An increase in only indirect bilirubin with a PCV < 25% indicates hemolysis.
- Physiologic icterus: If suspected, treat the primary cause; should resolve in 24–36 hours. Rarely, a healthy individual has persistent icterus and hyperbilirubinemia (indirect) associated with a conjugation defect.
- Hemolysis: If suspected, see p. 284.

LIVER FAILURE

Patients with liver failure may be examined on an emergency basis because of bizarre, maniacal behavior, blindness, severe depression, acute dermatitis (photosensitivity), discolored urine (bilirubinuria), or jaundice. Theiler's disease is one of the most common liver disorders requiring emergency care. Affected individuals may be either maniacal or obtunded and may demonstrate colicky signs.

Hyperlipemia in ponies and miniature horses is another common condition requiring immediate medical care. Affected individuals are generally depressed rather than maniacal, and edema of the ventral abdomen is a frequent finding.

Chronic active hepatitis and diseases that cause progressive fibrosis, e.g., pyrrolizidine alkaloid toxicosis and cholangiohepatitis, may cause a sudden demise, with severe depression, yawning, or maniacal behavior, necessitating emergency care. *Liver disease with elevations in serum hepatic enzyme activity is common with intestinal disorders and/or endotoxemia, but progression to liver failure is rare.*

FIGURE 28–1. Equine icterus/jaundice classification. AST, aspartate aminotransferase; GGT, gamma glutamyl transaminopeptidase; MCV, mean corpuscular volume; NH₃, ammonia; PT, prothrombin time; PTT, partial prothrombin time; PCV, packed cell volume; SDH, sorbitol dehydrogenase.

HEPATIC DISORDERS CAUSING LIVER FAILURE

Theiler's Disease (Serum Hepatitis)

General Information

- Disease of adults
- Often seen during late summer or fall
- May be more than one horse on a farm affected over a period of several weeks
- *May* have a history of previous tetanus antitoxin or other equine origin serum being administered 4–10 weeks earlier

> **In areas of the United States other than the western states, if you are called in late summer or fall to examine an adult with signs of acute encephalopathy without fever, the most likely diagnosis is Theiler's disease.**

Clinical Signs

HEPATOENCEPHALOPATHY

- Depression or bizarre behavior
- Blindness
- Ataxia

HYPERBILIRUBINEMIA

- Icteric mucous membranes—the neurologic signs may occur before the icterus in peracute cases.
- Discolored urine—bilirubinuria (with hemoglobinuria in some cases)

Laboratory Findings

- Marked elevations in serum hepatocellular-derived enzymes
  - ☐ Aspartate aminotransferase (AST): Usually > 1000 IU/L; more than 4000 IU/L is a poor prognosis.
- Moderate increase in biliary-derived enzymes
  - ☐ GGT usually between 100 and 300 IU/L
- Bilirubinemia—the direct (conjugated) bilirubin concentration is increased, but the most dramatic increase is usually in unconjugated bilirubin.
- Prolongation of prothrombin (PT) and partial thromboplastin (PTT) times (submit in blue top/citrate tube with a control sample)

Diagnosis

- Ultrasound examination
  - ☐ Usually cannot see the liver on the right side of the abdomen but it can be seen at the 7th–8th intercostal space low on the left. It may

look more anechoic than normal. (See indications for biopsy of liver on p. 283.)

Treatment

Supportive therapy for hepatic failure and hepatic encephalopathy, p. 283.

Cholangiohepatitis and Cholelithiasis

Signalment and Clinical Findings

- Cholangiohepatitis: Clinical findings most commonly include fever, jaundice, anorexia. Most common in adults.
- Cholelithiasis: Recurrent episodes of the above, plus *colic, weight loss*, and rarely neurologic signs. Middle-aged or older horses with cholangiohepatitis are more likely to have stones than are younger horses.

Diagnosis

- History, signalment, and clinical signs
- Laboratory findings:
  □ Marked elevation in GGT: 300–2500 IU/L
  □ Mild response in hepatocellular enzymes—AST usually < 1000 IU/L
  □ Liver function test: Increased bilirubin, often 50% or more is conjugated (direct) bilirubin; increased serum bile acids (normal < 12 μmol/L in an individual that is eating or < 20 μmol/L in an anorexic horse); PT, PTT are often normal.
  □ Increases often seen in WBC and neutrophil counts, fibrinogen, and total protein
  □ Biopsy reveals periportal fibrosis, dilation of bile duct, and inflammation. Culture usually shows gram-negative enteric organisms, if anything can be grown! **Positive cultures are obtained in only 50% of cases**.
- Ultrasound examination reveals:
  □ A subjectively enlarged liver
  □ Bile duct distention (Fig. 28–2) in some cases.
  □ Possible acoustic shadows (stones)
  □ Evidence of fibrosis, which can be severe in chronic cases.

Treatment

- For cholangiohepatitis:
  □ Antimicrobial therapy for those with fever and suspected cholangitis, or for prophylaxis—ceftiofur, 3.0 mg/kg IV or IM, q12h or trimethoprim-sulfa (TMP-S), 20–30 mg/kg PO q12h is a reasonable initial selection pending results of culture and sensitivity from the liver biopsy.
  □ Enrofloxacin, 5–7.5 mg/kg PO q24h, has also been used successfully. Add metronidazole, 15 mg/kg PO q8–12h, to any of the above if anaerobes are cultured.

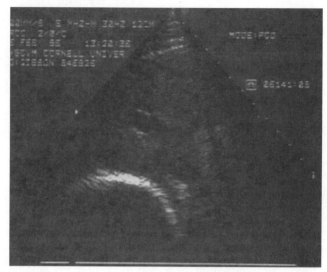

FIGURE 28–2. Bile duct distention. (From Divers TJ: Hepatic disorders. *In* Robinson NE: Current Therapy in Equine Medicine 4. Philadelphia, WB Saunders, 1997, p 217.)

- □ Administer vitamin K₁ IM or SQ for *chronic and severe* cholangitis. It may be ineffective if administered orally. **Do not administer IV**.
- □ DMSO 1 gm/kg as a 10% solution administered IV q24h for 5–7 days has the potential to dissolve calcium bilirubinate stones.
- □ Ursodeoxycholic acid should not be used.
- ■ Administer general treatment for liver failure when appropriate (see p. 283). **Hepatic encephalopathy is not as great a concern with cholangitis as in Theiler's disease, and some of the treatments for hepatic encephalopathy are usually not indicated when treating cholangiohepatitis, e.g., oral neomycin.**

Hyperlipemia

- ■ Occurs mostly in ponies, miniature horses, adults with pituitary adenomas, and less commonly in late pregnant and azotemic mares. It may affect foals or adults.
- ■ In ponies, most common in pregnant or early lactation mares. It is usually a disease of well-conditioned or fat ponies.
- ■ Characterized by fatty liver and serum that is cloudy due to accumulation of lipids
- ■ Any disease that decreases appetite or results in catecholamine release and lipolysis may initiate hyperlipemia.

Clinical Signs

- ■ Anorexia
- ■ Depression

- Diarrhea
- Ventral edema

Diagnosis (Laboratory Tests)

- Increased triglycerides, > 500 mg/dl
- Increased hepatocellular enzymes in the serum but liver function tests may not be markedly abnormal
- Whitish discoloration of the serum or plasma

Treatment

- Specific treatment for hyperlipemia in ponies:
  - □ Provide both IV and oral calories along with IV polyionic fluids, IV 0.45 NaCl and 5% dextrose or lactated Ringer's solution and 5% dextrose and additive KCL (20–40 mEq/L). Nasogastric intubation if the pony is not eating, with 0.5 gm/kg glucose as a 15% solution and 10–20 gm KCL. If appetite does not improve within 24 hours, start enteral feeding with either Osmolyte HN (Ross Laboratories, Columbus, Ohio) or Nutri Prime (Ken Vet, Ashland, Ohio) for adults or Nutrifoal (Ken Vet, Ashland, Ohio) for foals. Administer the enteral feeds in small volumes every 2 hours via an indwelling 18 Fr nasogastric tube (Ross Laboratories).
  - □ On the first day, give the adult patient 50 KCal/kg of Osmolyte and the foal 50 KCal/kg of Nutrifoal. If the feeds are well tolerated on day 1, increase to 75 KCal/kg on day 2 and 100 KCal/kg on day 3 and beyond. If the individuals do not tolerate enteral feeding (diarrhea or reflux), use IV nutrition if possible.
  - □ For individuals not tolerant to enteral feeding, use parenteral nutrition. This is one of the few indications for the emergency use of TPN in adults. Begin by placing a Mylar or Arrow catheter in the jugular vein. The TPN is formulated by mixing 50% dextrose and 4% branched chain amino acid solution (BranchAmin, Clintec, Deerfield, IL). The final solution should be <20% dextrose and administered at a rate of 2 ml/kg/h.
  - □ Monitor plasma glucose frequently; it should not be > 180 mg/dl. Feed the pony anything it will eat.
  - □ Heparin, 100 IU/kg IV q12h. This is of questionable benefit.
  - □ Flunixin meglumine, 0.25 mg/kg q8h for endotoxemia and/or to improve overall attitude
  - □ NOTE: Aggressively treat the primary disease.
  - □ NOTE: Administer pergolide, 0.0017–0.01 mg/kg PO for adults suspected of having a pituitary adenoma as an underlying cause. A low dose of 0.0017 mg/kg/day has recently been shown to be efficacious. If expense is a concern, the alternative is cyproheptadine, 0.25–0.5 mg/kg PO q12h. Pergolide may be more likely to suppress appetite.
  - □ Insulin is of questionable value but can be used if patients are being administered 10% dextrose IV. Protamine zinc insulin, 0.4 IU/kg SQ q24h, or ultralente insulin, 0.4 IU/kg IV q24h, may be used.
  - □ Ponies that have no appetite and cannot receive adequate nutritional support, have a primary disease that is difficult to treat, and/or have severe ventral edema have a very poor prognosis.

- Apply general principles for treating hepatic failure when appropriate, although fulminant hepatic encephalopathy is not common with hyperlipemia. It is important that affected individuals eat something even if it is a higher-protein feed!

Pyrrolizidine Alkaloid Toxicosis

Geographic Incidence

- Predominately a disease of the western United States
- The most common plants containing pyrrolizidine alkaloid are *Senecio jacobea* (Tansy ragwort), *Senecio vulgaris* (common groundsel), *Cynoglossum officinale* (hound's tongue), and *Amsinckia intermedia* (fiddleneck). *Crotalaria* (rattlebox) is a common plant of the southeastern United States containing pyrrolizidine alkaloid but is rarely ingested by horses.

Clinical Signs

- Although this is a chronic disease, most affected individuals have an acute onset of clinical signs.
- Central nervous system (CNS) signs are acute hepatoencephalopathic signs: depression, wandering, yawning, and so on.
- Icterus is mild to moderate.
- Photosensitization

Diagnosis

- Laboratory findings:
  - □ The AST is usually elevated. The GGT is consistently elevated and remains elevated for up to 6 months after removal of exposure to toxin in asymptomatic horses.
  - □ Bile acids are elevated.
- Ultrasound shows increased echogenicity (fibrosis).

Treatment

- Supportive therapy for fulminant liver failure and hepatic encephalopathy, p. 283.
- NOTE: What about other horses that have been exposed to pyrrolizidine alkaloids?
  - □ Monitor GGT and bile acids to determine whether the disease is progressing. If the individuals appear clinically normal at 6 months postexposure and GGT and bile acids are normal, the likelihood of developing hepatic failure from the exposure is minimal and they can be put back to work.

Tyzzer's Disease *(Clostridium piliformis)*

Signalment

Eight- to 42-day-old foal, usually only one foal on the farm affected, although farm problems may occur in certain areas, e.g., Oklahoma.

Clinical Signs

Acute death, depression, anorexia, hyper- or hypothermia, jaundice, convulsions, shock, diarrhea

Diagnosis

- Age and clinical signs
- Laboratory findings:
  □ Elevated AST and sorbitol dehydrogenase
  □ Abnormal liver function test: Bilirubinemia (both direct and indirect are increased)
  □ Hypoglycemia
  □ Severe metabolic acidosis
  □ Serology for recovered/suspect cases.
  □ Histopathology of the liver or PCR on feces.

Treatment

- Supportive therapy for fulminant hepatic failure and hepatic encephalopathy, p. 283.
- Additionally, antibiotics, either penicillin, 44,000 U/kg IV q6h, gentamicin, 6.6 mg/kg IV q24h (assuming the foal is urinating and is being treated aggressively with intravenous fluids) and metronidazole, 15 mg/kg PO q6–12h
- Additionally, aggressive treatment for septic shock
  □ Normalize blood pressure by a nonlactated polyionic crystalloid solution administered IV. If systemic arterial blood pressure cannot be normalized by fluid therapy and central venous pressure becomes elevated (> 11 cm H_2O), then administer alpha-adrenergic drug therapy—dopamine, 5–10 μg/kg/min—to normalize arterial blood pressure.
  □ Administer hyperimmune plasma incubated with 100 U heparin/L.
  □ Pentoxifylline, 8.4 mg/kg PO q8–12h
  □ Intranasal oxygen 5 L/min

Prognosis

Is grave!

Other Causes of Hepatic Disease That May Lead to Liver Failure

- Aflatoxicosis—rarely reported in horses
- Leukoencephalomalacia (moldy corn)—uncommon resulting in liver failure in horses, although it frequently causes liver disease.
- Obstruction of the bile duct—unusual
  □ Colon displacement: Suspect adults with mild persistent colic, afebrile, normal serum globulins, and plasma fibrinogen, with an abnormal

rectal examination and high bilirubin (usually > 12 mg/dl and GGT usually > 100 IU/L) of having a 180° ± displacement/volvulus of the large colon. A displaced colon in the horse occasionally obstructs the bile duct. Treatment is surgical correction. Bilirubin and GGT should decrease within 24–36 hours.

☐ Obstruction of the bile duct may also be seen in foals in association with healing duodenal ulcer and stricture. Serum GGT concentration is increased, and the foal may be icteric, but there is no retrograde movement of barium into the biliary ducts 2 hours after the oral barium study (1 liter/foal) as occurs with duodenal stricture posterior to the opening of the bile duct. Prognosis is very grave, although transposition of the bile duct and gastro- and/or duodenojejunostomy can be attempted.

- Portacaval shunts:
  ☐ Consider portacaval shunts in foals 2 or more months of age with an acute onset of blindness, seizures, coma, or other signs of bizarre behavior. Relapsing episodes are almost diagnostic. Foals rarely show clinical signs unless they are eating large amounts of grain or spring grass. Routine laboratory findings are often unremarkable. The liver enzymes are typically normal, AST and CK may be increased from seizure activity, and hypoglycemia may be present. Blood sample measurement of ammonia and bile acids are tests of choice to confirm the diagnosis.
  ☐ NOTE: Proper handling of the sample to measure blood ammonia is critical: the blood should be carefully (hemolysis interferes with the measurement) collected in a heparin tube, kept on ice, and taken to a laboratory within 1 hour. If this is not possible, harvest the plasma within 30 minutes and freeze it at − 20°C for measurement within 48 hours. Ideally, a control sample collected from an individual of similar age and diet should be submitted.
  ☐ Treatment—medical stabilization for hepatoencephalopathy, including polyionic crystalloid fluid therapy with 5–10 gm dextrose added per liter. Metronidazole, 15 mg/kg PO mixed with Karo syrup and administered three times 12 hours apart, may be as effective as neomycin in decreasing intestinal ammonia production. Sedation with a low-dose xylazine, 0.2 mg/kg, followed by pentobarbital or phenobarbital administration, 3.0–11.0 mg/kg or *to effect*, may be required to sedate a seizuring foal. *No diazepam!* Surgical correction can be performed following a diagnostic venogram to demonstrate the shunt location.
- Hyperammonemia and liver disease can occur in weanling Morgan foals. This syndrome appears to be familial and may be associated with a metabolic defect in urea synthesis.
  ☐ Diagnosis: Morgan breed, clinical signs (occur after weaning), diminished growth rate, and depression. Moderately elevated liver enzymes. Normal or only mildly elevated bilirubin. Blood ammonia levels are very high (>200 μmol/L).
  ☐ Prognosis: fatal to date.
- Klein grass and fall panicum
  ☐ Consider Klein grass as a cause of liver failure in those areas of the

country (southwestern United States) where the grass is grown. In the eastern United States, fall panicum may produce a similar syndrome.

- Alsike clover
  - □ Alsike clover poisoning is a cause of *photosensitization and jaundice* in horses in the northern United States and Canada. Outbreaks occur sporadically, likely associated with environmental conditions and increased growth of mycotoxin on the grass or a toxin (saponin) in the plant.
  - □ Diagnosis is based on history and exposure, clinical findings of liver disease/failure, and ruling out other causes of hepatic failure. With fall panicum, Klein grass, or alsike poisoning, multiple horses on the farm may have increases in GGT, although they may not have liver failure. Laboratory findings are similar to those with pyrrolizidine alkaloid poisoning (moderate increases in GGT and a mild to moderate increase in AST).
  - □ Treatment is supportive therapy and removal from the hay or pasture.
  - □ Prognosis for panicum and alsike toxicity is usually good.
- Iron intoxication may cause liver disease and occasionally failure. It may result from overzealous oral or more likely parenteral administration of iron sulfate. It may also occur in a few horses because of abnormal liver uptake and/or storage (hemochromatosis) rather than excessive administration.

Ultrasound Examination of the Equine Liver: To Biopsy or Not?

- Ultrasound examination of the liver is performed using a 5.0-MHz probe of the right abdomen beginning at the 10th intercostal space just above the point of the shoulder and continuing caudally and ventrally. Also scan the left cranial quadrant of the abdomen at the 7th–9th intercostal space in a line drawn from the point of the elbow and moving caudally.
- Liver biopsies or aspirates can be performed for diagnostic purposes, e.g., pyrrolizidine alkaloid toxicosis, suppurative cholangitis, culture, or for prognostic reasons, e.g., fibrosis. They are rarely needed as an emergency procedure and are not necessary for proper management in most cases. The biopsy can be performed using a true cut biopsy needle introduced into a section of liver viewed on ultrasound as relatively *avascular.* Only local anesthesia is required.

General Treatment of Fulminant Liver Failure and Hepatic Encephalopathy

- Tranquilize only if needed to control the individual, with low doses of xylazine (0.2 mg/kg IV as needed). NOTE: *Do not use diazepam.* If further sedation is required, pentobarbital or phenobarbital can be used to effect (generally 5.0–11.0 mg/kg IV).
- Minimize stress and *feed small amounts of grain* (preferably grain with higher amounts of *branched-chain** amino acids, e.g., sorghum and corn) *frequently.* Remove alfalfa hay and feed grass hay. Grazing of late

---

*A branched-chain amino acid paste is also available.

summer or fall nonlegume grasses is acceptable if performed in the evening to prevent photosensitization.

- Begin IV fluid therapy if dehydrated.
  - □ 0.45% or 0.9% NaCl with 2.5% dextrose and additive—40 mEq/L KCL. After volume deficits have been replaced, maintenance rates should be 80 ml/kg/day or greater. In many cases the PCV remains elevated despite apparent rehydration. Fluids containing acetate are preferred over lactate-containing fluids when treating hepatic failure.
- Administer 4–8 mg/kg neomycin sulfate orally q8h, mixed in molasses, when hepatoencephalopathy is present or a concern. This treatment may be continued at a lower daily rate for 3 days. Diarrhea may result with overzealous administration of neomycin.
- Special considerations:
  - □ *No diazepam!*
  - □ When hepatoencephalopathy is a major concern, do not pass a nasogastric tube unless needed to administer oral medication. Bleeding and swallowing of blood can worsen the hepatoencephalopathy.
  - □ NOTE: **Do not administer 5% dextrose as the sole source of fluid replacement because it does not sufficiently expand the intravascular space**.
  - □ Do not administer bicarbonate unless plasma bicarbonate is < 14 mEq/L. Rapid correction of the acidosis can increase ionized ammonia and exacerbate the CNS signs.
  - □ **Maintain adequate serum potassium (K^+) concentration because this is important in reducing the hyperammonemia**.
  - □ Do not leave affected individuals outside in the sun.
  - □ For primary hyperammonemia or fulminant hepatic failure with confirmed or suspected high blood ammonia concentration, metronidazole, 15 mg/kg q24h PO, mixed with molasses, is given *in addition* to the neomycin. Metronidazole is effective in decreasing enteric ammonia production, a good antimicrobial against anaerobic infections of the liver, and has anti-inflammatory and antiendotoxin properties.
  - □ For patients with severe and/or uncontrolled (using the preceding treatment) hepatoencephalopathy: flumazenil therapy (5–10 mg administered slowly IV to a 500-kg adult) can be attempted. The response is generally prompt. NOTE: **Expensive treatment**.
  - □ Administer B vitamins IV (slowly).
  - □ Consider parenteral nutrition for foals and adults with fulminant hepatic failure caused by an acute disease process. Use only formulations prepared for hepatic failure patients (Heptamine), and use a rate less than for routine TPN therapy. Experience with this form of therapy in acute hepatic failure is limited to a few cases.

HEMOLYTIC ANEMIA

General Diagnostic Statements

Collect blood in EDTA for direct Coombs test if an immunologic reaction is suspected, e.g., isoerythrolysis or recent penicillin administration. Ask for new methylene blue stain if a plant toxin, such as red maple, is a possibility. Collect serum for Coggins test and strep M protein antibody if edema and fever are present. Measure serum calcium if lymphoma is suspected. Examine thoroughly for other diseases (e.g., clostridial myositis) that may cause hemolytic anemia. For classification of anemia in horses, see Figure 28–3.

Toxic or Heinz Body Anemia

Acute hemolytic anemia may be caused by plant toxins or occasionally may be a direct effect of IV drug administration (DMSO, tetracycline, propylene glycol). It may also occur in association with clostridial bacterial toxins. Plants reported to cause intravascular hemolysis are wild onion and red maple. Red maple toxicity is most common during late summer and fall and results from ingestion of wilted leaves. It often occurs 3–4 days after a storm. Seen only in the middle or eastern United States.

Clinical Signs

- Depression
- Jaundice
- Discolored urine

Diagnosis

- History
- Clinical signs

Diagnostic Test

- PCV
- Total protein (TP)
- Bilirubin
- Urinalysis
- Methemoglobin*
- Red cell morphology
- Heinz bodies may be seen with meticulous searching in red maple poisoning. They are more commonly seen with onion poisoning. The PCV often drops to life-threatening values ($<$ 14%) with red maple toxicity; this is rarely the case with onion toxicity. Mean corpuscular volume (MCV) and mean corpuscular hemoglobin concentration (MCHC) may be increased, and plasma protein is usually normal or increased. The increase in serum bilirubin is mostly indirect.

Treatment

- Blood transfusion (see p. 294)
  - □ Transfuse if PCV drops to $<$ 18% within 24 hours.

---

*In some cases, the methemoglobin may be very high ($>$50%) and rapid death; the membranes are dark but not icteric, and the PCV may be normal. Methemoglobin can usually be measured at hospitals for humans. A new methylene blue stain and examination for Heinz bodies should be performed!

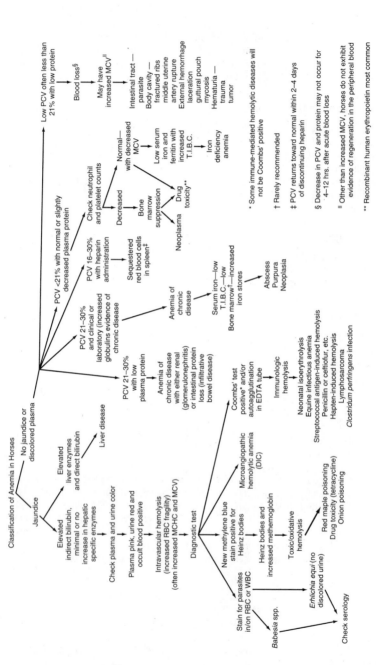

FIGURE 28-3 See legend on opposite page

Classification of Anemia in Horses

Jaundice
- Elevated liver enzymes and direct bilirubin → Liver disease
- Elevated indirect bilirubin, minimal or no increase in hepatic specific enzymes
  - Check plasma and urine color
    - Plasma pink, urine red and occult blood positive
      - Intravascular hemolysis (increased RBC fragility) (often increased MCHC and MCV)
        - Diagnostic test
          - Microangiopathic hemolytic anemia (DIC)
          - Coombs' test positive* and/or autoagglutination in EDTA tube
            - Immunologic hemolysis
              - Neonatal isoerythrolysis
              - Equine infectious anemia
              - Streptococcal antigen-induced hemolysis
              - Penicillin or ceftiofur, etc.
              - Hapten-induced hemolysis
              - Lymphosarcoma
              - Clostridium perfringens infection
          - New methylene blue stain positive for Heinz bodies
            - Heinz bodies and increased methemoglobin
              - Toxic/oxidative hemolysis
                - Red maple poisoning
                - Drug toxicity (tetracycline)
                - Onion poisoning
          - Stain for parasites in/on RBC or WBC
            - Babesia spp.
            - Ehrlichia equi (no discolored urine)
            - Check serology

No jaundice or discolored plasma
- PCV 21–30% with low plasma protein
  - Anemia of chronic disease with either renal (glomerulonephritis) or intestinal protein loss (infiltrative bowel disease)
- PCV 21–30% and clinical or laboratory (increased globulins) evidence of chronic disease
  - Anemia of chronic disease
    - Serum iron—low
    - T.I.B.C.—low
    - Bone marrow†—increased iron stores
      - Abscess
      - Purpura
      - Neoplasia
- PCV 16–30% with heparin administration
  - Sequestered red blood cells in spleen‡
- PCV <21% with normal or slightly decreased plasma protein
  - Check neutrophil and platelet counts
    - Decreased
      - Bone marrow suppression
        - Neoplasma
      - Drug toxicity**
    - Normal—with decreased MCV
      - Low serum iron and ferritin with increased T.I.B.C.
        - Iron deficiency anemia
- Low PCV often less than 21% with low protein
  - Blood loss§
    - May have increased MCV‖
      - Intestinal tract — parasite
      - Body cavity —
      - fractured ribs
      - middle uterine artery rupture
      - External hemorrhage
      - guttural pouch mycosis
      - Hematuria — trauma tumor

* Some immune-mediated hemolytic diseases will not be Coombs' positive

† Rarely recommended

‡ PCV returns toward normal within 2–4 days of discontinuing heparin

§ Decrease in PCV and protein may not occur for 4–12 hrs. after acute blood loss

‖ Other than increased MCV, horses do not exhibit evidence of regeneration in the peripheral blood

** Recombinant human erythropoietin most common

286

□ In cases with a slower decline in PCV, transfusion can be postponed until the PCV is < 12%.
- Isotonic fluids if there is clinical evidence of hypovolemia
- Oral vitamin C, 250 gm q12h for 2 days

Immune-Mediated Hemolytic Anemia

May result from either an autoimmune reaction or more commonly a result of another disease (lymphoma, EIA, *Clostridium perfringens*, or *Streptococcus* infection), or drug-induced hemolytic anemia (most commonly IV penicillin or ceftiofur)

Clinical Signs and Findings

- Lethargy
- Depression
- Edema, usually in the limbs and ventral body, may be the result of sludging of red cell complexes in the microcirculation.
- Pale mucous membranes
- In a few cases, red urine and fever

Diagnosis

- History of penicillin, ceftiofur, and so on administration within past 1–2 weeks
- Recent infection with *Streptococcus* sp. or less commonly *Clostridium perfringens*
- Suspicion of lymphoma

Laboratory Findings

- PCV decreased
- MCV and MCHC may be increased.
- Look for severe autoagglutination in the EDTA sample; the plasma may be either yellow or pink, depending on the duration of the hemolysis and whether it is intravascular or extravascular.
- Internal hemorrhage can be ruled out by history and normal or high plasma protein.
- Autoagglutination can be differentiated from normal rouleaux formation by diluting the sample 1:4 with 0.9% saline.

Additional Tests

- EIA—Coggins test (serology)
- Coombs test (required EDTA sample). If autoagglutination is obvious, there is no need to perform Coombs test.

FIGURE 28–3. Equine anemia classification. EDTA, ethylenediamenetetraacetic acid; MCV, mean corpuscular volume; PCV, packed cell volume; TIBC, total iron-binding capacity.

- Heinz bodies may be seen with oxidant-induced hemolytic anemia but not autoimmune hemolytic anemia.

Treatment

- Blood transfusion only if needed (see guidelines on p. 294) from donor compatible on the cross-match (see p. 295)
- Dexamethasone, 0.04–0.08 mg/kg IV q24h

Neonatal Isoerythrolysis (NI)

- Suspect in young foals, especially mule foals, <7 days of age with icterus, tachycardia, and weakness.
- The foal is usually a product of a multiparous mare.
- Urine is usually discolored in peracute cases: usually light red (hemoglobin), although it can be brown (bilirubin) in more chronic cases.
- *Remember, there are many causes of jaundice in young foals*, e.g., sepsis. NI can usually be separated from other causes simply by measuring the PCV, which is usually <20% in NI foals. Unrelated to the A or Q antigen in mules

Additional Tests

Use Coombs test with whole blood (EDTA) to confirm an immune reaction. Close examination of the sample may reveal autoagglutination (presence of clumps) in which case a Coombs test is not needed for confirmation.

Treatment

- If the foal is <48 hours of age, do not allow it to nurse unless the mare's colostrum has a colostrometer value of <1.03 and the colostrum added to the sire's red blood cells does not result in agglutination. Accomplish this with as little stress as possible to the foal (muzzle).
- Peracute severe cases with PCV <20% within 24 hours:

  □ Transfusion for horse foals from Aa and Qa negative donors. A cross-match (major and minor) is ideal. If a cross-match is not feasible, using a Aa/Qa negative donor is usually safe and effective. The mare's blood may be used if it is washed three times and suspended in saline before each transfusion, which is time consuming.

All equine practices should have Aa/Qa-negative donors identified for emergency purposes. Blood typing can be performed by sending samples of acid-citrate-dextrose anticoagulated blood to the Veterinary Genetics Laboratory, School of Veterinary Medicine, University of California, Davis, CA 95616; (916) 752 2211, or Equine Blood Typing Research Laboratory, University of Kentucky, Department of Veterinary Science, Lexington, KY 40546; (606) 257 3022. Donors should be free of Aa and/or Qa antigens and hemolytic or agglutinating Aa, Qa antibodies.

- □ Mule foals: If a female donor is used, use one that has not previously been bred by a donkey.
- IV fluids at maintenance level (approximately 60 ml/kg/day). *Administration of needed IV fluids lowers the PCV but does not reduce total RBC numbers and does not exacerbate hypoxemia.*
- Dexamethasone, 0.04 mg/lb (0.08 mg/kg), used only in peracute cases (foals 2 days of age or less with PCV <12%) and if donor cells cannot be administered immediately or if uncertain of compatibility.
- Intranasal oxygen (5 L/min) bubbled via a nasopharyngeal tube (see p. 40) in severely anemic foals.
- Antimicrobials-antibiotics for all NI foals to minimize sepsis. Despite evidence of passive transfer of colostral antibodies, NI foals can become septic. Valuable foals should be administered a combination of IV penicillin and amikacin or ceftiofur, whereas less valuable foals can be administered a combination of TMP/S (20 mg/kg PO q12h) and penicillin (22,000 IU/kg q12h IM).
- Antiulcer medication: Sucralfate, 1 gm PO q6h with or without an H_2 or proton pump blocker.
- Nutritional support (Land-O-Lakes) foal milk replacement, mare's milk, goat milk, at 20%–25% of body weight/day during the time* the foal is not allowed to nurse.
- Supportive care, e.g., keep the foal warm.
- Expect a second decline in PCV 4–11 days after the transfusion.

Other Causes of Hemolysis in Adults

Babesia *(Piroplasmosis)*

- *B. caballi* and *B. equi*
- *B. equi* is more pathogenic.
- Found in Americas, Europe, Russia, Asia, Africa, Middle East
- Clinical signs:
  - □ All horses are susceptible, older horses more severely affected. Once infected, survivors are carriers.
  - □ Incubation period is 5–28 days.
  - □ Fever 102°–107°F
  - □ Hemolytic anemia
  - □ Jaundice
  - □ Hemoglobinuria
  - □ Death
- Generalized signs: Depression, anorexia, incoordination, lacrimation, mucous nasal discharge, eyelid swelling, increased recumbency
- Differential
  - □ Equine granulocytic ehrlichiosis *(Ehrlichia equi)*
  - □ Equine infectious anemia (EIA)
  - □ Liver failure
- Diagnosis:
  - □ Serologic tests: Complement fixation (CF), indirect fluorescent anti-

---

*The foal should be 36–48 hours old before it is allowed to nurse (see p. 288).

body (IFA), cytologic identification of the organism on Giemsa-stained blood smear, although it may be negative in infected individuals even when the sample is drawn from a small-diameter vessel.

- Treatment:
  - □ *B. equi* is more refractory to treatment than *B. caballi*.
  - □ Imidocarb: For *B. caballi*: 2.2 mg/kg two times q24h; for *B. equi*: 4.0 mg/kg four times q72h. **CAUTION: Do not treat donkeys at the higher dosage—causes death**. Imidocarb may cause signs of colic.
  - □ Tetracycline, 6.6 mg/kg q12h slowly IV diluted.
- Prevention/control:
  - □ Tick control is key.
  - □ No effective vaccine available

Granulocytic Ehrlichiosis (a Differential Diagnosis for Babesiosis and Equine Infectious Anemia)

- General information:
  - □ Rickettsial disease (*Ehrlichia equi*)
  - □ Recovery (without treatment) is usually within 2–3 weeks.
  - □ The vector is believed to be a tick.
  - □ Disease is not contagious, but multiple cases may occur on the same premises.
  - □ Abortion is not an expected complication of granulocytic ehrlichiosis.
- Common in northern California and in parts of Connecticut and their surrounding states and has been reported in many other states
- Signs (typically worse if horse is over 3 years of age): fever (102°–107°F), icterus, depression, anorexia, limb edema, mucosal petechiae, ataxia, reluctance to move. Clinical disease is most common in the fall and winter in California.
- Diagnosis:
  - □ Cytoplasmic inclusions in neutrophils and eosinophils
  - □ Serologic test (Texas A&M Diagnostic Laboratory or University of California at Davis)
  - □ Leukopenia (mild to moderate)
  - □ Thrombocytopenia, anemia
- Treatment:
  - □ Supportive therapy
  - □ Benefit has been recognized with the administration of oxytetracycline, 6.6 mg/kg IV q12–24h, as it may shorten the disease course significantly.

Equine Infectious Anemia (EIA)

- General information:
  - □ A necrotizing vasculitis of the horse, donkey, and mule
  - □ Affected horses are carriers of the EIA retrovirus for life and may have periodic episodes of clinical signs.
  - □ Transmitted by the horsefly
  - □ Infected mares may abort at any stage of gestation.
  - □ Clinical EIA may be recognized in different stages: can be acute or

chronic. **Acute EIA is characterized by fever, depression, petechiae. The acutely affected individual may die in a few days.**
- ☐ **EIA IS A REPORTABLE DISEASE.**
- ■ Signs: Fever, anemia, icterus, ventral edema, weight loss, depression, petechiae (if acute)
- ■ Diagnosis:
  - ☐ Agar-gel immunodiffusion (Coggins test): Serum antibodies to EIA retrovirus. May be falsely negative in first 2 weeks following infection. May be falsely positive in foals born to infected mares. Use red top tube (clot tube) sample for Coggins test.
  - ☐ Anemia may be marked and progressive; Coombs test may be positive.
  - ☐ Mild lymphocytosis, monocytosis
  - ☐ Thrombocytopenia is common during febrile episodes.
- ■ Treatment:
  - ☐ Isolate as soon as possible (200 yards from other horses in a screened stall).
  - ☐ No treatment, other than supportive care, is successful in the carrier state. No treatment or vaccination specifically for EIA exists.
  - ☐ Remember EIA is a reportable disease. Contact the state veterinary medical office.
- ■ Other less common causes of hemolysis and icterus (also see discolored urine on p. 465):
  - ☐ Hepatic failure, p. 275.
  - ☐ Clostridial infections, p. 268.
  - ☐ Snake bite, p. 442.
  - ☐ Disseminated intravascular coagulation—a microangiopathic hemolytic anemia may occasionally be seen with DIC. Treatment is for the primary disease.
  - ☐ Renal failure, p. 462.
  - ☐ Leptospirosis—rarely causes hemolysis and/or hematuria.
  - ☐ NOTE: A common cause of acute anemia in the horse is *heparin* therapy. The PCV may drop as low as 14%. The anemia is a result of both spurious lowering of the PCV and increased sequestration of the red cells by the reticuloendothelial cells. Hemolysis does not occur, and PCV returns to prior level within 2–4 days after discontinuing heparin treatment.

HEMORRHAGE INTO BODY CAVITY

In adults, most often into the abdomen. May result from trauma (ruptured spleen or liver), foaling (ruptured middle uterine artery), postsurgically (e.g., ovariectomy), or from idiopathic causes. *Idiopathic causes are common, especially in older horses.* In the newborn foal, rib fractures and umbilical cord hemorrhage are most common.

Clinical Signs

Abdominal pain, increased respiratory rate, increased heart rate, pale mucous membranes, trembling, sweating, distress

Diagnosis

- Abdominocentesis:
  - □ Uniform stream of red fluid that does not clot, with a PCV often ranging from 8%–20%, is diagnostic for bleeding. Platelets are not seen and erythrophagocytosis is often present.
- Ultrasonography:
  - □ Perform ultrasound examination of the abdomen for detection of fluid in the abdominal cavity. Carefully inspect liver and spleen if trauma is suspected. Tears in the liver and spleen can be seen via ultrasound and usually require corrective surgery.

Treatment

Idiopathic

- Keep the patient quiet.
- Administer IV fluids (polyionic fluids), 20–80 ml/kg over several hours, depending on the degree of hypovolemia. Low normal blood pressure should be maintained.
- Epsilon-aminocaproic acid (Amicar): 10–20 mg/kg IV *mixed* in the IV fluids
- Analgesics as needed to control pain and anxiety
- Intranasal oxygen in severe cases
- Do not perform surgery unless the patient continues to deteriorate, because the bleeding is likely to stop in older individuals with no history of trauma.
- Transfusion if PCV declines to <15% in subacute cases or chronic cases. In peracute cases, transfusion may be required before a drop in PCV, p. 294.
- Autotransfusion is used if you are reasonably sure the bleeding is not associated with sepsis (traumatized bowel, liver abscess or tumor), p. 295.
- If bleeding into the abdomen or chest is so severe that it mechanically restricts ventilation, the blood should be removed. Otherwise, nonseptic blood should be left in the body cavity; the increased pressure helps promote clotting. It may be removed if an immediate transfusion is required.

Hemorrhage with Trauma

- Keep the patient quiet.
- Administer IV fluids (polyionic fluids), 20–80 ml/kg over several hours or more, depending upon the degree of the hypovolemia and blood pressure measurement.
- Epsilon-aminocaproic acid (Amicar): 10–20 mg/kg IV *mixed* in the IV fluids.
- Analgesics as needed to control pain and anxiety
- Intranasal oxygen in severe cases
- Consider exploratory surgery. If a tear in the liver or spleen is found, splenectomy is possible. Gel foam may be used for liver lacerations. Prognosis is guarded with liver lacerations.

Middle Uterine Artery Rupture (also see p. 424)

If the affected individual is very agitated, use acepromazine, 0.02 mg/kg, along with balanced crystalloids and blood transfusion. If the heart rate is > 100 beats/minute and the membranes are white, *do not* use acepromazine. Use hypertonic saline only if rapid deterioration appears imminent and temporary improvement in the blood pressure is needed to pursue a blood transfusion and/or surgery.

Rib Fractures

- General information:
  - □ Hemorrhage into the thorax is common in foals but not often recognized antemortem in adults.
  - □ Look for evidence of pneumothorax. Consider giving foal oxygen and perform thoracentesis; apply a Heimlich chest drain if dyspnea is severe. Keep the individual quiet and start antimicrobial therapy with a broad-spectrum antibiotic.
  - □ Any physical examination of a foal, especially a neonate, includes a careful examination of the thoracic wall. Rib fractures can cause severe pneumothorax/hemothorax and result in rapid death.
  - □ Keep the foal as quiet as possible.
- Signs of hemothorax:
  - □ Hemorrhagic anemia
  - □ Dyspnea
  - □ Painful chest, reluctance to move
  - □ Decreased or absent lung sounds ventrally, frequently recognized bilaterally
  - □ Possible jugular distention and/or jugular pulses
  - □ +/− Jaundice
- Diagnosis:
  - □ Physical examination
  - □ Ultrasound examination of the thorax reveals cellular pleural fluid.
  - □ Diaphragmatic hernia may occur simultaneously
  - □ Pleurocentesis reveals blood with no bacteria.
- Treatment:
  - □ *Keep foal quiet*—very important! Ideally, the foal is best lying on the fractured side to reduce fracture movement and laceration of a coronary artery.
  - □ Oxygen if dyspnea is severe.
  - □ Antibiotics: Broad-spectrum, especially if there is an open wound or evidence of pneumothorax.
  - □ Consider blood transfusion. See p. 294.
  - □ Pleurocentesis offers temporary improvement, but foal should be monitored carefully as the pleural cavity frequently fills rapidly.
  - □ Administer antiulcer medication (see pp. 172–173).
  - □ Surgical intervention should be considered if bleeding persists.

Ruptured Aorta

- Most common in older stallions during breeding.
- Often results in acute death (see p. 152)

Diaphragmatic Hernia

- Thoracic bleeding may occur with chest trauma or diaphragmatic hernias.
- Suspect this in a colicky horse with "negative" (or empty-feeling) rectal palpation and any evidence of respiratory compromise, especially if the lung sounds are quiet or absent, or gastrointestinal motility sounds are heard when auscultating the thorax.
  - □ Diagnosis by ultrasound examination of the thorax. Be careful performing a thoracocentesis because compromised bowel may be penetrated by even a teat cannula.
  - □ Treatment is corrective surgery.

Other Body Cavity Hemorrhage

- Bleeding from thoracic lymphosarcoma is common but rarely causes life-threatening anemia.
- Hemothorax may rarely develop following exercise and pulmonary hemorrhage. Conservative management to include treatment of the pneumothorax is often successful.

EXTERNAL HEMORRHAGE

Bleeding of a major vessel can be life threatening. This is most commonly a result of trauma, although occasionally cellulitis may erode through a major vessel and cause life-threatening hemorrhage. Whenever possible, either *pressure bandages* or *suturing of the vessel* is performed to prevent additional blood loss. If the heart rate is elevated and the patient appears to be in hypovolemic shock, a blood transfusion and administration of polyionic fluids is required. There may not be time for a cross-match; a horse known to be free of A and Q antigen and antibodies is ideal. *With acute hemorrhage, the individual can die without a decrease in PCV!*

Hemorrhage from the guttural pouch. This is most often a result of fungal infections and erosion of the external or internal carotid or maxillary arteries within the pouch. This should be confirmed by endoscopic examination. Surgery is performed ASAP. Plans for a transfusion should be made as soon as the diagnosis is confirmed because acute, severe bleeding can occur.

Other causes of epistaxis should be ruled out. Many require no specific treatment. Some can be managed medically (e.g., thrombocytopenia with immunosuppression therapy: dexamethasone, 0.01 mg/kg, and fresh blood transfusion collected in plastic), whereas others are corrected by laser surgery, or formalin injections, e.g., ethmoid hematoma.

GENERAL COMMENTS ON BLOOD TRANSFUSIONS

Perform when:

- PCV drops to < 20% in first 12 hours and hemorrhage or hemolysis is ongoing

- PCV drops to < 12% over 1–2 days, hemoglobin values < 5 gm/dl have a significant effect on tissue oxygenation.
- **In peracute cases, death from hemorrhage may occur without a decrease in PCV. In these cases, transfusion is based on severe tachycardia, white to gray mucous membranes, and evidence of severe bleeding.**

Choice of Donor

There are over 400,000 blood types in the horse, and there is no universal donor.

- If time permits, use a cross-matched donor; primary interest is in the major testing (donor RBC, plasma recipient). If the donor has not been previously tested for isoantibodies, perform a minor match. Most of the testing detects agglutination, although a few laboratories can test for lysis (need rabbit serum).
- If time does not permit, choose a gelding of the same breed and mix donor serum with patient RBC and vice versa looking for evidence of agglutination.
- Consider **autotransfusion**—body cavity bleeding **without sepsis**. Blood can be collected from the abdomen or chest by inserting a teat cannula and collecting the blood, using sterile technique, into a container with small amounts of ACD (approximately 1 part ACD/15 parts blood).
- Store autologous blood for rare elective procedures in which gross hemorrhage is anticipated, e.g., nasal surgery. Collect in citrate phosphate dextrose (CPD) rather than ACD—and can be stored at 4°C for several days.

Collection and Administration

- Collect blood using aseptic technique in 2.5%–4% ACD—9 parts blood to 1 part citrate.
- Use a blood collection set. 15%–20% of the blood volume (body weight in kg × 10% = liters of blood in the donor) from a healthy donor can be collected.
- Blood bags, bottles, and anticoagulant can be purchased from Animal Blood Bank, Box 1118, Dixon, CA; (916) 678 7350 or in the UK telephone 441977 681523.
- Administer with a blood administration set at a rate of 10–20 ml/kg/h, with close monitoring of vital signs. Filters should be replaced after 3–4 liters.
- Blood for transfusion should be warmed to body temperature.

Side Effects

If tachypnea, dyspnea, restlessness, piloerection, and fasciculation occur, stop or slow the transfusion and/or administer epinephrine, 0.005–0.02 ml/kg of 1:1000 (if severe anaphylaxis), or doxylamine succinate, 0.5 mg/kg IV very slowly. Doxylamine succinate may be administered SQ as prophylaxis before transfusion.

How Much Blood to Administer?

- At least 6–8 liters for an adult is an estimate.
- In addition, use polyionic fluids in the treatment of the hypovolemic shock.
- With more chronic hemolysis, use the following formula to estimate blood volume needed:

$$\frac{\text{Desired PCV} - \text{PCV recipient} \ (0.08 \times \text{Body wt in kg})}{\text{PCV of donor}} = \text{liters required}$$

There is no universal recommendation for a desired PCV. A measurement of venous oxygen (Vo) may provide an estimate. If the Vo is abnormally low, this may be an indication for increased hemoglobin.
  - ☐ Administer one third–one half of calculated volume at 10–20 ml/kg/h if there is no evidence of adverse reaction. The transfusion can then be slowed depending on the clinical conditions.
- Expected life span of transfused "compatible" RBCs is:
  - ☐ Autologous: at least 12–14 days
  - ☐ Allogenic: may be as little as 2–5 days (foals, 3–4 days longer)
- Blood collected in CPD maintains viable red cells for at least 2 weeks if refrigerated, but transfusion of stored whole blood increases chance of reaction.

Other Therapy

- Dexamethasone, 40 mg q 24h, for adult with immune-mediated hemolytic anemia. As the PCV stabilizes, dexamethasone can be decreased.
- Isotonic fluids if the individual is hypovolemic. Although the PCV decreases, it actually improves oxygen-carrying capacity. Nonisotonic fluids are not recommended.
- Intranasal oxygen is indicated if the individuals are severely hypoxic.
- An alternative to whole blood transfusion if a compatible donor cannot be found is Bovine Hemoglobin (Biopure Corp., Boston), administered at 30 ml/kg. The half-life is approximately 2 days.

SUGGESTED REFERENCES

George LW, Divers TJ, Mahaffey EA, Suarez MJH. Heinz body anemia and methemoglobinemia in ponies given red maple leaves. Vet Pathol 1982;19:521–533.

Maxson AD, Giger U, Sweeney CR, Tomasic M, Sack JE, Donawick WJ, Cothran EG. Use of bovine hemoglobin preparation in the treatment of cyclic ovarian hemorrhage in a miniature horse. J Am Vet Med Assoc 1993;203:1308–1311.

Moore BR, Abood S, Hinchcliff KS. Hyperlipemia in nine miniature horses and miniature donkeys. J Vet Intern Med 1994;8(5):376–381.

Oryan A, Asiani MR, Rezakhani A, Maleki M, Shad-del FA. *Babesia caballi* and associated pathologic lesions in a horse. Equine Pract 1994;16:33–36.

Robbins RL, Wallace SS, Brunner CJ, Gardner TR, Defranco BJ, Speirs VC. Immune mediated hemolytic disease after penicillin therapy in a horse. Equine Vet J 1993;25:462–465.

Traub-Dargatz JL, McClure JJ, Koch C, Schlipf JW. Neonatal isoerythrolysis in mule foals. J Am Vet Med Assoc 1995;206:67–70.

29 Musculoskeletal

Pamela Wagner von Matthiessen and
James A. Orsini

Equine orthopedic emergencies include

- **Fractures**
- **Luxations**
- **Lacerations of supporting structures**
- **Lacerations of major peripheral blood vessels**
- **Punctures of synovial structures, including joints, bursae, and tendon sheaths and/or infections of these structures**

Most of these injuries cannot be treated easily in the field and require transport of the patient to another environment or referral to a surgical facility.

The horse is frequently anxious as it attempts to use the injured limb, causing additional secondary soft tissue injury *that complicates later repair efforts.*

Emergency Steps

- Calm the patient using tranquilization, sedation, and pain relief.
- Cursory examination to determine whether repair is feasible
- Application of protective splints, bandages, or a cast
- Further diagnostic examination
- Transport to an equine hospital

TRANQUILIZATION, SEDATION, AND PAIN RELIEF

- There is a choice of sedative drugs and at least one tranquilizer (acetylpromazine) to calm the patient.
- Several opioid agonists (morphine, meperidine [Demerol]) and agonist-antagonist preparations (butorphanol, pentazocine) can be used to treat pain.

The goal is relaxation without ataxia. Table 29–1 lists suggested regimens to reduce anxiety with readily available drugs. The most commonly used are xylazine plus butorphanol and detomidine plus butorphanol; additional combinations are available. They provide sufficient time to stabilize the limb, assess the degree of bony involvement, and radiograph before transporting.

TABLE 29–1. **Drug Combinations and Dosages Useful in Equine Orthopedic Emergencies**

Combination	IV Dosage	Effects
Xylazine (Rompun)[1] plus	0.3–1.1 mg/kg (average, 2 ml/500 kg)	Produces sedation and analgesia for up to 30 minutes
Butorphanol (Torbugesic)[2]	0.02–0.05 mg/kg (average, 1.5 ml/500 kg)	Useful for limb stabilization and early transportation
Xylazine (Rompun)[1] plus	0.3–0.6 mg/kg (average, 2 ml/500 kg)	May cause profound hypotension in the face of excitement or high blood loss
Acetylpromazine (Acepromazine)[3]	0.02–0.03 mg/kg (average, 1.5 ml/500 kg)	Horse may fall due to a dramatic decrease in arterial blood pressure
Detomidine (Dormosedan)[4] plus	0.01–0.02 mg/kg (average, 0.5 ml/500 kg)	Ataxia is present at higher dosages, making control more difficult
Butorphanol (Torbugesic)[2]	0.02–0.05 mg/kg (average, 1 ml/500 kg)	Sedation is profound, allowing more painful manipulation. May have to delay trailering for more than 1 h

Concentrations:
[1] Rompun—100 mg/ml (Miles, Inc., Shawnee Mission, KS)
[2] Torbugesic—10 mg/ml (Fort Dodge Animal Health, Fort Dodge, IA)
[3] Acepromazine—10 mg/ml (Fort Dodge Animal Health, Fort Dodge, IA)
[4] Dormosedan—10 mg/ml (Pfizer Animal Health, Exton, PA)

COMMON ORTHOPEDIC EMERGENCIES

- Sedate or restrain patient enough to examine the injury.
- Cursory examination allows the general category of the injury to be determined.
- For **nonweight-bearing** lameness, the common ruleouts are
  □ **Displaced fractures**
  □ **Luxations**
  □ **Infection**
- Orthopedic emergencies allowing some degree of **weight bearing** include
  □ **Lacerations**
  □ **Puncture wounds**
  □ **Nondisplaced fractures**
- *Determining whether the patient can bear weight allows an initial decision to be made on how to proceed.*

FRACTURES

- Emergency treatment focuses on calming or restraining the horse.
- Assess the severity of the fracture.
- Protect the injured limb to prevent further damage.

- Horses attempt to bear weight on even a grossly unstable leg. Protection of that limb with splints or casts is needed before
  - □ Radiographic examination
  - □ Transportation to a surgical facility
- Fractures can occur in many different situations and should be suspected when
  - □ Acutely nonweight bearing
  - □ A loud crack is heard before onset of lameness.
  - □ The limb is grossly unstable.
- Physical examination determines the level of the suspected fracture.
  - □ *Forelimb fracture divisions:*
    Level 1—Phalanges and distal metacarpus
    Level 2—Midforearm to distal metacarpus
    Level 3—Mid and proximal radius
    Level 4—Proximal to the cubital (elbow) joint in the forelimb
  - □ *Hindlimb fracture divisions:*
    Level 1—Phalanges and distal metatarsus
    Level 2—Mid and proximal metatarsus
    Level 3—Tarsus (hock) and tibia
    Level 4—Femur and above

Immobilization

- Closed fractures at **levels 1 and 2** have the best prognosis for repair and are treated with a cast or splint immediately to *protect the soft tissues* from further damage.
- **Level 3** fractures, i.e., of the mid and proximal radius and the tibia, carry a grave prognosis and are often open fractures and difficult to immobilize for transport.
  - □ In foals, splinting and transport to a hospital for repair is feasible.
  - □ In adults, because of the poor prognosis, euthanasia is often recommended.
- **Level 4** fractures are surrounded by a large muscle mass and provide protection against an open fracture.
  - □ Little is done to splint or support these fractures.
  - □ Front limb splintage of the carpus allows the patient to balance on the limb for transport.

A splint-cast is recommended before transporting the patient with a fracture of the digit or the distal metacarpal/metatarsal bones (level 1).

Materials for a Splint-Cast

- Leg bandage materials
- Polyvinyl chloride (PVC) splint, 40–45 cm (~16–18 in) long
- 4–6 rolls of 4–5 inch fiber glass casting material

Procedure

- After application of a light cotton bandage to the limb from carpus/tarsus to coronary band, elevate the limb and have an assistant hold it proximal to the carpus or tarsus.

- Maintain the leg in this position until the splint-cast application is complete and the cast material cures.
- Place a PVC or wood splint on the dorsal surface of the forelimbs or the plantar surface of the hindlimbs (Figs. 29–1 and 29–2).
- PVC splints are constructed by cutting the appropriate length of 4-inch PVC pipe (available at any hardware store) into thirds longitudinally and rounding the edges.
- Incorporate PVC pipe into a fiber glass cast and allow it to set.
- Padding is minimal to prevent cast slippage during transport.
- With the limb in a cast, the patient is able to support weight on the toe without additional damage.
- Incorporation of the foot with the heel elevated requires more cast material and helps the horse maintain better balance during transport.

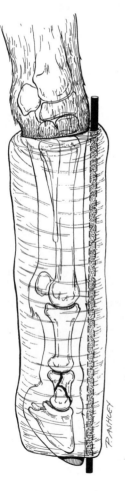

FIGURE 29–1. Splint-cast placement for a **level 1** fracture of the foreleg. The splint is placed on the dorsal surface of the limb, over minimal padding, and secured with cast material.

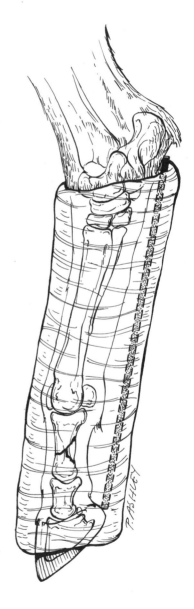

FIGURE 29–2. Splint-cast placement for a **level 1** fracture of the rear limb. The splint is placed on the plantar aspect of the limb.

Radiographs taken through the cast provide a more accurate prognosis regarding the injury and treatment options.

- An alternative limb immobilization is the use of a preformed splint that holds the leg in a slight degree of flexion and allows weight bearing on the toe. The Leg-Savr brace is an aluminum splint secured to the limb with Velcro straps (Kimzey Inc., 164 Kentucky Avenue, Woodland, CA 95695; (916) 662 9331; fax (916) 662 9178).

Fractures at level 2, proximal metacarpus to distal radius and proximal metatarsus, are supported with a Robert Jones bandage with splints caudal and lateral.

- Restrain the patient.
- Apply heavy cotton bandage to stabilize the limb and prevent fracture fragment shifting.
- Bandaging also serves to reduce edema and hematoma formation at the fracture site.
- With this support, the patient can use the limb for balance, even though not fully weight bearing, which helps reduce anxiety.

Materials for a Robert Jones Bandage

- 6–8 rolls of 1-pound-roll cotton
- 4–6 gauze bandages or elastic tape, 6-inch
- 1–2 Ace bandages, 6-inch
- 2–4 broom handles or wood splints
- Duct tape, 2-inch

Procedure

- Apply multiple layers of cotton directly to the limb if the fracture is closed and over a sterile dressing if there is a skin wound.
- After application of two rolls of cotton, place a 6-inch gauze or elastic bandage with enough pressure to hold the cotton securely in place.
- The internal pressure of the bandage protects the overlying soft tissues. In the forelimb, the resultant bandage extends from elbow to ground and is three times the diameter of the limb when completed.
- In the rear limb, the bandage extends from tuber calcaneus to the ground and is two times the diameter of the limb.
- If splints are used, they are incorporated into the last layer of cotton and gauze.
- The outermost layer of tape is inelastic material, i.e., duct tape (available at any hardware store), for rigidity.

Fractures at level 3, mid and proximal radius, tarsus, and tibia, are difficult to splint because of abduction of the lower portion of the limb.

- The lateral muscles of the upper forearm pull the lower portion of the limb outward, displacing the fracture fragments medially.
- A long extension of the lateral splint to the shoulder or hip after place-

ment of a Robert Jones wrap is used to neutralize lower limb abduction (Figs. 29–3 and 29–4).

- The splints are applied with nonelastic tape to minimize slippage during transporting.

Transportation of the Patient

- Loading should be as atraumatic as possible and is facilitated by bringing the trailer as close to the patient as possible.
- Adults do best when trailered in a confined space; they use the space for support.
- The patient is tied loosely, or not at all, allowing use of head and neck for balance.
- For a forelimb fracture, it is helpful to trailer the patient facing backward so the individual can support itself and use the rear limbs when stopping.
- If the individual has never trailered before, the added anxiety may not warrant this approach.

FIGURE 29–3. Robert Jones bandage plus splint for a fore limb **level 3** fracture. The extended splint helps reduce lower limb abduction.

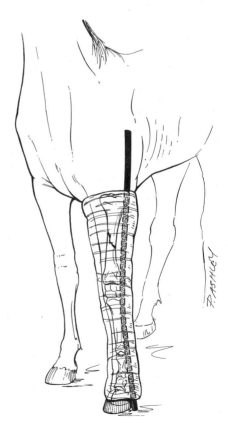

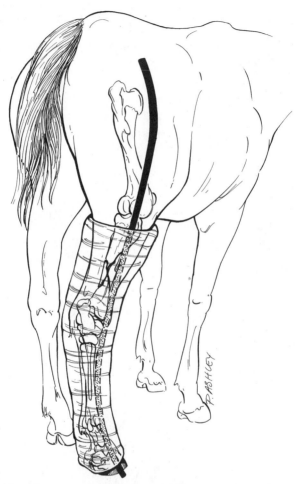

FIGURE 29–4. Robert Jones bandage plus splint for a rear limb **level 3** fracture.

- A hindlimb fracture is best transported with the patient facing forward, and extreme care is needed during unloading to protect the injured limb.
- A large stock trailer with a partition is best for a mare and injured foal. The mare is restrained on one side so she can see the foal. The bedding is deep on the foal's side for comfort.
- Having an assistant cradle the foal's head and prevent struggling is helpful.

Prognosis of Long Bone Fractures

- *The prognosis for successful repair decreases as age and weight increase.*
- Owners frequently base their decisions on whether to transport a horse for surgery on the veterinarian's advice.

- The prognosis for return to athletic function or, as a minimum, reproductive function is often the basis for the decision.
- After general evaluation and limb stabilization, take radiographs of the affected area to determine treatment options.
- Consult the nearest surgical facility treating long bone fractures for experiences and costs.
- Some owners pursue all possibilities and therefore should be referred as soon as a splint is in place; radiographs can be taken at the referral center.
- Open fractures have a poorer prognosis than closed fractures.
- Fractures more proximal on the limb have a poorer prognosis than those more distal.
- Each fracture must be considered in regard to:
  □ The owner's intended use of the horse
  □ Temperament of the horse
  □ Surgical expertise available
  □ Economics
- Specific prognoses for fractures and their treatments are summarized in Table 29–2.

Incisive Bone, Mandible, and Premaxilla Fractures

These are common; the mandible is the most frequently occurring fracture in the head.

Etiology

- Unilateral or bilateral
- Occur when teeth are caught on a fixed object
- Iatrogenic during tooth extraction/repulsion or pathologic as a result of chronic alveolar periostitis
- Interdental space most common site

Diagnosis

- Malocclusion of the incisor teeth
- Pain on palpation
- Crepitation
- Food packed into open fracture
- Fetid odor if fracture several days old
- Salivation, dysphagia, tongue protruding
- Radiographs—lateral, dorsoventral, and oblique projections

Treatment

- Horizontal and vertical fractures generally do not require surgical intervention because soft tissues support rami (pterygoid and masseter muscles)
- Stable, nondisplaced unilateral fractures generally use conservative approach.
- Fractures involving deciduous teeth require removal of involved teeth.

TABLE 29–2. **Treatment and Prognosis for Return to Former Use for Various Equine Fractures**

Fracture Location	Fracture Type	Treatment	Prognosis
Distal phalanx	Articular	Medical or surgical	Guarded
	Nonarticular	Medical	Good
Middle phalanx	Comminuted	Medical or surgical	Guarded
Proximal phalanx	Comminuted	Surgical	Guarded to poor
	Noncomminuted	Medical or surgical	Good
Proximal sesamoids			
Apical	Small/large fragments	Surgical	Good
Midbody	Displaced	Surgical	Guarded
Abaxial	Small fragments	Surgical	Fair to Good
Basilar	Small fragments	Medical/ surgical	Guarded to Poor
Comminuted/ biaxial	Several fragments	Medical/surgical	Poor
Sagittal	Complete	Medical/surgical	Poor
Metacarpal/tarsal III			
Condyle (lateral)	Nondisplaced	Surgical	Good
	Displaced	Surgical	Guarded
Condyle (medial)	Articular	Surgical	Good
Dorsal cortical	Nonarticular	Surgical	Good
Transverse	Displaced	Surgical	Poor
	Nondisplaced	Surgical	Good
Small metacarpals/ tarsals	Distal	Surgical	Good to excellent
	Proximal	Surgical	Good
Carpal bones	Chip	Surgical	Guarded to excellent
	Slab	Surgical	Poor to guarded
Tarsal bones			
Talus	Trochlear Ridges	Surgical	Good
	Sagittal	Surgical	Good
	Comminuted	Surgical	Poor
Calcaneus	Small/large fragments	Medical or surgical	Guarded
	Calcaneal tuberosity	Surgical	Guarded
	Comminuted	Medical or surgical	Fair
Central and third tarsal fractures	Slab	Surgical	Favorable
Ulna	Open	Surgical	Fair
	Closed	Surgical	Good
Radius	Open	Surgical	Poor
	Closed (<400 lb)	Surgical	Good to fair
	Closed (>400 lb)	Surgical	Poor
Humerus	Stress	Medical	Excellent
	Complete	Medical	Poor
Scapula			
Supraglenoid tubercle	Displaced	Surgical	Fair
Neck/body	Complete	Surgical	Grave
Tibia	Physeal	Surgical	Good
	Diaphyseal	Surgical	Guarded to poor
Patella			
Sagittal	Displaced	Surgical	Fair to good
Comminuted	Displaced	Surgical	Fair to good
Femur	Physeal	Medical or surgical	Guarded to poor
	Diaphyseal	Surgical	Guarded to poor

- Unstable fractures need surgical management:
  - Intraoral wire fixation
  - Orthopedic pin and wire fixation
  - Lag screw fixation
  - External thermoplastic brace
  - Intraoral U-bar technique
  - Intraoral acrylic splint
  - Intramedullary pinning
  - External skeletal fixation device
  - Dynamic compression plating

Prognosis

- Generally good.
- NOTE: Requires adequate immobilization

Temporomandibular Fractures

- Unusual occurrence
- Surgical intervention when
  - Fractures enter joint
  - Septic arthritis secondary to lacerations or puncture wounds
  - Osteoarthritis secondary to fracture healing

Clinical Signs

- Soft tissue swelling overlying the joint
- Crepitation
- Inability to open mouth
- Masseter muscle atrophy

Diagnosis

- Physical examination
- Radiographs—including oblique projections

Treatment

- Conservative approach if nondisplaced fracture
- Mandibular condylectomy—unilateral/bilateral

Prognosis

- Guarded outcome because secondary arthritis may affect mastication.

Cranial Fractures

Etiology

- Result from trauma:
  - Halter breaking

□ Trailering
□ Kick
□ Impacting a fixed structure

Clinical Signs

- Increase in intracranial pressure via edema and hemorrhage:
  □ Ataxia
  □ Anisocoria
  □ Nystagmus
  □ Head tilt
  □ Bradycardia
  □ Depressed respiration
  □ Hyperthermia
  □ Altered state of consciousness
- Hemorrhage from nose and ears

Diagnosis

- Two most common types:
  □ Dorsal/dorsolateral fractures
  □ Basilar skull fractures
- Radiographic examination of all suspected fractures of the skull

Treatment

- Nonsurgical management:
  □ Corticosteroids: 0.25 mg/kg aqueous dexamethasone IV
  □ Dimethyl sulfoxide (DMSO), 1 gm/kg as a 10%–20% solution of 0.9% saline
  □ Furosemide, to decrease circulating blood volume and pressure.
  □ Broad-spectrum antimicrobials
- Surgical management:
  □ Closed, nondisplaced fracture associated with hemorrhage and edema
  □ Open fracture with brain trauma
    Class I—does not penetrate dura mater
    Class II—inner portion of fracture penetrates dura, resulting in hemorrhage
    Class III—injury to dura mater and brain parenchyma

Prognosis

Guarded to poor if surgery is required.

Orbital and Periorbital Fractures

Clinical Signs

- Pressure on globe may result in permanent eye damage.
- Periorbital soft tissue structures may be distorted.

Diagnosis

- Physical examination and palpation
- Swelling, heat, and pain around eyelids
- Chemosis and subconjunctival hemorrhage
- Strabismus
- Radiographs, including oblique projections

Treatment

- Surgical reduction
  - □ Open technique
  - □ Closed technique

Prognosis

- Cosmetic appearance and functional status generally good
- Older and more severe fractures—poorer prognosis
- Injuries resulting in neuropathies to eye, edema, and severe trauma to globe, and fractures with injury to nasolacrimal system—guarded to poor prognosis

Nasofacial Fractures

Clinical Signs

- Common injury to the horse, involving maxilla, nasal, and frontal bones
- Marked respiratory compromise if severe bony displacement with significant soft tissue swelling obstructing the airway
- Facial deformity

Diagnosis

- Physical examination
- Facial bone asymmetry
- Local pain on palpation
- Subcutaneous emphysema
- Bone crepitation
- Epistaxis
- Soft tissue disruption overlying the fracture
- Radiographs—not always conclusive

Treatment

- Surgical treatment preferred to minimize potential sequelae:
  - □ Permanent facial deformity
  - □ Bone sequestration
  - □ Chronic sinusitis
  - □ Upper respiratory tract compromise

Prognosis

- Generally good
- Monitor for sinus infection and/or bone sequestrum formation

LUXATIONS

- Luxation results after disruption of one or more support structures of the joint.
- Clinical presentation ranges from complete instability to full weight bearing in normal alignment.
- Luxation confirmed by gross instability or severe pain when attempting weight bearing
- The interrupted soft tissue structures include:
  - ☐ Collateral ligaments
  - ☐ Intra-articular ligaments
  - ☐ Joint capsule
  - ☐ Synovium
- The luxation may be open if the skin is torn over the joint.
- The luxation can spontaneously reduce and recurs with weight bearing.
- In the most extreme cases, the joint remains dislocated.
- The prognosis depends on:
  - ☐ The degree of instability
  - ☐ Whether the luxation is open or closed

Diagnosis

- **After tranquilizing the patient, the severity of damage to the collateral support structures is evaluated by palpation, plain radiographs, stress radiographs, and ultrasound examination of the supporting soft tissues**.
- Palpation of the limb helps determine the level of the luxation if it has spontaneously reduced.
- Stress radiographs with the limb manipulated to open the affected joint space aid in determining which soft tissue structures are involved.
- If needed, ultrasound confirms complete disruption of a supporting structure.

Types of Luxation

- **Lower limb luxations**
  - ☐ Require reduction and external coaptation
  - ☐ If the luxation is open, copious lavage of the joint is required before cast application.
  - ☐ If the patient is to be transported to another facility for treatment, protect the limb as described for fractures.
- **Luxations of the scapulohumeral/shoulder joint** (rare) involve rupture of some or all of the soft tissues that stabilize this joint. These include:
  - ☐ Biceps brachii
  - ☐ Supraspinatus muscles

- □ Tendon of insertion of the infraspinatus muscle
- □ Joint capsule
- **Stifle luxation** involves damage to at least one collateral ligament in addition to one or more cruciate ligaments.
    - □ Damage to the menisci often occurs.
    - □ The prognosis for use is very poor, with degenerative joint disease a common sequela.
    - □ The exception is **patellar luxation** that is surgically managed and is usually not a traumatic event requiring emergency treatment.
- **Luxations of the hip/coxofemoral luxations** usually result in disruption of the surrounding joint capsule and the round and accessory ligaments of the femur.
    - □ Anesthesia is needed to reduce the luxation, and maintaining reduction is difficult in all but the smallest patients.
    - □ Arthritis is generally the sequela.

Prognosis

- Closed luxations of the distal tarsal, metacarpo/metatarsophalangeal, and proximal interphalangeal joints are successfully managed with long-term (12 weeks) external coaptation (cast application).
- The limb is cast in normal alignment; the foot included in the cast. General anesthesia is required for correct limb orientation. *Arthritis is a potential sequela*, so advise the owner of this.
- Individuals treated with external coaptation are often functional.
- Luxations of the distal interphalangeal joint are rare and associated with advanced degenerative joint disease and biaxial neurectomy used in treating chronic pain. Prognosis is poor. Arthrodesis is difficult.
- Affected individuals with luxations of the shoulder/hip that spontaneously reduce usually recover function of the joint.
- Patients requiring manual reduction of the luxation under general anesthesia have a guarded prognosis for a pain-free joint.
- If reduction of the luxation is not maintained, the joint becomes nonfunctional and arthritis results; euthanasia is recommended.
- Luxations of the stifle generally have severe damage to supporting structures, with limb instability making treatment impossible.

INFECTION

- Nonweight-bearing lameness indicates infection in:
    - □ A joint
    - □ Bursa
    - □ Tendon sheath
    - □ Other soft tissue structure
- Sepsis is often secondary to a laceration or puncture wound that occurred before and was not diagnosed or treated early and aggressively to prevent contamination progressing to infection.
- Lacerations, punctures, and management of secondary infections are covered in the following section.

Summary

A patient unable or unwilling to bear weight on a limb requires rapid intervention to reduce anxiety and prevent further damage to the limb.

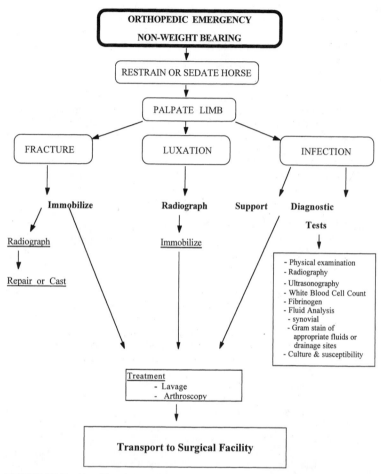

FIGURE 29–5. Algorithm for emergency management of nonweight-bearing problems.

Figure 29–5 summarizes the steps required to minimize damage, obtain a preliminary diagnosis, and prepare for referral to a medical facility.

LACERATIONS

- **One of the most common reasons for emergency assistance**.
- The initial and most important first step: determine which structures are involved.
- **Adequate treatment is impossible until all affected structures are identified**.

- The patient is restrained for evaluation, then treated or referred to a surgical facility if needed.
- Referral is based on whether the injury requires facilities or expertise not available locally and is made after the initial examination.
- Lacerations requiring special treatment include:
  □ Tendons and tendon sheaths
  □ Extensive degloving injuries
  □ Periosteum
  □ Veins and arteries
  □ Coronary band and hoof wall
  □ Joints
- Lacerations involving less critical structures are cleaned, debrided, and sutured primarily or bandaged for several days and then sutured (delayed primary closure).
- **With any laceration, adequate *tetanus prophylaxis* and appropriate antibiotic therapy is mandatory.**

Lacerations Requiring Special Care

Lacerations to Flexor Tendons and Their Sheaths

- Tranquilize the patient and assess the damaged structures.
- The depth and etiology of the laceration determines which structures are injured or severed.
- Superficial lacerations cause damage to the flexor tendon sheath only.
- Deeper lacerations affect first the superficial digital flexor tendon, next the deep digital flexor tendon, and then the suspensory ligament.
- Degree of damage, contamination, duration of injury, temperament, and extended use contribute to the prognosis. **The best prognosis is if:**
  □ **Blood and nerve supply are intact**
  □ **Contamination is minimal**
  □ **Injury is located outside the tendon sheath**
- If a flexor tendon or the suspensory ligament is completely severed, changes in the axial and flexure alignment of the limb are useful in determining the degree of damage.
- A complete laceration of the superficial flexor tendon causes the fetlock to drop slightly. When both the superficial and deep flexor tendons are severed, the fetlock drops slightly and the toe dorsiflexes—**elevates with weight bearing**.
- *Severe* loss of fetlock support results from severance of the superficial and deep flexor tendons *and* the suspensory ligaments, accompanied by toe elevation.
- "Breakdown injuries" (traumatic disruption of the suspensory apparatus—TDSA) demonstrate the same bony malalignment and are due to rupture of the suspensory ligament, distal sesamoidean ligaments, and/or biaxial fracture of the sesamoid bones. Radiographs determine the involved structures.

To transport, apply a splint to minimize hyperextension of the limb.

- This limits tendon end distraction and preserves blood and nerve supply. Several commercially produced splints can be used:

☐ Leg-Savr, Kimzey, Inc., Woodland, CA
☐ A board splint using readily available materials

Materials Needed for a Board Splint

- Leg bandages
- 1 roll of cotton padding
- Elastic tape
- 1 hardwood board, 40 cm long × 12 cm wide × 2 cm thick
- Hand drill
- Steel drill bit
- Heavy wire

APPLICATION OF THE BOARD SPLINT

- After cleaning the laceration, place a nonadherent dressing on the wound and cover the limb from coronary band to the carpus or tarsus with a cotton wrap. Place a 2-cm-thick hardwood board, 12 by 40 cm, flat on the ground. Drill holes through the horses' hoof at the toe and matching holes in the board at one end (Fig. 29–6A). If a shoe is in place, leave

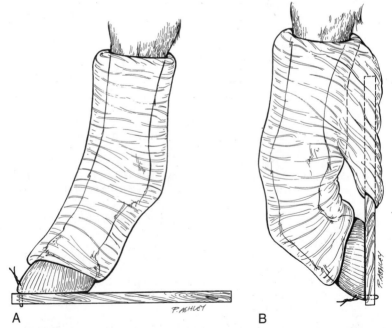

A   B

FIGURE 29–6. *A,* A flexor tendon laceration splint can be fashioned by wiring a hardwood board to the toe and flexing the limb to reduce tension on the severed tendon. *B,* The board is then incorporated into the bandage.

the shoe intact and drill holes through the shoe. Secure the board to the toe using heavy wire (16/18 gauge). Pad the board and flex the limb at the fetlock, bringing the board parallel to the caudal aspect of the cannon bone, and incorporate it in the bandage (Fig. 29–6B).

- The patient bears weight on the toe, sparing the flexor tendons, and can be safely transported to a hospital facility.
- The splint can be used as a conservative treatment, with the wraps changed as needed by lowering the splint and replacing it after wound dressing.
- If both flexor tendons or a tendon sheath is involved, *the prognosis is guarded* for return to athletic soundness.
- Perform general anesthesia and surgical debridement, reapproximation of tendon ends, and flushing of the tendon sheath (lavage of the tendon sheath using a balanced crystalloid solution with or without antibiotics added).
- If the laceration is surgically repaired, clean the site meticulously, debride the tendon ends to healthy tissue, and use heavy monofilament absorbable suture to reappose the tendon ends.
- The potential for tendon sheath infection is high, and adhesions usually occur as the tendon heals.
- Even minor tendon lacerations of the tendon sheath are expensive to manage properly, so prepare the owner for this before undertaking treatment.
- Perform cultures of the lacerated area at surgery. Start broad-spectrum antibiotic therapy immediately and make adjustments when results of the culture and sensitivity are final. Intrathecal antibiotics can be injected into the tendon sheath to increase tissue levels of the drugs. Broad-spectrum antibiotic regimens recommended for orthopedic emergencies are given in Table 29–3.

TABLE 29–3. **Broad-Spectrum Antibiotic Regimens for Orthopedic Emergencies**

Combination	Dosage	Route and Frequency
Penicillin G plus	22,000–44,000 IU/kg	IM, IV q6h
Gentamicin or	2.2 mg/kg 6.6 mg/kg	IM, IV q6–8h IM, IV q24h
Amikacin	6.6 mg/kg 15–25 mg/kg	IM, IV q8h IM, IV q24h
Ampicillin sodium plus	25–100 mg/kg	IV q6h
Gentamicin or	2.2 mg/kg 6.6 mg/kg	IM, IV q6–8h IM, IV q24h
Amikacin	6.6 mg/kg 15–25 mg/kg	IM, IV q8h IM, IV q24h
Ceftiofur (Naxcel)	1–4 mg/kg	IM, IV q12–24h
Trimethoprim/sulfa	20–30 mg/kg	PO q12h
Ticarcillin/clavulanic acid	100 mg/kg loading dose then 50 mg/kg	IV, q6h

Lacerations to Extensor Tendons

- These injuries rarely involve a tendon sheath and have a better prognosis than flexor tendon injuries.
- Frequently they can be cleaned, bandaged, and maintained in an extensor splint and heal well without primary reapposition of the severed tendon ends.
- An extensor splint is fashioned by drilling two holes in the toe of the hoof with the shoe in place.
- A splint is made of heavy PVC the length of the limb from toe to just below the carpus or tarsus.
- Holes matching those on the hoof are drilled in one end of the splint.
- Clean and debride the wound, then dress and bandage.
- Wire the splint to the cranial aspect of the limb, bring it up over the bandage, and secure it in place with elastic tape (Fig. 29–7).
- Lower the splint periodically for wrap changes during healing.

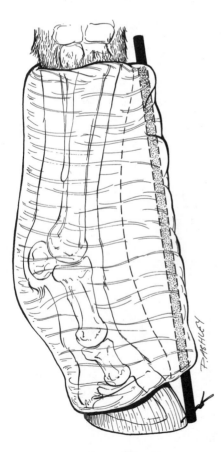

FIGURE 29–7. An extensor tendon laceration can be protected by wiring a polyvinylchloride splint to the toe, extending the digit, and incorporating the splint into the bandage.

- This splint prevents knuckling of the foot during walking and helps insure that the extensor tendon heals in the normal position.

Degloving Injuries

- Lacerations that remove large amounts of tissue from the lower limb are referred to as **degloving injuries** because the superficial tissues pull away like a glove from the hand.
- Assessing tissue viability when the wound is first examined is difficult.
- Clean, dress, and bandage the wound.
- Start broad-spectrum antibiotic therapy (see Table 29–3) immediately. If the degloving injury is extensive, use general anesthesia to debride and reapproximate the tissues.
- Meticulously remove dirt, and use large mattress sutures to reappose the injured tissues.
- A cast is advisable for 7–10 days to immobilize the injured tissues, reduce edema, and promote revascularization.
- **Large areas of skin can be salvaged by rapid cleaning and cast immobilization**.
- After the cast is removed, which tissues are viable and which need to be debrided is apparent.
- Debride dark brown or black, leathery tissue back to healthy, pink, and bleeding tissue.
- Skin grafting may be needed later to cover unepithelialized areas.
- When a degloving injury has exposed bone, osteitis, osteomyelitis, and bone sequestration are frequent sequelae.
- Suspect these conditions if healing of the original injury is slow, or if the wound reopens after closing.
- Obtain radiographs of the limb if healing does not progress as expected, to determine whether a sequestrum or other bony problem exists.
- If the bone shows areas of lysis, periostitis, or sequestration, additional debridement and/or antibiotic therapy is needed before the overlying tissues will heal.

Large Vessel and Nerve Lacerations

- If a large vessel of the distal limb is lacerated, it is possible, but uncommon, for exsanguination to occur.
- The bleeding is reduced/stopped by compression, using pressure wraps over the bleeding area, padding the area heavily, and reinforcing the bandage with elastic tape.
- If the severed vessel is the major blood supply to the area, perform suture repair under general anesthesia.
- Leave the pressure bandage in place until the patient is under anesthesia, to minimize additional blood loss.
- Lacerations of major arteries such as the brachial and femoral **can** be rapidly fatal and usually accompany fractures of the humerus or radius (brachial artery) or femur and pelvis (femoral artery). Repair is usually not feasible.
- Lacerations to nerves in the lower limb are more common than clinically

recognized (unless neuromas form during healing) and generally cause few problems.

- Severance of major nerves high in the limb is caused by fractures of the humerus or femur and is not repaired.
- Complete severance of nerves is difficult to distinguish from nerve trauma (neuropraxia) that resolves with time.
- When in doubt, use nonsteroidal anti-inflammatory drugs (NSAIDs) to decrease edema and inflammation around the nerve. An improvement in the limb is seen within several days with neuropraxia, and no change if the nerve is severed.
- In most cases, damage to large nerves is recognized clinically by a change in limb carriage:
  - ☐ Damage to the main trunk of the radial nerve interrupts innervation of the triceps muscle, causing the elbow to drop, and is most common with a fracture of the humerus.
  - ☐ Damage to lower branches of the radial nerve cause stumbling or poor placement of the foot and is due to an injury to the antebrachium.
  - ☐ Damage to the femoral nerve supplying the quadriceps muscles causes the affected individual to be unable to fix the stifle or bear full weight on the limb.
  - ☐ Damage to the tibial and peroneal nerves results in stumbling and the inability to extend the digit.

Coronary Band and Hoof Wall Lacerations

- The coronary band supplies blood to the germinal tissue of the hoof wall; any interruption in its integrity results in a permanent hoof wall defect.
- Clean lacerations of the coronary band carefully and place a large, horizontal mattress suture of #1/2 nonabsorbable suture material to bridge the defect.
- Minimizing the gap in the coronary band defect minimizes the hoof wall defect.
- If a portion of the coronary band is displaced, repair it at the time of injury.
- If such a wound heals by second intention, the abnormal hoof wall growth requires lifelong hoof wall management caused by the defect.
- Lacerations of the hoof wall are examined for
  - ☐ Depth of the defect
  - ☐ Instability of the hoof capsule
  - ☐ Involvement of the distal interphalangeal joint and soft tissues
- To evaluate deep lacerations properly, use local or general anesthesia.
- To transport, place a clean, well-padded bandage around the foot, including the sole, and extend it to the fetlock joint.
- If bleeding is excessive, use several layers of cotton applied over the initial bandaging material.
- Placing a plastic bag between cotton layers helps confine the hemorrhage, keeps the outer layers from becoming blood-soaked, and minimizes contamination during transport.
- When the wrap is complete, impervious tape (duct tape) is placed over the outside to waterproof and provide wear resistance until repair.

- Broad-spectrum antibiotic therapy (see Table 29–3) and tetanus prophylaxis are recommended.
- After cleaning and debriding a hoof wall laceration, achieve stability by using a "slipper" cast (Fig. 29–8) or by using a bar shoe and bandages.
- Hoof wall lacerations require 4–8 months to heal by new hoof formation rather than healing from side to side.

Joint Lacerations

- A joint laceration is an emergency and is confirmed if bone and cartilage are seen.
- Even if the joint surface is not seen, the proximity of the laceration to the joint may suggest involvement.
- If joint involvement is even suspected, broad-spectrum antibiotics (see Table 29–3) are started immediately, followed by additional diagnostic procedures to rule out joint involvement.
- Techniques to determine joint involvement:
  □ Sedate the patient.
  □ Surgically prepare the opposite side of the joint, inject sterile saline intra-articularly, and check if it communicates with the laceration.
  □ Sterile methylene blue dye can be used.
  □ Alternatively, inject sterile contrast medium and take a radiograph focusing on the lacerated area to determine whether the joint capsule is open.
- *If the joint is involved, place the patient under general anesthesia and lavage the affected joint copiously*:
  □ After sterile preparation, place a 14-gauge needle intra-articularly opposite the laceration.

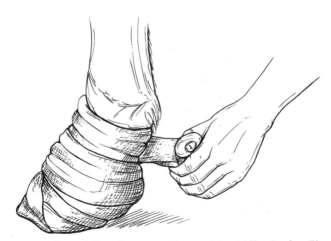

FIGURE 29–8. Short "slipper" casts can be used to stabilize hoof wall/coronary band lacerations. The cast can be applied with the horse standing and should extend to just beneath the fetlock joint.

□ Infuse a continuous ingress flow of lactated Ringer's plus 10% DMSO through the joint during debridement of the wound.

□ Infusion of an antibiotic solution after lavage is advocated in addition to broad-spectrum systemic antibiotics.

□ Avoid antibiotics with a low pH; they are irritating to the synovium.

□ Crystalline penicillin (1×10^6 IU) or a solution of gentamicin (50 mg/ml) or amikacin (250 mg/ml) buffered with sodium bicarbonate (1 mEq/ml) is safely infused after a thorough lavage.

□ Gentamicin is supplied at a pH of 2.0, and a near-normal pH is achieved by adding 2 ml of sodium bicarbonate to 1 ml of gentamicin.

□ If the laceration is clean and can be closed primarily, maintain a closed suction drain for 2–4 days.

□ Apply antibiotic ointment at the drain exit site and cover the area with a sterile bandage.

□ When fluid is removed from the suction system, be careful not to contaminate the drain and the exit portal.

□ Superficial contamination may lead to an ascending infection and therefore requires careful monitoring.

□ After drain removal (<10 ml q6–8h), leave sterile wraps in place until joint fluid is no longer evident on the bandage.

- *If the patient becomes progressively more lame as the laceration heals, suspect infection.*
- Aspiration of joint fluid for cytology and culture and susceptibility testing is essential in determining etiology.
- A white cell count >30,000 cells/dl in synovial fluid is presumptive evidence of infection.
- Repeat culture and sensitivity testing of the fluid until sepsis is ruled out.
- If antibiotic therapy had been discontinued, reinstitute it.
- Sequential joint lavages, with continuous suction drainage between, reduces the bacterial count and joint destruction caused by the septic inflammation.
- Joint lacerations carry a guarded prognosis: **early, aggressive** diagnosis and treatment maximize the chance for recovery.

PUNCTURE WOUNDS

- **Punctures into synovial structures, including joints, tendon sheaths, and bursae**, are emergencies:
  □ Introduction of bacteria into these closed spaces can result in life-threatening infections.
  □ Joint and tendon sheath punctures are treated as small lacerations to these structures.
  □ Aspiration of synovial fluid for culture and sensitivity, meticulous cleaning of the area, copious lavage, broad-spectrum antibiotic therapy (see Table 29–3), and bandaging are recommended.
- **Puncture wounds of the sole of the foot**, with injury to the frog or the bars, are likely to involve deeper structures such as the digital cushion, navicular bursa, deep digital flexor tendon and sheath, and distal interphalangeal joint.

- If these structures are involved, **conservative treatment with soaking and systemic treatment alone are NOT sufficient to prevent infection**.
- If a puncture wound is found in this area, aggressive diagnosis and treatment are required.
- Radiograph the foot with the penetrating object in place if possible to give an indication of the depth of penetration.
- If the object has been removed, locate, open, and clean the tract and introduce a sterile probe before taking the radiograph. **Do NOT force** the probe into the deeper tissues.
- Extension of a tract can be delineated using contrast medium.
- If radiographs indicate that the navicular bursa, deep digital flexor tendon sheath, or distal interphalangeal joint has been entered, synovial samples of these structures are confirmatory for involvement:
  - ☐ Distal interphalangeal joint fluid is obtained by aspiration 1 cm above the coronary band, 1 cm medial or lateral to the extensor tendon (Fig. 29–9b).
  - ☐ Flexor tendon sheath fluid is obtained by aspiration of the most fluctuant area of the sheath (Fig. 29–9a).
  - ☐ Navicular bursa fluid is difficult to aspirate. Aseptically prepare the area on the lateral aspect of the pastern proximal to the collateral cartilage; insert a 20-gauge, 1.5-inch needle palmar to the second phalanx and dorsal to the deep digital flexor tendon. Advance the needle toward the sole of the medial hoof (Fig. 29–9c).
- If the white cell count is increased with degenerate neutrophils, suspect infection and lavage the joint or tendon sheath—best accomplished with the patient under general anesthesia.
- If the navicular bursa is involved, create a surgical window into the bursa from the frog and establish ventral drainage (Fig. 29–10). This is referred to as a "street nail" procedure.
- Punctures are misleading because they appear benign when first encountered; thus aggressive therapy is frequently delayed until clinical signs of infection occur.
- *At this point the prognosis is guarded for return to athletic function.*
- When penetration is suspected, aggressive treatment is recommended.

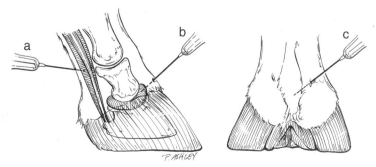

FIGURE 29–9. Placement of needles for centesis of the deep digital flexor tendon sheath (a), distal interphalangeal joint (b), and navicular bursa (c).

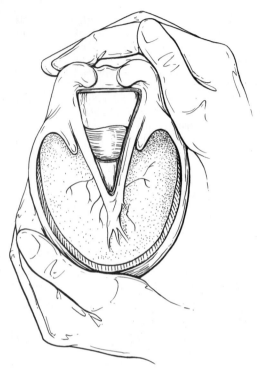

FIGURE 29–10. With punctures in the middle third of the frog, damage to the navicular bone and/or its bursa should be suspected. A "street nail" surgery to drain the bursa and see the navicular bone may be needed.

- Perform lavage with the patient standing, using xylazine and butorphanol sedation (see Table 29–1); however, most cases require general anesthesia.
- Post lavage bandaging includes sterile dressings over the puncture site, and, if a portion of the sole or frog is removed, bandaging is needed until horn tissue covers the area. Fabricate a treatment or "medicine plate" shoe, allowing easy bandage changes to minimize the work and cost of daily treatment.
- Keep the foot dry and clean and limit exercise until the wound is covered with granulation tissue and a cornified layer forms.

Summary

- Many equine orthopedic emergencies present with the patient bearing all or some weight on the affected limb.
- This is true in cases of minor, or incomplete, fractures, lacerations, and puncture wounds.

- Because the patient appears to be in less distress, the injury is not viewed as serious or requiring emergency care.
- *If treatment is not initiated soon after injury, the sequela can be life threatening.*
- Figure 29–11 provides guidelines for treating injuries in which the patient presents with an injury that allows weight bearing and is managed as an emergency.

LAMINITIS (FOUNDER)

Acute Laminitis

- Inflammation and degenerative changes of the lamina along the dorsal aspect of the foot, arising from metabolic events that reduce blood flow to the laminae.
- Changes within the foot include vasoconstriction, arteriovenous shunting, microthrombosis, resulting ischemia, and edema.
- Platelet aggregation may be an early event.
- Systemically, tachycardia, hypovolemia, hypertension, and mild metabolic acidosis are usually observed.
- The forefeet are more commonly affected, but laminitis may involve just one digit or all four feet.
- Always consider acute laminitis an *emergency* condition. Irreversible degenerative changes to the foot can result from treatment delays.

Advanced/Refractory Laminitis

- Severe pain and lameness
- Distal phalangeal rotation
- Vertical distal phalangeal displacement (sinking)
- Digital sepsis and necrosis
- Hoof wall detachment
- Digital abnormalities:
  □ Abnormal hoof growth seen as rings on hoof wall
  □ Long toes
  □ Overgrown heel
  □ Dropped sole with flat or convex foot
  □ Distal phalanx penetrates sole.
- Recurrences of acute laminitis

Precipitating Factors

- Carbohydrate overload (excess grain, lush pasture)
- Obesity
- GI disease or endotoxemia, including:
  □ Colic
  □ Enteritis/colitis including NSAID toxicity
  □ Strangulation/obstruction of small intestine
  □ Also, retained placenta, metritis, abortion, pleuritis
- Abdominal surgery

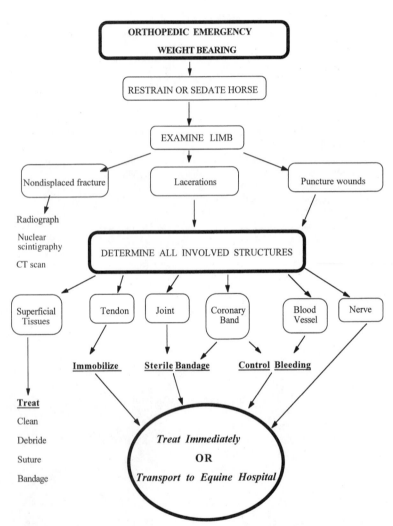

FIGURE 29–11. Algorithm for emergency management of weight-bearing problems.

- Corticosteroid therapy (particularly triamcinolone acetate)
- Hypothyroidism
- Excessive exercise on hard surface (road founder, usually subacute, self-limiting)
- Exposure to black walnut wood shavings (usually subacute, self-limiting)
- Excessive cold water intake when overheated
- Equine Cushing's disease/pituitary gland adenomas (7–40 years)

Preventive Measures for Individuals at Risk

- Eliminate exposure to precipitating factors
- Mineral oil via nasogastric tube in cases of ingested toxins/ overload
- Maintain hydration
- Support frog
- Treat sepsis or other underlying disease
- Anti-inflammatory drugs, e.g., phenylbutazone, flunixin meglumine, ketoprofen, or carprofen
- Anticoagulant therapy: aspirin (11–20 mg/kg); heparin advocated by some (40–150 IU/kg q8–12h)
- Appropriate nutrition
- Pentoxifylline, 8.4 mg/kg PO q12h
- Nitroglycerine ointment, 15 mg/digital artery/day

Diagnosis

SIGNS

- Increased digital pulse—in most cases
- Heat felt over hoof wall—in most cases
- Pain evident with hoof testers over toe—in most cases
- Pain noted when digital pressure is applied to the coronary band
- Edema in the pastern region—in some cases
- Signs of pain and lameness:
  - Lifting feet constantly while standing (Obel grade 1)
  - Stiff or stilted gait (Obel grade 2)
  - Refusal to allow foreleg to be lifted (Obel grade 3)
  - Recumbent, unwilling to move (Obel grade 4)
- Digital abnormalities (suggesting rotation):
  - Depression at base/toe of coronary band
  - Sole flat rather than concave
- Systemic hypertension common
- Signs of endotoxemia common

RADIOGRAPHIC ASSESSMENT

Use baseline and serial lateral radiographs of affected digit to monitor therapy. Signs of progression include:

- Separation of distal phalanx from dorsal hoof wall
- Distal displacement of distal phalanx

- Rotation of distal phalanx away from dorsal hoof wall
- Rotation and sinking of distal phalanx
- Soft tissue defect along dorsal coronary band
- Accumulation of gas beneath hoof wall (suspect infection)
- Pedal osteitis or osteomyelitis in chronic laminitis
- Spur formation on tip of distal phalanx in chronic laminitis

Treatment

Goals

- Restore blood flow to foot.
- Control pain and inflammation.
- Normalize blood pressure.
- Protect foot from further injury—both physiologic and mechanical.
- Prevent or treat infection.
- Prevent or correct rotation.
- Prevent displacement of distal phalanx.

MEDICAL TREATMENT

- Mineral oil to remove or block uptake of intestinal contents (1–3 treatments, 2 hours or longer apart, 4 liters for a 500-kg adult)
- Hyperimmune plasma incubated with 100 U heparin to activate antithrombin III (AT III) and decrease hoof edema
- Phenylbutazone, 4.0 mg/kg IV initial dose, then orally 4.0 mg/kg q24h, gradually tapering dose when stabilized
  or
- Flunixin meglumine, 1.1 mg/kg IV q8h for several days; analgesic effect is not as good as phenylbutazone; anticoagulant and vasodilating effects via inhibition of prostanoids may be greater.
- Antihypertensive/vasodilating agents, such as:
  □ Phenoxybenzamine (0.8 mg/kg IV in two divided doses, 12 hours apart)
  □ Acepromazine, 0.02–0.06 mg IV or IM 3–6 times daily, 1–3 days, preferred unless hypovolemia present
  □ Isoxsuprine, 1.2 mg/kg orally q12h indefinitely
- Aspirin, 11–20 mg/kg every other day, can be used in combination with other NSAIDs.
- DMSO, 10% solution, 1.0 gm/kg IV, can be used in combination with NSAIDs.
- *Treatment* of *accompanying disease* (e.g., *metritis, diarrhea, colic*)
- Contraindicated: corticosteroids
- Nerve blocks sometimes used to alleviate pain, but there is risk of further mechanical injury with increased weight bearing.
- Insulin and glucose therapy sometimes used in obese individual or when laminitis follows steroid treatment

- Lidocaine infusion for refractory pain: 9 vials/20% lidocaine in 1 liter fluids = 16.5 mg/ml; maintenance dose (ml/hr): (0.05 mg × kg) × 60 (min) ÷ 16.5; this equals 0.05 mg/kg/min.
- Nitric oxide—nitroglycerine patches, 60 mg/day topical dose, approximately equivalent to 0.3 mg/kg q24h (1-inch strip = 15 mg)

PHYSICAL AND NUTRITIONAL THERAPY

- Stand affected individual in sand, or bed in sand topped with fine wood chips.
- Pack sole with evenly distributed resilient material, e.g., silicone, tar and oakum, gauze, cast material; if sinking occurs, support frog only.
- Moderate exercise on soft surface to improve digital blood flow, if pain is not too severe; *forced exercise may contribute to digital abnormalities.*
- Avoid exercise if rotation or sinking is present.
- *IV fluids if needed to prevent dehydration*—avoid overhydration.
- Feed grass hay, or grass and alfalfa hay, with little or no grain.
- Potassium chloride orally, 30 gm q12h; withhold sodium chloride.
- Oral methionine, 30 gm daily, and biotin, 15–100 mg daily, to help restore normal hoof
- Multivitamin and trace mineral supplementation
- Wrap limbs to prevent edema, which may inhibit venous return.
- If the feet are hot, continue standing in cold water to decrease tissue oxygen requirement and preserve cellular integrity when used with medical therapy.

THERAPEUTIC TRIMMING AND SHOEING

Goals
- Trimming—reverse distal phalanx rotation and provide nonpainful weight-bearing surface.
- Shoeing—prevent further tissue destruction or distal phalanx rotation, provide support to painful areas, and enhance healing of digit.

Options and Considerations
- Debride abscesses and soak foot in dilute povidone-iodine and Epsom salt solution.
- Trim to shorten and roll toe and to lower heel.
- Multiple trimmings at 4-week intervals may be needed.
- Hoof wall resection or selective decompression by drilling may be needed to expose necrotic tissue or drain infected laminae, or to relieve pressure produced by sinking.
- Support frog with padding.
- Lower heel with pad.
- Silicone rubber inserts between pad and sole.
- Shoe should provide frog or sole support; recommendations include glue-on shoes, adjustable and nonadjustable heart bar shoes, frog pads with steel or aluminum treatment plates.
- Frequent adjustments by a skilled farrier are generally needed.

SURGICAL TREATMENT

- Deep digital flexor tenotomy—reserved for refractory laminitis, usually a salvage procedure for breeding individuals.
- Inferior check ligament desmotomy

PROGNOSTIC INDICATORS

- Good:
  - □ Response to therapy evident after 24–48 hours
  - □ Normalization of blood pressure
  - □ No signs of rotation or sinking
  - □ Low Obel grade at time of diagnosis/treatment
  - □ Less than 5.5° of rotation
  - □ Normalization of endocrine dysfunction
  - □ No progression evident radiographically over 8 weeks of treatment
- Poor:
  - □ More than 11.5° of rotation
  - □ All four feet affected
  - □ Decrease in size of distal phalanx
  - □ Transverse fractures of distal phalanx
  - □ Significant sinking of distal phalanx
  - □ Concurrent chronic disease (e.g., chronic infection, liver, renal, or GI disease, or hypertension)
- Guarded:
  - □ No response in 24 hours to appropriate anti-inflammatory therapy

PEDIATRIC ORTHOPEDIC EMERGENCIES

- The principles for emergency treatment of foals parallel those for adults:
  - □ Sedate or tranquilize the patient.
  - □ Examine the injury.
  - □ Apply protective splints or bandages.
  - □ Consider the advisability of and options for further treatment.
- Compared with adults, fractures in foals respond to treatment well and heal more rapidly.
- Internal fixation is more successful than with the adult because of lower body weight.
- With open fractures or puncture wounds, the foal may be more prone to complications of septicemia and/or focal infection due to:
  - □ Greater blood flow to the growing bone
  - □ The immaturity of the immune system

Splints and Casts

- A splint can be constructed from half-shell PVC pipe applied over sufficient cotton wrapping.
- Remove and reset twice a day to prevent pressure sores from developing.
- If used, a cast should leave the foot free (sleeve/cylinder cast).
- Full-leg casts can produce osteopenia and severe flexor laxity.
- Two products that can be adapted for treating orthopedic injuries in foals:
  - □ A semirigid support-wrap (Scotchrap, Animal Care Products, 3M Health Care, St. Paul, MN 55133-3275 (800) 228-3957)
  - □ A one-step splint (Scotchcast, 3M Animal Care Products)
- When rigid immobilization is not required, use a semirigid support.

- The one-step splint consists of:
  - □ Multiple layers of knitted fiberglass fabric impregnated with polyurethane resin.
  - □ One side has an air- and moisture-permeable nonwoven fabric, and the other is padded with a permeable open-cell foam.
  - □ After it sets on exposure to water, the splint is lightweight, strong, and radiolucent and conforms to the limb.

Tendon Rupture

- Bilateral extensor tendon rupture can occur in a foal with flexural contracture that is straining to keep up with the mare at pasture.
- Most often seen in large foals with mildly bucked knees and marked by a soft, fluid-filled swelling on the carpus
- Heavy wraps reduces the swelling but may cause tendon laxity.
- Larger foals require more rigid support, and for them, splints or fiberglass-reinforced wraps are added to the support wraps.
- Surgery is usually not required to reappose the tendon ends, which reunite over the course of several months.

Rupture of the Gastrocnemius Tendon

- Rare in the foal and usually occurs in foals <1 week old; believed more common in the premature or dysmature foal struggling to rise, particularly on slippery floors.
- Occurs at the muscle-tendon junction of the gastrocnemius rather than at the insertion and therefore heals rapidly.

Diagnosis

Common clinical signs:

- Large hematoma on caudal aspect of the affected hind limb
- It is possible to flex the hock without flexing the stifle.

Ancillary testing to confirm the diagnosis:

- Ultrasound
- Radiography—to rule out avulsion fractures

Treatment

NOTE: **Treat as an emergency**.

- Apply Schroeder-Thomas splint ASAP.
- Assist foal in standing on three legs to:
  - □ Nurse
  - □ Prevent decubital sores
- After 5–7 days, apply an external coaptation bandage, i.e., Robert Jones bandage with splint; reset every 2–3 days.
- Remove Schroeder-Thomas splint after a maximum of 10–12 days to prevent severe contracture and problems with soft tissues.

Prognosis

Good for use as a pleasure horse, and poor for use as a performance athlete.

Prevention

Avoid slippery surfaces, especially if foal is weak. Assist/support the weak individual and improve footing.

Luxation of the Superficial Digital Flexor (SDF) Tendon

- Reported in adults due to trauma; rare in foals and presumed to be traumatic in origin or due to overexercise in rapidly growing foals
- Due to disruption of the supporting structure of tendon; may be bilateral

Diagnosis

- Large swelling uni- or bilaterally in area of tuber calcaneus
- Acute lameness that improves with symptomatic treatment
- Ultrasonography diagnostic procedure of choice:
  - □ Disruption of medial attachment with tendon displaced laterally most common
  - □ Disruption of lateral attachment with tendon displaced medially
  - □ SDF splits longitudinally with a portion of tendon on each side of tuber calcaneus

Treatment

- Conservative
  - □ Stall confinement
  - □ External coaptation
  - □ NSAIDs
- Surgical correction
  - □ Mesh onlay graft to repair disrupted tissue

Prognosis

Varies with expectations for athletic use.

Fractures

Management

- Fractures of any bone of the hind- or forelimb are relatively common in foals, due to their playful disposition and the vulnerability of the growing bone to the effects of a kick or a fall. In most cases treatment is surgical.
- Compared with adults, foals respond well to methods of internal fixation because:
  - □ Bone remodeling and periosteal growth are more rapid.
  - □ Their body weight approximates that of adult humans, for whom the orthopedic implants were originally designed.

□ They are more easily restrained after reduction and fixation, making refracture less likely during recovery from anesthesia.
- Fractures to the third metacarpal/metatarsal bone require immediate stabilization because of the sparse soft tissue covering; prognosis depends on the success and stability of fixation.
- Suspensory disruption or breakdown injury occasionally occurs as a result of biaxial fracture of the proximal sesamoid bones in youngsters that are overexercised (Fig. 29–12).
- Management with splints has generally been more successful than surgical treatment.

Physeal Fractures
- The physis is the vulnerable point in the immature skeleton.
- It is weaker than the mature bone, joint capsule, ligaments, or tendons;

FIGURE 29–12. Biaxial fractures of proximal sesamoid bones; dorsal palmar view.

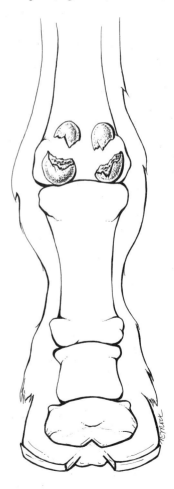

sufficient shearing or avulsion force often results in a fracture through the cartilaginous cells in the growth plate.

- Physeal fractures are the *most common* fracture in foals; suspect them in any foal showing signs of joint fracture or dislocation.
- Considered more serious than diaphyseal fractures because of the risk of disturbed growth patterns and of involvement of adjoining articular surfaces.
- Early recognition and treatment are essential to prevent development of angular limb deformity or arthritis.
- The Salter-Harris classification (Fig. 29–13) is a useful guide to determine prognosis and treatment options.
- In general, the prognosis worsens as the classification number increases, but other relevant prognostic factors include:
  □ Severity of the trauma to the growth plate
  □ Integrity of the vasculature
  □ Location of the physis
  □ Foal's age
  □ Time elapsed after injury before treatment is initiated.
- Types I and II are the most common physeal fractures, with a relatively good prognosis for healing without lameness, and involve metacarpal/metatarsal III.

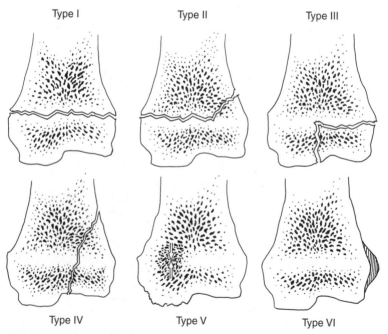

FIGURE 29–13. Salter-Harris fracture classification. (Adapted from Salter RB, Harris WR: Injuries involving the epiphyseal plate. *In* Stashak TS: Adam's Lameness in Horses. Philadelphia, Lea & Febiger, 1987, p 298, with permission.)

- Femoral capital physeal fractures or proximal femoral physis fractures are among the most common of types I and II and are generally managed more successfully with internal fixation than with stall confinement.
- Proximal femoral fractures have a better prognosis than those to the distal femoral physis because the contour of the distal femur makes repair difficult and the strength of the available implants is often inadequate.
- Younger foals appear to have better prospects for achieving a sound, straight limb than older ones.
- Physeal fractures heal rapidly, in approximately half the time required for metaphyseal fractures.
- Commonly occurring complications:
  □ Infection
  □ Flexor muscle/atrophy
  □ Tendon contracture
  □ Cast sores
  □ Gluteal muscle atrophy in the affected limb
  □ Stretched flexor tendons
  □ Angular limb deformity in the contralateral limb
- Premature closure of the growth plate may occur regardless of the method of treatment.

Infection

- Infection can cause serious physeal damage and leads to instability and failure in repaired fractures.
- The extensive vasculature of equine long bones promotes bacterial spread, septic arthritis, osteomyelitis, and physitis, which are often present concurrently.
- For this reason, assume foals with septic arthritis and osteomyelitis in one or more joints to be septicemic, though there may be few clinical signs of systemic infection.
- Because of increased blood flow to the developing bone, septicemia quickly spreads to involve the joints, with bacteria carried across the growth plates by the transphyseal vessels that supply the area.
- Bacterial penetration of the physis is followed by an acute inflammatory reaction, with subsequent ischemia and bone necrosis.
- Once significant necrosis has occurred, antimicrobial therapy alone is not adequate. Debridement and drainage of the inflammatory by-products from the joint by through-and-through lavage are needed.
- The most common sites of focal infection (osteomyelitis or septic arthritis):
  □ Medial and lateral femoral condyles
  □ Tibial tarsal condyles
  □ Lateral styloid process of the radius
  □ Distal tibia
  □ Patella
  □ Distal metacarpal/metatarsal III
- Foals with septic arthritis or osteomyelitis have:
  □ Lameness
  □ Pain
  □ ± ↑ Rectal temperature

- □ Warmth and swelling in the affected joints
- □ Involvement of more than one joint also supports a diagnosis of septic arthritis or osteomyelitis.
- ■ Radiographically:
  - □ Osteomyelitis is recognized by bone lysis with or without associated soft tissue swelling.
  - □ Septic arthritis appears as soft tissue swelling and widening of the joint space and is distinguished from incomplete ossification primarily by the physical signs of swelling and warmth in the affected joints.
- ■ Infection in epiphyseal bone is marked early on by:
  - □ Swelling at the level of the physis and sensitivity to point pressure at this site
  - □ Radiographic signs may not be present for 3–7 days, at which time the prognosis has worsened considerably.
  - □ Suspect septic epiphysitis (and septic arthritis) in any foal with lameness, synovial fluid WBC > 40,000 cells/μl, total protein > 2.5 g/dl, and bacteria isolated from the joint.
- ■ Musculoskeletal infections in newborns and foals are most frequently caused by:
  - □ Gram-negative organisms; gram-positive pathogens are sometimes isolated in foals with septic arthritis.
  - □ Broad-spectrum antibiotic treatment is indicated, pending results of culture and sensitivity studies.
  - □ A combination of an aminoglycoside (gentamicin or amikacin) with a penicillin or cephalosporin provides broad, relatively safe coverage pending culture results.
  - □ Foals are believed to be more sensitive to the nephrotoxic effects of aminoglycosides because of their slower rate of elimination.
  - □ If use of an aminoglycoside is contraindicated by the presence of renal disease, a third-generation cephalosporin provides the needed gram-negative coverage.
  - □ Dosage guidelines are presented in Table 29–4.
  - □ Polymethylmethacrylate (PMMA) antibiotic impregnated beads placed at the site of infection increase tissue concentration of drugs (e.g., gentamicin and amikacin).

Angular Limb Deformity

Not considered an orthopedic emergency but important to recognize early in any foal with "crooked" legs. Three major types:

TABLE 29–4. **Antibiotic Treatment for Infection in Newborns and Foals**

Agent	Dose	Route and Frequency
Procaine penicillin G	22,000–44,000 IU/kg	IM, q12h
Sodium/potassium penicillin G	22,000–44,000 IU/kg	IV, q6h
Gentamicin	2.2 mg/kg/6.6–8.8 mg/kg	IM, IV q6–8h/q24h
Amikacin	6.6 mg/kg/15–25 mg/kg	IM, IV q8h/q24h
Ceftiofur	1–4 mg/kg	IM, IV q12h
Ticarcillin/clavulanic acid	50–100 mg/kg	IV, q6h

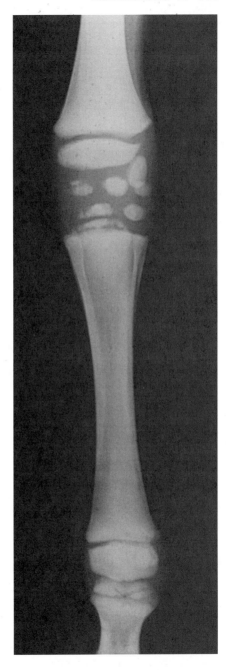

FIGURE 29–14. Dorsopalmar radiograph of the carpus, demonstrating incomplete ossification of cuboidal bones. Note the wide joint spaces surrounding small, rounded bones.

- Laxity of the periarticular supporting structures:
  - ☐ Usually knock-kneed (valgus deformity)
  - ☐ MUST differentiate from incomplete ossification of the cuboidal bones, using radiographic evaluation
  - ☐ Responds with moderate exercise over 7–10 days
- Incomplete ossification of cuboidal bones of the carpus and tarsus:
  - ☐ MOST COMMONLY recognized in the premature, dysmature, or twin foal
  - ☐ Radiographic evaluation *essential* to confirm incomplete ossification (Fig. 29–14)
  - ☐ Affects cuboidal bones of carpus and tarsus primarily
  - ☐ Results in permanent deformity and early degenerative joint disease if not recognized EARLY in life
  - ☐ Treatment includes external coaptation with well-padded splints or tube casts.
- Disproportionate growth of epiphysis/metaphysis:
  - ☐ A growth imbalance above the affected joint
  - ☐ Generally seen in foals several weeks of age or older
  - ☐ Differentiated by radiographic evaluation of epiphysis
  - ☐ Treatment is designed to promote growth on affected side.

Summary

- Orthopedic emergencies are not uncommon in foals, whose immature bones are vulnerable to kicks, falls, infection, and the ill effects of overfeeding and inappropriate exercise.
- Foals respond to treatment more readily and rapidly than do adults.
- Internal fixation is most often the preferred treatment option.
- Infection should always be a concern with any trauma to the bone or joint.

SUGGESTED REFERENCES

Bramlage LR. Emergency first aid treatment and transportation of equine fracture patients. *In* Auer JA, ed: Equine Surgery. Philadelphia, WB Saunders, 1992, pp 807–811.

Embertson RM, Bramlage LR, Gabel AA. Physeal fractures in the horse: Management and outcome. Vet Surg 1986;15:230.

Holland M. Preanesthetic medication and chemical restraint. *In* White NA, Moore JN, eds: Current Practice of Equine Surgery. Philadelphia, JB Lippincott, 1990, pp 59–64.

Honnas CM. Surgical treatment of selected musculoskeletal disorders of the forelimb. *In* Auer JA, ed: Equine Surgery. Philadelphia, WB Saunders, 1992, p 1036.

Nixon AJ. Tendon lacerations. *In* White NA, Moore JN, eds: Current Practice of Equine Surgery. Philadelphia, JB Lippincott, 1990, pp 455–461.

Orsini JA. Pharmacotherapy of the critically ill neonate. *In* Higgins AJ, Wright IM, eds: The Equine Manual. London, WB Saunders, 1995, pp 755–763.

Orsini JA, Kreuder C. Musculoskeletal disorders of the neonate. Vet Clin North Am Equine Pract 1994;10:137–166.

Richardson DW. Unit IX fractures. *In* White NA, Moore JN, eds: Current Practice of Equine Surgery. Philadelphia, JB Lippincott, 1990, pp 589–686.

Stashak TS. Wounds. *In* Stashak TS, ed: Adams' Lameness in Horses. Philadelphia, Lea & Febiger, 1987, pp 767–768.

Stashak TS. Adams' Lameness in Horses. Philadelphia, Lea & Febiger, 1987, p 675.

Todhunter RJ. Therapeutic principles for joint disease and repair of articular tissues. *In*

Stashak TS, ed: Adams' Lameness in Horses. Philadelphia, Lea & Febiger, 1987, pp 883–901.

Turner TA. Abscesses and Punctures of the Foot. *In* White NA, Moore JN, eds: Current Practice of Equine Surgery. Philadelphia, JB Lippincott, 1990, pp 399–401.

Watkins JP. Treatment principles of tendon disorders. *In* Auer JA, ed: Equine Surgery. Philadelphia, WB Saunders, 1992, pp 916–924.

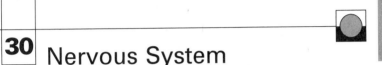

30 Nervous System

Cynthia A. Jackson and Thomas J. Divers

Neurologic disorders frequently have an acute onset, may rapidly worsen, and often require emergency diagnostics and therapeutics.

The *first goal* of the examination is to determine that the nervous system is involved in causing the clinical signs.

The *second goal* is to determine the anatomic location that is dysfunctional within the nervous system and shortens the list of differential diagnosis. Incoordination or ataxia suggests involvement of the long tracts in the spinal cord. A problem with balance suggests a vestibular or on rare occasion a cerebellar problem. Change in mentation indicates a cerebral or brain stem disorder. If the brain stem is involved, cranial nerve deficits and ataxia may be observed. Always consider metabolic disorders as a potential cause of change in mentation, e.g., hepatic or uremic encephalopathy. When evaluating horses with acute neurologic disorders, it is important to consider rabies. Weakness without ataxia causes a support problem and is characteristic of neuromuscular or ventral motor neuron disease.

The *third goal* is to be able to complete the examination and provide reasonable diagnostics and therapeutics without further bodily injury to the horse, humans, or facilities.

ACUTE ATAXIA

Ataxia (incoordination) results from loss of the ability to sense the position of the limbs in space. It is the hallmark of spinal cord disease in the horse but can also be a feature of vestibular disease.

Physical Examination

- Proceed with caution to avoid injury to the patient and personnel. Use of an open grassy area with a slight incline is ideal.
- Observe the animal for inappropriate circumduction, adduction, or abduction of the limbs; basewide stance; delay in protraction of the limbs; scuffing or abnormal wear of the hooves; and striking one limb with

another. Tight circles, backing, and serpentines often exaggerate these deficits.
- Careful examination of the cranial nerves is helpful in formulating a differential diagnosis.

Equine Protozoal Myelitis (EPM)

EPM may present as an acute onset of ataxia with or without cranial nerve deficits (vestibular disturbance and facial paresis are the most common cranial nerve deficits).

Diagnosis

- Signalment is useful in arriving at a diagnosis, because the disease is most common in horses between 15 months and 4 years of age, although it may affect individuals of *any* age.
- EPM appears to affect performance horses more frequently and seems more prevalent in the eastern United States.

Clinical Signs (Acute Onset)

- *Depression—if present, often serves to separate EPM from many other spinal cord diseases*
- Ataxia (often asymmetric) may progress to recumbency. In some cases the ataxia is symmetric, and then it is virtually impossible to separate EPM from equine degenerative myelopathy (EDM) or cervical stenotic myelopathy (CSM) by clinical examination.
- Trembling (one or two limbs)—can be mild to severe (rare) and indicates lower motor neuron involvement. Trembling appears similar to that seen with botulism.
- Head tilt
- Facial paralysis
- Difficulty managing food or swallowing
- Dragging one or more limbs
- Blindness is rare but may occur.
- Seizures, as the only clinical sign, have been reported.

Laboratory Testing—Serology

A serum and/or cerebrospinal fluid (CSF) sample (see p. 86) can be sent to EBI, A153 Astecc Building, University of Kentucky, Lexington, KY 40502–0286; (606) 257 2300, Ext. 226; FAX (606) 257 2489; or Neogen Corp., 628 East 3rd Street, Lexington, KY 40505 (800) 477 8201 for measurement of antibodies against *Sarcocystis neurona* or for polymerase chain reaction to determine the presence of *S. neurona* DNA. A negative serum antibody test has a good negative predictive value, but a positive serum antibody test *does not* have a strong predictive value of disease. It is estimated that 45%–60% of the equine population has serum antibody against *S. neurona*. Blood-contaminated CSF or blood-brain barrier abnormalities, such as occurs with herpes myelitis, lowers the positive predictive value of the CSF test for EPM.

Treatment

- Dimethyl sulfoxide (DMSO), 1 gm/kg IV in saline or other polyionic fluid as a 10% solution, administered over 30–60 minutes once per day for 5 days
- Sulfadiazine, 20–30 mg/kg PO q12–24h, alone
with:
- Pyrimethamine, 1.0 mg/kg orally q24h (do not mix with feed or administer at time of feeding). A 2.0 mg/kg dosage may be used for the first week in nonpregnant mares.
- Treat individuals that show improvement for a minimum of 12 weeks. Test all pregnant and treated mares for plasma folic acid concentration and supplement with folinic acid if needed.
- Diclazuril, 5 mg/kg PO q24h, is another treatment alternative.

Supportive Therapy

- Feed patients that cannot eat or drink with a gruel at least twice daily by stomach tube.
- Apply ophthalmic ointment to the eye of patients with facial paralysis four times daily.
- **Corneal ulcers that develop as a result of facial nerve paralysis can be refractory to treatment**.
- Long-term use of corticosteroids is contraindicated. Short-term (1 or 2 days) dexamethasone at an anti-inflammatory dosage (0.1–0.2 mg/kg) in severe cases may improve clinical signs, but is recommended only in cases that are rapidly progressing to recumbency.
- Flunixin meglumine, 0.5–1.0 mg/kg IM q12–24h if signs are more severe after treatment is started

Prognosis

- Fair for return to function for individuals receiving early and appropriate treatment
- **Poor for individuals with dysphagia or recumbent**

Cervical Stenotic/Compressive Myelopathy

Horses with cervical stenotic myelopathy (CSM) or cervical compressive myelopathy may present on an emergency basis due to a traumatic accident that acutely worsens the underlying compressive disease.

Signalment

- Often a young, rapidly growing individual; may have a history of clumsiness suggesting a pre-existing condition
- Trauma can exacerbate clinical signs to the point of extreme ataxia or recumbency.
- Males are more commonly affected.

Clinical Signs

- Symmetric ataxia (in the majority of cases) involving all four limbs. Deficits in the thoracic limbs may be subtle.
- No cranial nerve deficits unless secondary to trauma
- Neck pain infrequent; abnormal resistance to neck flexion may be seen.
- Most patients are bright and alert with no depression.

Diagnosis

- Survey radiographs may *suggest* CSM characteristics: vertebral canal stenosis (minimal sagittal diameter ratio <0.5)* and osteoarthritis of the articular processes.
- Obtain definitive diagnosis through myelographic demonstration of impingement on the spinal cord (>50% impingement of the dorsal column).
- CSF is usually normal.

Treatment

- Dexamethasone, 0.1–0.2 mg/kg IV once per day for 1–2 days, and DMSO, 1 gm/kg IV as a 10% solution in saline or lactated Ringer's solution, once per day for 5 days, may provide transient improvement in cases made abruptly worse by trauma.
- Long-term dietary and exercise restrictions may help stop the progression of the disease in some youngsters.
- Surgical arthrodesis may benefit some individuals, determined by neurologic status, myelographic findings, and duration of clinical signs.

Prognosis

Fair to poor, depending on the site(s) of compression, age of the individual, and severity of signs.

Equine Herpes Virus-1 Myeloencephalitis

EHV-1, or rhinopneumonitis, causes respiratory disease and abortion as well as neurologic disease. The neurologic form occurs sporadically, often as a sequela to either of the other two forms.

Signalment

- Most commonly adults (rarely occurs in foals)
- Race track, breeding farm, or training facility
- Often multiple cases on the same farm within a short time period. Isolated cases have been reported.
- No seasonality
- May be a risk factor in individuals housed with donkeys or mules.

---

*Determined by comparing the narrowest dorsal-ventral measurement of the cranial vertebral canal with the widest dorsal-ventral measurement of the corresponding cranial vertebral body

Clinical Signs

- Abrupt onset of (usually) symmetric ataxia and paresis that may progress rapidly to recumbency
- Neurologic deficit of pelvic limbs is worse than thoracic limbs in most cases.
- *Urinary bladder paralysis with urine dribbling is a common clinical sign.*
- Hypotonic tail and fecal retention in only a few cases
- May have vestibular signs and other cranial nerve deficits
- Fever may be detectable early in the disease course. Asymptomatic individuals on the same farm may be febrile.

Diagnosis

> **Multiple individuals from the same farm with an acute onset of hindlimb ataxia and bladder paralysis and an episode of prior respiratory disease on the farm is the classic presentation.**

- Hematology and serum biochemistry profile are usually unremarkable.
- CSF may be normal or have an elevated protein with few nucleated cells. The CSF may be yellow (xanthochromia).
- Fourfold rise in serum neutralization titer in samples drawn 10 days apart is highly suggestive of EHV-1 infection but is not always present in neurologically affected individuals.
- Virus isolation from the buffy coat, CSF, or neurologic tissue from the neurologically affected is rarely successful. Immunocytochemistry demonstrating herpes antigen in the CNS vascular endothelium is the preferred post mortem test.
- Nasal/pharyngeal swabs for virus isolation in horses with respiratory or neurologic disease should be attempted and are helpful if positive. Adjacent asymptomatic horses should also be tested.
- Many affected individuals have relatively high serum neutralization titers (1:640 or >) at the onset of clinical signs.

Treatment

- DMSO, 1 gm/kg IV as a 10% solution mixed in saline or any isotonic polyionic fluid once per day for 5 days
- *Urinary bladder catheterization and drainage three to four times per day in cases with dysuria and bladder distention*
- Bethanechol, 0.04 mg/kg SQ q8h for treatment of bladder distention. Injectable bethanechol is expensive and, therefore, not an option in some cases. Bethanechol tablets, for oral administration (0.2–0.4 mg/kg PO q8–12h) are not as expensive and not as effective as the parenteral product.
- Antibiotics (for cystitis, which is inevitable with frequent catheterization).

- Trimethoprim-sulfa, 20 mg/kg PO q12h, or ceftiofur, 2.2–4.4 mg/kg IV q12h.
- Urine culture is recommended as resistant infections may develop despite antibiotic therapy.
- *Administer corticosteroids in progressive or severe cases*; use caution as it may potentiate secondary bacterial infections.

The potent anti-inflammatory effects of short-term (1–2 days) dexamethasone, 0.1–0.2 mg/kg IV, may prove lifesaving to a recumbent patient. Corticosteroids should be used in those individuals that are rapidly progressing and/or acutely recumbent.

- Supportive care: Protective leg wraps, a laxative diet, IV or oral fluids to maintain hydration, topical care of decubital ulcers, and avoidance of urine scalding. Note: *Do not overhydrate!*

Prognosis

Highly variable—many individuals make a full recovery, others are left with residual deficits; some are euthanized due to paralysis and secondary complications. Nursing care can be very intensive. Full recovery may take months. Prognosticating the outcome at the beginning of the clinical course is often difficult. Bladder dysfunction may be the last clinical problem to resolve in many cases.

Management of an Outbreak

- Quarantine the facility for at least 30 days after confirming the *last* case.
- Minimize movement of individuals within the facility to avoid spread of the virus.
- Specific personnel should care for affected individuals and should not handle healthy horses.
- Monitor temperature (twice per day) of all at-risk individuals in order to detect a fever that generally precedes clinical disease by 5–9 days.
- Steam cleaning and phenol- or the iodophor-based disinfectants kills the virus.
- *Vaccination in the face of an outbreak is not known to be useful and potentially could exacerbate the problem.*
- There is no reported recurrence of the neurologic syndrome in a recovered individual.
- Individuals that have to be moved into a stable that has had EHV-I should be vaccinated, but the vaccines may not protect against the neurologic form of the equine herpes virus.

Vestibular Disease

Clinical Signs

The vestibular system controls balance and maintains orientation of the head, eyes, and trunk. Ataxia is often a manifestation of an acute vestibular disturbance.

- Low-grade fever
- Head tilt
- Staggering, leaning, drifting sideways
- Abnormal nystagmus—quick phase away from the affected side
- Strabismus (especially when the head is elevated)
- If severe, recumbency and inability to maintain sternal recumbency
- Blindfolding exacerbates balance loss.
- Other cranial nerve deficits
- History of ear rubbing or head shaking

Differential Diagnosis

- Cranial trauma (see p. 363)—common
- Otitis media and interna with or without temporohyoid osteoarthropathy is common.
- EPM (see p. 338)—common
- Polyneuritis equi (cauda equina)
- Space-occupying mass
- Encephalitis (viral/hepatic) (see p. 358)
- Guttural pouch mycosis with extension to the middle ear
- Idiopathic vestibular disease

The distinction between a peripheral (outside the brainstem) and central (within the brainstem) lesion is summarized here:

Peripheral	**Central**
normal mentation	depressed
no proprioceptive deficits	proprioceptive deficits
normal strength	weakness (paresis)
possible involvement of the 7th cranial nerve	possible involvement of multiple cranial nerves

Diagnosis

- Palpate the base of the ear for any signs of pain.
- Skull radiographs: lateral, oblique, and ventrodorsal (most useful) views. Evaluate stylohyoid bone, tympanic bullae, petrous temporal bone, and guttural pouch.
- Endoscopic evaluation of upper airway and guttural pouch. In the guttural pouch, look for proliferative changes (bulging) of the proximal stylohyoid bone or the temporohyoid joint.
- Careful aural examination and culture of any exudate.
- CSF analysis, including *S. neurona* antibody titer to rule out EPM (see p. 339)
- CT scans may be needed for confirmation in some cases.

- Those few individuals with drainage from the ear most often have *Staphylococcus aureus* infection. *Streptococcus* and *Actinobacillus* have also been isolated from infected ears.

Treatment

- DMSO, 1 gm/kg IV as a 10% solution in saline, or any isotonic fluid intended for IV administration, once per day for 5 days.
- Trimethoprim-sulfa, 20 mg/kg PO q12h for 30 days. **This is the treatment of choice for most staphylococcal infections in the horse!**
- Phenylbutazone, 2.2 mg/kg PO once or twice daily for 7–10 days.
- Corticosteroids: 0.05–0.1 mg/kg dexamethasone IV q24h. Judicious use is advised and not recommended unless the vestibular dysfunction is *traumatic* and/or *rapidly progressive*.
- Supportive care: **Ophthalmic ointment for cases with facial nerve paralysis**, protective leg wraps, good footing, and easy access to food and water.
- Surgical resection of the mid-section of the stylohyoid bone is indicated in cases of osteoarthropathy that do not respond to medical treatment.

Prognosis

- Fair to good for otitis media and interna
- Uncontrolled and/or fracture cases can progress to meningitis.
- Fair to poor for central vestibular disorders
- Cases of idiopathic vestibular disease resolve without treatment over several days.

Rabies

> **As rabies becomes endemic throughout certain areas of the United States, serious consideration of this disease in cases with a change in mentation, acute ataxia, and recumbency is essential**.

The antemortem diagnosis of rabies is difficult due to the wide spectrum of clinical signs and the lack of an accurate antemortem diagnostic test. Individuals are usually infected by the bite of a rabid wild animal, but physical evidence of such a wound is often not discovered. The incubation period can vary from 2 weeks to several months, but once clinical signs develop there is usually a short (average, 3–5 days) course of progressive neurologic deterioration culminating in death.

Signalment

- No gender, breed, or age predilection.
- Young individuals, being more inquisitive, may be at increased risk.
- Although vaccination is thought to be highly protective, the consideration

of rabies in any horse with an acute onset of neurologic signs is recommended regardless of vaccination status!

Clinical Signs

Highly variable. See Table 30–1.

Rapid progression of clinical signs is a feature of equine rabies. Most cases are terminally recumbent within 3–5 days after the onset of clinical signs, although one individual remained ambulatory for 9 days after the onset of clinical signs.

Diagnosis

- CBC and serum biochemistry supply little useful information. Severe hyperglycemia may occur due to stress.
- CSF: May be normal or of low cellularity, with the predominant cell type being lymphocytes. Total protein may be normal or elevated in the CSF.
- No accurate antemortem test available
- **CAUTION**: Handle any bodily fluid from a rabies suspect with care. **Label specimens appropriately and inform laboratory personnel**.

Precautions in Dealing with a Rabies Suspect

- Reduce human exposure, especially people with open wounds.
- Wear gloves.
- Wash hands thoroughly—virus is relatively fragile and is killed by most detergents.
- Keep a list of all people who come in contact with the suspect.

Treatment may not be advisable for cases highly suggestive of having

TABLE 30–1. **Clinical Signs of Rabies**

Common	Less Common
recumbency	head tilt
ataxia and paresis	circling
hyperesthesia	teeth grinding
muscle tremor	blindness
lameness	pharyngeal paralysis
anorexia	tenesmus
loss of tail and anal tone	drooling
loss of hindlimb sensation	roaring
fever	sweating
colic	paddling while recumbent
depression	abnormal vocalizations
convulsions	
aggressiveness	
paraphimosis	

rabies. Postmortem diagnosis is imperative due to zoonotic implications. Vaccination of horses after a bite has occurred may not be effective. Individuals that have been vaccinated and later bitten by a rabid animal should be vaccinated again two to three times, 4 to 7 days apart, and quarantined for 6 months. Unvaccinated individuals bitten by a proven rabid animal should be euthanized or quarantined for at least 6 months.

Submission of Rabies Material to State Diagnostic Laboratory

- Brain stem and cerebellum are the brain samples of choice. Do not submit the entire head.
- Appropriate samples can be obtained with minimal contact through the foramen magnum. Latex gloves, surgical mask, and glasses should be worn during sample collection.
- Remove the head and using a hacksaw remove the back of the calvaria. DO NOT use power saws (including Stryker saws), which may aerosolize the virus.
- Refrigerate specimens before shipment. Tissues must *not* be fixed with chemical preservatives.
- Place specimens in at least two separately sealed plastic bags with gel-type cold packs in a Styrofoam-insulated cardboard box.
- Test results are generally reported within 24–48 hours of laboratory receipt.
- All instruments and surfaces are disinfected with a 10% solution of household bleach in water.

Veterinarians are encouraged to undergo rabies prophylaxis. Human serum for assessing current titer status may be submitted to Kansas State University; (913) 532 5660. Titer assessment is recommended before boostering. *With proper precautions*, the chance of humans acquiring rabies from large animals is low. In fact, there are no reported human rabies cases in the United States that have been transmitted from large animals.

Verminous Encephalitis

May cause acute ataxia and/or change in mentation. *Halicephalobus (Micronema) deletrix* is the most common non-sarcocystis parasite causing verminous encephalitis.

Verminous encephalitis due to *Strongylus vulgaris* is rare and causes profound neurologic disease, which results from the migration of larvae within the brain or the thrombosis of multiple small arteries to the brain. The thrombosis is due to embolism of pieces of the verminous plaque, which may originate at the bifurcation of the brachycephalic trunk. The lesion is asymmetric, and in the case of a thromboembolism, results in clinical signs that most closely resemble an intracarotid injection (see p. 370) or acute, severe EPM (see p. 338). In one report, more than one individual on a farm was affected. Rare episodes of CNS migration by the cattle bots fly *Hypoderma bovis* or *H. lineatum* and by *Setaria* sp., a filarial nematode commonly found in the peritoneal cavity, have been reported in the horse.

Clinical Signs

- *Micronema* encephalitis most often results in signs resembling cerebellar ataxia (hypermetria, head tremors).
- Hematuria and signs of renal disease may be present along with the ataxia.

Diagnosis

- It is unlikely that a confirmatory diagnosis can be made antemortem unless there is a lesion elsewhere in the body that can be biopsied, e.g., kidney, bone.
- CSF may have a pleocytosis, suggestive of inflammatory disease, but this could also be seen with EPM.

Treatment

- May be attempted with fenbendazole, 10 mg/kg PO q24h for 5 days, along with corticosteroids: dexamethasone, 0.04–0.16 mg/kg IV q24h on days 1 and 2, with tapering dosage thereafter.
- There are no reports of known successful treatment in horses with CNS infection.
- Use of ivermectin, 0.22 mg/kg PO in a single dose is controversial and may cause a worsening of neurologic signs.

Plant-Induced Ataxia

In certain areas of the United States (especially the south), during certain summers (probably associated with environmental conditions), ataxia may occur in one or more individuals at pasture when grazing rye, Bermuda grass, or fescue grass.

Clinical Signs

- Affected individuals are usually adults.
- Ataxia may be severe.
- Head tremors and hypermetria may occur.
- Occurs more commonly with individuals on pasture than those being fed hay
- NOTE: Sorghum/Sudan grass and black locust bark can also cause ataxia.

Distinctive clinical signs are:

Sorghum/Sudan Grass	**Black Locust Bark**
dribbling urine	posterior paresis
abortion	anorexia, depression
arthrogryposis in utero	mild colic
stringhalt-like gait	irregular heart beat

Treatment

- No specific treatment for Sorghum/Sudan grass and black locust bark other than removal from the source of poisoning.
- Treat with DMSO, 1 gm/kg IV, as a 10%–20% solution in saline or any isotonic fluid q24h for 3–5 days, and/or dexamethasone, 0.04–0.08 mg/kg IV q24h for 1–2 days, with a tapering dose.
- Affected individuals often return to normal within 5 days.

Other Causes of Acute-Onset Ataxia

Spinal Cord Trauma. See p. 366.

Fibrocartilaginous Emboli. Rare, but may cause acute hemiparesis and ataxia without evidence of vertebral pain.

Equine Ehrlichiosis. Affected individuals are frequently ataxic, depressed, jaundiced, and febrile and have petechiations. The organism can be seen in neutrophils. Treatment is tetracycline, 6.6 mg/kg IV q12h.

Grove Poisoning. A syndrome causing ataxic and convulsion-like signs, with oral mucous membrane congestion, is reported to occur in adults in proximity to large crop farms or orchards. A toxicity is suspected. Signs may wax and wane, and affected individuals may recover. There is no known treatment.

TREMBLING IN HORSES

Causes include weakness, pain, shock, adverse drug reactions, hypothermia, or toxicity. Diseases presented here are neurologic and/or neuromuscular diseases causing trembling. Trembling from pain, shock, and the like, is discussed in Chapter 36.

Physical Examination

A careful physical examination reveals whether the trembling is a result of weakness, pain, shock, or other causes. In conditions with generalized weakness, eyelids, tongue, tail, and anus are all weak. Botulism, equine motor neuron disease, and severe cachexia cause affected individuals to stand with all four feet closer together than normal. If the weakness is a result of electrolyte abnormalities, hypocalcemia, or periodic paralysis, a tetanic appearance may be seen. Trembling associated with abdominal pain or endotoxemia is also common and can be detected by a complete clinical examination. Sweating may occur with either weakness or pain. Trembling due to primary muscle disorders may be difficult to separate from other causes of trembling.

Botulism

Signalment

FOALS

- Are often 2–8 weeks of age (most of these are 21–28 days old)
- Generally occurs because of toxicoinfectious botulism
- Most common in foals in Kentucky, Maryland, Pennsylvania, and New Jersey

ADULTS

- Most often a result of ingestion of a preformed toxin (although it is rarely found)
- Rarely, associated with a closed wound
- Endemic in the mid-Atlantic states (*Clostridium botulinum* type B is common in the soil)
- Outbreaks of *Clostridium botulinum* types C or D have been reported in other parts of the country associated with contamination of the feed with dead animals.

Clinical Signs

- Generalized (and therefore symmetric) weakness
- Decreased tail, eyelid, and tongue tone (the tongue may easily be pulled from the mouth and held with two fingers).
- Trembling
- Lying down
- Dysphagia
- Standing with all four limbs close together
- The disease often progresses to severe paresis, with inability to stand and subsequent respiratory failure.
- The onset is usually acute, with rapid progression within 18–48 hours, although some cases may progress more slowly or even stabilize without treatment.

Diagnostic Tests

- The diagnosis of botulism is made by consideration of the signalment, clinical signs, and geographic location.
- Anaerobic culture of soil, feed, or wounded tissue for identification of *Clostridium botulinum* and its toxin may be submitted to support the diagnosis in adults to Dr. R. H. Whitlock, University of Pennsylvania, New Bolton Center, Kennett Square, PA 19348–1692; (610) 444 5800. In foals, the presence of organisms in the feces is considered diagnostic if appropriate signs are present.
- Muscle enzymes are normal or only slightly elevated (unless the individual has been recumbent).
- Endoscopy often reveals a displaced soft palate, even in mild cases.
- Arterial or venous pCO_2 > 70 mm Hg (suggests hypoventilation and a poor prognosis).

Treatment

- **DO NOT STRESS!**
- Remove hay and water; muzzle if individual attempts to eat the bedding.
- Administer polyvalent botulism antiserum IV (costs up to $1500/foal and $2500/adult). Contact Dr. R. H. Whitlock; (610) 444 5800.
- Broad-spectrum antibiotics: Ceftiofur, 4.4 mg/kg IV q12h or potassium penicillin, 22,000 IU/kg IV q6h.

> **Procaine penicillin, aminoglycosides, and tetracycline should
> NOT be administered because of their affect on the neuro-
> muscular system.**

- **Debride wound (in the unusual case of wound botulism).**
- Supply feed and water or milk by *nasogastric* intubation (see Nutritional Guidelines, Chapter 43). *In acutely affected adults, passage of a nasogastric tube may be postponed, to reduce stress, until the antitoxin has been administered (at least 24 hours).*
- In foals, the standard 22% ± of milk/kg body weight/day is usually not required since the activity levels of these foals is markedly decreased and abdominal distention should be prevented.

Prognosis

FOALS

- **Foals that can stand** have a fair to good prognosis with antitoxin therapy.
- **Recumbent foals** without respiratory distress have a guarded prognosis.
- **Foals with respiratory distress and $pCO_2 > 70$ mm Hg** have a poor prognosis without ventilatory support, which is costly and requires 2–3 weeks of hospitalization. These foals can be maintained by intranasal intubation and an Ambu bag until they can be admitted to an intensive care facility for ventilatory support.

ADULTS

- **Adults that have a 2–3-day history of weakness and are still standing** have a fair to good prognosis—sometimes even without antitoxin treatment.
- **Adults that cannot stand or have a peracute course of the disease** have a poor prognosis.

Equine Motor Neuron Disease

Affects adults, are usually in a management situation where there is little or no pasture and poor hay quality—most commonly in the northeastern United States.

Diagnosis

Clinical signs provide a tentative diagnosis:

- Weight loss of 150+ lb (70 kg)
- Trembling
- Weakness of the limbs and neck
- Generalized muscle atrophy
- Standing with all four limbs close together
- Increased periods of recumbency
- Good appetite

- NO *dysphagia, ataxia, or weak tail*
- Raised tailhead

Definitive diagnosis may be obtained by:

- Laboratory test (suggestive, not diagnostic). Serum (creatine kinase, CK) is mildly or moderately elevated (500–2000 μ/l) in about 90% of cases.
- Muscle biopsy of the sacrocaudalis dorsalis medialis (tailhead) muscle. This is the most superficial muscle on either side of midline at the base of the tail. To biopsy: sedate with xylazine and administer local anesthesia SQ and into the muscle. Make a 3-inch skin incision, dissect through any SQ fat to the muscle. Undermine the muscle before cutting to obtain a 1-inch-long by 0.25-inch-wide specimen. Collect 2 specimens. Place one in formalin; wrap the second in gauze sponges *lightly* moistened with saline, and ship to a pathologist experienced in the evaluation of equine muscle.
- Biopsy the ventral branch of the spinal accessory nerve (submitted in formalin)—approximately 94% accurate in predicting the disease in the hands of an experienced pathologist.

Treatment

- None known. Possibly vitamin E (6000 IU vitamin E—*without added selenium*—PO q24h).
- Buckeye Feeds produces a supplement, sold only to veterinarians, that contains vitamin E, folic acid, and thiamine.
- Prednisone, 0.5–1 mg/kg PO q24h, appears to improve the signs in acute, severely affected individuals.

Prognosis

- Poor for return to prior function
- Some affected individuals begin to stabilize after 2–4 weeks.
- Not enough is known to speculate on suitability as breeding animals.

Tetanic Hypocalcemia in Horses

Causes

- Lactation: More common in draft horses
- Blister beetle toxicity (see p. 223)
- **Idiopathic: Most common**
- Transport and stress
- Hypoparathyroid: More common in foals (frequently 2–5 months of age)
- Diarrhea and colic in adults or exhaustion syndrome in endurance horses.
- Farm problems may occur, in which case low dietary magnesium as a cause of diminished parathyroid hormone (PTH) activity should be investigated.
- Excessive bicarbonate administration

Clinical Signs

- Generalized stiffness
- Trismus
- Trembling
- Dysmetric flared nostrils
- **Synchronous diaphragmatic flutter**
- Prolapsing third eyelids
- Respiratory distress
- Stringhalt or goose-stepping gait
- Recumbency
- Dilated pupils
- Sweating
- Elevated heart rate
- Hyperesthesia
- Choke
- Elevated temperature
- Seizures in foals

Laboratory Findings

- Ca usually < 5.0 mg/dl
- Mg < 1.0 mg/dl
- May be alkalotic and hypochloremic due to sweating, which further aggravates the hypocalcemia

Treatment

- 11 gm (500 ml) 23% calcium borogluconate **slowly IV** over at least 15 minutes for a 450 kg adult. The calcium borogluconate can be mixed in 4–5 liters of 0.9% NaCl and administered over 30–45 minutes. Adults with severe distress may be administered 200 ml calcium borogluconate slowly IV without fluid dilution.
- Monitor heart rate and rhythm.
  - ☐ The expected cardiovascular response is an increase in the intensity of the heart sounds.
  - ☐ An infrequent extrasystole may be expected, but pronounced change in rate or rhythm is an indication to discontinue the treatment immediately.
- Complete recovery from hypocalcemia may require several hours to days. Retreatment may be needed.

Prognosis

Good except for those individuals with hypoparathyroidism, which is most common in foals. Laboratory samples for parathyroid hormone (to diagnose hypoparathyroidism) can be sent to the Endocrine Diagnostic Section, Animal Health Diagnostic Laboratory, Michigan State University; (517) 353 0621. Blood samples must be clotted, centrifuged, and sent overnight on ice. Normal values are reported to be 0.25–2.0 picomoles/L. Prognosis is poor for foals with hypoparathyroidism.

Hyperkalemic Periodic Paralysis

HYPP is a defect in muscle membrane transport that is inherited via an autosomal dominant gene.

Signalment

Quarter Horses, Appaloosas, and Paints that are descendants of the Quarter Horse sire "Impressive."

ADULTS

- Typically 2–4 years of age at initial episode
- Some are older when they first exhibit clinical signs.

FOALS

- May be neonates to weanling age.
- Dam may have no history of clinical disease.

Clinical Signs

ADULTS

- Anxious attitude; remains alert
- Episodic muscle tremors, often seen first in the muscles of the face and neck, then progress to diffuse body tremors
- Swaying, staggering
- Dog-sitting posture (hindquarter paresis), which may progress to involuntary recumbency
- Prolapse or "flash" of the third eyelid
- Usually completely normal after recovery from an episode
- Signs may develop after a stressful episode (e.g., colic), cold weather, anesthesia or after feeding.
- Increased respiratory rate and noise

FOALS

- Loud inspiratory noise
- Respiratory distress
- Collapse
- Most often exhibit respiratory signs when exercised, restrained, or nursing
- These foals are usually homozygous for the gene.

Diagnosis

Signalment, clinical signs, endoscopy in foals, laboratory data, and response to treatment provide a tentative diagnosis. HYPP genetics testing provides identification of homozygous and heterozygous individuals.

Laboratory Data

- Hyperkalemia (5–12.3 mEq/L) *during an episode*. Both affected adults and foals are rarely reported to be *normokalemic* during clinical episodes.
- Muscle enzymes (CK and aspartate transaminase [AST]) may be elevated. Muscle biopsy is not diagnostic.
- DNA testing has eliminated the need for the potassium chloride challenge test.
- HYPP testing by the Veterinary Genetics Laboratory at the University of California, Davis, CA; (916) 752 2211; in Canada: Dr. Doug Nickel, Health Science Center, 3330 Hospital Drive, Calgary, Alberta, Canada TZN 4N1. Submit 5–10 ml of blood in an EDTA (purple top) tube. Results available in 3–5 working days.

Treatment

FOALS

- DO NOT STRESS!
- Tracheotomy may be required in foals with excessive laryngeal edema.

ADULTS AND FOALS

- 23% calcium gluconate (0.2–0.4 ml/kg) in 1–2 liters of 10% dextrose *or* 250 ml 50% dextrose *or* sodium bicarbonate (0.5 mEq/kg), administered IV over 30 minutes.
- Milder cases respond to dextrose or Karo syrup and/or sodium bicarbonate (baking soda) administered orally or via nasogastric tube.
- Acetazolamide, 2.2 mg/kg orally q12h. This is a potassium-wasting diuretic, used to reduce the incidence of clinical signs.
- Decrease potassium content of diet. Change from alfalfa to grass hay but not brome grass. Feed oats instead of sweet feed or pellets. Avoid supplements (e.g., molasses, Litesalt, kelp) that contain potassium.

Prognosis

- Acetazolamide therapy and dietary changes control clinical signs in the majority of affected individuals.
- Recurrent episodes are reported in some individuals that initially responded to treatment.
- Sudden death is occasionally reported.
- Discourage breeding of individuals that test positive for the disease (even those with no clinical signs).

Tetanus

Tetanus is caused by an exotoxin produced by *Clostridium tetani* that blocks the release of inhibitory neurotransmitters and results in spasticity of skeletal muscles.

Signalment

- Any unvaccinated horse is susceptible.
- Clostridial organisms are usually introduced via a soft tissue or hoof wound.

Clinical Signs

- Initial signs are colic and vague stiffness.
- Trembling, spasm, and paralysis of voluntary muscles. Masseter muscle is commonly affected.
- Protrusion of the third eyelid—especially when menaced
- Eyelid retraction, flared nostrils, and erect ear carriage
- Sawhorse stance, stiff spastic gait, may progress to recumbency.
- Inability to open jaw, difficulty swallowing, aspiration pneumonia
- Raised tailhead

> All of these signs are exacerbated by activity or excitement. Stimulation of an individual with tetanus may precipitate panic, recumbency, and subsequent long bone fracture or other secondary trauma.

Diagnosis

- By clinical signs in an unvaccinated individual
- There are no diagnostic blood tests.
- Anaerobic culture of *C. tetani* from the inciting wound may be attempted.

Treatment

- Provide a quiet environment with good footing.
- Pad stall walls to reduce chance of injury.
- Minimize stimulation—darken stall and stuff cotton in the ears.
- Deep bedding with straw, especially if recumbent
- Provide muscle relaxation/tranquilization.
  - □ Acepromazine, 0.05 mg/kg IM or IV q6h. Increasing doses or shorter intervals may be required with time. Or use phenobarbital, 6–12 mg/kg slowly IV, followed by oral phenobarbital, 6–12 mg/kg q12h. Or haloperidol, 0.01 mg/kg, once every 7 days IM, may be used as a long-acting tranquilizer.
  - □ Eliminate the source of infection.
  - □ Debride the wound, do not suture.
  - □ Infiltrate wound with procaine penicillin.
  - □ Administer potassium penicillin, 22,000 IU/kg IV q6h for a minimum of 7 days.
- Neutralize unbound toxin.
  - □ 100–200 U/kg tetanus antitoxin, IV or IM, should bind circulating residual neurotoxin but does not cross the blood-brain barrier to neutralize toxin in the CNS.
  - □ Intrathecal administration of antitoxin: Remove 50 ml of CSF via atlanto-occipital aspirate (30 ml in a foal), replace with an equal volume of tetanus antitoxin. Anesthetize with xylazine and ketamine for the CSF collection.
- Maintain hydration and nutritional status.

- ☐ Place food and water off the ground in an easily accessible location.
- ☐ IV fluids may be necessary to maintain hydration.
- ☐ Oral fluids and gruel may be administered through a small-bore naso-gastric tube in some cases. Intubation may be difficult due to muscle spasms and pharyngeal paralysis. Feed at peak tranquilization periods to reduce stress.
- ▪ Establish active antitoxin immunity.
  - ☐ Amount of toxin necessary to produce disease is often insufficient to stimulate an immune response. Vaccinate with tetanus toxoid in a separate site from the antitoxin administration.

Prognosis

Fair to poor.

- ▪ Contingent on the severity of clinical signs and the attitude of the affected individual.
- ▪ Clinical signs may persist for weeks.
- ▪ Secondary complications include aspiration pneumonia, myopathy, and long bone or pelvic fracture.
- ▪ If the affected individual cannot stand, the prognosis is grave; if ambulatory after 5 days of clinical signs, the prognosis is fair to good.

Myopathy/Myositis

Trembling may also occur with myositis or myopathy. These conditions include:

- ▪ Nonselenium-deficient tying-up syndrome. Rule out glycogen storage if a draft horse, Warmblood or Quarter Horse is affected (see polysaccharide storage myopathy below), and rule out other specific causes of myopathy.

If the myopathy is believed to be caused by exertion and unrelated to the specific causes listed, treatment includes:

- ☐ Fluids to correct dehydration and electrolyte abnormalities. Remember, most individuals with mild to moderate myopathy and/or exhausted individuals are likely to be hypochloremic and alkalotic. Therefore, 0.9% NaCl with 20–40 mEq KCl/L is often the preferred fluid. Fluid diuresis may also prevent myoglobinuric nephropathy. Hypertonic saline can also be used.
- ☐ Analgesic: 2.2 mg/kg phenylbutazone IV q12h for 1–2 days.
- ☐ Acepromazine, 0.02 mg/kg IV or IM q6h
- ☐ Hot packs for affected muscles
- ▪ *Compartmentalization syndrome* associated with ischemia (localized myositis from trauma). Treatment is similar to the foregoing, but if the disease is progressive and severe swelling occurs in areas of important nerves like the radial nerve, perform a fasciotomy to release the pressure.
- ▪ *Selenium-deficient tying-up.* Consider this in certain areas of the United States (e.g., northeast and north central) and Canada, especially (but not always) if the horses are poorly fed.
- ▪ *White muscle disease* (selenium deficient myopathy) most commonly occurs in foals from birth to 60 days of age; most common in the US northeast and northwest. If the cardiac muscle is affected, death may occur without clinical signs. With skeletal muscle involvement, dyspnea,

dysphagia, recumbency, or stiff gait are characteristic. Hyponatremia, hypochloremia, hyperkalemia, and marked elevations in muscle enzymes are typical biochemical abnormalities.

□ Diagnosis: Clinical signs, increased serum muscle enzyme activity, serum selenium < 10 mg/dl. NOTE: If selenium has already been administered and confirmation of the diagnosis is needed, blood can be collected in an anticoagulant tube and submitted to Michigan State Diagnostic Laboratory for glutathione peroxidase activity. After selenium administration, several days are required before the selenium molecule is incorporated into the red blood cell glutathione peroxidase. Repeated intramuscular injections of selenium, 0.06 mg/kg IM, may be required for treatment.

- Purpura hemorrhagica myositis
- Parasitic myositis *(S. fayeri)*—rare
  Clinical findings:
  □ Acute trembling and stiffness
  □ Elevated muscle enzymes
  □ Diagnose by muscle biopsy and confirmation of the organism.
  Treatment:
  □ Phenylbutazone, 2.2 mg/kg PO q12–24h
  □ Trimethoprim-sulfa, 20 mg/kg PO q12h
  □ Pyrimethamine, 0.5 mg/kg PO as a loading dose, then 0.25 mg/kg PO q24h
- Polysaccaride storage myopathy in horses (may progress to recumbency and death)
  □ Appears to be a glycogen storage disease
  □ Common in draft horses, Warmbloods and Quarter Horses
  □ Trembling and stiffness that can progress to recumbency
  □ Serum selenium may be normal or abnormal.
  □ No response to treatment with selenium
  □ Recurrent episodes and/or persistent elevation in muscle enzymes may be reported.

Diagnosis: Muscle biopsy sample of semimembranous or semitendinosus is placed on tongue depressor and then submerged in formalin or placed in a *slightly* damp 4×4 for overnight (chilled) shipment to Univesity of Minnesota or Cornell University. The muscle enzyme activity in the serum is high in severely affected cases but *may* not be dramatically elevated as this is not a myositis.

Treatment: Mild to moderate cases, 2 cups vegetable oil PO q24h (usually via nasogastric tube). Severe recumbent cases, 2 cups vegetable oil PO and IV intralipid, 0.2 gm/kg, administered slowly over 1–2 hours. Rice bran (1–5 lbs/day) (natural glow, Wolcott Farms, Willows, California) is an excellent source of fat.

Other Causes of Trembling

There are many other causes of acute trembling besides those presented here, including trauma, hypothermia, cachexia, drug reactions, etc.

- White snake root poisoning: Signs of weakness leading to recumbency in horses eating white snake root. Frequency of urination is commonly observed.

- Acute lead poisoning: Trembling, depression, ataxia. *Laryngeal paralysis may not be present with acute lead poisoning!*
  □ Diagnosis: Exposure, clinical signs, and blood lead level > 0.3 PPM
  □ Treatment: Ca EDTA, 110 mg/kg in 5% dextrose, administered IV q24h for 2 days. Further interval treatment may be required.
- Muscle spasms, sweating, prolapse of the third eyelid and "colic-like" signs have been associated with ear tick *(Otobius megnini)* infestation. On percussion, some muscles have prolonged and severe contracture. The muscle enzymes are usually mild to moderately elevated. The spinose ear tick can be found in the ear of affected individuals, and signs resolve within 24–96 hours after treatment of the ticks with the pyrethrin piperonyl butoxide.
- Aortic-iliac thrombosis (saddle thrombus). Although most cases are chronic and intermittent, a few individuals may have acute onset of trembling of the rear limbs, violent shaking of the limbs, and weakness in the hindlimbs. Diagnosis is by transrectal ultrasound (7.5-linear-MHz probe). Palpation of limbs for decreased pulse is inconsistent.
  □ Treatment: Pentoxifylline, 8.4 mg/kg PO q12h, can be attempted but is not proven; aspirin 15 mg/kg PO EOD. In severely affected cases surgical removal via the femoral artery should be attempted.

CHANGE IN MENTATION

A change in the demeanor or behavior of a horse may be the first neurologic clinical sign recognized by an owner and suggests cerebral dysfunction. Erratic behavior or depression combined with ataxia or apparent blindness can be a sign of bacterial, viral, or metabolic diseases that affects the CNS.

Hepatic Encephalopathy

Hepatic encephalopathy is perhaps the most common cause of acute cerebral signs in the adult (see p. 276).

Mycotoxic Encephalopathy

Known by many pseudonyms (moldy corn poisoning, blind staggers, leukoencephalitis, foraging disease), mycotic encephalopathy is caused by a toxin elaborated by the mold *Fusarium*, a common contaminant of corn. The clinical syndrome is highly variable and depends on the dose of toxin ingested, species of *Fusarium*, duration of the exposure, and individual susceptibility.

History

- Highest incidence in late fall to early spring, and incidence varies from year to year.
- Contaminated corn is part of the diet for at least 2 weeks.
- Multiple horses on the farm are often affected.
- Death occurs within 1–3 days of onset of clinical signs.

Clinical Signs

NEUROLOGIC SYNDROME

- Afebrile
- Behavioral changes (depression to mania)

- Ataxia and weakness—may proceed to recumbency
- Blindness
- Asymmetric cranial nerve deficits
- Seizures
- Coma and death

No consistent pattern of neurologic signs is typical, due to the variability of the CNS lesion produced.

HEPATOTOXIC SYNDROME (see p. 276)

- Severe icterus
- Swelling of the muzzle and nose
- Difficulty in breathing
- Coma and death
- Associated with high dose of the toxin

Diagnosis

- History of feeding corn contaminated with *Fusarium* and multiple individuals with sudden onset of bizarre neurologic signs.
- Laboratory data is usually nonspecific, with a stress leukogram and normal to elevated liver enzymes.
- CSF analysis may be normal or show a neutrophilic pleocytosis with increased protein.
- Postmortem finding of focal areas of liquefaction necrosis of cerebral white matter is diagnostic.
- Feed can be quantitatively analyzed for *Fusarium*.
- Feed may look grossly normal.

Differential Diagnosis

- Hepatic encephalopathy
- Viral encephalopathy
- Trauma
- Equine protozoal myeloencephalopathy
- Cerebral abscess
- Rabies
- Space-occupying mass
- Botulism
- Herpes myelitis

Treatment

- Remove the source of the corn.
- DMSO, 1 gm/kg IV as a 10% solution in saline or any isotonic fluid, once a day for 5 days
- Maintain hydration with IV fluids.
- Corticosteroids, 0.1–0.2 mg/kg dexamethasone IV once per day for 1–2 days
- Broad-spectrum antibiotic therapy
- Thiamine, 10 mg/kg in IV fluids q12h
- Good nursing care

Prognosis

Poor. Because of extensive CNS damage, few survive.

Equine Viral Encephalitides

ALPHAVIRUSES

The *Alphavirus* subcategory of the family Togaviridae is the classification of eastern (EEE), western (WEE), and Venezuelan (VEE) equine encephalitides. These diseases, clinically indistinguishable, present with an acute onset of fever and depression followed by diffuse CNS signs.

Signalment

- Any age, breed or either sex. Not common in foals less than 3 months old.
- Disease occurs most commonly at the height of the vector (mosquito/tick) season. In the southeastern United States, this can be year round.
- EEE and WEE—usually one individual in a herd
- VEE—morbidity up to 50%. Last American outbreak of VEE was in 1971.

Clinical Signs

- High fever
- Malaise
- Colic
- Anorexia

Neurologic Signs

- Depression—may progress to somnolence
- Dementia—compulsive walking, excitability, aggression
- Head pressing
- Hyperesthesia
- Ataxia
- Blindness
- Circling
- Seizures
- Head tilt
- Recumbency
- Paralysis of pharynx, larynx, and tongue
- Irregular breathing
- Cardiac arrhythmias

Diagnosis

- Fourfold rise in serum titer over 2–3-week period.
- CSF analysis: Leukocytosis, elevated total protein, xanthochromia. Most

dramatic CSF changes with EEE, less dramatic with WEE and VEE. May be able to isolate virus from the CSF
- Histopathology of the brain and spinal cord: No gross lesions characteristic of the disease. Best microscopic lesions in the cerebral cortex, thalamus, and hypothalamus. Submit fresh or frozen brain specimen for virus isolation.

> Caution: *Sufficient viral particles for human infection may be present in the CNS (especially with VEE). Use caution at postmortem. Do not use power tools.*

Treatment

- No specific treatment effective
- DMSO, 1 gm/kg IV, as a 10% solution in saline or lactated Ringer's solution once per day for 5 days
- Dexamethasone, 0.1–0.2 mg/kg IV, once or twice per day for 1–2 days
- NSAID: Phenylbutazone, 2.2 mg/kg IV or PO q12h
  or flunixin meglumine, 0.25–0.5 mg/kg IV or PO q12h
- Anticonvulsants: Diazepam, 0.1–0.4 mg/kg IV for a 450-kg adult
  phenobarbital, 3–12 mg/kg IV or to effect
- Monitor hydration
- Laxative diet
- Supply nutrients.
- Protect from self-induced trauma.

Prognosis

- EEE: 75% to 100% mortality, complete recovery is rare.
- WEE: 20% to 50% mortality, persistent neurologic deficits common
- VEE: 40% to 80% mortality, may be viremic for 3 weeks after recovery—keep isolated

Report cases of EEE, WEE, or VEE to health officials. The affected individual is not a source of WEE and EEE for human infection, whereas VEE can be readily transmitted to humans directly or via mosquitoes.

OTHER VIRUSES

In Canada and the Western United States, *Bunyavirus* encephalitis has been reported. Recovery is possible. Other unidentified viruses may also sporadically produce encephalitis with recovery.

Cerebral Abscess

Signalment

- Usually a young foal, 3 months of age or older
- Often a history of strangles, pneumonia, or cranial trauma a few weeks before the onset of signs

Clinical Signs

- Acute onset, may be febrile
- Depression progressing to stupor
- Often episodes of violent behavior, head pressing, or circling
- Hindlimb ataxia, falling, acute recumbency
- Unilateral or bilateral blindness
- Often multiple cranial nerves affected
- Head tilt and signs of neck pain common
- Seizures and coma

Signs frequently wax and wane—affected individuals may improve with treatment and then suddenly worsen despite treatment.

Etiology

- *Streptococcus equi* and *S. zooepidemicus* are the organisms most frequently reported.
- Access to CNS via hematogenous spread from suppurative lesion (bastard strangles), *OR* extension of suppuration from sinus, nasal cavity, guttural pouch, or middle ear, *OR* direct seeding of a variety of organisms from penetrating wound or fracture

Diagnosis

- History
- Clinical signs
- CSF sample (elevated protein and nucleated cells, culture of spinal fluid)
- Brain scan (CT or radioisotope imaging)

Differential Diagnosis

- Neoplasia
- Intracranial hematoma
- Cholesterol granuloma—middle-aged overweight adult
- Equine protozoal myeloencephalitis
- Rabies
- Hepatic encephalopathy
- Vestibular disease
- Encephalitis

Treatment

- Potassium penicillin, 22,000 IU/kg IV q6h
- Trimethoprim-sulfa, 20 mg/kg PO q12h
- DMSO, 1 gm/kg IV as a 10% solution in saline or any isotonic fluid
- Flunixin meglumine, 0.5 mg/kg IV q12h
- Dexamethasone, 0.1–0.2 mg/kg IV, single dose, if necessary to reduce cerebral edema
- Phenobarbital to effect, 3–12 mg/kg IV, as needed to control seizures

Prognosis

Medical treatment in reported cases has been uniformly unsuccessful even if aggressive. Surgical drainage combined with long-term antibiotic therapy is considered heroic but may be the only hope of success.

Fungal Meningitis

Cryptococcus is the most common fungal infection of the CNS. Affected individuals may have predominantly cerebral or spinal cord signs. Fever is usually present. The CSF has a marked neutrophilic pleocytosis (generally greater than the clinical signs would indicate). The organism can be identified on *close* inspection of the CNS.

Treatment

Itraconazole, 2.6 mg/kg PO q12h

Equine Self-Mutilation Syndrome

A self-mutilating behavior described as biting at the flank area, tail, or lateral thoracic wall, often precipitated by stress (anticipation of eating or interaction with others), and equated with Tourette syndrome in humans. Males are seven times more likely than females to develop the condition, which most often starts during the first 2 years of life. Heritable factors, inactivity or confinement, and stimulation of endogenous opioids may be involved in the development of the behavior. Castration, change in diet, stabling changes, and the use of opioid antagonists (nalmefene) are used to treat the behavior with partial success. Imipramine, a tricyclic antidepressant drug, 1 mg/kg PO q12h, has been successfully used.

SUDDEN COLLAPSE

Examining a horse that has suddenly collapsed is a formidable diagnostic and therapeutic challenge. Metabolic, respiratory, cardiovascular, and orthopedic causes for sudden collapse must be considered, as well as the neurologic differential list presented. Prognosis for future use is often the determining factor in many of these cases, and an accurate anatomic diagnosis is the first, and sometimes the most difficult, step. *Always consider the possibility of rabies* (see p. 344).

Cranial Trauma

Cerebral edema is the most deleterious manifestation of cranial trauma and the primary lesion to treat. Clinical signs are most severe within 12 hours, but uncontrolled cerebral edema can result in progression of intracranial signs.

Causes

- Collisions
- Penetrating wounds

- Falls: Over a jump; rearing and falling over backward
- Injury:
  - □ Direct injury to neural parenchyma radiating from the point of impact
  - □ Indirect injury by displacement of basioccipital and basisphenoid bones into the overlying brain stem

Clinical Examination

- Obtain an accurate history.
- Do as complete a physical examination as possible. Look for hemorrhage or leakage of CSF from wounds, ears, and nose; respiratory distress (abnormal respiratory patterns); evidence of laryngeal injury. Do an ophthalmic examination (fixed, dilated pupils are a poor prognostic finding). Retinal detachments may occur following head trauma, although optic nerve injury is more common.
- Stabilize the medical condition.
  - □ Maintain a patent airway—it is very important that the $PaCO_2$ be maintained at a low normal or low range because elevations in $PaCO_2$ increase cerebral blood flow and edema.
  - □ Intubate if necessary; supply oxygen.
  - □ Control blood loss and hyperventilate to lower $PaCO_2$.
  - □ Keep the head elevated 30° if possible and do not occlude jugular veins.
- Assess for signs of shock and institute treatment.
  - □ IV fluids
  - □ Corticosteroids—see Treatment section.

Neurologic Examination

- Assess mentation (alert, depression, stupor, coma).
- Cranial nerve examination—especially pupil size, symmetry, pupillary light response, menace response (a severely depressed individual may not menace even though it is visual), presence of nystagmus, strabismus, or dysphagia
- Voluntary limb movement/quality of the gait. Evaluate for concurrent spinal cord or orthopedic injury.
- Pain perception, withdrawal and patellar reflexes
- Abnormal body position or head tilt
- Keep an accurate written record of all observations; serial reassessment is crucial to evaluate progress and modify therapy.

ANCILLARY PROCEDURES

If feasible, the following may prove valuable:

- Skull radiographs
- CSF aspirate and analysis—if blood is grossly contaminated, think a fracture and a grave prognosis. Cisternacentesis (aspirate) and removal of a small volume of fluid should be done with *caution*.
- Upper airway and guttural pouch endoscopy

Treatment

- Dexamethasone, 0.1–0.2 mg/kg IV q6–8 h for the first 24 hours postinjury, then q24h for 2–3 days (of questionable value for cerebral injury)
- DMSO, 1 gm/kg IV, as a 10%–20% solution in saline or other polyionic fluid q12–24h for 5 days
- Mannitol* 0.5–2 gm/kg IV SLOWLY as a 20% solution, repeated once or twice at 4–8-hour intervals. One treatment for a 450-kg adult = 36 (50 ml) bottles of 25% mannitol.
- Furosemide, 1 mg/kg IV q12h for 1–2 days. Potent diuretic; monitor for electrolyte imbalances and maintain hydration, especially when combined with mannitol. Do not overhydrate.
- Broad-spectrum antibiotics—especially if palpable fracture or evidence of hemorrhage!
- Vitamin E, 20,000 units PO q24h for an adult
- Hypertonic saline can be administered to increase cardiac output and may decrease intracranial pressure.
- Fracture repair

If sedation is necessary (try to assess neurologic status before sedation):

- Xylazine 0.1–0.2 mg/kg IV, may *transiently worsen* intracranial hemorrhage due to hypertensive effects, and if the individual is standing, may cause *lowering of the head and worsening of the cerebral edema.*
- Diazepam, 0.1–0.2 mg/kg (5–15 mg) IV for foals
- Phenobarbital to effect, 3–12 mg/kg IV. May have a protective effect on the brain.
- DO NOT use phenothiazines (acepromazine), which may potentiate convulsions.

CT imaging and exploratory craniotomy are available at select academic centers.

Poor Prognostic Indicators

- Deterioration in vital signs
- Altered respiratory patterns (brain stem injury)
- Slow pulse rate, decreasing blood pressure (medullary lesion)
- Unresponsive dilated pupils (midbrain lesion)
- Miotic pupils that become mydriatic (midbrain edema/compression)
- Deterioration of mental status
- Tetraparesis/paraparesis
- Progressive loss of cranial nerve function (compression/hypoxia)
- Opisthotonos (cerebellum, midbrain)
- Vestibular signs (head tilt, circling, inability to maintain sternal recumbency, truncal torsion, abnormal nystagmus) *combined with* abnormal

---

*Use of mannitol if hemorrhage in the cranial cavity has not been controlled, i.e., if there is bleeding from the nose or ears or a palpable skull fracture or a grossly bloody CSF sample, controversial.

mental status and other cranial nerve abnormalities (central vestibular lesion)
- Intensifying seizures

Basisphenoid/Basioccipital Fractures

Fractures of one or both of these bones are especially common in individuals that flip over backward. Often hemorrhage is seen in both the nose and ear.

If the displacement is minimal, clinical signs may improve and the individual recovers or is left with a mild residual head tilt. Minor displacement can be difficult to recognize on standard radiographs. If the displacement is severe, cerebral hemorrhage occurs and the affected individual does not recover.

A hemorrhagic CSF sample may or may not be seen with cerebral hemorrhage, depending on the location of the hemorrhage in the brain.

Some individuals that flip over backward may rupture the muscles within the guttural pouch with a fracture. Hemorrhage and a mild head tilt occur as a result of the muscle rupture.

As with most traumatic injuries of the CNS, DMSO may be administered.

Spinal Cord Trauma

Causes

- Fall, including over a jump and rearing over backwards
- Collision with an immovable object
- Pathologic fracture secondary to osteomyelitis—diskospondylitis—(especially *R. equi* or *Streptococcus equi* in 2–10-month-old foals)

Clinical Signs

- Acute ataxia after an injury or often unassociated with a traumatic event with discospondylitis. The ataxia may be posterior ataxia, tetra-ataxia, or hemi-ataxia depending upon the location of the lesion.
- Progression to recumbency may be rapid.
- Perform a complete physical examination: The affected individual may be unmanageable due to pain.
- Remember that spinal cord trauma may or may not be associated with a fracture.

Stabilize Medical Condition

- Support ventilation.
- Control hemorrhage.
- Treat shock with IV fluids (e.g., hypertonic saline and corticosteroids).
- Assess and treat other injuries—assess for orthopedic injuries.

Neurologic Assessment

- *If standing*, evaluate attitude, posture, and gait. Look for ataxia—are forelimbs involved or only hindlimbs? Examine for palpable cervical abnormalities and neck pain.

- *If recumbent*, carefully assess whether the individual can become sternal, rise with assistance, or support weight.

Localizing the Lesion

C1–C3—can only lift head.

- Hyperactive reflexes all four limbs
- May prefer to lay on one side.

C4–C6—can elevate head and neck but is tetraparetic.

- Hyperactive reflexes all four limbs

C6–T2—tetraparesis/tetraparalysis

- Decreased spinal reflexes and tone in forelimbs
- Normal or hyperactive reflexes and tone in the pelvic limbs

T3–L3—may be able to dog sit.

- Thoracic limbs are normal.
- Pelvic limb paresis to paralysis
- With severe lesion, bladder paralysis and loss of anal and tail tone
- May have patchy sweating along the trunk from damaged sympathetics

L4–L6—may dog sit.

- Pelvic limb paresis or paralysis
- Loss of patellar reflex

Sacral fracture—bladder paralysis with severe lesion

- Possible pelvic limb gait deficit
- Pain on rectal palpation and manipulation of the tail
- Fecal retention and decreased anal and tail tone may be evident.
- Hyperesthesia of perineum, anus, and tail may be evident.

> Schiff-Sherrington syndrome rarely occurs in the horse.
> Horner syndrome may result from a severe cervical spinal cord lesion or a T1–T3 lesion involving the sympathetics. Signs are ipsilateral facial, neck, or truncal sweating; miosis; ptosis; and third eyelid prominence to the side of the lesion.

Diagnosis

- Radiographs
- **Gross blood in CSF = poor prognosis.**
- Myelogram
- CT imaging

General anesthesia should be undertaken with caution. Death can result from respiratory failure in severe cervical spinal cord lesions. Relaxation of muscle tone can cause displacement of fractures and exacerbate neurologic injury.

Treatment

- Dexamethasone, 0.2–0.4 mg/kg IV q12h for the first 1–2 days
- DMSO, 1 gm/kg IV, as a 10% solution in saline or LRS
- Broad-spectrum antibiotics if recumbent or wounds present
- Maintain hydration and nutrition.
- Catheterize and drain bladder if necessary.
- Good nursing care
- Surgery—decompression or stabilization

Prognosis

Many weanlings or foals that fall over backwards recover completely within a few days. Adults seem to be more predisposed to fractures and therefore have a poorer prognosis. Fractured sacrum may result in a cauda equina syndrome. Blindness is a common sequela in all age adults suffering an acute head injury.

Seizures

May be either generalized or localized (partial seizures). *Generalized seizures* are characterized by tonic-clonic muscle activity, involuntary recumbency, and loss of consciousness. Postictal blindness and depression are common.

Partial seizures have localized clinical signs such as facial or limb twitching, compulsive circling, self-mutilation of a particular area, or excessive chewing.

The diagnostic goal is to uncover a treatable underlying etiology for the seizures, if one exists.

Etiology

Seizures can be classified as a manifestation of a structural brain disease, a metabolic disease, or idiopathic.

STRUCTURAL BRAIN DISEASE

- Neoplasia
- Abscess
- Parasitic (EPM)
- Embolism (due to *Strongylus*)
- Encephalitis (viral, bacterial, fungal)
- Meningitis
- Secondary to trauma
- Intracarotid injection
- Other masses—cholesterol granuloma
- Ischemic/hypoxic damage

If the lesion is in a quiet area of the brain, the affected individual is normal in the interictal periods. If the lesion is in an active area of the brain, the individual shows signs of depression or some cranial nerve or proprioceptive deficit in the interictal period.

METABOLIC DISEASE

- Hypoglycemia
- Neonatal maladjustment syndrome
- Hepatic encephalopathy—especially portosystemic shunt
- Renal encephalopathy
- Hyperlipemia/hyperlipidemia
- Hyperkalemia (HYPP)
- Hyperthermia
- Intoxication:
  □ Organophosphates
  □ Lead
  □ Arsenic
  □ Strychnine
- Hypocalcemia/hypomagnesemia
- Hyponatremia

IDIOPATHIC

- Idiopathic epilepsy of foals
  □ Onset usually 3–9 months of age
  □ Generalized seizures with or without involuntary recumbency
  □ May be hereditary in Egyptian Arabians
  □ Responds well to anticonvulsants
  □ Usually outgrow the problem
- Seizures during estrus in mares
  □ Related to elevated estrogen levels
  □ Occur during estrus only
  □ Underlying etiology is unknown.
  □ Control with progesterone or ovariectomy
- Primary cerebral vascular disease (stroke) that is not traceable to an infectious or traumatic cause has been seen in one case.
- On a rare occasion, acute and extensive (rostral) thrombosis of the jugular vein may cause seizures and circling.

Differential Diagnoses for Seizures

- Colic
- Exertional myopathy
- Syncope—cardiac, problems such as severe bradycardia, obstruction of cerebral blood flow, and so on
- Upper airway problems, such as laryngeal obstruction or acute pulmonary edema
- Narcolepsy/cataplexy—especially common in Miniature horses and Shetland ponies
- Tetanus
- A normal sleeping foal may exhibit eyelid, lip, and limb movements that new owners misinterpret as seizure activity.

Diagnosis

- Laboratory tests (immediately after a seizure if possible)
- Obtain an accurate description of the seizure.
- Interictal examination—closely examine cranial nerves.
- CSF sample and analysis
- Skull radiographs
- Fundic examination
- Brain scan (CT or radioisotope imaging)

Treatment

TO STOP A SEIZURE

- Diazepam, 5–20 mg IV for a foal.
- Phenobarbital (administer IV to effect: approximately 6–15 mg/kg).
- Xylazine, 0.5–1.0 mg/kg IV—not recommended as the first choice. Decreases cerebral blood flow and may increase intracranial pressure, thereby potentially exacerbating seizures. It can be used as a last resort or if only a small-volume injection is possible.

ANCILLARY TREATMENTS

- DMSO, 1 gm/kg IV, as a 10% solution in saline or any other isotonic fluid once a day for 3–5 days
- Flunixin meglumine, 0.5 mg/kg IV q12–24h. Potentially ulcerogenic in foals.
- Antibiotics—if a bacterial etiology is suspected
- 10% dextrose IV for hypoglycemia, HYPP, and hepatic encephalopathy

MAINTENANCE THERAPY

- Phenobarbital, 5–10 mg/kg PO q12h (wide individual variation in dosage). May take 2–3 weeks to acclimate to dosage. Reduce if individual is too sedated.

Prognosis

Depends on the etiology—i.e., if there is a treatable intracranial or extracranial condition. Poor prognostic signs include: increasing frequency of seizures, increasing intensity of seizures, and poor response to maintenance therapy.

Drug-Induced Hyperexcitability, Seizure, or Collapse

Due to inadvertent intracarotid injection, procaine penicillin reaction, drug-induced hypotension.

Inadvertent Intracarotid Injection

- Onset during injection or a few seconds postinjection
- Acute seizure with recumbency and paddling
- May be preceded by facial twitching and wide-eyed appearance

- Severity of signs depends on volume injected, properties of the drug, and individual sensitivity.
- **CAUTION**: It is very difficult to distinguish between arterial and venous (blood) puncture when using a 20-gauge needle to administer IV medication.

If drug is water soluble (xylazine, acepromazine):

- The affected individual can usually stand in 5–60 minutes.
- The individual is usually clinically normal in 1–7 days if no secondary injuries occur.
- May see the following clinical signs in addition to collapse:
  □ Contralateral blindness
  □ Nasal septum hypalgesia
  □ Subtle hemiparesis
- Treatment may not be necessary as most recover on their own.

TREATMENT

- DMSO, 1 gm/kg IV as a 10% solution in saline
- Dexamethasone, 0.1–0.2 mg/kg IV q12h for the first 24 hours
- Phenobarbital to effect, 3–12 mg/kg IV q12 or 24 h

If the drug administered intracarotid is insoluble or oil-based (e.g., phenylbutazone, procaine penicillin, trimethoprim-sulfa):

- Acute death often occurs.
- Recovery is usually unsatisfactory.
- Seizure is more severe.
- Persistent stupor or coma may occur.
- Condition usually warrants euthanasia.

Reaction to Procaine Penicillin Injected IM

- Result of rapid intravenous absorption of procaine penicillin after IM administration
- Reaction may occur even with correct injection technique.
- Reaction is most frequent after several IM injections in more vascular areas.
- Reaction usually starts after injection has been completed or nearly completed.
- Patient acts as if it is "seeing spooks"—wildly circles the stall and snorts or bangs around in the stall, then collapses and seizures.
- KEEP AFFECTED INDIVIDUAL CONFINED! Often the most serious outcome is self-inflicted trauma, which can escalate if the patient is loose.
- *Acute death can occur if a large volume is absorbed IV.*
- Treatment is generally not possible. If the individual has collapsed and appears in a stupor, administer dexamethasone, 0.1–0.2 mg/kg IV.

Drug-Induced Hypotension

- Usually occurs with acepromazine administered IV
- May be hypotensive from blood loss or shock

- Drug potentiates hypotension and collapse.
- Does not seizure.
- Treat with IV fluids, hypertonic saline, or blood transfusion (if hemorrhage is a predisposing factor).

Drug-Induced Hyperexcitability

- Butorphanol produces bizarre head tremors in some horses, especially when xylazine is not given a few minutes beforehand. No treatment required, although naloxone may reverse signs.
- Abnormally high plasma and CSF concentrations of aminophylline results in bizarre behavior.
- Treatment: Discontinue aminophylline, provide fluid therapy, and control any seizures with xylazine.

Bizarre Behavior

- May occur following treatment with the long-acting tranquilizer fluphenazine decanoate (Prolixin)
- The reaction appears to be idiosyncratic.
- Treatment: Antihistamines such as diphenhydramine, 0.5–2.0 mg/kg slowly IV or IM, may be helpful, but pentobarbital, 5–15 mg/kg IV, may be required to quiet the individual. Phenobarbital, 5–15 mg/kg PO, may be required for several days to keep from injuring itself.
- Gross overdosing of piperazine may cause recumbency and dementia.
- Treatment: Supportive

DYSPHAGIA

Dysphagia (difficulty in swallowing) has many possible etiologies, such as oral **irritation**/injury, esophageal obstruction, a brain stem disease, or peripheral **damage to cranial nerves IX, X, XI, or XII. Individuals with a cerebral disease and severe depression may also have decreased tongue function—the tongue may remain protruded or be slow to return to the mouth.**

Differential Diagnoses

- Choke (see p. 166)
- Oral foreign body/irritation (see Salivation, p. 164)
- EPM (see p. 338)
- Guttural pouch disease—mycotic plaques in dorsomedial compartment or melanoma of the pouch.
- Botulism (see p. 348)
- Yellow star thistle intoxication (see following)
- Viral encephalitis (see p. 360)
- Cerebral abscess (see p. 361)
- Pharyngeal swelling/obstruction (see p. 435)
- Rabies (see p. 344)
- Organophosphate/lead intoxication
- Grass sickness (exotic)

- White muscle disease
- Neonatal maladjustment syndrome and/or soft palate dysfunction (see p. 482)
- Fractured mandible or stylohyoid bone (see p. 305)

Yellow Star Thistle Intoxication

Signalment

- Any age or breed or either sex
- Access to plant (pasture or hay) for several weeks
- *Centauria solstitialis*—yellow star thistle
- *Centauria repens*—Russian knapweed

Clinical Signs

- Weight loss
- Depression
- Acute rigidity in the muscles of mastication
- Purposeless chewing
- Inability to open or close the mouth completely

Death results from starvation. There is no treatment.

Fractured Jaw

- This may also result in purposeful head tilt, tongue protrusion, and salivation.
- Diagnosis can be made by physical examination, inability to properly align teeth, and radiographs.
- Consider surgical treatment if signs are severe.

Trauma and Fracture of Stylohyoid Bone

- May also cause uncontrolled head tilt and facial paralysis if the most dorsal area of the bone is fractured (see p. 343).
- Diagnosis is by endoscopy of the guttural pouch and radiographs.

Treatment

- Medical therapy to alleviate damage to the nerves (e.g., DMSO, 1 gm/kg q24h).
- Antibiotics: Trimethoprim sulfa, 20 mg/kg PO q12h, and procaine penicillin, 22,000 U/kg IM q12h.
- Ophthalmic treatment to prevent exposure keratitis.
- Additional nursing care (e.g., nutritional support, and so forth)
- Surgical removal of a section of the bone (see p. 344)

Prognosis

Guarded for return to normal function after acute fracture of the stylohyoid bone.

PERIPHERAL NERVE DISEASE

Suprascapular Nerve (Sweeny)

- Almost invariably caused by trauma:
  - □ Collision with a solid object or a kick
  - □ Ill-fitting driving collar in draft horses
- Other possible causes:
  - □ Peripheral nerve neoplasm or abscess compressing C6 nerve or suprascapular nerve
  - □ Equine protozoal myelitis
- Atrophy of supraspinatus and infraspinatus muscles results in an abnormal gait.
  - □ Initial stumbling, dragging of the toe
  - □ Abduction (popping) of the shoulder on weight bearing
- If neurapraxia (nerve contusion), function returns in days to weeks.
- If severance of the nerve has occurred, regrowth of the nerve down the fibrous framework is at a rate of 1 mm/month.
- Wait at least 2–8 weeks post-trauma; if no improvement, surgery is advised to explore the area and relieve any entrapment due to adhesions or fibrosis. Removal of a portion of the cranial edge of the scapula is advised to decrease compression of the suprascapular nerve.
- Electromyelograms can be useful 2–4 weeks postinjury to detect involvement of other nerves.
- Anesthetic recovery can be mechanically difficult in any individual with nerve injury, muscle atrophy, and/or disuse of a limb!

Radial Nerve

- May accompany humeral fractures:
  - □ Evaluation before surgery may be difficult as there is no reliable autonomous zone for skin sensation. The dorsolateral aspect of the leg receives sensory innervation from the radial nerve and should be evaluated for sensation. Examine nerve at the time of surgery.
- May be due to prolonged lateral recumbency:
  - □ Most likely a combination of ischemic myopathy and ischemic neurapraxia.
- Direct trauma is less likely due to protection by surrounding muscle.
  - □ If trauma is the known etiology, more likely it is a brachial plexus contusion/avulsion (see following).
- Affected individual unable to bear weight with paralysis due to lack of elbow, carpus, and fetlock extension. Elbow dropped during locomotion, toe drags, pectoral muscles may be able to move leg forward half a stride. When standing, leg rests on the dorsum of the toe. May be able to paw with the limb.
- Limb must be supported with a splint or cast to avoid further injury as well as muscle contracture.

- Recovery, in cases of neurapraxia, may take several weeks. If no improvement in 6–8 weeks, prognosis is poor. Radial nerve damage/severance combined with humeral fracture warrants an extremely guarded prognosis.
- Rule out septic arthritis of the elbow, fracture, EPM, rupture of medial collateral ligament of the elbow using ultrasound, and focal myopathy.

Brachial Plexus Avulsion

Many cases of shoulder injury with signs of radial paralysis are probably caused by damage to the roots of the brachial plexus.

- Carriage of the limb is almost identical to that described for radial nerve paralysis.
- Total avulsion results in flaccid paralysis of the entire limb and sensory loss distal to the elbow.
- Damage to the median and ulnar nerves without radial nerve damage results in a stiff, goose-stepping gait with hyperextension of the lower limb. Analgesia may be present over the lateral aspect of the cannon bone and pastern.
- Individuals that have suffered contusions progressively improve over 6 to 18 months. Physiotherapy (especially swimming) has been useful in returning to function. Return to racing after brachial plexus injury has been reported.
- Neoplasia (nerve sheath) and EPM may have identical clinical signs.
- Prognosis, though, in general is guarded to poor.
- The opposite limb should be bandaged for mechanical support.

Femoral Nerve

- Nerve is well protected from external trauma but may be damaged by:
  - Penetrating wound to the caudal flank
  - Abscess/neoplasia
  - Aneurysm in the region of the external iliac arteries
  - Secondary to dystocia (hip or stifle lock) in a newborn foal
  - Femoral or pelvic fracture (rare)
  - Secondary to compression during anesthesia and complicated by myopathy (may be bilateral)
  - EPM
- Individual is unable to support weight if femoral paralysis is present. The limb is advanced with difficulty. When the horse attempts to bear weight, the stifle collapses (flexes), and the hock and fetlock flex due to the reciprocal apparatus.
- At rest, all the joints are flexed.
- Atrophy of the quadriceps is evident in 2–4 weeks.
- Patellar reflex is depressed or absent.
- Hypalgesia may be evident over the medial thigh if the saphenous nerve or the femoral nerve dorsal to the iliopsoas muscle is involved.
- Prognosis is guarded regardless of etiology.

Sciatic Nerve

- In foals, may occur due to *Salmonella* osteomyelitis of the sacrum and pelvis or, more commonly, from intramuscular injection into the caudal thigh. Damage to the nerve occurs because of:
  - ☐ Needle puncture of the nerve
  - ☐ Irritation due to the drug injected—penicillin, diazepam, and chlorpromazine causing widespread axonal degeneration after intrafascicular injection
  - ☐ Pressure from a hematoma
  - ☐ Scarring around the nerve
- In adults, damage to the sciatic nerve may occur owing to:
  - ☐ Pelvic fracture (especially ischium)
  - ☐ Coxofemoral luxations
  - ☐ Other injuries (kick)—especially the peroneal branch of the sciatic nerve
  - ☐ Postfoaling—dystocias with delivery of a large foal
  - ☐ EPM
- Gait and posture
  - ☐ Can support weight if the limb is positioned under the body
  - ☐ At rest, limb held behind, with stifle and hock extended and fetlock flexed, with the dorsum of the foot rolled forward
  - ☐ The toe is dragged as limb flexion is poor.
  - ☐ Hypalgesia exists over most of the limb, except the medial thigh.
  - ☐ Postfoaling mares with sciatic damage may be unable to stand completely on the hind legs.

PERONEAL PARALYSIS

Because the peroneal nerve is involved in sciatic nerve paralysis, the clinical findings are similar. In peroneal paralysis, hypalgesia may exist over the craniolateral gaskin, hock, and metatarsus. Paresis of the peroneal nerve is common after extended recumbency, and recovery generally occurs within 1–3 days; frequently the individual is found standing.

TIBIAL PARALYSIS

This is less common than peroneal nerve paralysis. The gait in tibial nerve paralysis resembles stringhalt. Flexion of the hock and extension of the digit is unopposed, so that the individual overflexes the limb and raises the foot higher than normal. The hock is flexed (dropped hock), and the fetlock knuckles forward at rest. Sensation may be reduced in the caudal and medial coronet region.

Treatment is generally supportive, including bandaging of distal limbs to prevent excoriations of the dorsal aspect of the limb and support-wraps on the opposite limb. If a recognizable mass is compressing the nerve (e.g., hematoma, fracture), surgical decompression is indicated. Treat postfoaling mares with sciatic nerve damage aggressively, with DMSO, 10% IV, mild sedation if anxiety is a problem, and physical support (e.g., tail-tie) for short periods of time to enable the mare to stand. If the mare cannot stand with this therapy, administer a single dose of dexamethasone, 0.2–0.4 mg/kg, IV. Postfoaling mares that cannot stand are difficult to manage and often develop severe myopathy secondary to the recumbency.

Cranial Gluteal Nerve

Damage to this nerve results in profound atrophy of the gluteal muscles of the rump. There is little alteration in gait. May be seen with pelvic fracture or EPM involving L6 ventral gray column.

Lumbar, Sacral, and Caudal Roots

Most commonly injured secondary to vertebral fracture.

- L6, L7, S1—appear as sciatic nerve paralysis
- S1, S2, S3—inability to close anus, analgesia of anus and perineum, distention of bladder and rectum
- Caudal nerves—analgesia of perineum and penis but not prepuce, and inability to move tail

Polyneuritis of the cauda equina also affects the same nerves, but the onset of signs is insidious with a slow progression.

Facial Nerve

Facial nerve paresis/paralysis may result from *vestibular syndrome* (see p. 343), *EPM* (see p. 338), trauma, polyneuritis equi, or may be idiopathic. If the facial nerve is affected at the nucleus (e.g., EPM) or as it courses through the middle/inner ear, all branches (auricular, palpebral, and buccal) are involved. With more distal injury, only one or two branches are usually involved (e.g., injury to the buccal branch caused by halter pressure during anesthesia).

Injury to Buccal Branch of Facial Nerve

CLINICAL SIGNS

Lower lip droop and decreased nostril diameter on affected side, and deviation of nose to the contralateral side

TREATMENT

Apply ice compresses to the affected side of the face for the first 24 hours. Corticosteroids can be administered but, unless there is a skin laceration and severance of the nerve, recovery usually occurs in a couple of weeks.

Idiopathic Paralysis

- This often involves both the buccal and palpebral branches and is usually permanent. **With any cause of facial paresis involving the palpebral branch, monitor closely to prevent corneal ulceration.**
- If no corneal ulcer is present at the initial examination, apply ophthalmic ointment (Lacri-Lube) q6h for 1–2 weeks. Most affected individuals

compensate for the paresis after a period of time and do not require further ophthalmic treatment.
- For corneal ulceration, see p. 390.

SUGGESTED REFERENCES

Cervical Stenotic/Compressive Myelopathy
Moore BR, Reed SM. Equine spinal ataxia: Ancillary diagnostic tests. Proc Am Assoc Equine Pract 1993:107.

Vestibular Disease
Blythe LL, Watrous BJ, Pearson EG, et al. Otitis media/interna in the horse—a cause of head shaking and skull fractures. Proc Am Assoc Equine Pract 1990:517–528.

Rabies
Green S. Equine rabies. Vet Clin North Am Equine Pract 1993;9(2):337.

Verminous Encephalitis
Ruggles AJ, Beech J, Gillett DM, Midla BS, Reef VB, Freeman DE. Disseminated *Halicephalobus deletrix* infection in a horse. J Am Vet Med Assoc 1993;203:550–552.

Acute Ataxia
DeLahunta A. Veterinary Neuroanatomy and Clinical Neurology. 2nd ed. Philadelphia, WB Saunders, 1983.
Mayhew IG. Large Animal Neurology. Philadelphia, Lea & Febiger, 1989.

Equine Motor Neuron Disease
Divers TJ, Mohammed HO, Cummings JF, et al. Equine motor neuron disease: Findings in 28 horses and proposal of a pathophysiological mechanism for the disease. Equine Vet J 1994;26(5):409–415.

Myopathy/Myositis
Traub-Dargatz JL, Schlipf JW, Granstrom DE, Ingram JT, Shelton GD, Getzy DM, Lappin MR, Baker DC. Multifocal myositis associated with *Sarcocystis* sp. in a horse. J Am Vet Med Assoc 1994;205(11):1574–1576.

Causes of Trembling
Madigan JE, Valberg SJ, Ragle C, Moody JL. Muscle spasms associated with ear tick (*Otobius megnini*) infestations in five horses. J Am Vet Med Assoc 1995;207:74–76.

Cerebral Abscess
Raphel CF. Brain abscess in three horses. J Am Vet Med Assoc 1982;180:874–877.

Equine Self-Mutilation Syndrome
Dodman NH, Normile JA, Schuster L, Rand W. Equine self-mutilation syndrome (57 cases). J Am Vet Med Assoc 1994;204:1219–1223.

31 Ophthalmology

Nita L. Irby

EQUINE OCULAR EMERGENCIES

Many problems involving the horse's eye are true emergencies:

- Corneal or eyelid lacerations
- Corneal ulcerations or stromal abscesses
- Uveitis
- Glaucoma
- Blunt head trauma
- Acute blindness or visual disturbance
- Other traumatic injury to the eye

These cases need to be seen immediately by a veterinarian or veterinary ophthalmologist because *long-term prognosis for vision and even retention of the globe* depend on immediate, accurate diagnosis and treatment.

Because many drugs administered systemically do not reach adequate levels in the eye, the owner should be prepared to administer topical medication to injured eye every hour. Cases requiring frequent medication benefit by placement of a transpalpebral lavage apparatus (see p. 83).

DIAGNOSTIC AND THERAPEUTIC AIDS TO TREATMENT

Auriculopalpebral Nerve Block

- The horse has a powerful orbicularis oculi muscle and can overcome any attempt to open its eyelid; therefore, use this block routinely for any examination of the equine eye that requires manipulation of the eyelids or is painful.
  - □ The auriculopalpebral nerve can be palpated as it crosses the bony orbit rim dorsolateral to the eye.
  - □ Cleanse the area and inject 1–2 ml of local anesthetic subcutaneously (SQ).
- A properly performed block results in almost complete akinesia of the upper eyelid and greatly facilitates examination of the eye.
- **Never attempt to forcefully open the closed eyelids of an individual without eyelid akinesia; this could rupture a deep corneal ulcer or eviscerate an eye with a laceration.**

Frontal Nerve Block

- This nerve block also provides very good to excellent akinesia of the upper lid.

- Local anesthetic instilled SQ in the area of the supraorbital foramen (located on the orbital rim in the supraorbital process of the frontal bone dorsal to the medial canthus of the eye) results in anesthesia to the majority of the upper eyelid.
- Preferred block for routine examination purposes because the patient does not feel the manipulations of the lid, tending to resist examination much less.

Topical Anesthesia

- Proparacaine (0.5%), tetracaine (0.5%), and other topical anesthetic agents cause mild stinging when placed in the eye and result in hyperemia of the conjunctiva. Complete your initial examination before instillation.
- Apply via a spray from stock solution placed in a tuberculin syringe, needle hub attached but *with the needle broken off.*
- Repeated applications of topical anesthetic every 15–30 seconds for 3–5 minutes greatly enhances the depth of topical anesthesia.

TRAUMA TO THE HEAD

- Traumatic injuries to the orbit and globe, self-inflicted or induced, are common in the horse due to the prominent lateral position of the eye, the high-strung, nervous temperament of many individuals, and the powerful reflex throwing of the head.
- Always treat ocular and orbital traumatic injuries as emergencies.
- Once an injury has occurred, immediately restrain the individual's head to avoid additional self-induced injury that occurs from rubbing the eye against the stall, the wall, or the individual's forelimb.
- Avoid examination or manipulation of the ocular and periocular tissues until adequate restraint and tranquilization are completed.

Blunt Trauma to Head

- Commonly results from individual rearing and flipping backward
- May cause sudden unilateral or bilateral loss of vision from partial or complete shearing of the optic nerve from the brain as it exits from the optic canal
- Pupillary light reflexes, menace responses, obstacle course evaluation, and complete ophthalmic examination, including examination of the fundus, must be performed in all cases of blunt head trauma.

Acute Findings

- Partial or complete unilateral or bilateral blindness
- Normal or abnormal pupillary light reflexes (almost always abnormal if the eyes are significantly visually impaired)
- Possible optic disc edema and/or hemorrhage (usually not seen due to the injury occurring near the brain and not near the eye)

Chronic Cases

- Optic nerve atrophy as evidenced by pallor, darkening, and decreased size of the nerve head
- Decreased retinal vasculature
- Peripapillary retinal and choroidal atrophy

Prognosis

- Some cases of partial blindness, indicating some optic fibers still intact, improve with time and aggressive treatment for central nervous system (CNS) trauma (systemic corticosteroids, IV dimethyl sulfoxide [DMSO], and so on—see p. 366).
- Most cases are permanently visually impaired.
- Prognosis is guarded to grave in all cases, and visual loss may progress for several days after the injury.

Blunt Trauma to Eye Without Laceration or Rupture

- Always perform careful physical, neurologic, and ophthalmic examinations, including fundus examination; the eye may appear normal or have any combination of injuries.
  - □ Indirect ophthalmoscopy is more likely to allow examination of the fundus through a cloudy media.
  - □ Some cases may be normal; others have a mild to severe optic nerve hyperemia with or without peripapillary retinal and choroidal edema.
- Perform fundus examinations at 1, 3, 6, and 12 months post-injury because some cases develop "butterfly lesions" (areas of peripapillary choroidal disturbance and atrophy), possibly as a result of compression of the back of the eye around the stalk of the optic nerve (Fig. 31–1, see Color Plate 1). Visual disturbance has not been documented in these cases.
  - □ Butterfly lesions may be associated with recurrent uveitis, an unsoundness in the horse.
  - □ Document butterfly lesions to prevent any question of an unsound condition being present later in life.

Bony Trauma

- The dorsal (frontal bone) and temporal (temporal and zygomatic bones) regions of the bony orbit are most commonly injured.
- The bones may be contused or fractured.

Clinical Signs

- Edema, swelling, pain, blepharospasm of the eyelids, coupled with lid or face lacerations in some cases
- Subcutaneous and/or orbital emphysema if the frontal sinus is fractured (Fig. 31–2, see Color Plate 1).

- Palpable disruption of the normal bony contour if a displaced fracture has occurred.
- Abnormal nasal discharge
- Strabismus or displacement of the globe
- Enophthalmic, exophthalmic, or normally positioned globe
- Upper eyelid function may be impaired due to lid swelling or injury to the auriculopalpebral nerve.

Diagnosis

- Generally straightforward if a known traumatic injury has occurred
- Rule out orbital cellulitis (see later).
- Complete physical and neurologic examination and palpation of the affected site once it has been determined that the patient can be safely tranquilized and topically anesthetized
- Any combination of skull radiographs, oblique views, ultrasonography, computed tomography; primarily in cases with strabismus or displacement of the globe that may be surgical candidates

Treatment

- Most cases with no major ocular injury, displacement or evidence of periocular muscle entrapment, or significantly displaced fractures: treat symptomatically with cold compresses, topical ocular lubricants, analgesics, and anti-inflammatory agents.
- Do NOT use systemic corticosteroids unless there is damage to the optic nerve.
- Use hot compresses after the first 12 hours for 5–10 minutes q2h.
- Use broad-spectrum antibiotics for skin wounds or sinus fractures.
- Skin or corneal wounds may require surgical repair.

- Repair the bony orbital fracture, if significantly displaced, resulting in ocular displacement, optic nerve compression, or cosmetically unacceptable result.
- Surgical repair is easiest in the first 24–48 hours and is accomplished by digital or mechanical manipulation, bone traction, or more extensive orthopedic procedures.
- Repair the fracture as an emergency if optic nerve compression is suspected.

EYELID EMERGENCIES

Acute Blepharitis

Etiology

- Possible known causes include:
  □ Allergic reactions
  □ Exposure to noxious plants

□ Insect stings
□ In most cases a cause is never determined.

Clinical Signs

- Swelling, edema
- Blepharospasm
- Epiphora
- Secondary exposure keratitis due to the improper contact between the eyelid and the cornea

Diagnosis

- Careful history: Has this occurred before? What has the individual been exposed to recently? and so on.
- Careful examination of the head and eye, including conjunctival surfaces of the lids and nictitating membrane:
  □ Requires a lid block and application of topical anesthetic
  □ Remove any foreign material(s) that may be present.

Treatment

- Most cases require only symptomatic therapy.
  □ Cold compresses
  □ Sterile ophthalmic lubricant (such as Lacri-Lube) until the lid(s) has returned to normal
  □ Treat any secondary ulcers that may develop from the exposure keratitis.

Facial Nerve Damage

Local or central facial nerve injury may result in inability to close the eyelids, which results in exposure keratitis and possible corneal ulceration.

Diagnosis

Absence of a blink response to either eyelid touch or with corneal stimulation

Treatment

TEMPORARY TARSORRHAPHY

- Horizontal mattress sutures placed split-thickness in the eyelids may suffice for 1–3 weeks.
- Semipermanent tarsorrhaphies can be performed at a later time, if warranted.

Prognosis

Guarded. Partial to complete function usually returns over a 6–12 month period, sooner if due to local injury from swelling or trauma.

Eyelid Lacerations

- Most common involving the upper eyelid
- Any periocular injury necessitates a complete ocular examination.
- Make sure the eye is lubricated and protected from self-mutilation before and during the examination.
- If the etiology is unknown, skull radiographs are indicated to rule out metallic foreign bodies. Carefully explore the wound before closure.

Etiology

- Usually occur because the individual has caught the upper or lower eyelid on a hook, nail, or other pointed object
- May be a result of blunt compression or trauma

Diagnosis

- Usually obvious!
- May be a simple laceration perpendicular to the lid margin; a flap of eyelid hanging from a pedicle; a laceration that has removed the lid margin—uncommon
- The wound is usually edematous and bloody.
- Blood, tears, and mucoid to mucopurulent ocular discharge are seen on the lid and periocular area, moist or dry depending on the time since injury.
- The individual is usually in mild to moderate pain.
- A fluorescein dye test MUST be performed to assess the integrity of the cornea. Treat any corneal injury appropriately.

Treatment

> ANY EYELID LACERATION THAT BREACHES THE EYELID MARGIN MUST BE SURGICALLY REPAIRED! NEVER REMOVE SEEMINGLY REDUNDANT EYELID TISSUE OR EYELID FLAPS THAT HAVE OCCURRED AS A RESULT OF A LACERATION!

- Eyelids are heavily vascularized and very "forgiving" of injury if properly repaired.
- Tissue appearing hopelessly desiccated, inflamed, and/or infected may heal well if properly repaired.
- No tissue in the body can substitute for lost eyelid margin.
- Removal or improper repair of an eyelid margin leads to chronic corneal disease from irritation by eyelid hairs (trichiasis), exposure keratitis due

to improper spreading of the tear film over the cornea, and chronic conjunctivitis due to an inability of the eye to cleanse itself properly.

ANESTHESIA AND WOUND PREPARATION

- Perform repair following local anesthesia and sedation if the patient is cooperative and the repair is a simple one.
- Use general anesthesia in all cases of complicated repairs or if the patient is difficult to manage.
- In either case, topical anesthetic application is a useful adjunct to repair.
- Avoid clipping the lid hair around the wound because the small cut hairs are difficult to eliminate from the wound. Wounds that extend into the longer hair of the lid or face may require clipping.
- Meticulously and repeatedly cleanse the wound with sterile saline or a 1:10 dilution of povidone-iodine *solution*. Avoid detergent cleansers as they are highly toxic to ocular tissues (e.g., chlorhexidine).
- Debride the wound margins with sterile gauze until the cut surfaces are bleeding freely. Avoid sharp debridement in order to preserve the maximum amount of eyelid tissue.

ACUTE INJURIES (<12 HOURS OLD)

- 4-0 or 5-0 absorbable suture material on a small needle is preferred.
- Perform a two-layer closure on all full-thickness lacerations.
- Examine the deeper layers of the eyelid until the thin connective tissue layer of the eyelid is identified. This is the layer in which to place subcutaneous sutures.
- The first suture placed is the most important—it should exactly appose the eyelid margin.
  - ☐ The first suture is a buried figure 8/mattress-type suture that securely closes the subconjunctival tissue and leaves the knot deeply buried beneath the conjunctiva and well away from the eyelid margin.
  - ☐ If placement is not exact and a *"step"* develops in the eyelid margin, remove and replace the suture.
- Place additional subcutaneous/subconjunctival sutures, as necessary, depending on the length of the laceration.
- The surgeon should confirm that subcutaneous suture(s) **DO NOT** penetrate the conjunctiva.
- Skin closure is routine—simple interrupted sutures using 4-0 or 5-0 absorbable material; use synthetic absorbable sutures in the skin as well.
  - ☐ Make certain that the cut ends of the skin sutures *do not* contact the cornea.
- Severe lacerations may benefit by stent support and can be stented to the opposing eyelid via tarsorrhaphy, using split-thickness horizontal mattress sutures in the eyelid margins.
  - ☐ If the eyelids must be closed, plan ahead and place a transpalpebral lavage apparatus for administration of topical medications before closure of the lids (see p. 83).

Postoperative Medical Management
- Warm compresses, if possible, 10 minutes every 2–3 hours for 2 days
- Avoid topical corticosteroids.

- Topical broad-spectrum antibiotic six times a day for 24 hours, then four times a day for 7–10 days
  - □ Avoid placing unnecessary tension or stress on the eyelid during the application of topical medications.
  - □ If this is not possible, then topical ophthalmic antibiotic solutions may be sprayed onto the cornea via medication in a tuberculin syringe with the needle hub attached, but *with the needle broken off* the hub. This makes a very effective, simple, medication "squirt gun."
- If the cornea is injured, administer topical medications more intensively and choose more judiciously.
- Systemic antibiotics may be indicated if the wound is heavily contaminated.
- Systemic anti-inflammatories/antiprostaglandins are indicated depending on the degree of inflammation and discomfort. Minimally, administer phenylbutazone, 2.2–4.4 mg/kg PO q12h, for 3–5 days.
- Administer tetanus toxoid.
- Gently cleanse the periocular area as often as exudate and discharges accumulate.
- Following cleansing and drying, coat the drainage area of the face beneath the eye with a film of petrolatum jelly to prevent hair loss from irritation by ocular secretions.

SUBACUTE TO CHRONIC LACERATIONS (>12 HOURS OLD)

- Postpone repair for a few days, if needed, to stabilize the patient if other injuries are present or to allow any infection to be controlled by medications.
- Topical and medical management are as just noted.
- The wound edges are sharply restored by scarification with a #15 scalpel blade, taking care not to remove tissue, only to restore a liberally bleeding surface.

EMERGENCIES INVOLVING THE GLOBE

Acute Exophthalmos

ALWAYS AN EMERGENCY!

Clinical Signs

- The eye protrudes any abnormal degree from the orbit.
- The nictitating membrane is protruding or recessed.
- ±Fever
- Pain, redness, swelling, and discharge of purulent material vary, depending on the duration and etiology.

Differential Considerations

ORBIT INFLAMMATION

- Infection/cellulitis:
  - □ May be a result of foreign body penetration

□ May be an extension from an infected tooth root or sinus infection
□ May occur secondary to penetrating injury
□ Myositis
□ Rare in the horse

GLAUCOMA

- Rarely an acute problem in the horse but may have gone unrecognized for long enough that exophthalmos is the first presenting sign.
- The eye usually has obvious abnormalities (see Glaucoma, p. 403.)

ORBITAL NEOPLASIA

- Numerous neoplasms have been reported in the horse, both primary and as extensions from adjacent regions, particularly sinus and the nasal cavity.
- Rarely an acute problem
- Usually accompanied by clinical disease other than the eye

Diagnosis

- Complete physical and ophthalmic examination
- Further diagnostics determined by the physical examination and include
  □ Radiographs
  □ Ultrasound
  □ Endoscopy of the upper airway and medial orbital regions
  □ Computed tomography
  □ Anesthesia and exploration

Treatment

Immediate therapy:

- Prevention of self-mutilation
- Careful cleansing of the eye and periocular tissues with sterile saline or a sterile eye wash. Contact lens solutions in squeeze bottles are commonly available and may be used.
- Determine whether the cornea has any abrasion or ulceration due to exposure.
- If the eye needs treatment other than lubrication, place a transpalpebral lavage apparatus because the eyelids may be temporarily closed as part of the therapy (see p. 83).
- Following cleansing, heavily lubricate the eye and any exposed periocular tissues with a sterile ophthalmic lubricant such as Lacri-Lube.
- Perform a temporary tarsorrhaphy to keep the eyelids closed.
  □ Extreme care is taken in placement of tarsorrhaphy sutures so that they do not rub the cornea and create additional problems. They should split the thickness of the lids, exiting from the eyelid margins. They should be firmly, but not tightly, apposed.

Further therapy varies with the etiology.

Lacerations and Ruptures of the Fibrous Coat

> If there is any suspicion that a laceration of the cornea or sclera has occurred, instruct the owner that the individual must be prevented from self-mutilating the eye. Any examination of the eye or periocular area by the owner or veterinarian should await heavy sedation and akinesia of the lids. Failure to follow these guidelines can result in a simple laceration becoming a hopeless evisceration. Also instruct the owner that NOTHING (particularly ointments) should be instilled into the eye.

LACERATIONS OR RUPTURES WITH POOR PROGNOSIS

- The injury has resulted in *extensive laceration*, with prolapse of intraocular contents other than iris tissue (lens, vitreous, retina). Do not consider repair (other than placement of an intraocular prosthesis) because the end result is almost always phthisis bulbi (a small, shrunken, and often painful or irritating eye).
- *Lacerations that extend across the limbus* into the sclera have a poorer prognosis if uveal tissue has prolapsed through the wound.
  □ Uveal tissue in these cases usually includes the ciliary body.
  □ Damage to the ciliary body results in decreased aqueous humor production, hypotony, and phthisis bulbi.
  □ Enucleation or prosthesis implantation is often indicated in these cases.
- *Lacerations with associated severe intraocular hemorrhage*
- *Lacerations in which the anterior chamber has collapsed* and not re-formed

LACERATIONS WITH A GOOD PROGNOSIS

- Those with a formed anterior chamber
- Those with a small amount of hemorrhage or fibrin and uveal tissue closing the wound, with minimal distortion of uveal structures
- Simple lacerations with minimal contamination and minimal iris prolapse

At no time during the examination or surgery should ophthalmic ointments be placed on the eye! ONLY solutions should be used.

Full-Thickness Lacerations

> - **All full-thickness lacerations of the equine eye require immediate surgical repair under general anesthesia.**
> - **Referral to a veterinary ophthalmologist is recommended for all but the most simple cases. Do not attempt surgery unless standard ophthalmic surgery instruments and appropriately sized suture are available. The operations are often more difficult than expected.**

- Clinical signs are generally obvious:
  - Decreased intraocular pressure
  - Decreased depth or total collapse of the anterior chamber
  - Fibrin, hypopyon, and/or hyphema in the anterior chamber
  - Visible lesion, usually plugged with uveal tissue
  - If fluorescein is applied to the cornea, fluorescence of the aqueous humor may occur if the wound is not yet sealed.
- **Do not** use ketamine for general anesthesia.
- Wound apposition should be precise, with the surgeon assisted by binocular magnification if possible.
- *Gently* lavage, cleanse, and carefully replace prolapsed uveal tissue (iris, usually) into the anterior chamber whenever possible, with the surgeon understanding that postoperative uveitis is proportional to the degree of uveal damage/handling.
  - Carefully debride necrotic, desiccated, or otherwise devitalized uveal tissue.
  - Uveal excision can result in severe hemorrhage—be prepared.
- Suture material: 6-0 to 8-0 monofilament absorbable
- Suture placement: 1–2 mm apart, carefully positioned to extend at least two thirds thickness but NOT full thickness of the cornea
- Wound may be reinforced with adjacent conjunctiva as a conjunctival flap.
  - This is usually not necessary unless the security of the wound closure is in doubt.
  - Flap placement almost always results in a dense, opaque corneal scar postoperatively.
  - The eye should *NOT* be covered by a tarsorrhaphy or membrana nictitans flap because these often develop complications, potentially increase intraocular pressure, which results in wound leakage, and preclude direct examination of the globe, which is important postoperatively.
- The anterior chamber should be reformed as soon as the wound is securely closed.
  - Balanced salt solution is preferred for reinflation, but sterile saline may be used instead.
  - Air may be injected into the chamber.
- Postoperative care
  - The eyes should be closely monitored for 7–10 days; usually they develop profound secondary uveitis and may become infected.
  - Treatment is facilitated by placement of a transpalpebral lavage apparatus while the patient is under general anesthesia.
- Medications
  - Topical 1% atropine solution, to effect, to maintain pupil dilation
  - Topical broad-spectrum antibiotic solutions q1–2h × 24h, then q2h × 3 days, then q4–6h depending on the condition of the eye
  - Systemic broad-spectrum antibiotics with a good gram-positive spectrum
  - Systemic nonsteroidal anti-inflammatory agents until the wound is healed and any associated uveitis controlled

Partial-Thickness Lacerations

- If the wound margins have separated more than 1 mm, repair by suturing under general anesthesia (as noted)
- Treat less severe lacerations like corneal ulcers, but carefully monitor every 1–2 days for secondary infection, particularly if the laceration is caused by plant matter.
- Medications:
  - ☐ Topical 1% atropine to effect to maintain pupil dilation
  - ☐ Topical broad-spectrum antibiotics q1–2h × 24h, then, q2–6h depending on the condition of the eye
  - ☐ Systemic nonsteroidal antibiotics until the wound is healed and any associated uveitis controlled

Partial-Thickness Flaps

- Repair flap wounds of varying thickness that are still attached to the cornea-like lacerations.
- Flaps that are very thin with minimal edema: Carefully replace over the wound bed, press firmly in place by rolling over the flap with a cotton swab and secure at the wound edges with points of tissue adhesive, or excise. Preserve corneal tissue whenever possible.
- Medications—as for uncomplicated ulcers

CORNEAL ABRASIONS AND ULCERS

- The cornea of the horse is approximately 0.8 mm thick, with the peripheral cornea approximately 1 mm thick. It fills the entire palpebral fissure, prominently protrudes from the side of the face, and is easily traumatized.
- Corneal ulcers are self-induced or from numerous external causes.
- **Any corneal lesion that breaches the corneal epithelium is an emergency** because:
  - ☐ The cornea is an avascular tissue, and the corneal defense mechanisms are reduced compared with other well-vascularized parts of the eye or body.
  - ☐ The cornea is continually exposed to environmental contaminants, bacteria, and fungi.
  - ☐ The maximum thickness of the cornea in the horse is approximately 1 mm, and therefore a superficial ulcer becomes a perforated one in a short period of time.

Clinical Signs

- The individual should be examined IMMEDIATELY if *any* of the following are observed:
  - ☐ Pain (squinting, tearing, reluctance to maintain the eye fully open, rubbing the affected eye). The severity of the problem and degree of pain are not directly proportional. An individual with a superficial corneal abrasion may exhibit more signs of pain than one with a perforated ulcer.

□ Swelling of one or both eyelids
□ Redness and swelling of the conjunctiva lining the eyelids and covering the sclera and third eyelid
□ Corneal clouding from edema or inflammatory cell infiltrate

Diagnostic Generalities

- The classic hallmark of corneal abrasions or ulcerations is the uptake of fluorescein stain by the cornea. The examiner should be careful, however, because dye uptake does not occur in all cases.
  □ Stromal ulcerative processes can occur with active infection, stromal dissolution, and necrosis in the presence of an intact, overlying epithelium (Fig. 31–3, see Color Plate 1). The cornea in these cases does not retain fluorescein dye. General guideline: If the eye looks like it has an ulcer, treat it as such even if it does not stain with fluorescein.
  □ Deep ulcers that extend to Descemet's membrane retain stain only in the circumferentially adjacent stroma, and perhaps not even in this region if the stroma is covered by healing epithelium.

Diagnostic Steps

- Before touching the patient, determine whether tear production is adequate and lid function appears normal.
  □ Dry eye is rare in the horse but is seen. If the eye is painful and an ulcer is suspected, then the patient should be reflexly tearing—if not, suspect decreased tear production as a cause of the ulcer.
  □ Abnormal lid function, due to facial nerve dysfunction or to a decrease in corneal sensation with resultant failure of reflex blinking, causes corneal disease. *Assess the palpebral response*—be *sure* to do this before the lids are blocked. *Assess the corneal sensation*—generally wait until the patient is sedated.
- The patient is tranquilized, restrained, and the eyelid paralyzed.
- Obtain a culture of the cornea using a premoistened Culturette.
  □ This is unnecessary for simple ulcers of known cause when wound contamination is not expected.
  □ However, obtain an initial culture at the start; it can always be discarded if not needed.
- Carefully examine the cornea, conjunctiva, sclera, nictitating membrane, and eyelids, using a bright, focal light.
  □ Make a thorough examination, particularly if the etiology is unknown.
  □ Examination of these tissues is performed with magnification, concentrating in the areas of conjunctiva, nictitans, and eyelid that correspond to the position of the ulcer. Evert the corresponding area of eyelid over your finger to examine carefully.
  □ Careful examination of these areas in ulcer cases with unknown etiologies frequently discloses a foreign body, plant awn or spicule, or aberrant hair (trichiasis) as the cause of the problem.
- Apply fluorescein stain to the eye, making sure that it covers the entire cornea; lavage excess fluorescein from the eye, if necessary, and look for dye retention in the cornea.

☐ If dye retention is not obvious, an ultraviolet light source or illumination through a cobalt blue filter (standard on many veterinary ophthalmoscopes) enhances the dye fluorescence.

☐ **Perform this examination meticulously because failure to detect even a focal erosion has serious consequences, particularly if corticosteroids are then administered to the eye.**

■ Record the size, position, and depth of the corneal wound and note the amount of corneal edema present (the amount helps the novice examiner assess the depth of a corneal lesion).

☐ *Corneal abrasions* (surface epithelium lost but underlying basement membrane intact):

Patient in great pain

Lesion is not usually visible to the naked eye

No change in contour of the cornea

Little to no corneal edema because the basement membrane serves as a barrier to fluid uptake by the corneal stroma

Fluorescein dye uptake patchy to strong depending on the amount and depth of epithelial loss

Corneal ulcers (extend through epithelium into the underlying stroma):

Affected individuals in great pain (but some patients with deep ulcers are less so as superficial nerve endings are lost to necrosis)

Lesion usually readily visible

Corneal edema obvious within and adjacent to the ulcer bed

Intense fluorescein dye uptake

■ Be sure to show the lesion to the owner and instruct the owner on signs indicating a worsening problem (Fig. 31–4, see Color Plate 1)

☐ *Any increase in edema*

☐ Change in contour

☐ Change in color

Originally clear cornea:

turning white (edema) or

turning yellow-white (inflammatory cell infiltrate)

Originally cloudy cornea:

turning whiter (increasing edema)

turning yellow-white (inflammatory cells increasing)

turning clear (may indicate that a descemetocele is developing)

developing a black spot (descemetocele or impending iris prolapse)

☐ Decrease in the size of the pupil

☐ Purulent ocular discharge

☐ Ulcer beginning to develop a mucoid appearance. This means that keratomalacia is occurring. Remember—this can occur under intact epithelium!

Pseudomonas is commonly blamed as a culprit in melting ulcers, but keratomalacia actually develops with a number of gram-positive or -negative bacteria, with fungal infections, or with corneal ulcers secondary to alkali injuries.

Any corneal disease resulting in a rapid influx of neutrophils or has rapid keratolysis occurring, develops keratomalacia

Other changes indicating complications but that the owner may not be able to see include *poor epithelial regrowth* and *corneal neovascularization*.

- Apply topical anesthetic to cases with ulcers and obtain a corneal sample via scraping for cytologic interpretation and culture.
  - □ 4–6 applications of topical anesthesia over a 5-minute period greatly enhances the depth of topical anesthesia.
  - □ The noncutting end of a sterile scalpel blade makes an excellent sampling instrument.
  - □ Remove surface debris before scraping.
  - □ Obtain 3–4 samples from stroma at the wound margins and smear them on 3–4 precleaned glass microscope slides.
  - □ Cover the slides to prevent environmental contamination.
  - □ Place a final scraping on a moistened Culturette for bacterial and fungal culture.
  - □ Cytologic samples are assessed rapidly for presence and Gram's classification of bacteria and for fungi. Any initial treatments are adjusted based on the cytologic interpretation.
- Microorganisms invading the corneal stroma are generally resident conjunctival flora, most of which are gram-positive bacteria (usually staphylococci and streptococci). Following treatment with antibiotics or corticosteroids, isolated flora are predominantly gram-negative.
- Simple, superficial ulcers may develop complication mandating *follow-up examination* by a clinician or ophthalmologist.

Simple Ulcers

Treatment

- Simple abrasions/erosions are treated simply with topical antibiotics, four to six times a day for 24–48 hours, then tapering if the lesion is resolving.
  - □ A broad-spectrum antibiotic ointment or solution is used. Solutions are preferred because they are easily applied by simple spray devices (discussed earlier), cleaner to use, and less likely to result in injury to the eye from a medication tip.
  - □ Triple antibiotic combinations (such as bacitracin-neomycin-polymyxin) are the drug of choice for uncomplicated abrasions or erosions.
  - □ Chloramphenicol is not recommended for routine use because it is bacteriostatic and less effective than other drugs against routine bacterial isolates.
  - □ If there is a suspicion that the wound is contaminated, use a topical aminoglycoside (topical tobramycin or 33 mg/ml fortified gentamicin).
- Mydriatics—cycloplegics
  - □ 1% atropine solution, once or twice to effect the first day for cycloplegia, is usually sufficient to relieve the pain caused by the ciliary body spasm and resultant pupil constriction.
  - □ If more frequent usage is needed, it may indicate that the ulcer is progressing.
- Systemic nonsteroidal anti-inflammatory drugs (NSAIDS): Usually only necessary for 1–2 days in uncomplicated abrasion cases

□ Phenylbutazone, 2.2–4.4 mg/kg IV q12h
□ Flunixin meglumine, 0.5–1.0 mg/kg IV, IM q12h

Complicated Ulcers

Treatment

- Require more aggressive treatment: Antibiotics q1–2h until there are no signs that the ulcer is progressing
  □ Recommended empirical regimen for suspected bacterial ulcers until the offending organism and sensitivities are identified: cefazolin, 133 mg/ml, hourly, in combination with tobramycin, 14 mg/ml, hourly. Gentamicin, 33 mg/ml, may be used instead of tobramycin. (93.4% of *Pseudomonas* isolates from deep corneal scrapings from horses are reported to be sensitive to amikacin, 85.1% to gentamicin, and 86.7% to tobramycin.)
  □ When culture results are obtained, alter treatment, if necessary, based on results. Recommended drugs for *gram-positive organisms*: Ticarcillin, erythromycin, cefazolin, ciprofloxacin; for *gram-negative isolates*: amikacin, tobramycin, gentamicin (only at >33 mg/ml concentrations), polymyxin B, neomycin
- Mydriatics—cycloplegics
  □ 1% atropine topical ophthalmic solution four to six times a day, occasionally more often if the pupil does not dilate. Instruct the owner to monitor GI motility based on bowel sounds and fecal output. If these diminish, discontinue atropine until motility is normal and monitor the individual carefully for signs of colic.
- Acetylcysteine and other anticollagenase and antiprotease drugs (EDTA, heparin) are reported to be beneficial in some cases of "melting" ulcers:
  □ Acetylcysteine (10%), 1–2 drops q1–2h in acute cases, tapering as the ulcer stabilizes
  □ Progressive keratomalacia is an indication that the ulcer needs to be re-evaluated.
- Systemic NSAIDs:
  □ These drugs are invaluable to control the severe secondary uveitis that often develops in complicated ulcers.
  □ Flunixin meglumine is subjectively more effective than phenylbutazone in these cases.
- Systemic antibiotics

Ulcer Debridement

- Very beneficial in cases of melting ulcers (Fig. 31–5, see Color Plate 1).
  □ Decreases necrotic material and therefore likely decreases numbers of bacteria and proteolytic enzymes
  □ May enhance drug penetration
  □ Helps maintain a more even corneal contour, which facilitates the spread of tear film
- Perform under tranquilization, lid block, and repeated administration of

topical anesthetic, using toothed forceps to pick up the malacic cornea and small corneal or eyelid scissors to excise it.

Surgical Intervention for Severe Cases

- Conjunctival flap placement:
  - □ A routine procedure that provides an immediate blood supply to the ulcer to aid healing, as well as a source of fibrovascular tissue to reinforce the wound.
  - □ Use judiciously and only when necessary for ulcers located in the central cornea, because the resulting scar is dense and permanent.
- Corneoscleral transposition, lamellar keratectomy, and penetrating keratoplasty are recommended as possible surgical aids to healing.
  - □ Useful in some severe cases.
  - □ May result in more severe scar.
  - □ May require referral to veterinary ophthalmologists trained in the procedure(s).
- Third eyelid (membrana nictitans) flaps or tarsorrhaphies are NEVER recommended. The resultant increase in heat and potential for increased rate of bacterial growth, the inability to constantly monitor the eye covered by a flap, as well as the possibility that the flap may cause additional problems completely preclude their use.

FUNGAL ULCERS

Only rarely present as emergency cases, occurring instead as secondary infections of primary ulcers, as chronic stromal abscesses, or as chronic primary ulcers. For complete discussion of fungal keratitis, please consult standard ophthalmology references.

Diagnosis

- Corneal scraping
- Culture

Treatment

- Cautery
- Itraconazole

EOSINOPHILIC KERATITIS

A frustrating type of corneal ulcerative disease, usually seen in the summer months, and can take 1 to many months to resolve.

Similar lesions previously have been attributed to ocular onchocerciasis, but this parasite is not found in these cases. May affect both eyes and recur in same individual.

Clinical Findings (Fig. 31–6, Color Plate 2)

- One or multiple, acute, *superficial* corneal ulcers
- Usually found in the *peripheral, perilimbal cornea*
- Usually covered partially to completely with a firmly *adherent, caseous white plaque* that may be thin and translucent or several millimeters thick and opaque
- The ulcers tend to *extend along the limbus* but may encroach upon the central cornea as they increase in size.
- The ulcer may or may not have associated neovascularization, depending on the duration of the disease.
- Minimal corneal edema around the ulcers—probably because they are located extremely superficial in the cornea.
- Pain, blepharospasm, epiphora, conjunctival hyperemia, and chemosis are also variably present.
- There may be a copious, caseous ocular discharge.

Diagnosis

- Fluorescein dye may be difficult to interpret because of the large amount of surface debris. Remove debris and restain.
- Exfoliative cytology—characteristically, large numbers of eosinophils with some mast cells and neutrophils, amorphous cellular debris, and degenerated epithelial cells are abundant. Bacteria and fungi are rarely seen but may be present as contaminants in the debris.
- Culture should be performed after all surface debris is removed, usually negative.
- Perform histology of excised lesion.

Treatment

- Prophylactic triple antibiotic q6–12h
- Topical corticosteroids (0.1% dexamethasone or 1% prednisolone q4–6h). These are the *only* times when topical steroids should be used in the presence of a corneal ulcer. Do not use corticosteroids unless
  □ The diagnosis is certain.
  □ Bacterial and fungal cultures are negative.
  □ Daily re-examinations are possible for the first 7–10 days of treatment to make certain that the ulcers do not worsen with steroid treatment.
- Refractory cases require lamellar superficial keratectomy.

Prognosis

- The ulcers may increase in size and number for several days following the onset of the disease.
- They rarely increase in depth. Depth may be subjectively monitored by noting the degree and extent of corneal edema adjacent to the ulcer.
- Neovascularization or the ulcers develop slowly or very rapidly and can be quite extensive in some cases (Fig. 31–7, see Color Plate 2).
- Some cases heal slowly in 4–6 weeks. Healing is usually accompanied

by intense corneal neovascularization and granuloma formation; other cases remain unchanged for 6 weeks or longer, in spite of rigorous therapy. Lamellar superficial keratectomy is recommended in chronic cases or in selected acute cases to speed disease resolution (the cornea usually heals 10–14 days postoperatively).

CORNEAL FOREIGN BODIES

Etiology

Plant materials are most common. Metal, glass, gunshot, and numerous other types have been reported. Occasionally, one of the patient's own eyelashes may become a foreign body after a traumatic injury.

Clinical Signs

- Similar to corneal ulcers
- Signs vary with the size, location, nature, and extent of the injury and the type of foreign body.

Diagnosis

- Sedation, eyelid block, and topical anesthesia are necessary for diagnosis since most cases are painful, with intense blepharospasm.
- Corneal foreign bodies can be readily apparent or small and difficult to see even with magnification.
- Examine the iris and anterior chamber carefully for evidence of penetration.
  - □ Flare, fibrin, hyphema, and so on are obvious or very subtle.
  - □ Foreign body penetration into the anterior chamber has a guarded prognosis.

> BE AWARE—small black bodies in the cornea that appear as foreign bodies may instead be a piece of iris or corpora nigra sealing a penetrating injury. Approach with caution because disturbing them may cause the aqueous humor to leak. Careful anterior chamber and iris examination is diagnostic.

Treatment

- Regardless of the treatment used, it is critical to make certain that all foreign material is removed. This requires a very bright focal light source and magnification.
- Cases with large or deep foreign bodies are referred to a specialist trained in microsurgical technique who is capable of managing a potential perforation.
- After removal, send foreign particles for bacterial and fungal cultures.
- Medical management is as for complicated ulcers.

SUPERFICIAL, NONPENETRATING FOREIGN BODIES

- Remove under topical anesthesia, sedation, and a lid block using a sharp stream of sterile saline directed tangentially at the particle.
- Removal is aided by a 25-gauge needle or small-toothed forceps.

DEEP, NONPENETRATING FOREIGN BODIES

- Frequently require general anesthesia and surgical removal
- Generally the safest approach in case the anterior chamber is entered during removal

PENETRATING FOREIGN BODIES

- Refer to a specialist.
- Prognosis is guarded, particularly if perforation by plant material or hair.

ACUTE CORNEAL EDEMA

- Poorly understood condition; etiology or etiologies generally unknown
- Any age individual may present with partial to complete corneal edema of mild to severe degree; one or both eyes may be affected.
- Affected cornea appears to bulge significantly because it is severely swollen from edema.
- Etiology often unknown, but blunt cornea trauma with disruption of endothelial cell function is a known cause, as is venous stasis due to jugular thrombosis
- Viral endotheliitis is suspected as a cause in group outbreaks in young individuals. Retinal detachments occur in some of these cases, either when the edema develops or during subsequent weeks; affected individuals require regular fundus examinations (Fig. 31–8, see Color Plate 2)
- Anterior uveitis

Diagnosis

Complete ocular and systemic examinations, ultrasonography if the cornea is opaque.

Treatment

- Unrewarding if the edema is extensive.
- Topical corticosteroids are useful if the corneal epithelium is intact and likely to remain so (affected cases frequently develop corneal bullae or blisters as the edema accumulates under the tight junctions of the epithelium—steroids should be used with extreme CAUTION in these cases because the bullae rupture and turn into ulcers).
- Topical hyperosmotic agents such as 5% NaCl 4–6 ×/day are useful in some cases.
- Use topical broad-spectrum antibiotics because of the likelihood of epithelial slough.

- Topical NSAIDS are beneficial:
  - Flurbiprofen
  - Suprofen
- Systemic NSAIDs are indicated for 7–10 days.
- Systemic antihistamines may be beneficial in rare cases.
- Tarsorrhaphy may be indicated if sizable bullae develop in the cornea.

Prognosis

Guarded. If fibrovascular ingrowth from the limbus develops, it serves to reinforce and reorganize the swollen cornea.

ACUTE HYPHEMA

Etiologies include trauma, penetrating injuries, uveitis, glaucoma, intraocular neoplasia, retinal detachments, blood dyscrasias, or congenital anomalies.

- Small amount of hemorrhage or the entire globe may be filled with blood.
- Clotted red blood is usually the result of recent trauma.

Treatment

Controversial, at best

- Repair the cause.
- Mydriatics—prevent synechiae but may occlude drainage angle
- Miotics—may facilitate synechiae formation but may increase drainage and expose a larger iris surface to enhance fibrinolysis
- Anti-inflammatory drugs
  - Topical corticosteroids
  - Systemic and topical NSAIDs
- Rest—include tranquilization if necessary.
- Restrict head movement.
- Monitor intraocular pressure frequently, watching for development of glaucoma.
- Surgical intervention is possible in severe cases:
  - Refer to a veterinary ophthalmologist.
  - Tissue plasminogen activase may be used as an aid to clot dissolution.

Nonclotted blood is resorbed in 5–10 days, clotted in 15–30 days.

Prognosis

- Varies, depending on the amount of blood and the etiology
- Hyphema occupying more than half the anterior chamber has a poor prognosis.
- Recurring hyphemas have poorer prognosis.
- Possible sequelae include synechiae, cataracts, blindness, glaucoma, phthisis bulbi.

LENS LUXATION

Rarely an emergency since the great majority of cases occur secondarily to anterior uveitis, but may be presented as such.

See following section on Anterior Uveitis.

UVEITIS

- Along with corneal ulcers, uveitis (usually nongranulomatous anterior uveitis with the inflammation confined to the anterior and posterior chambers) is the most common ocular complaint in the horse and is the leading cause of blindness.
- Unfortunately, many cases of equine uveitis do not present as emergencies when, in fact, they truly are. Rapid and prolonged treatment may prevent future recurrences and disastrous long-term sequelae.
- The horse's uveal tissue has a profound ability to become inflamed after seemingly mild ocular insults.
- The potential for loss of vision in uveitis cases is enormous. Not only is vision reduced in the acute case but the sight-threatening sequelae of inflammation are common:
  - □ Corneal decompensation and edema
  - □ Glaucoma
  - □ Cataracts
  - □ Vitreal opacities, hemorrhages, and liquefaction
- In many cases the eye being examined as an "emergency" has likely had subclinical disease for days to weeks, and therefore treatment results are less than expected.
- All cases require aggressive initial therapy (q1–2h topically); therefore, use a transpalpebral lavage system (see p. 83).
- Any case of acute uveitis may turn into recurring uveitis, an unsoundness. Obtain a thorough history and complete ocular examination, including fluorescein staining of the cornea, along with a general physical examination.

Etiologies

Infectious

- Any number of bacterial agents that cause septicemia can result in uveitis (*Rhodococcus equi, Leptospira, Salmonella),* as can endotoxemia.
- Most common in neonatal foals and usually bilateral

Noninfectious

- Traumatic—blunt or penetrating
- Idiopathic
- Immune-mediated
- Phacoanaphylaxis
- Neoplastic

Clinical Signs

- Examine BOTH eyes!
- Examination usually requires heavy sedation, eyelid akinesia, and topical anesthesia.

Acute

- Pain—lacrimation, blepharospasm, photophobia
- Hyperemia of the conjunctiva and scleral vessel engorgement
- Intraocular pressure is reduced.
- Corneal changes:
  - Edema—mild and focal to severe and diffuse
  - May have keratic precipitates on the endothelial surface (white dots coalescing to greasy yellow-white plaques)
  - May have early corneal vascular ingrowth from the limbus
- Anterior chamber findings:
  - *Aqueous flare is a hallmark of anterior uveitis.*
  - Flare results from the presence of protein and/or cells in the normal cell and protein-poor aqueous. Flare is usually subtle and is assessed in a totally dark room with a focal light directed into the eye at an angle from the examiner's line of view.
  - More severe cases have fibrin, hypopyon, or hyphema present in the anterior chamber.
- Pupil—*miotic*
- Iris changes:
  - May be none or swollen in appearance with loss of the fine surface architecture of the normal iris
  - The iris color may be dulled to profoundly abnormal in light-colored irises.
  - Corpora nigra are normal to swollen with rounded, rather than normal, spiculated, contours.
  - The iris is slow to respond to mydriatic agents.
- Fundus findings:
  - The fundus is poorly seen due to the anterior segment inflammation.
  - Examination is facilitated by the use of indirect ophthalmoscopy, which is much more effective in penetrating hazy media.
  - Vitreous liquefaction and "floaters"
  - Possible choroiditis, retinal edema, and focal to diffuse nonrhegmatogenous retinal detachment

Chronic

- Corneal changes:
  - Diffuse edema, ± fibrosis
  - Fibrovascular ingrowth from the limbus, focal or diffuse
  - Focal to multifocal superficial erosions
- Iris changes:
  - Posterior synechia formation with resultant dyscoria
  - Loss of corpora nigra
  - Hyperpigmented

- Lens changes:
  - Cataract
  - Lens luxation
- Other findings:
  - Secondary glaucoma
  - Retinal detachment with or without vitreous degeneration and traction bands
  - Retinal and optic nerve degeneration and atrophy
  - Blindness
  - Phthisis bulbi

Treatment

Aggressive, prolonged medical treatment reduces the incidence of secondary complications. Treatment should not be discontinued prematurely but should continue on a tapering schedule for 4–6 weeks beyond the time when there is no evidence of aqueous flare and the eye looks normal. Life long treatment may be necessary.

Medications

- Corticosteroids, topically, periocularly, and/or systemically, are the basis of therapy in most cases.
  - Topical 1% prednisolone acetate (NOT succinate) solution is the steroid of choice; 1.0% dexamethasone ointment is also very effective. Either medication is administered six to eight times/day.
  - Subconjunctival steroids administered under the bulbar conjunctiva may be used but ONLY when the cornea is healthy.
- Mydriatic agents:
  - Topical 1% atropine solution, 1–2 drops or a small spray two to three times/day to effect (every few hours in acute flare-ups to every few days as inflammation subsides)
- Topical NSAIDs:
  - Flurbiprofen, 0.03%, or suprofen, 1% q2–6h
  - May be indicated if the corneal integrity is in question, precluding the use of topical corticosteroids
  - May be used in combination with topical corticosteroids
- Cyclosporine may be useful because of its inhibition of T cell function. Obtain owner's consent.
- Systemic anti-inflammatory agents:
  - Phenylbutazone, 2.2–4.4 mg/kg, or flunixin meglumine, 0.5–1.0 mg/kg, not longer than 1–2 weeks
  - Systemic corticosteroids
  - Aspirin, 20–25 mg/kg PO

Continue medications 10–14 days beyond the time when clinical signs have resolved, and then taper slowly. Continue topical corticosteroids q12h for 4–6 weeks. Before discontinuing them, carefully examine the eye for signs of uveitis and then re-examine weekly for a month. Advise the owner to monitor the eye daily for signs of inflammation (redness, miosis) and request re-examination immediately if abnormalities develop.

GLAUCOMA

Etiology

- Acute glaucoma is rare.
- Most cases of glaucoma occur secondarily to
  - Chronic iridocyclitis (anterior uveitis) and angle closure due to fibrosis
  - Trauma
  - Acute anterior displacement of a luxated lens (the usual cause is trauma or chronic uveitis)

Clinical Signs

- Pain—absent to severe; lacrimation, photophobia, blepharospasm, small convulsive jerking movements of the head during rest
- Hyperemia of the conjunctiva and episcleral vein engorgement
- Corneal changes:
  - Edema—mild, focal to severe, diffuse
  - Linear white lines traversing the cornea in any direction. These are usually a chronic change associated with breaks in Descemet's membrane and disruption of adjacent endothelial cell function.
  - Focal to diffuse superficial ulcers if corneal edema is severe
- Pupil—midposition to dilated, and slowly to nonresponsive to bright light stimulus
- Iris:
  - Normal in an acute, primary case (rare)
  - Usually an abnormal dark chocolate brown color, or a darker color than normal for the eye
  - Corpora nigra absent or abnormally smooth in contour due to previous bouts of inflammation and fibrosis
- Vision likely impaired but not clinically evident in all cases
- If the glaucoma is secondary to an anterior lens luxation the (often cataractous) lens is readily seen in the anterior chamber. If corneal edema prevents examination of the anterior chamber, ultrasound examination is indicated.
- The eye may be slightly to grossly enlarged (buphthalmic)

Diagnosis

- If available, perform applanation tonometry.
  - The patient is tranquilized and topical anesthetic applied to both eyes.
  - The eyelids are held open with pressure on the bony rim, taking care that pressure is not transmitted to the globe.
  - Normal intraocular pressures for the horse are approximately 18–25 mm Hg
- If tonometry is not available, a gross assessment of intraocular pressure is made by gently pressing the index and middle fingers alternately back

and forth on the dorsal portion of the globe, through the closed eyelid. Use the patient's other eye or the examiner's own as a control. In these cases, referral to a specialist for confirmation is recommended ASAP.

Treatment

- Generally unrewarding, and the condition slowly progresses in spite of medical treatment.
- Acute and some chronic cases show improvement in the short term.
- Ophthalmic beta-blockers such as timolol maleate, 1–2 drops of 0.5% q8h, in combination with topical and systemic therapy, as for anterior uveitis, is recommended. Topical atropine is considered to enhance uveoscleral outflow of aqueous.
  □ The cornea is stained before therapy and topical corticosteroids are generally not used if there is evidence of corneal epithelial loss.
- Systemic control of intraocular pressure in the horse, other than that which is obtained by reducing intraocular inflammation via NSAID administration, is difficult and complicated. Systemic carbonic anhydrase inhibitors require large doses, become very expensive to use, and cause numerous side effects. Systemic hyperosmotic agents, such as mannitol or glycerine administered per os, may result in severe diarrhea with or without colic, and their use is not recommended.
- Surgical control of intraocular pressure requires referral to a highly equipped tertiary facility with veterinary ophthalmologists on staff.
  □ Argon laser for trabeculoplasty
  □ Filtration surgery
  □ Destruction of the ciliary body

SUGGESTED REFERENCES

Bony Trauma

Caron JP, Barber SM, Barley JV, et al. Periorbital skull fractures in 5 horses. J Am Vet Med Assoc 1986;188:280–284.

Corneal Abrasions

van der Woerdt A, Gilger BC, Wilkie DA, et al. Effect of auriculopalpebral nerve block and intravenous xylazine on intraocular pressure and corneal thickness in the horse. Am J Vet Res 1995;56(2):155–158.

Corneal Ulcers

McCarthy PH. The zygomatic branch of the auriculopalpebral nerve. Anat Histol Embryol 1996;25(1):7–10.

Moore CP, Collins BK, Fales WH. Antibacterial susceptibility patterns for microbial isolates associated with infectious keratitis in horses: 63 cases. J Am Vet Med Assoc 1995;7(207):928–933.

Sweeney CR, Irby NL. Topical medical therapy of *Pseudomonas* sp.-infected corneal ulcers in horses: 66 cases (1977–1994).

32 Reproductive System

Robert B. Hillman, James A. Orsini,
and Thomas J. Divers

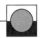

2

STALLION BREEDING INJURIES

Paraphimosis

The inability to retract the penis into the sheath is most frequently seen following trauma that occurs while the stallion is attempting to breed an uncooperative mare. Other factors that result in paraphimosis include:

- Large lesions of the glans penis
- Edema of the prepuce following castration
- Myelitis
- Spinal injuries
- Viral infections
- Physical exhaustion
- Inanition
- Paralysis of the retractor muscles following tranquilization

Physical examination includes evaluation of the sensation of the penis and prepuce as well as the stallion's ability to move the penis. Institute therapy as soon as possible to limit the formation of edema, cellulitis, hematoma, thrombosis, and gangrenous necrosis of dependent structures.

TREATMENT

- Treat the inciting cause when possible.
- Prevent further trauma to penis and prepuce.
  - Clean the penis and prepuce with mild cleansers, rinse, and dry thoroughly by blotting gently with nonirritating material.
  - Liberally apply a lanolin-based antibiotic cream to entire penis and prepuce. Petroleum jelly can also be used. Repeat cleaning and local treatment daily.
- Reduce swelling:
  - With acute trauma, use cooling techniques (cold water showers, applying a plastic sleeve filled with crushed ice or snow).
  - After acute phase, gently massage with alternating cold and hot showers and/or an air splint may be placed on the distal end of the penis and inflated for a maximum of 15–20 minutes.
  - Swelling can also be reduced by covering the penis with an elastic bandage beginning at the distal end of the penis and wrapping proximally. The bandage is left in place for 15–20 minutes.
- Nonsteroidal anti-inflammatory drugs (NSAIDs):
  - Flunixin meglumine, 1 mg/kg IV or IM q12–24h

☐ Phenylbutazone, 2.2 mg/kg PO q12–24h
- Prophylactic antibiotics to prevent infection and abscess formation. Use either:
  ☐ A combination of potassium penicillin, 22,000 U/kg IV q6h
  OR
  procaine penicillin, 22,000 U/kg IM q12h
  AND
  gentamicin, 6.6 mg/kg IV or IM q24h (use gentamicin only if creatinine is normal, stallion is urinating, and hydration is assured)
  ☐ Ceftiofur, 3.0 mg/kg IV/IM q12h
- Diuretics:
  ☐ Furosemide, 1 mg/kg IM
- Support:
  ☐ Support of the penis and prepuce is *very* important to avoid additional vascular impairment and increased edema. Place a support around the penis and prepuce to hold the penis in the sheath. Use nylon mesh attached by rubber tubing or gauze (Fig. 32–1). This material permits urination without retaining moisture and does not chafe the skin.
  ☐ Daily cleaning and treatment of the penis and sheath, combined with massage, are essential.
  ☐ Once the swelling is reduced sufficiently to return the penis within the prepuce, it can be retained by a pursestring suture at the preputial orifice, or a retention device can be fabricated from a 500-ml narrow-neck plastic bottle. Remove the bottom of the plastic bottle, pad the edges with tape, and place the bottle over the end of the penis with the urethral process at the neck of the bottle. The bottle is held in place by rubber tubing or gauze attached to the neck and tied in a pattern similar to that used for the nylon mesh.

Penile Hematomas

Most hematomas are from damage to the erect penis by direct kicks from unreceptive mares or trauma during collection. Superficial vessels of the penis/

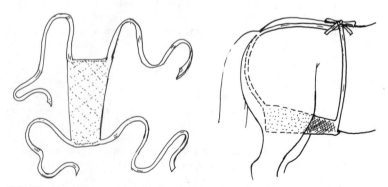

FIGURE 32–1. Support placed around the penis and prepuce to hold the penis in the sheath.

prepuce or, less commonly, small leaks in the corpus cavernosum penis are the source of the hematoma. Swelling may be rapidly progressive and can result in paraphimosis.

TREATMENT

Early treatment is important to prevent permanent dysfunction.

- Control swelling:
  □ Ice packs or cold hydrotherapy for at least 30 minutes a minimum of three times daily
- Antibiotics for 7–10 days. Use either:
  □ A combination of potassium penicillin, 22,000 U/kg IV q6h
    OR
    procaine penicillin, 22,000 U/kg IM q12h
    AND
    gentamicin, 6.6 mg/kg IV or IM q24h (use gentamicin only if creatinine is normal, stallion is urinating, and hydration is assured)
  □ Ceftiofur, 3.0 mg/kg IV/IM q12h
- NSAIDs
  □ Flunixin meglumine, 1 mg/kg IV or IM q12–24h
  □ Phenylbutazone, 2.2 mg/kg PO q12–24h
- Diuretics:
  □ Furosemide, 1 mg/kg IM PRN*
- Supportive care of the penis and prepuce:
  □ See earlier section on Paraphimosis.
  □ Check frequently
  □ Clean and lubricate often
- Management:
  □ Keep the stallion isolated from any exposure to mares in estrus.
- Surgery:
  □ If vessels need to be ligated or if the tunics of the penis are ruptured (recognized by continued enlargement of the hematoma), refer to a surgical facility for repair as soon as possible.
  □ In less complicated cases, delay surgery for 7–10 days to allow the hematoma to organize.

PROGNOSIS

Early and appropriate therapy is crucial to prevent secondary reproductive dysfunction, such as fibrosis that may cause deviation of the penis, thermal damage to the testes, nerve damage, or paraphimosis. The prognosis for return to function is better assessed after 3 weeks of rest by exposing the stallion to a mare and doing a complete reproductive examination.

Paralysis of the Retractor Muscle Following Tranquilization

TREATMENT

Administer 8 mg/450 kg benztropine mesylate (Cogentin) IV slowly as soon as possible after the inciting drug, along with immediate institution of conservative therapy as listed earlier.

---

*PRN = according to circumstances

Large Lesions of the Glans Penis

- Carcinoma of the penis usually requires referral for phallectomy.
- Cutaneous habronemiasis is seen primarily in warm months as granulo-matous growths on the urethral process but can involve the glans, pre-puce, and scrotum. Biopsies are required to confirm this diagnosis and to eliminate the possibility of a more serious primary lesion, such as squamous cell carcinoma. Oral administration of ivermectin, 0.2 mg/kg and corticosteroids, dexamethasone powder, 5 mg PO, often results in rapid reduction in the size of the lesion. Supportive therapy as described earlier is also indicated.

Paraphimosis Secondary to Inanition or Debility

- Requires dietary supplementation as well as a complete physical exami-nation to eliminate the other causes of hypoproteinemia (parasitism, bad teeth, chronic disease). Maintain supportive therapy, combined with mild exercise, for a long period until the edematous swelling of the penis and prepuce is resolved, allowing the penis to return to its normal position.
- Penile dysfunction is a common sequela. Treatment failure leaves the penis insensitive and cold to the touch. Thrombi form within the cavern-ous spaces, and the tissues fibrose. These tissues are very prone to continued trauma and excoriation if left untreated. If the paraphimosis is permanent, refer the individual for phallopexy after castration.
- NOTE: Continued service of some stallions has been accomplished through diligent supportive care and retraining the stallion to ejaculate with manual assistance and/or the modified use of an artificial vagina. This is not appropriate management for all affected stallions. To be successful, the stallion must possess appropriate breeding behavior and penile sensation, and all personnel must be dedicated to the care, han-dling, and retraining of the stallion.

PROGNOSIS

Varies with the inciting cause but is generally regarded as poor to fair.

OTHER REPRODUCTIVE INJURIES

Ruptured Corpus Spongiosum Penis

This structure is rarely damaged in the breeding stallion housed alone but can be injured by kicks sustained a few centimeters below the anus in stallions that are turned out with a band of mares or other horses. Hematoma formation in this area can have disastrous complications, including obstruction of the urethra, with consequent rupture of the urinary bladder and death.

Diagnosis

- Based on history of trauma to the region and identification of the hematoma—evident as a painful, fluctuant swelling below the anus.
- Investigate integrity of the bladder by a rectal examination if the patient tolerates it, but this is often quite painful. If not possible, use abdomi-

nocentesis to diagnose uroperitoneum following rupture of the urinary
bladder (see p. 55).
- Catheterization is often difficult because it is painful to pass the catheter
past the region of the hematoma.

Treatment

Immediate therapy for controlling inflammation and preventing potentially fatal
sequelae while stabilizing the individual for transport to a referral surgery center.
- Anti-inflammatory drugs:
  - □ Corticosteroids: dexamethasone, 0.05–2.0 mg/kg IV
  - □ Flunixin meglumine, 1 mg/kg IV q12–24h, provides analgesia as well.
- Hydrotherapy:
  - □ Ice packs or cold water hosing for a minimum of 30 minutes at a time

PROGNOSIS

Poor for return to service

Abrasions and Lacerations

Trauma to the skin of the penis and prepuce may result from mare tail hairs,
breeding stitches, stallion rings, artificial vaginas, kicks, whips or leadropes
striking the erect penis (as in disciplining of show and racing stallions to
discourage arousal at inappropriate times), or from breeding mares through a
wire fence.

Due to the vascularity of this region, open wounds in the penis and prepuce
bleed profusely.

**As with other traumatic injuries to the penis and prepuce, early treat-
ment is essential to prevent sequelae that may interfere with reproductive
performance.**

Diagnosis

- Careful physical examination; this entails thoroughly cleaning the wound
to identify involved structures.
- Subtle lesions that may interfere with breeding performance or precipitate
more serious problems must be identified (e.g., trauma involving the
urethra, inflammation near the scrotum).

Treatment

- Clean the wound gently to remove debris and blood, rinse, and dry
thoroughly.
- Apply a lanolin-based cream, with an antibiotic such as tetracycline, to
the entire penis to prevent dryness and infection.
- Reduce swelling:
  - □ Low-pressure cold hydrotherapy
  - □ Ice packs
- Support the penis and prepuce as soon as possible if paraphimosis
develops—see Paraphimosis section.

Testicular Trauma

- Thermal injury of spermatogenic cells within the testicles is an added complication in testicular trauma.
- Emergency care is to treat the primary injury and protect the testicular parenchyma from inflammatory hyperthermia and subsequent testicular degeneration and atrophy.
- As with trauma to other external genitalia, testicular trauma can result in paraphimosis.

Diagnosis

- Physical examination:
  - □ Unilateral or bilateral heat, pain, or swelling (swelling may be minimal due to the nonelastic tunica albugineae)
- Ultrasound:
  - □ May identify hematoma formation (anechoic or hypoechoic regions) or fibrosis (hyperechoic) that indicates prior injury

Treatment

- Reduce swelling:
  - □ Ice packs or cold hydrotherapy
- Anti-inflammatory drugs:
  - □ Flunixin meglumine, 1 mg/kg IV or IM q12–24h.
- Antibiotics; use either:
  - □ A combination of potassium penicillin, 22,000 U/kg IV q6h
    OR
    procaine penicillin, 22,000 U/kg IM q12h
    AND
    gentamicin, 6.6 mg/kg IV or IM q24h (use gentamicin only if creatinine is normal, stallion is urinating, and hydration is assured)
  - □ Ceftiofur, 3.0 mg/kg IV/IM q12h
- Prophylactic hemicastration to protect the unaffected testicle in unilateral injuries
- Sexual rest for a minimum of 3–6 weeks

POSTCASTRATION COMPLICATIONS

Immediate Complications

Hemorrhage

- Etiology:
  - □ Improperly applied emasculator
  - □ Reversing emasculator
  - □ Testicular vessels insufficiently crushed because scrotal skin included in emasculator
- Signs:
  - □ Blood dripping for several minutes after surgery is not unusual. **CAUTION:** Continuous bleeding for 15–30 minutes

□ Testicular artery usual source
- Treatment:
  □ Grasp *anesthetized* cord and reapply crushing forceps or emasculator.
  □ Reanesthetize patient, if needed, to crush end of cord safely.
  □ Sterile gauze tightly packed into the inguinal canal and scrotum closed with sutures or towel clamps.
  □ *Leave packing in place for a minimum of 24 hours.*
  □ Topical coagulants are of questionable value and are not recommended.

Evisceration

- UNCOMMON/POTENTIALLY FATAL
- Standardbreds and Tennessee Walking Horses are more commonly affected.
- Generally occurs within hours after castration but can occur days later
- IMMEDIATELY ANESTHETIZE—minimizes contamination and damage to prolapsed intestine (see p. 646)
- Administer IV fluids, hypertonic saline, 4 ml/kg IV, to minimize hypotension.
- Clean, irrigate, and replace prolapsed intestine.
- Ligate spermatic cord and vaginal tunic proximally.
- Superficial inguinal ring closed or packed with sterile gauze for 24–48 hours
- Start parenteral broad-spectrum antimicrobial agents and fluid therapy along with NSAIDs
- Refer to surgical facility if resection of devitalized intestine needed.
- Prolapse of the greater omentum through scrotal incision after castration generally is not an immediate emergency but signals potential evisceration.

Delayed Complications

- Edema is most common complication.
  □ Treatment: Open incision, hydrotherapy, antimicrobial(s)
- Funiculitis—inflammation of the spermatic cord
- Infection—*Clostridium* spp.
- Peritonitis
- Penile injury
- Hydrocele

MARE REPRODUCTIVE EMERGENCIES: DYSTOCIA

Due to the severe abdominal press (straining) and early detachment of the placenta, dystocia in the mare is life-threatening both for the mare and the fetus and requires immediate obstetric assistance. Before the arrival of the obstetrician, advise the owner to keep the mare walking to reduce straining. Placing a nasogastric tube in the trachea so the glottis cannot close also reduces the ability of the mare to generate an abdominal press.

Perform obstetric manipulations in an area large enough to allow a thorough examination and to administer corrective actions to a standing or recumbent mare. NOTE: Avoid stocks if possible. Restraint should be the minimum required to ensure the safety of the clinician while not alarming the mare. Frequently, a holder standing at the head on the same side as the obstetrician is all that is required. A nose twitch can be utilized if necessary. Rarely a rope side line may be indicated to control the mare's rear legs, but the danger of the mare becoming entangled must be remembered. Use drugs (tranquilizers or anesthetics) with *caution* if the fetus is alive, because they sedate the fetus and the mare.

Obtain a complete history while disinfecting the perineal region and performing a genital examination. *Remember:* BE CLEAN, BE GENTLE, AND USE LOTS OF LUBRICATION!

Treatment

Once a diagnosis is made and a plan of action formulated, it may be necessary to administer epidural anesthesia, 5–8 ml of 2% lidocaine (see p. 11). If the required manipulation is simple, do not perform epidural anesthesia because the mare can assist the delivery once the corrective action is performed. Nearly all manipulations to correct the abnormalities in presentation, posture, or position require some repulsion of the fetus in order to gain working room. Standing the mare with her hindquarters elevated assists corrections.

Straining can be reduced by:

- Keeping the mare walking (but this complicates manipulations)
- Placing a nasogastric tube in the trachea
- Pulling out the tongue to prevent closing the glottis, or
- Administering epidural anesthesia.

If initial manipulations are unsuccessful, general anesthesia can be induced (xylazine, 0.5–1.0 mg/kg, and ketamine, 2.2 mg/kg) to stop the straining and allow elevation of the rear quarters to provide more room for repositioning of the fetus.

While the mare is anesthetized, a hoist may be used to elevate the rear quarters. If this is to occur, the mare should have an IV catheter placed and receive guaifenesin (formerly called glyceryl guaiacolate), 100 mg/kg IV total, as a 5% solution, 50 gm/L, to prevent struggling.

After the guaifenesin, monitor respiratory and cardiac effects closely because of the weight of the pregnant mare's organs on her diaphragm.

If practical, administer oxygen intranasally to the mare at 15 L/min (see p. 40). If the foal's head is in the pelvis, oxygen can also be administered to the foal as long as it does not impede manipulations to deliver.

Common Causes of Dystocia and Their Corrective Measures

Fetotomy equipment:

- Thygensen fetotome
- Wire saw
- Wire saw sounding wire

- Wire saw leader
- Handgrips for the wire saw
- Double-jointed hook of Krey-Shottler
- Obstetric snare
- Eye hooks
- 3 Obstetrical chains (60 inches)
- Obstetrical chain handles
- Lubricant (J-lube), stomach pump and nasogastric tube

All equipment should be up-to-date and in good repair.

RETENTION OF HEAD AND NECK

- Secure the head with eye hooks or a head snare before repelling the body to allow for more room to extend the head and neck.
- If repositioning is unsuccessful and a living fetus is present, cesarean section is indicated.
- If the fetus is dead, a partial fetotomy (transection of the neck) saves time and reduces trauma resulting from extensive manipulations.

CARPAL FLEXION

- Repel the fetus and extend the leg while pushing the carpus in a dorsolateral direction and bringing the flexed fetlock in a ventral and medial direction, guarding the hoof to prevent uterine trauma.
- If the fetus is dead, it may be less traumatic and time-saving to do a partial fetotomy (transect the leg through the carpus, leaving part of the carpus on the forearm to allow application of chains for traction).

SHOULDER FLEXION

- Elevate the shoulder to produce carpal flexion and proceed as above. This is difficult to achieve, so if both legs are involved and the fetus is alive, cesarean section is indicated if the correction cannot be accomplished after anesthetizing the mare and lifting the hindquarters.

FOOT-NAPE POSTURE

- Can result in third-degree perineal laceration if not corrected as the leg extends dorsally when elbow contacts the pelvic brim as the mare strains.
- Repel the fetus, shift the legs to a position under the head, and apply traction.

FLEXED HOCK POSITION

- Repel fetus, push hock in dorsolateral direction while bringing flexed fetlock in a medioventral direction, guarding the hoof and extend the leg. Repeat on second leg and apply traction.
- If the fetus is dead, a partial fetotomy (cutting through the hock just below the point of the hock) usually saves time and trauma to the reproductive tract.

BREECH POSITION (BILATERAL HIP FLEXION)

- Repel fetus and position legs in a bilateral flexed hock position and proceed as above. Completely extending one leg before flexing both hocks allows the fetus to enter the mare's pelvic area, making it very difficult to flex the second hock.

TRANSVERSE PRESENTATION

- When the fetus is alive, a cesarean section is advised.
- With a small fetus in a dorsotransverse position (back of fetus presented to the cervix), it may be possible to repel the anterior portion of the fetus and grasp the base of the tail to produce a bilateral flexed hip position and proceed as above.
- A transverse ventral presentation is best resolved by cesarean section. Must be differentiated from twins

TWINS

- This must be distinguished from transverse ventral presentation, which can be difficult, because the clinician may not be able to reach far enough to touch the abdomen.
- Repel one foal while extracting the other one. If both keep pulling into the pelvis, suspect a transverse presentation. Check orientation of feet.

Notes on Fetotomy

- Fetotomy is indicated if the fetus is dead and the procedure results in reduction of time, effort, and trauma during delivery. Fetotomy in the horse is complicated by the mare's strong tenesmus and the delicate nature of the equine reproductive tract. The procedure is best accomplished by experienced clinicians using specialized equipment because extensive or prolonged fetotomies frequently cause trauma to the cervix and/or uterus that results in subfertility or infertility.
- The mare should be well restrained with the hind quarters elevated. Epidural anesthesia should be administered to diminish abdominal straining (see p. 11). Tranquilizing the mare with a combination of xylazine (0.15 mg/kg) and acepromazine (0.04 mg/kg) administered intravenously reduces contractions.
- Transverse and oblique cuts are made by introducing the head of the fully threaded fetotome to its desired position in the dorsum of the genital tract and then advancing the wire around the part to be removed. Cuts are made keeping the head of the fetotome in the hollow of the hand and maintaining finger contact with the fetus at all times.
- The number of incisions should be kept to the minimum needed to deliver the fetus without extensive trauma to the mare's reproductive tract.
- Flexed extremities are transected through the joints (avoiding cutting long bones) by advancing the wire from a partially threaded fetotome with a wire saw leader around the limb or neck. The wire saw is then slid through the second tube of the fetotome and the fetotome is adapted to the fetal part to be sectioned. Solid fixation is also important. It is necessary to cut through the flexed joint, leaving part of the carpus or tarsus on the fetus so that traction can be applied without the chains slipping off. Check the wire after each cut to make sure none of the strands are broken, because broken strands can traumatize the endometrium and/or cause the wire saw to break during subsequent cuts. Keep

entrance to and maneuvering in the genital tract to the minimum needed to perform the fetotomy to prevent trauma and contamination. *Remember,* BE CLEAN, BE GENTLE, AND USE LOTS OF LUBRICATION.

Postdystocia/Fetotomy Treatment

- Involution of the uterus is often delayed postfetotomy. Use oxytocin to aid in involution, 20 IU/450-kg mare IV, IM, or SQ every 2 hours.
- Use systemic antibiotics because of the increased incidence of retained placentas and endometritis following fetotomies, particularly if the uterus is atonic. Use either:
  □ Potassium penicillin, 22,000 U/kg IV q6h, or procaine penicillin, 22,000 U/kg IM q12h, and gentamicin, 6.6 mg/kg q24h (use gentamicin only if creatinine is normal, mare is urinating, and hydration is normal)
  OR
  □ Ceftiofur, 3.0 mg/kg IV or IM q12h and metronidazole 15 mg/kg PO q8h
- Flushing the uterus with 2–4 liters of physiologic saline, followed by infusion of the uterus with chemotherapeutic agents (e.g., 2.0 gm oxytetracycline in 100–200 ml saline), is recommended if it is unresponsive to oxytocin.

Postfoaling Colic

Mares frequently exhibit mild colic following delivery of their foal as the uterus contracts to expel the placenta. Walking the mare for 10 minutes or so frequently resolves the problem. If colic persists or becomes acute, check the mare for a ruptured uterine artery or a gastrointestinal problem, e.g., ruptured cecum and/or rupture of another organ.

UTERINE TORSION

- Usually occurs in mares from 8.5 months of gestation to term
- No known predilections, and often no known cause can be ascertained
- Less than 50% of torsions occur at parturition.

Diagnosis

CLINICAL SIGNS

- Colic in the third trimester
  □ Discomfort is mild in most cases and usually is temporarily responsive to analgesics.
  □ Depression, pawing, flank watching, kicking, rolling

> Pain is proportional to the degree of torsion and the involvement of the GI tract.

PHYSICAL EXAMINATION

- Normal to slightly increased temperature, pulse, respirations (TPR)
- Normal or decreased gastrointestinal sounds

RECTAL EXAMINATION

- Carefully palpate the uterine wall to identify uterine tears or ruptures.
- Carefully palpate other abdominal structures to identify any concurrent or associated GI involvement.
- Broad ligaments are pulled tightly downward.
- Asymmetry of the broad ligaments indicates direction of the torsion (this often is not easy to determine).
  - □ Clockwise (from rear): right tighter than left, left crosses over top of uterus
  - □ Counterclockwise (from rear): left tighter than right, right crosses over top of uterus.

Treatment

NONSURGICAL

Manipulation per Vagina at Term

> **CAUTION:** In late gestation with partial torsions, traction applied to the foal can cause a uterine rupture that can result in fatal hemorrhage in the mare or peritonitis. CORRECT THE TORSION FIRST!

When diagnosed at term, 80% of uterine torsions at term can be corrected this way:

- Keep the mare standing! (No SEDATIVES—use an epidural (see p. 11) to minimize straining.)
- Elevate the mare's hindquarters (stand her on a ramp or hill).
- Try to get through the cervix (if torsion is <270°).
- Manually correct the torsion:
  - □ Grasp the fetus as far in as possible (upper forearm or body)
  - □ Rock back and forth and use momentum to attempt derotation (may have to repeat to complete derotation).
- When derotated, mare should spontaneously begin second-stage labor.
  - □ May be delayed because of decreased uterine contractility, secondary to edema or vascular congestion
  - □ Induce if necessary with 20–40 IU oxytocin.

Rolling with Plank in the Flank (Fig. 32–2)

- Anesthetize the mare (see p. 646).
  - □ Drop the mare in lateral recumbency on the side to which the torsion is directed.
- Place a board (3–4 m long × 20–30 cm wide) across the recumbent mare's upper paralumbar fossa (see Fig. 32–2).

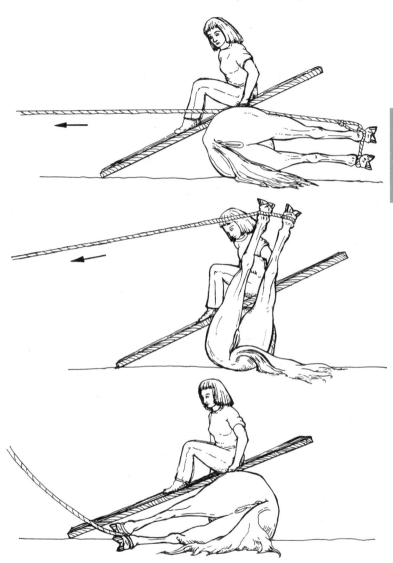

FIGURE 32–2. Rolling with plank in the flank.

- Have an assistant kneel on the board.
- Roll the mare SLOWLY to decrease the risk of rupture, e.g.:
  - □ Dx: Clockwise torsion (torsion is to the right). Counterclockwise torsion (torsion is to the left)
  - □ Tx: Lay the mare down in right lateral recumbency and rotate her clockwise. Lay the mare down in left lateral recumbency and rotate her counterclockwise

- Assess the progress by rectal examinations.
- Repeat if necessary.

SURGICAL

- Refer to a surgical facility as soon as possible (see p. 211).
- Intubate the mare with a nasotracheal tube to prevent glottis closure required for abdominal press.
- Surgery is performed standing through a flank incision.
- Incision is made on the side toward which the torsion has occurred, and the gravid uterus is gently lifted back into normal position.

Prognosis

FOR CURRENT PREGNANCY

- Nonsurgical correction—85% success rate
- Surgical correction—73% success rate

Complications
- Premature placental separation, resulting in death or abortion
- Uterine wall necrosis and rupture
- Peritonitis
- Endotoxic shock
- Recurrence of the torsion within the same pregnancy

FOR FUTURE PREGNANCIES

- Good for the mare to conceive and carry another pregnancy. Worsens with:
  □ Cesarean section
  □ Uterine rupture
  □ Torsions in late gestation
  □ Extensive torsion
  □ Delay in diagnosis and treatment

Uterine Rupture

- In the peripartum period, most often result from mutation and/or fetotomy.
- Earlier in gestation, can be due to violent intrapartum movement or occur as sequela to hydrops or uterine torsion.

Diagnosis

HISTORY

- Moderate to severe abdominal pain during the third trimester or within hours to 3 days after foaling

CLINICAL SIGNS

- May show no pain after rupture until signs of peritonitis develop
- Exsanguination may occur, but external hemorrhage is rare.

PREPARTUM RECTAL EXAMINATION

- Try to identify the uterus and the fetus.
  - □ The fetus may not be palpable if it has slipped down into the abdomen.
  - □ The uterus may still be twisted or feel corrugated and thick as involution begins immediately.
  - □ If tear is small and dorsal, a rectal examination may identify a localized peritonitis by the presence of fibrin on the uterine surface and in the peritoneal aspirate.

ABDOMINOCENTESIS

- Large volumes of clear to blood-tinged fluid are obtained at multiple sites. If peritonitis is present, white blood cells (WBC) and debris are abundant.

ULTRASOUND

- Transabdominal is performed to identify the fetus in the abdomen.
- Transrectal is usually unrewarding.

LAPAROTOMY

- Laparotomy is the only means by which a definitive diagnosis can be made if the lesion cannot be reached by a careful endometrial digital examination.

Treatment

POSTPARTUM

- Refer to surgical hospital for a ventral midline laparotomy (see p. 211).
- Administer fluids and antibiotics

PREPARTUM

- Refer to a surgical hospital for a ventral midline laparotomy.
- Per vagina. If the fetus can be extracted per vagina and the tear is small, dorsal, and close to the cervix, the uterus can sometimes be repaired by placing sutures reaching through the vagina and cervix.

HYDROPS OF FETAL MEMBRANES

DEFINITION

Hydramnion: Hydramnios or hydrops of the amnion
Hydrallantois: Hydrops allantois

Excess fluid accumulation (hydrops) in either the allantoic or amniotic cavity is not a common occurrence in the mare but can lead to the mare's demise if not diagnosed and treated rapidly. Hydramnion is most often seen in pregnancies with congenitally abnormal foals and hydrallantois is due to abnormal chorioallantoises. The location of the fluid can be distinguished clinically but does not alter the therapeutic regimen.

Diagnosis

HISTORY

- Normal pregnancy until 7.5–11 months of gestation

CLINICAL SIGNS

- Increased uterine fluid over 10–14 days
  - □ Hydrallantois accumulates fluid more rapidly.
  - □ Abdominal discomfort
  - □ Difficulty in walking
  - □ Difficulty in breathing
  - □ Recumbency if condition is severe enough

PHYSICAL EXAMINATION

- Distention of the uterus
- Inability to palpate the fetus
- Complications:
  - □ Severe ventral edema
  - □ Abdominal pain
  - □ Rupture of the abdominal muscles
  - □ Rupture of the prepubic tendon
  - □ Inguinal herniation
  - □ Uterine rupture

Treatment

INDUCE ABORTION

Fluid Therapy
- Very important to provide IV fluids as the uterine fluid is removed in order to prevent cardiovascular collapse. The hydrops often contains 30–50 gallons of fluid. Hypertonic saline (5%–7%) with or without hetastarch is a good choice.
- Induce abortion by gradual dilation of the cervix over 15–20 minutes.
- Drain fetal fluids slowly.
- Forced extraction of the fetus is often necessary because uterine inertia is usually present.

INDUCE PARTURITION

- Induction of parturition with oxytocin, 20–40 IU is effective in some but not all cases. Oxytocin may be useful if the fetus is near term.
- Treatment with corticosteroids, 20 mg dexamethasone, 24 hours before induction helps mature the fetal lungs in a fetus close to term.
- Administer fluid therapy as discussed above.

FOLLOW-UP CARE

- Uterine involution usually occurs normally.
- Follow-up with ultrasound examination and repeated drainage if necessary

Prognosis

Prognosis for further reproductive performance varies depending on uterine involution. Because most cases of hydramnion are due to congenitally abnormal foals, it is recommended that the mare be rebred to a different stallion.

Induction of Parturition

This is being successfully utilized in many practices, but it is not without risk.

Before induction, each mare must be carefully evaluated to ensure fetal maturity in order to avoid delivery of a premature foal that mandates prolonged neonatal intensive care with its required extensive commitment of time and expense. When the proper preinduction criteria are strictly adhered to, an essentially normal birth occurs and a healthy foal is delivered.

If it becomes necessary to induce a mare before full term, neonatal intensive care facilities, equipment, and personnel must be available if the foal is to survive. Induction of parturition requires professional assistance at the time of delivery.

INDICATIONS FOR INDUCTION AT FULL-TERM

- History of premature placental separation
- Previous delayed parturition due to uterine atony
- Mares that have suffered injuries or tears at previous foalings
- Mares that have produced icteric foals (neonatal isoerythrolysis), in order to prevent ingestion of colostrum until it can be checked for compatibility with newborn foal's blood
- Teaching and research investigations
- Placentitis or placental thickening, nonresponsive to medical treatment, resulting in abnormal heart rate and movement.

INDICATIONS FOR INDUCTION BEFORE TERM
(REQUIRES NEONATAL INTENSIVE CARE!)

- Preparturient colic
- Excessive ventral edema with impending rupture of the prepubic tendon
- Hydrops of the amnion
- Severe injury to mare (e.g., fracture)
- Imminent death of mare
- Severe placental dysfunction nonresponsive to treatment and resulting in deterioration of the foal.

INDUCTION CRITERIA

- Length of gestation—minimum of 330 days
- Enlarged udder with teats distended with colostrum
- Relaxation of sacrosciatic ligaments
- Electrolyte changes in colostrum as indicated by test strips for increased calcium content
  - □ Predict-a-Foal test (Animal Health Care Products, Chino, CA)
  - □ Sofchek teat strips (Environmental Test Systems, Elkhart, IN)
  - □ Titrets calcium hardness test kit (CHEMetrics, Inc., Calverton, VA)

Induction Protocol

- Oxytocin, 20–40 IU IM, 2.5–10 IU IV, repeated every 15–20 minutes until delivery completed, or 40–100 IU IV in a liter of saline over 30–60 minutes for approximately 450-kg mare. Foaling is usually complete by 60 minutes using any of these methods.
- Once induction is started, monitor delivery until complete.

Complications

- *Premature placental separation.* Occasionally the red, velvet-like allanto-chorion with its cervical star appears at the vulvar lips. **Open the membrane immediately to allow passage of the amnion containing the fetus.** If the allantochorion is not ruptured, the membrane separates from the endometrium, resulting in the birth of a severely hypoxic or potentially dead foal.
- *Malpresentation of the fetus.* Rarely the foal presents with a malalign-ment. If delivery does not appear to be progressing normally (no sign of the amnion with the feet present) by 20–30 minutes after administration of oxytocin, a clean exploration of the reproductive tract reveals a malalignment, and correction is usually easily accomplished before the beginning of strong abdominal contractions forcing the fetus into the pelvic canal.
- *Delivery of a premature foal.* If induction criteria are strictly adhered to, this rarely occurs. If the mare must be induced before term, this must be anticipated.
- *Neonatal maladjustment syndrome* (see p. 491).

VAGINAL/VESTIBULAR HEMORRHAGE

Postpartum Hemorrhage

Hemorrhage due to trauma from foaling is seldom life threatening, even with third-degree perineal lacerations.

Treatment

- Tetanus toxoid
- Medical neglect: Most vaginal/vestibular bleeding requires no treatment.
- Profuse hemorrhage:
  - □ If possible, ligate the affected vessel.
  - □ Pack vagina/vestibule with a large tampon and/or ice packs (tampons can be made of rolled cotton secured using umbilical tape).
  - □ Cover tampon with petroleum jelly or an oil-based antibiotic prepara-tion (mastitis preparations work well).
- Hematomas: **Do not drain.**
  - □ May be drained at a later date, after the vessel has clotted and the hematoma organized.
  - □ May cause difficulty in defecating. Continue laxative diets (bran and/or mineral oil) until the hematoma resolves or is drained.
  - □ Antibiotics for large hematomas

Hemorrhage During Late Pregnancy

Hemorrhage occurring late in pregnancy of older mares is often due to the presence of varicose veins at the vulvovaginal junction.

- In most cases, hemorrhage is minimal and is best treated by benign neglect.
- If hemorrhage is persistent and copious, ligating the affected vessel(s) may be required.
- Hemorrhage from varicose veins must be differentiated from hemorrhage from the cervix, which may signal an impending abortion.

Vaginal Hemorrhage Following Natural Service

- Minimal hemorrhage in maiden mares may result from perforating a persistent hymen and does not require treatment and must be differentiated from vaginal rupture.
- Vaginal rupture may occur when a small mare is bred to a large stallion.
- *Clinical signs* include mild to moderate bleeding, on rare occasions tenesmus, and/or protrusion of the small intestines from the vulvar lips.

Diagnosis

- Perform careful speculum examination of the vagina. A tube speculum may provide an adequate view of the injury, but a Caslick speculum is preferred for a more complete evaluation of the injury.
- A careful, clean (sterile gloves and lubrication) digital examination can determine whether the peritoneal cavity is penetrated.
- A peritoneal aspirate may reveal the presence of peritonitis and/or spermatozoa.

Treatment

WOUND NOT ENTERING THE PERITONEAL CAVITY

- Gentle lavage with sterile saline
- Infusion of a local antibiotic (e.g., nitrofuranzone [Furacin])
- A tetanus booster
- If tenesmus is present:
  - □ Flunixin meglumine, 1.0 mg/kg q12–24h IV or IM
  - □ Epidural anesthesia—5–8 ml 2% lidocaine (see p. 11)
- Systemic antibiotics for at least 1 week. Use either:
  - □ A combination of potassium penicillin, 22,000 U/kg IV q6h
    OR
    procaine penicillin, 22,000 U/kg IM q12h
    AND
    gentamicin, 6.6 mg/kg q24h (use gentamicin only if creatinine is normal, mare is urinating, and hydration is assured)
    OR
  - □ Ceftiofur, 3.0 mg/kg IV or IM q12h
    AND
    metronidazole for vaginal anaerobes, 15 mg/kg PO q8h

WOUND ENTERING THE PERITONEAL CAVITY

- Tetanus booster
- Local and systemic antibiotics (as described)
- Peritoneal lavage with large volume of sterile physiologic saline solution (PSS)
- Wash herniated intestines with sterile saline and replace through the laceration.

NOTE: If extensive trauma to herniated small intestines or gross contamination of the peritoneal cavity, refer the mare for surgery. In this case, treatment consists of cleaning and replacing the herniated intestine and suturing the vulvar lips closed for transport to the referral center. If the mare is showing signs of shock (depression, cold extremities, elevated heart rate, pale mucous membranes) administer IV fluids (see p. 539) before shipment.

Following surgery or whenever there has been a perforation of the abdominal cavity through the vagina, it is recommended that the mare be cross-tied for at least 5 days to prevent lying down.

ARTERIAL RUPTURES (UTERINE ARTERY, EXTERNAL ILIAC ARTERY)

- More common in older mares and/or multiparous mares
- Usually occurs after parturition and leads to sudden death
- Once a mare has a history of periparturient hemorrhage, the mare is more likely to bleed in future pregnancies.
- Hemorrhage may occur into the abdomen or into the broad ligament.

Diagnosis

CLINICAL SIGNS

- Colic; sweating; increased heart rate; anemia; death
- Can occur anytime from 30 minutes to several weeks postpartum
- NOTE: Clinical signs may be masked early after parturition by normal postpartum colic.

RECTAL EXAMINATION

- Hematomas in the broad ligament or uterine wall may be palpable per rectum and are usually painful.

Treatment

NONSURGICAL

- Keep the mare quiet.
  □ Administer a small dose of acepromazine, 0.01–0.02 mk/kg, only if the patient is anxious.
  □ Keep foal from under mare so she does not injure it.
  □ Blood transfusion or plasma therapy (see p. 294). An autotransfusion is possible (see p. 295).

□ Oxytocin, 20 IU IM every 30 minutes
□ Oxytocin decreases bleeding from the myometrium and/or intraluminal bleeding only. **Does not affect hemorrhage from the external iliac or uterine arteries; do not administer if there is a hematoma in the broad ligament.**
- Analgesics:
  □ Flunixin meglumine, 1 mg/kg IV or IM q12–24h

SURGICAL

- Surgical correction is unlikely to be successful due to the acute and rapidly progressive bleed.

ANTIBIOTICS

- Administer ceftiofur or penicillin/gentamicin, and metronidazole for large vaginal/broad ligament hematomas.

INTRAVENOUS FLUIDS

- Administer if the mare is hypotensive (based on increased heart rate, poor pulse quality, and cold extremities or by measuring blood pressure using a Doppler tail cuff with systolic pressure <80 mm Hg). Do not use hypertonic saline unless the mare is rapidly deteriorating!
- Aminocaproic acid (Amicar), 10–20 mg/kg, is administered slowly IV in the fluids or by slow infusion if fluids are not being administered.
- NOTE: Iliac artery rupture is also a common sequela to displaced pelvic fracture. A progressive swelling in a rear limb is generally noted.

Prognosis

Poor with any treatment option if there is uncontrolled bleeding into the abdominal cavity

Retained Placenta

- Placenta normally expelled within an hour and a half of foaling; retention beyond 3 hours is considered abnormal.
- Institute treatment immediately to prevent serious complications, which include metritis, septicemia, laminitis, and/or death.

Signs

Protrusion of the fetal membranes from the vulva is the most obvious indication of a retained placenta and alerts the clinician to the possibility of the complications described. However, the same complications can result from the undetected retention of a small piece (i.e., tip of the horn) of placenta tissue, which emphasizes the need for careful examination of all fetal membranes after foaling so that appropriate therapy can be instituted immediately if a portion of the placenta is retained.

Treatment

- If the membranes protruding from the vulva extend below the hocks, it may stimulate kicking and endanger the foal. Therefore, tie the membranes in a knot above the hocks. Do not cut the protruding placenta because the weight assists in the cleaning process.
- Administer oxytocin using one of the following protocols:
  - 20–40 units as a bolus IM.
  - It is generally recommended to administer 20 units IM at 3 hours postpartum and repeat the dose with another 20 units every 1–1.5 hours for three additional injections if necessary.
  - 10–100 units of oxytocin in a liter of saline administered slowly IV over 30–60 minutes
- If the retained membranes are not expelled by 12 hours after foaling, expand treatment to include:
  - Systemic antibiotics (ceftiofur, 3.0 mg/kg IM or IV q12h, or penicillin, 22,000 U/kg IV q6h, or procaine penicillin, 22,000 U/kg IM q12h, and gentamicin, 6.6 mg/kg q24h) (only if hydration normal and mare is urinating).
  - NSAIDs (flunixin meglumine, 0.3 mg/kg q8h)
  - Infusion of the allantochorionic space with 10–12 liters of 1%–2% povidone-iodine solution by stomach tube and then tying the opening of the fetal membranes closed. The distention of the uterus, cervix, and vagina stimulates release of endogenous oxytocin, which in turn stimulates uterine contractions. Distention of the uterine wall also allows the uterine crypts to release the fetal villi. Using this technique the membranes are usually passed within 30 minutes.
- If fetal membranes are still present after this, maintain the mare on systemic antibiotics and NSAIDs until they are passed. Gentle manual removal can be attempted but should never exceed 10 minutes. Successful techniques include:
  - Gentle tension on the protruding membranes.
  - Carefully sliding the hand between the chorion and the endometrium massaging to free the membrane.
  - Twisting the exposed fetal membranes to form a tight cord. This technique is sometimes combined successfully with the slow IV administration of oxytocin described previously.
- Tetanus toxoid
- NOTE: Monitor for signs of laminitis (see p. 323).

Acute Septic Metritis

- In most cases, occurs when there is extensive trauma and resulting contamination of the reproductive tract during difficult dystocias.
- Incidence is increased when corrective manipulations take an extended period of time, excessive force is employed for extraction, or prolonged fetotomies are required.
- Retention of the fetal membrane, if untreated, can also result in septic metritis.

Signs

- Septicemic signs include increased TPR, anorexia, injected mucous membranes, dehydration, and perhaps beginning signs of shock (cold extremities, and so on).
- Vaginal discharge is usually not copious in the mare, but a thin, watery discharge with a variable smell (sweet to putrid depending on the organisms involved) may be seen. The vaginal walls are inflamed.
- Rectal examination reveals an enlarged, usually thin-walled uterus distended with fluid.

Treatment

- Systemic antibiotics as dictated by culture and sensitivity. Penicillin, gentamicin, and metronidazole can be used until laboratory results are reported.
- Flunixin meglumine, 0.3 mg/kg IV or IM q8h
- IV fluids to combat dehydration and shock
- Uterine lavage with large volumes of warm saline

One lavage technique employs a "Bovine Uterine Drain catheter."* This 5.5-foot-long catheter is made of soft tygon and has six side openings at one end. The soft consistency of the tube allows it to bend easily, so it is unlikely to traumatize the compromised uterine wall.

One or two liters of warm (45–47° C) saline is placed in a plastic sleeve knotted just above the hand to prevent the fluid from running down into the fingers. The tail is wrapped and the perineal region disinfected before the fenestrated end of the catheter is carefully passed through the cervix. While the catheter is being placed, the exposed end is crimped to prevent aspiration of air into the uterus.

With the catheter in position (6 to 8 inches within the uterus), the exposed end is placed inside the sleeve containing the saline. The sleeve is then clamped tightly around the end of the catheter, inverted, and elevated to allow the saline to run into the uterus. When the saline infusion is almost completed **but before it is finished,** lower the sleeve below the level of the uterus; the saline and uterine contents siphon back into the sleeve. If a clear plastic sleeve is used, it is easy to examine evacuated uterine contents.

The lavage is repeated until the recovered fluid is reasonably clear. The uterus can then be treated locally with the appropriate antibiotics.

Because fluid may continue to accumulate with toxemia and until the infection is controlled, careful monitoring is needed. Removal of the toxic uterine fluid should improve systemic signs. A lack of improvement dictates repeated flushings and continued treatment.

> *Universal Medical Instrument Corp., 2906 Route 9, Ballston Spa, NY 12020-3990.

- *Early* treatment for laminitis (p. 323). Preventive treatment includes
  - ☐ Soft footing
  - ☐ Comfortable frog support
  - ☐ Aspirin, 90 grains/450-kg horse PO q48h
  - ☐ Antibiotics and fluid therapy
  - ☐ Pentoxifylline, 8.4 mg/kg PO q12h
  - ☐ Nitroglycerine cream, topically, q12h
  - ☐ Flunixin meglumine, 0.3 mg/kg q8h

VENTRAL RUPTURES

Include rupture of the prepubic tendon and/or of the abdominal musculature; occur most often in late gestation. Although any breed is affected, there is a higher incidence among draft breeds. Individuals at higher risk include older mares, sedentary mares (because of decreased muscle tone), and mares with hydrops or twins. However, in many cases no identifiable predisposing factors or causes are found.

Diagnosis

Definitive diagnosis can be made only on postmortem evaluation.

Clinical Signs

- Abdominal pain; can be differentiated from other causes of colic by noting increased pain on palpation of the caudal abdomen
- Reluctance to walk
- Dependent abdomen or a discrete bulge of the ventrolateral abdomen
- THICK plaques of ventral edema that do not decrease with exercise. Plaques are from the increased pressure of the uterus on the caudal epigastric and caudal superficial epigastric veins or from trauma to the musculature.
- Elevation of the tuber ischii; this occurs when the prepubic tendon ruptures and the udder moves cranially.
- Blood in the milk is due to rupture of vessels.

Treatment

- Repair of abdominal muscle ruptures (see p. 211) is difficult and is performed only if the cause (hydrops or external trauma) is unlikely to recur.
- Extensive edema and/or hydrops with or without rupture of the prepubic tendon:
  - ☐ *If gestation is >330 days:* Induce parturition using oxytocin, 20 IU/450-kg mare IM, or as drip, 20–100 IU over 30–60 minutes.
  - ☐ Pretreat with corticosteroids, 20 mg dexamethasone, 24 hours before induction to stimulate fetal lung maturity.

- ▫ If gestation is <330 days and the mare is stable:
- ▫ Support abdomen until parturition is safely induced using belly band or wrap with wide adhesive tape

Uterine Prolapse

When this occurs (rarely), it requires prompt treatment to prevent additional trauma, shock, and/or even death of the mare. Before arrival, advise the owner to restrain the mare and if possible cover the everted uterus in a moistened sheet or towel to prevent further trauma or dehydration of tissues. Elevating the uterus helps to decrease edema.

Treatment

- ■ Sedate the mare as needed. **CAUTION:** Large doses of some tranquilizers (acepromazine) may accentuate signs of shock.
- ■ Administer epidural anesthesia, 1 ml 2% lidocaine/75 kg or 0.25 mg xylazine/kg mixed in 8–10 ml saline.
- ■ Clean and replace the uterus. Use large volumes of warm, mild antiseptic solution to cleanse the endometrial surface thoroughly. Before attempting replacement, carefully palpate to confirm that the bladder is not within the everted uterus. Presence of a distended bladder requires drainage before replacement. This can sometimes be done by passing a soft rubber stallion catheter through the urethra. If this is not possible, empty the bladder by placing a 2-inch, 14-gauge needle through the uterine wall into the bladder and apply gentle pressure.
- ■ Replace by applying firm, gentle pressure with the flat of the hand and the fingers closed or using a clenched fist. Apply pressure first near to the cervix, gradually working the everted uterus back through the cervix. It is important to gently work all sides evenly, being careful to use a flat surface (flat of hand) to prevent poking holes through the uterus. Having an assistant elevate the everted uterus on a tray or sling assists replacement. Once the uterus is passed through the cervix, it is important to be sure the tips of the horns are not inverted. If an arm is not sufficient to reach the tip of the uterine horn, an empty clean wine bottle can be grasped by the neck and the flat base of the bottle carefully extended to the tip of the horn.
- ■ Once the uterus is replaced, flush with 2–3 liters of warm saline solution a minimum of two times (see p. 427 for siphoning technique). Then place 2 gm of tetracycline powder in the uterus.
- ■ Systemic treatment includes 20 IU oxytocin IM to involute the uterus and systemic antibiotics (ceftiofur or combination penicillin and gentamicin) and 0.30 mg/kg flunixin meglumine; tetanus toxoid, and other recommended treatment (see p. 323) to prevent metritis and laminitis.

MASTITIS

Clinical Signs

- ■ Swollen udder, usually unilaterally (possible for only one lobe to be involved)

- Pain on udder palpation
- Ventral edema
- Fever
- Depression
- Anorexia
- Only half of clinical cases are found in lactating mares, and one quarter of clinical cases have signs within 8 weeks of weaning.

Diagnosis

Based on gross examination and culture of the milk for Gram stain. Obtain milk in a sterile vial after swabbing the teat with alcohol. *Streptococcus zooepidemicus* is frequently the cause. An aseptic cause of mastitis is avocado poisoning.

Treatment

- Strip the gland frequently (using lubricant) and hot pack the gland several times per day.
- Penicillin if small, gram-positive organisms are cultured. Trimethoprim-sulfadiazine (TMP-SDZ) or gentamicin if gram-negative rods are cultured. Confirm with sensitivity test as soon as possible.
- Intramammary infusions q12h–q24h or after milking (commercial bovine preparations)
- Flunixin meglumine, 0.25 mg/kg q8h if systemically ill.

Prognosis

Usually very good. Mares do not commonly have a recurrence after a single episode.

AGALACTIA

- Occasionally observed in a mare in any geographic region; it is most common where fescue pasture is contaminated with the fungus *Acremonium coenophialum*.
- In addition to agalactia; mares grazing infested pasture may have increased gestational length, increased incidence of stillbirths and retained placentas, increased placental thickness, and decreased prolactin and progesterone concentrations.
- Agalactia is an emergency since foal death occurs from sepsis if prompt treatment is not provided.

Treatment of Foal

- 2 liters of high-quality colostrum (specific gravity 1.080 or >) if foal is <24 hours of age. Administer colostrum in smaller amount, if foal is >24 hours of age, to provide IgA.
- Administer 1–2 liters of equine plasma IV to all foals born to agalactic

mares unless the colostrum can be given within 2–3 hours after birth, and IgG determinations at 14–18 hours demonstrate adequate serum IgG (>800 mg/dl).

- Feed foal appropriately and keep warm and dry.
- Administer antibiotics, e.g., ceftiofur, 3.0–4.0 mg/kg IV q8–12h, if the foal is several hours old when found.
- Sucralfate, 1 gm PO q6h
- Provide routine postnatal care:
  □ Clinical examination
  □ Dip navel with 1% chlorhexidine.
  □ Enema with *soft* rubber tubing and warm water, adding a small amount of Ivory or green soap.

Treatment of Mare

- Administer doperidone, 1.1 mg/kg PO q24h, a dopamine receptor antagonist that does not cross the blood/brain barrier and is effective in many cases. The drug is not approved; information is available through D. L. Cross, Department of Animal Dairy and Veterinary Sciences, Clemson University, Clemson, South Carolina 29631 (864) 656 5155.
- An alternative is perphenazine, 0.3–0.5 mg/kg PO q12h, which is available through your local pharmacy.
- Treat any factors that may cause agalactia, such as malnutrition, water deprivation, and concurrent illness.

FOAL REJECTION

Occurs primarily in primiparous mares; more common in certain families or breeds. The Arabian breed appears to be over-represented.

Treatment

- Rule out medical conditions that cause a painful udder. If no udder pathology, gently restrain the mare with *low*-dose acepromazine, 10 mg/ 450-kg mare. Feed the mare grain during the bonding process to entice the mare to let the foal nurse. Hand-milking the mare and feeding the foal by bottle held under the mare's udder reinforces a positive experience for mare and foal. Avoid painful restraint of the mare if possible, although a twitch is used if other methods fail. After tranquilizing the mare, place the mare in stocks to prevent sideways movement.
- A final approach, although more dangerous, is to place the mare and foal in a large paddock with other horses to encourage maternal behavior in the mare. Observe closely and continuously! Proper attention to the foal regarding adequate serum antibody titers and nutrition (see p. 430) is essential during the adjustment period.
- If these treatments are not successful in a few days, the foal should be bonded with a nursemare or fed as an orphan (see p. 689). Nursemare farms are listed (see below).

Nursemare Directory

Indiana
For-rest Hill Farm
Stephen and Margaret Kaiser
6250E 550N
Lafayette, IN 47905-9762
765/589-3838

Kentucky
C & G Partnership
Clinton and Garnett Porter
PO Box 177
Soldier, KY 41173
606/286-2367

Gail Curtsinger
1820 Clintonville Rd.
Winchester, KY 40391
606/745-6122

Horse Play Farm
Emmett R. Davis, Jr.
PO Box 52
Paris, KY 40361
606/987-3399

Mountain View Farms
Paul Stamper
PO Box 89
Ezel, KY 41425
606/725-5635

Pinecrest Farms
E.R. Stevens
PO Box 276
Millersburg, KY 40348
606/484-2281

Don and Judy Roseberry
Rt. 1, River Road
Box 162
Butler, KY 41006
606/472-5421

Walton Hills
Estill Walton
319 Walnut St.
Carlisle, KY 40311
606/289-5273

Maryland
Dolly Pouska
2720 Biggs Hwy.
Northeast, MD 21901
410/658-5062

New York
Milfer Farm, Inc.
Jonathan Davis, DVM
Joel Reach, Farm Manager
RD 1, Box 201
Unadilla, NY 13849
607/369-9408 or 607/369-9100
FAX 607/369-2406

North Slope Farm*
Sandy Kistner
PO Box 4
Trout Creek, NY 13847-0004
607/865-7926 or 607/865-7927

Debra Pease
67 Austerlitz St.
Chatham, NY 12037
518/799-6874

---

*Colostrum bank also available
From Modern Horse Breeding, February 1995, p 29.

SUGGESTED REFERENCES

Stallion Breeding Injuries

Varner DD, Schumacher J, Blanchard TL, Johnson L. Diseases and management of breeding stallions. Gotea, CA, American Veterinary Publications, 1991, pp 276–277.

Wilson DV, Nickels FA, Williams MA. Pharmacologic treatment of priapism in tow horse. J Am Vet Med Assoc 1991;199:1183–1184.

Dystocia

Vandeplascche M. Dystocia. *In* McKinnoon AO, Voss JL (eds): Equine Reproduction. Philadelphia, Lea & Febiger, 1993.

Uterine Torsion—Nonsurgical

Wichtel JJ, Reinertson EL, Clark TL. Nonsurgical treatment of uterine torsion in seven mares. J Am Vet Med Assoc 1988;193:337–338.

Uterine Torsion—Surgical

Pascoe JR, Meagher DM, Wheat JD. Surgical management of uterine torsion in the mare: A review of 26 cases. J Am Vet Med Assoc 1981;179:351–354.

Arterial Ruptures

McKinnon AO, Voss JL. Equine Reproduction. Philadelphia, Lea & Febiger, 1993.

Mastitis

McCue PM, Wilson DW. Equine mastitis—a review of 28 cases. Equine Vet J 1989;21(5):351–353.

Foal Rejection

Houpt KA. Foal rejection and other behavior problems in the postpartum period. Comp Cont Educ 1984;6:S144–S150.

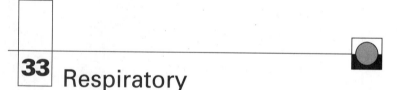

33 Respiratory

Thomas J. Divers

Emergencies of the respiratory system are generally diseases causing respiratory distress, and in some cases the disease can be life threatening without producing distress, e.g., pleuropneumonia, and therefore is treated as an emergency.

The initial diagnostic goal when evaluating an individual with respiratory distress is to determine whether the problem is an upper respiratory disorder (obstruction) or a lower respiratory problem (pulmonary edema, bronchoconstriction, pneumothorax, and so on). Upper respiratory obstruction, including tracheitis, can usually be determined by the noise the individual is making when breathing, especially on inspiration. Lower respiratory disease causing respiratory distress can usually be determined by auscultation of the thorax. Inspiratory dyspnea is often more pronounced than expiratory dyspnea with upper airway obstruction, whereas the reverse is true with lower airway obstruction, e.g., heaves.

Life-threatening respiratory infections without respiratory distress requiring emergency care, such as pleuropneumonia or aspiration pneumonia, can usually be determined by history, auscultation of the thorax, and routine diagnostics, e.g., ultrasound and tracheal aspirate.

RESPIRATORY DISTRESS WITH RESPIRATORY NOISE, AIRWAY OBSTRUCTION

- *Labored breathing* usually producing *noise*
- The list of differentials is long; therefore, perform a complete physical examination with ancillary diagnostic equipment to identify clinical features that narrows the possible causes.
- *Important to remember that acute respiratory obstruction is often rapidly progressive for two reasons:*
  □ The primary disease process, e.g., edema, is often progressive.
  □ Constant turbulence of air flow against the compromised airway leads to increased edema.
  □ Increased negative pleural pressure caused by increased effort against an obstructed airway may lead to pulmonary edema.
- Therefore, consider any acute respiratory noise an emergency.

Laryngeal Obstruction

Nasotracheal intubation may be difficult to perform on a distressed individual; in most cases a tracheotomy is preferred. If the instruments to perform the tracheotomy are not readily available, attempt nasotracheal intubation! If the patient collapses, then perform nasotracheal intubation because it is faster. *Secondary pulmonary edema is a common occurrence with acute severe upper airway obstruction; routinely administer furosemide in these cases.*

Laryngeal Edema—Anaphylaxis

Etiology is often unknown, but it can be due to an *anaphylactic reaction* to vaccine antigens and can accompany *purpura hemorrhagica*.

DIAGNOSIS

- Endoscopic examination is the best diagnostic tool: edema and collapse of the tissues around the larynx are seen. *Avoid tranquilization if possible.*
- Administer acepromazine, 0.02–0.04 mg/kg IV, and butorphanol, 0.01–0.02 mg/kg IV, for sedation if necessary to better examine the larynx endoscopically.
- Do not administer acepromazine if systemic anaphylaxis is a possibility.
- Do not use xylazine as it increases upper airway resistance.

TREATMENT

- If due to **anaphylactic** reaction: **Epinephrine**, 3–7 ml/450-kg adult (1:1000 as packaged), administer **slowly IV**. If time permits, dilute in 20–30 ml of 0.9% saline. Similar doses of epinephrine may be administered IM or SQ in less severe cases. If respiratory stridor is noted, suggesting 80%

or more compromise of the airflow, pass a nasotracheal tube to prevent further obstruction and the need for tracheotomy.

- If severe: Tracheotomy (see p. 44).
- If pulmonary edema has developed (crackles on auscultation or froth at the nostril), *begin* furosemide, 1 mg/kg IV, therapy and see p. 445.
- Dexamethasone, 0.25 mg/kg, IV bolus; dimethyl sulfoxide (DMSO), 1 gm/kg IV in 3 liters of 0.9% saline.
- For systemic anaphylaxis, both crystalloid and colloid fluids because affected individuals are hypotensive.

PROGNOSIS

Generally good but the condition may persist for several days or recur.

Arytenoid Chondritis

In most cases, the chondritis has been present for a long time, and the obstruction may be acute. If noise is apparent at rest, there is probably 80% or more compromise of the airway.

DIAGNOSIS

Endoscopic examination

TREATMENT

- Tracheotomy (see p. 44 for procedure)
- Surgical removal (arytenoidectomy) of the diseased cartilage.

Hypocalcemia

Hypocalcemic patients can have laryngeal paresis and consequently laryngeal obstruction.

DIAGNOSIS

- History is important, such as lactation in a mare, but idiopathic cases have occurred not associated with lactation.
- Other clinical signs: *Trismus of facial muscles, thumps, and trembling.*
- Confirm all presumptive cases by serum calcium levels. Serum calcium concentration is usually <6.5 mg/dl in adults with severe clinical signs. Profuse sweating, hypochloremia, and resultant alkalosis further exacerbate hypocalcemia.

TREATMENT

- Calcium borogluconate (NOTE: Safer than calcium chloride): 11 grams *SLOWLY IV* over 20 minutes to an adult (450 kg) while monitoring heart rate and rhythm.

> *Do not administer subcutaneously!*

If clinical signs do not abate, a second treatment may be required. Administer additional calcium diluted with polyionic fluids at a slower rate.

Acute Guttural Pouch Empyema

Often associated with *Streptococcus zooepidemicus* or *equi* infection.

DIAGNOSIS

- Endoscopic examination of pharynx, larynx, and guttural pouch
- Radiographic findings of a fluid line in the guttural pouches
- Nasal discharge
- Swelling and pain behind ramus of mandible

TREATMENT

- Tracheotomy is rarely needed.
- Appropriate antibiotic(s) (penicillin), administered systematically and through an indwelling catheter in the guttural pouch, serves to improve drainage.
- Pass a Chambers catheter into the guttural pouch for drainage and lavage with 1 liter of **nonirritating** polyionic fluid (warm saline with potassium [K] penicillin), after acepromazine, 0.02 mg/kg IV, and butorphanol, 0.01 mg/kg IV, for sedation. If the respiratory obstruction is not severe, substitute xylazine for the acepromazine to lower the head during the flushing procedure and improve drainage.

Laryngeal Spasms or Temporary Paresis

Frequent postanesthetic complication and therefore a problem at referral centers performing general anesthesia. Commonly occurs after removal of the endotracheal tube during recovery. Pulmonary edema quickly follows the obstruction and is a factor in the prognosis. More common in adults with laryngeal paresis, e.g., Draft breeds.

TREATMENT

- Tracheotomy (see p. 44) or pass a nasotracheal tube
- Furosemide, 1 mg/kg IV
- DMSO, 1 gm/kg IV in 3 liters of 0.9% saline, plus dexamethasone, 0.25 mg/kg, in cases of pulmonary edema

Proximal Esophageal Choke

On rare occasions can cause respiratory distress if the obstruction is in the proximal esophagus.

DIAGNOSIS

- Endoscopic examination
- Dorsally collapsed larynx
- Feed material may be seen at the esophageal opening or immediately on entering the esophagus.

TREATMENT

- Passage of a nasogastric tube to relieve the esophageal obstruction. If unsuccessful, a tracheotomy is performed.

Pyrollizidine Alkaloid Toxicity

Acute laryngeal paralysis is rarely seen in cases of pyrollizidine alkaloid poisoning. Clinical and biochemical evidence of liver disease is present.

TREATMENT

- Tracheotomy relieves the respiratory distress, but the prognosis is poor because of the potential for liver failure.

Strangles with Involvement of the Retropharyngeal Lymph Nodes in Foals

Obstruction is usually due to the septic lymphadenopathy. In most cases, there is not a "mature" abscess to be drained. *These cases are difficult to manage*, although the prognosis for life is good. Dysphagia may be a presenting complaint.

TREATMENT

- Tracheotomy (see p. 44). NOTE: Expect a purulent discharge from the tracheotomy site with soft tissue reaction around the area.
- Drain lymph node if abscessed.
  - □ Anatomy is complicated—Use ultrasound guidance to identify the abscess, although this is rare.
  - □ A 12-gauge teat cannula inserted through a stab incision into the lymph node may drain the abscess. NOTE: With or without drainage, laryngeal paralysis or dysfunction is often seen on endoscopic examination months later.
  - □ Penicillin: Clinical improvement may take 1 week or more. IV penicillin: 44,000 U/kg q6h is preferred in the initial stages of treatment to speed the recovery. If a tracheotomy is performed, place the IV catheter as far from the tracheotomy site as possible. If aspiration occurs broader spectrum antibiotics are indicated.

Idiopathic Laryngeal Paralysis in Foals

HISTORY

A young foal with stertorous breathing with no other physical abnormalities

DIAGNOSIS

- Endoscopy
- Rule out other causes in young foals:
  - □ Hyperkalemic periodic paralysis (HyPP) in Quarter Horses with "Impressive" breeding homozygous for the defective gene. There should be both laryngeal and pharyngeal collapse with HyPP. Does not usually cause clinical signs in newborn foals
  - □ Transient displacement of the soft palate in newborn foals. Milk reflux is more a problem than respiratory obstruction.
  - □ Selenium deficiency may also cause collapse of the airways and respiratory noise with distress in very young foals. Consider this in areas

(primarily northern United States and Canada) known to be selenium-deficient. Administer selenium *IM (NOT IV)* if a deficiency is suspected.

TREATMENT

Tracheotomy—for acute relief (see p. 44).

PROGNOSIS

- Very poor for idiopathic cases—most cases show little improvement.
- For other differentials—good

Hyperkalemic Periodic Paralysis

Airway obstruction occurs in homozygously affected foals. A loud fluttering sound may be made during episodes, with a persistent noise after treatment. Most do not require tracheotomy and can be managed medically. Stressful events such as weaning or excitement may precipitate onset or worsening of clinical signs.

DIAGNOSIS

- Young Quarter Horse foals usually (<5 months)
- Endoscopically, there is collapse of the soft palate, pharynx, and larynx. Do *not* use xylazine for sedation as this increases upper airway resistance.
- Direct descendant of "Impressive" on both sides of lineage
- Confirm homozygous status for the defective gene by DNA evaluation:
  - *Collect*: 1 EDTA tube (5–10 ml) of blood labeled with the patient's name. Do not freeze or separate.
  - *Send to*: Veterinary Genetic Laboratory/HyPP Test
    School of Veterinary Medicine
    University of California
    Davis, CA 95616-8744

CLINICAL CHEMISTRY FINDING

Serum potassium (K) is often normal, slight elevations are found in some foals. Some individuals can have elevated creatine kinase, but this is not uniform.

TREATMENT

- 50 ml of 50% dextrose IV if hyperkalemic. Do not use if the individual is collapsed and is believed to have suffered hypoxic brain damage. The high concentration of dextrose can aggravate central nervous system (CNS) intracellular acidosis as the dextrose is metabolized anaerobically to lactic acid. The benefit of glucose is to stimulate insulin release and move K intracellularly. Insulin is elevated within 5 minutes after glucose infusion and causes an immediate intracellular shift.
- 1 mEq/kg 7.5% or 8.4% $NaHCO_3$ IV over 5–10 minutes to shift K intracellularly. Use dextrose over $NaHCO_3$ because $NaHCO_3$ lowers ionized calcium, which has a "cellular protective" activity against hyperkalemia. $NaHCO_3$ may contribute to respiratory acidosis. Paradoxic CNS acidosis may also be caused by the administration of $NaHCO_3$ although evidence for this is not strong in the horse.

- Acetazolamide, 2.2 mg/kg PO, q12h
- Remove alfalfa hay, molasses, and electrolyte supplement.

Selenium Deficiency

Can cause a variety of signs in foals and adults. In young (sometimes newborn) foals, pharyngeal and laryngeal paresis results in respiratory noise and/or milk reflux.

DIAGNOSIS

- Geographic location and clinical signs (may be involvement of the skeletal muscles resulting in weakness, abnormal gait, and so on)
- Serum creatine kinase levels are variable but if elevated should arouse suspicion. Collect blood for selenium determination (<10 mg/dl supports the diagnosis).

TREATMENT

IM injection of selenium (*NOT IV*). Repeat in 3 days.

Tracheal Collapse

May occur from trauma or progressively enlarging masses (e.g., hematoma, thyroid, cyst, abscess) dorsal to the trachea. Most common in *adult* (usually > 10 years old) Miniature horses and Shetland ponies. The collapse generally occurs throughout the cervical and thoracic area.

CLINICAL SIGNS:

- Respiratory noise
- Respiratory distress
- Cyanosis

DIAGNOSIS

Confirmed by endoscopic examination of the upper airway and trachea. Provide intranasal oxygen during the endoscopic examination. The edges of the flattened trachea may be palpated in the jugular furrow in some cases. Radiographs and/ or ultrasound are useful in cases resulting from impinging mass.

TREATMENT

The extent of the collapse in Miniature horses and Shetland ponies makes repair difficult. If the collapse is in only a single area of the neck, extraluminal prosthetic devices can be implanted to increase tracheal diameter. Surgically drain or incise compressing masses.

A rare cause of tracheal collapse is a mediastinal abscess/tumor (e.g., *Streptococcus equi* abscess) or severe pneumomediastinum. Diagnosis is based on radiographs, endoscopy, and/or ultrasound. Treatment requires *both* a tracheotomy and placement of an endotracheal tube through the tracheotomy site.

Tracheal/Bronchial Foreign Body

Rarely, horses inhale foreign bodies (e.g., sticks or twigs) down the trachea lodging in a primary bronchus. This results in acute onset of coughing with variable respiratory distress.

Diagnosis: Endoscopic examination

Treatment: Removal via endoscopy is difficult. Referral and a surgical approach for removing the foreign body may be required.

Epiglottitis

May cause a respiratory noise and on *rare* occasions produce respiratory distress similar to croup in humans. In horses, a tracheotomy is rarely needed for epiglottitis.

Guttural Pouch Tympany

In foals, this may cause a respiratory noise and predispose to pneumonia but rarely causes respiratory distress.

Nasal Obstruction

To cause respiratory distress, both nares must be compromised. The most common causes of acute, bilateral nasal obstruction:

- Trauma
- Anaphylaxis
- Snake bite
- Acute obstruction of the jugular vein, along with low head carriage (depression and/or tranquilization).

Trauma of the Nasal Cavity

Can occur when a healthy individual runs into an object in the field or in an individual with cerebral disease that may be continuously head pressing. Also, in severely depressed individuals that keep their heads lowered and are frequently stomach tubed.

TREATMENT FOR BLUNT TRAUMA (INJURY TO THE NOSE)

- *Keep affected individual as quiet as possible* but *do not use xylazine or any tranquilizer that causes lowering of the head* or an increase in upper airway resistance.
- Apply ice packs to the external nasal surface.
- Spray lidocaine with epinephrine (25 ml in each nostril per adult) into the nasal cavity. Phenylephrine spray (10%) can also be used.
- If progressive nasal swelling expected, a small 9–15-mm-diameter, 4–8-cm-length tube can be sutured in the nostrils to help maintain a patent nasal airway. This is easier than performing a tracheotomy, but nasal mucosal necrosis may result from the pressure of the tube.
- Tracheotomy may be needed in some cases.
- Try to keep the head level or elevated.

- Begin antibiotics (e.g., penicillin).
- Suture any wounds.
- Administer tetanus toxoid.

Thrombosis of Jugular Veins

Bilateral thrombosis of the jugular veins occurs in severely ill patients receiving medications (especially hypertonic fluids or acidic or alkaline drugs) via the jugular vein. Unfortunately, many of these individuals are often depressed and hold their heads lower than normal because of the primary disease. Progressive nasal edema can result. With medical treatment, a tracheotomy can be avoided if the individual can maintain its head in a normal position.

TREATMENT

- Medical treatment is primarily antiedema therapy (e.g., DMSO, 1 gm/kg IV q12h administered slowly and diluted in 3 liters of sterile polyionic fluid). Administer further IV treatments via the lateral thoracic vein or cephalic vein.
- If one jugular vein is patent with a catheter in place, remove the catheter and place it elsewhere (e.g., lateral thoracic vein) if possible.
- Begin aspirin, 60–120 grains/450-kg adult PO along with pentoxifylline, 8.4 mg/kg PO q12h. Give aspirin every 2–3 days for its antiplatelet effect. Pentoxifylline has both antiplatelet aggregation and anticytokine effects, in addition to making red blood cells more deformable.
- If hypoproteinemia is compounding the problem, administer plasma (fresh or fresh frozen). Consider cost and expected benefit. If plasma is administered, add 100 U heparin to the plasma to stimulate antithrombin III activity before administration.

Bee Sting

Bee stings or vaccine reactions can produce acute severe nasal edema.

TREATMENT

- Cold compresses
- Antihistamines, e.g., doxylamine succinate, 0.5 mg/kg—*administered slowly IV*
- Dexamethasone if the edema is progressive and severe: 0.02 mg/kg q24h IV
- Epinephrine, 3–5 ml of a 1:100 solution IV to a 450-kg adult if the swelling is rapidly progressive or if there are signs of systemic hypotension (tachycardia, poor pulse quality)
- Tracheotomy if needed (see p. 44)
- Keep the head level.

Snake Bite

- Venomous snakes may bite horses and cause severe tissue necrosis.
- The nose is a common site for a bite, and severe swelling results.
- Swelling is marked with rattlesnake bites.

The swelling is initially warm, then becomes cool as the skin becomes necrotic. Shaving the area may be needed to see the fang marks.

The most frequent sequelae:

- Airway obstruction when bitten on the nose
- Severe cellulitis often associated with *Clostridium* sp.
- Hemolytic anemia rarely occurs.

Severe systemic effects from the venom are not common in adults. In foals, systemic effects include hypotension and/or shock, which should be treated appropriately with IV fluids and/or inotropic/pressor drugs, e.g., dopamine, 5–10 µg/kg/min or dobutamine, 5–15 µg/kg/min. Remember that foals do not have as dramatic increase in blood pressure in response to pressor drugs as adults do. Change in heart rate should be monitored in foals receiving β- and α-agonist combination drugs, and >40% increase in heart rate is a signal to slow the rate of drug administration.

TREATMENT

- If the airway becomes obstructed, perform a tracheotomy.
- If the nose is bitten and airway obstruction has not developed, keep the head level or elevated to minimize severe swelling. Pass a nasotracheal tube, shortened stomach tube or syringe case and leave in place to prevent airway obstruction.
- Flunixin meglumine is administered to decrease inflammation and diminish systemic effects caused by proinflammatory prostanoids. It has little effect on platelet function.
- Administer penicillin in all cases, 22,000–44,000 U/kg, preferably IV q6h, or 22,000 U/kg IM q12h.
- Metronidazole, 15 mg/kg q8h PO, and gentamicin, 6.6 mg/kg IV q24h (if hypotension is absent or minimal signifying dehydration), penicillin can be added to the treatment to improve anaerobic coverage. Substitute ceftiofur, 3.0 mg/kg IV or IM q12h, for gentamicin if hydration and/or renal function is a concern.
- Tetanus toxoid for adults or toxoid and antitoxin in foals
- If hypotensive therapy needed: Administer fluids, including hypertonic saline, plasma, and dopamine, if the fluids do not correct the hypotension (see systemic shock, p. 538).
- Antivenin (equine origin) is not recommended unless given within the first 8 hours of the bite. It may benefit foals bitten by coral snakes.

RESPIRATORY DISTRESS WITHOUT NOISE

Pneumothorax

Severity depends largely on the inciting cause and the completeness of the mediastinum. Inflammatory causes, e.g., pneumonia, rarely result in bilateral pneumothorax, whereas traumatic pneumothorax can be unilateral or bilateral and idiopathic pneumothorax (no evidence of trauma but probable lung rupture) is often bilateral or has such a marked increase in intrapleural pressure on the affected side causing the opposite side to be compromised.

Traumatic Pneumothorax

If the mediastinum is complete then the pneumothorax is unilateral. The affected individual has a rapid respiratory rate but should remain stable. If bilateral, signs are more severe, with progressive respiratory distress.

DIAGNOSIS

- The individual exhibits signs of respiratory distress (flared nostrils and increased respiratory rate).
- Auscultation reveals little or no movement of air dorsally (either bilaterally or unilaterally).
- Confirm findings with radiographs or ultrasound.
- Perform a diagnostic aspirate using a 3.5-inch needle or catheter with stylet. Attach a short extension tube to the needle or catheter, place 3–5 ml of sterile saline into the tubing, and hold proximally as the needle is advanced into the dorsal thorax (usual depth 2 inches). If a pneumothorax is present, the saline "bubbles" back as the thorax is entered and the air is forced out. If negative pressure is still present, the saline is sucked into the thorax.

TREATMENT

- Administer intranasal oxygen, 10–20 ml/kg/min, via nasopharyngeal tube. Even with unilateral pneumothorax, the other side of the lung can be physically compromised owing to the positive pressure on the mediastinum.
- Close any wounds and suture as soon as possible.
- Remove the air in the thorax after the wounds are closed. Use an 18-gauge needle or a 4-inch teat cannula.
- Start broad-spectrum antibiotic therapy for all forms of externally induced pneumothorax: Potassium penicillin, 44,000 U/kg q6h IV, and gentamicin, 6.6 mg/kg IV q24h, or ceftiofur, 3.0 mg/kg IV q12h.
- Administer analgesics.

Pneumothorax Secondary to Pneumonia

Generally unilateral because the mediastinum is usually complete with inflammatory disease. Alveoli rarely rupture associated with a severe pneumonia, or air leaks into one side of the chest from a chest drain, resulting in pneumothorax. Unilateral pneumothorax in patients with pneumonia may cause severe respiratory distress because the pneumothorax is compounded by bilateral lung disease and the pressure of the pneumothorax forces the mediastinum to the opposite side.

TREATMENT

- Replace leaking chest valve if a problem.
- Place a 3.5-inch, 16-gauge IV catheter HIGH in the 13th intercostal space, and as soon as the chest is entered pull the stylet back a quarter inch. Using a 60-ml syringe and three-way stopcock or vacuum pump (*make certain the pump is set on suction*), aspirate the air.

Idiopathic

Affected individuals have no evidence of external trauma nor do they have pneumonia. They often present with bilateral pneumothorax or bilateral compromise, are in severe respiratory distress, and may die acutely. Tension pneumothorax is suspected in these cases.

TREATMENT

- Bilateral: With severe respiratory distress, decompress the thorax as described and place a oneway chest tube Heimlich valve HIGH on the chest wall. *This must be done quickly!* Affected individuals have tension pneumothorax; therefore, an incision into the thorax may reduce the internal thoracic pressure.
- Unilateral: If stable, no need to suction thorax unless pressure in the hemithorax is compromising the opposite side of the thorax.

Pneumomediastinum

Commonly found radiographically after tracheal aspiration but rarely needs treatment. Occasionally tracheal perforation (most often from kicks) or severe axillary wounds results in a pressure pneumomediastinum that can severely affect preload (venous return) to the heart, causing life-threatening hypotension with respiratory distress. The diagnosis is confirmed radiographically and endoscopically.

TREATMENT

- *Tracheal perforation*—endoscopy of trachea reveals point of perforation; perform repair via a ventral cervical incision in the standing individual. Do not close the skin incision.
- *Axillary wound*—cross-tie the patient to decrease movement, and pack the wound to prevent more air from entering the wound.
- In both situations, administer intranasal oxygen, 10–20 ml/kg/min, and administer fluids to improve venous return and cardiac preload. In severe cases of tracheal perforation, surgery is required.

Pulmonary Edema

Acute pulmonary edema frequently arises from conditions that increase the pulmonary vascular pressure, such as left-sided heart failure, or alter the permeability of the pulmonary vascular endothelium, such as endotoxic shock, adverse drug reactions, or anaphylaxis. Other causes of pulmonary edema include:

- Smoke inhalation (see p. 447)
- Toxins
- Acute airway obstruction
- Neurogenic
- Iatrogenic overzealous administration of IV fluids in recumbent neonates or adults with anuric acute renal failure

Pulmonary edema usually occurs with acute problems and is rarely observed in hypoproteinemic patients with glomerulopathy or protein-losing enteropathy in spite of severe subcutaneous edema.

Diagnosis

Physical examination and the presence of a pre-existing disease such as acute heart failure, endotoxic shock, or anaphylaxis.

Treatment

- Treat the primary disease.
- Reduce the edema.
- Provide oxygen support until adequate ventilation is restored.
- NOTE: If anxiety is present, sedate with diazepam, 0.05–0.2 mg/kg IV or IM.

Pulmonary Edema Secondary to Endotoxic Shock/Systemic Inflammatory Syndrome* Response

TREATMENT

- Low-dose flunixin meglumine, 0.25 mg/kg IV; DMSO, 1 gm/kg IV diluted in 3 liters of 0.9% saline or 5% dextrose; dexamethasone, 0.25 mg/kg IV bolus
- Furosemide, 1 mg/kg IV (monitor systemic blood pressure because it may lower cardiac output)
- Intranasal oxygen, 10–15 L/min/450-kg adult
- Pentoxifylline, 8.4 mg/kg PO q8–12h
- Cardiac output is usually low; treat with plasma and dobutamine, 2–10 μg/kg/min. Steroids are controversial.
- Hypertonic saline is the fluid of choice when intravenous fluids are required with pulmonary edema and hypotension.

Pulmonary Edema Secondary to Heart Failure

TREATMENT

- Digoxin, 1 mg IV/450-kg adult
- Furosemide, 1 mg/kg IV
- Intranasal oxygen, 10–15 L/min
- Arterial vasodilator to decrease afterload, hydralazine, and the like

Pulmonary Edema Secondary to Anaphylaxis (Adverse Drug Reaction)

TREATMENT

- Epinephrine, 3–5 ml for adults, diluted in 20–30 ml of saline and administered slowly IV and in less severe cases, IM or SQ

---

*A shocklike syndrome similar to endotoxic shock but without evidence of endotoxemia.

- Dexamethasone, 0.25 mg/kg IV bolus
- Furosemide, 1 mg/kg IV
- Intranasal oxygen, 10–20 ml/kg/min
- IV plasma or synthetic colloid (hetastarch)

Purpura Hemorrhagica

Rarely causes acute pulmonary edema

TREATMENT

- Dexamethasone, 0.25 mg/kg IV; furosemide, 1 mg/kg IV q24h; intranasal oxygen

Fluid Therapy in Patients at High Risk for Developing Pulmonary Edema

High-risk patients:

- Septic foals
- Septic and recumbent foals
- Equine endotoxic shock
- Generalized anaphylactic diseases causing rapid protein loss

Fluid therapy for hypovolemia is required for many of these patients.

TREATMENT

- Hypertonic saline initially, 4–8 ml/kg, to improve cardiac output and blood pressure and to decrease pulmonary arterial pressures
- Oncotic plasma expanders, equine plasma, or hetastarch may decrease lung fluid volume and are recommended, but are expensive.

Airway Obstruction

TREATMENT

- Perform an immediate tracheotomy or pass a nasotracheal tube.
- Furosemide, 1 mg/kg IV

Smoke Inhalation

Horses may be seriously affected or die from smoke inhalation in a barn fire. They can die without skin burns. Three pulmonary consequences can occur in association with smoke inhalation:

- Carbon monoxide poisoning—immediate
- Pulmonary edema—hours later
- Pneumonia—hours to days later

Smoke inhalation and pulmonary edema are the immediate primary concerns when affected individuals are examined after a fire.

Diagnosis and Clinical Findings

Respiratory signs following smoke exposure:

- Coughing
- Labored breathing
- Polypnea
- Frothy exudate

Other clinical findings:

- Tachycardia
- Widespread wheezes and crackles
- Cyanosis

Treatment

- Treat pulmonary, laryngeal, or pharyngeal edema. NOTE: If skin burns are present, avoid corticosteroids! (See Pulmonary Edema, p. 445.)
- Prevent airway obstruction from fibrin debris: Suction via endoscope is preferred. Perform a tracheotomy only if life-threatening laryngeal edema is occurring. The tracheotomy prevents the patient from coughing up necrotic casts.
- Oxygen therapy. Humidified, 10–15 liters/min for adults, administered intranasally or through tracheotomy; continue oxygen during suctioning!
- Alleviate bronchoconstriction:
  - ☐ Albuterol, 0.016–0.032 mg/kg PO q12h
    OR
  - ☐ Clenbuterol, 0.8–1.6 μg/kg IV or PO q12h (may be nebulized: 10 ml containing 0.03 mg/ml)
    OR
  - ☐ Atropine, 0.014–0.02 mg/kg IV *once or twice only* (7 mg/450-kg adult)
- Prophylactic treatment for shock. In spite of pulmonary edema, fluid therapy is needed to maintain tissue perfusion. Fluid therapy is essential in patients receiving furosemide to treat pulmonary edema.
  - ☐ Polyionic fluids to prevent shock: Maintenance rate, 1–2 liters/hour (adult). Add additional KCl (20–40 mEq/L) if renal function normal and if serum K normal or low.
  - ☐ *Plasma*, 1–2 liters with antiendotoxin antibodies. Larger volume in severe cases and/or synthetic colloids, e.g., hetastarch.
  - ☐ NSAIDs: Flunixin meglumine, 0.25 mg/kg q8h *or* ketoprofen, 1 mg/kg q12h
- Treatment for sepsis: Administer **broad-spectrum bactericidal antibiotics** to those patients believed to be septic (fever or the presence of intracellular bacteria on examination of tracheal sputum). If deep burns exist on the body or if a tracheotomy is performed, administer antibiotics:
  - ☐ Ceftiofur, 3 mg/kg q12h *or*
  - ☐ Penicillin, 22,000 IU/kg IV q6h, and amikacin, 15–25 mg/kg IV q24h *or* enrofloxacin, 7.5 mg/kg PO q24h
  - ☐ Metronidazole, 15 mg/kg PO q8h.

Chronic Obstructive Pulmonary Disease (Heaves)

Individuals with chronic obstructive pulmonary disease (COPD) often develop respiratory distress following exposure to allergens and/or an infectious agent. COPD airways appear to be hyperactive to particulate matter (e.g., dust, mold spores, noxious fumes, and even high humidity), predisposing individuals to respiratory crises despite good management. Increased mucus production and decreased lung function provide the ideal environment for secondary infections that frequently trigger episodes of respiratory distress. Fever of 103–104° is often present in patients with bacterial bronchitis and heaves.

Diagnosis

- Clinical findings
- Auscultation: Fine crackles and wheezes are usually heard over most lung fields. The lungs are sometimes abnormally quiet (especially ventral) in severe episodes.

  This is confused with ventral consolidation (pneumonia) or pleural effusion, but horses with pleuropneumonia infrequently present for respiratory distress and when they do, they usually have signs of sepsis (injected, discolored mucous membranes; severe depression, commonly with a hemorrhagic or fetid discharge from the nostrils).
- Response to treatment is often a useful diagnostic test if heaves is thought to be the problem. A marked response to a single injection of atropine supports this.
- Tracheal sputum examination: The sample can be collected via an endoscope for both culture and cytology.* It is important that the procedure be performed rapidly to prevent oropharyngeal fluid flowing down the trachea and contaminating the sample. *If the patient is in severe respiratory distress, do not perform a transtracheal wash as severe pneumomediastinum can occur.*
- Sedation may be needed for the endoscopic procedure: Xylazine, 0.3 mg/kg IV, and butorphanol, 0.01 mg/kg IV.

Treatment

- Atropine, 0.014–0.02 mg/kg (7–10 mg IV/450-kg adult), for immediate relief unless severe tachycardia (>80 BPM) is present. NOTE: Atropine decreases intestinal motility, so advise owners to monitor for signs of colic, although unusual when this dose is used once.
- Corticosteroids
  □ Prednisone, 1–2 mg/kg *or*
  □ Dexamethasone, 0.02–0.04 mg/kg PO or parenterally q24h until a clinical response is seen

---

*A Darien microbiology aspiration catheter, Mill Rose Labs Inc., Mentor, OH, can be used if culture is required, and sterile polyethylene 205 tubing with an adapters, from Intramedic and Intramedic Luer Stud Adapter, Becton Dickinson, Parsippany, NJ 07054, works well for sample collection for cytology and culture.

- Antibiotics: If there is a fever and/or bacterial bronchitis is suspected as the underlying cause for heaves: Ceftiofur, 3 mg/kg q12h.
- Glycopyrrolate; 0.005 mg/kg IV, IM, or SQ q8–12h, can be used instead of atropine but is not as effective. Higher doses may result in GI atony, gas distention, or small colon impactions in some individuals.

> **CAUTION:** If the patient has a high heart rate (>80 bpm), do not administer atropine or glycopyrrolate. Be cautious when administering other bronchodilators to individuals with severe tachycardia.

- Intranasal oxygen: 10–15 liters/min via nasopharyngeal catheter sutured at the nostril. Bubble the oxygen through warm water if possible.
- Use nebulization as additional therapy or in chronic cases. *It should not be used solely for therapy in acute severe cases.* Clenbuterol (10 ml containing 0.03 mg/ml), ipratropium bromide (200 µg [10 puffs]), or beclomethasone (3750 µg [14 puffs]) may be delivered with an aeromask.
- Furosemide, 1.0 mg/kg IV or IM improves lung function but generally without noticeable clinical improvement.
- *Do not use NSAIDs in patients with COPD,* unless another disease requires their administration because these drugs may decrease prostaglandin E_2 and its bronchodilatory effect.
- Maintain adequate hydration because dehydration thickens the mucous plugs in the airways. Provide fresh, clean water and electrolyte/glucose supplement. In some cases it may be necessary to administer fluids by nasogastric intubation or IV.

Prognosis

Good in most cases. However, satisfactory clinical improvement may require 3–5 days. Do not expect improvement in individuals with COPD and concurrent bacterial bronchitis until corticosteroid therapy is added to the antimicrobial therapy. Some older patients with prolonged histories of COPD with severe parenchymal disease may not respond to this treatment, especially if they are not responsive to a test dose of atropine.

Management

Management of COPD involves minimizing contact with allergens by changing feeds (generally best to prevent hay exposure) and bedding (newspaper can be used) so that the mold count and dust are decreased.

Most affected individuals should be kept outside 24 hours a day if possible. If not, it is best to move them to the end of the barn (or an area with the best ventilation) and outside at haying time and during bedding change.

In southeastern United States, some individuals develop respiratory signs of COPD while at pasture (pasture-associated COPD) and may improve within 24 hours simply by housing them in a barn.

Intradermal skin testing and radioallergosorbent testing (RAST) may be used to identify the allergen. RAST appears more reliable for detecting the allergen. Perform both tests if desensitization is considered.

Viral (or Postviral) Respiratory Distress Syndrome

Most often seen in *young adults* and rarely foals exposed to viral infections of the upper respiratory tract. Incidence in horses affected with viral upper respiratory infections is low.

Affected individuals initially have a fever (often as high as 106° F) associated with the viral infection, and within 1–3 days develop severe tachypnea with labored breathing.

The pathophysiologic mechanism of the syndrome is undetermined and is believed to be an overreactive airway triggered by the virus and/or irritants. This syndrome is distinctly different from pleuropneumonia (see p. 456) which results in severe weight loss.

Diagnosis

- History: Includes recent arrival from a sale barn or recent exposure (show) to a large group of young horses
- Fever up to 106° F
- Auscultation: Wheezes and crackles are heard but are less dramatic than the clinical signs; lung sounds are quiet for the effort expended in breathing.
- Transtracheal aspirate is usually nonseptic, although bacteria, e.g., *Pasteurella* spp., may be occasionally cultured.
- Generally affected individuals are not toxic, and have a normal appetite but labored breathing.
- Affected individuals may appear like heavey patients, except age (foals and young adults) and history are different.
- Radiographs and ultrasound show abnormalities (e.g., interstitial pattern, or alveolar edema and roughening of the pleura), but they are not severe!

Treatment

- Bronchodilators:
  - Clenbuterol, 0.8–1.6 µg/kg PO for 2–3 days *OR*
  - Albuterol, 0.016–0.032 mg/kg PO (8–16 mg/450-kg adult) q12h for 2–3 days (make sure potassium intake is adequate as β-adrenergic drugs can decrease serum potassium)
    AND
  - Glycopyrrolate, 1–3 mg/450-kg adult SQ q12h for 2–3 days
- Intranasal oxygen: 10–20 ml/kg/minute continuously
- Antimicrobial therapy: Ceftiofur, 3.0 mg/kg, for bacterial infections, especially *Pasteurella* spp.

Prognosis

Despite respiratory distress for 3–6 days, the prognosis is good. *In rare cases, such as unvaccinated horses or mules not previously exposed to influenza, rapid progression to death may result* from the influenza virus.

Rhodococcus equi Pneumonia in Foals

Generally affects foals between 2 weeks and 3 months of age and rarely individuals over 4 months, present with acute respiratory distress. *Rhodococcus equi* infection must be differentiated from bronchointerstitial pneumonia, due to viral etiology or unknown causes, because it also results in respiratory distress in nursing foals.

Diagnosis

Based on:

- The age of the foal (2 weeks–4 months)
- A history of previous *Rhodococcus equi* infections on the farm
- Swollen joints without severe lameness occur in approximately 25% of affected individuals
- Geographic location (increased prevalence in some areas of the country, e.g., dry, dusty, warm areas)
- Season—most commonly affects foals in the late spring
- Clinical presentation—acute respiratory distress, a high fever, and minimal cough
- Auscultation:
  □ Harsh lung sounds are heard diffusely, except for the caudal tip, which is generally loud but normal.
  □ The lung sounds are often less musical than with other bacterial infections.
- Tracheal aspiration: Use the least traumatic method of collection—percutaneous transtracheal wash with an Intracath or similar catheter (see p. 36). The Intracath does not require local anesthesia or an incision and therefore is less stressful. If sedation is needed, use 5 mg of diazepam.
  NOTE: This method of performing tracheal aspirates is more costly than other diagnostic methods
  Culture and *Gram-stain* the aspirate. *R. equi* shows small, pleomorphic, gram-positive rods (see p. 676).
- Chest radiographs: Use standard units and 400-speed film/screen combination, and 80 KVP at 20 MA 0.2 to 0.3 sec nongrid. *R. equi* infection produces a "white out" of the lungs, except for the caudal tips of the diaphragmatic lung lobes, which remain black.

Treatment

- Antibiotics:
  □ Erythromycin, 30 mg/kg PO q 8–12h
  AND
  Rifampin, 5 mg/kg PO q12h

NOTE: Most foals are in severe respiratory distress, so compliance by owners is important to ensure that the entire dose is swallowed.

- Trimethoprim-sulfa, 20 mg/kg PO q12h for *Pneumocystis carinii*
- Vancomycin, 5–7 mg/kg, diluted and administered slowly IV q8–12 h, if the foal is unable to swallow oral medications.
- Intranasal oxygen, 10–20 ml/kg/min continuously (see p. 40).
- IV fluid therapy: Polyionic fluids may be required at a maintenance rate of 40 ml/kg IV over 24 hours if dehydration is present and foals are unable to nurse. DMSO, 1 gm/kg slowly IV diluted in 1 liter of 0.9% saline, is useful in acute, severe cases.
- β_2-Specific bronchodilators; Clenbuterol, 1.6 μg/kg PO q12h, or albuterol, 0.016–0.032 mg/kg PO q12h. *Do Not Use* aminophylline—rarely efficacious and potential drug interaction with erythromycin, toxic levels of aminophylline can result and cause seizures in foals.
- Ulcer prophylaxis: Ranitidine, 6.6 mg/kg PO q8h and sucralfate, 1–2 gm q6–8h—do not combine or administer simultaneously with antibiotics, bronchodilators, famotidine, or other H_2-antagonists.

NOTE: On hot days, some foals on erythromycin develop high fevers, 106–110°. Cool with alcohol or cold water bath, and fans, place in the shade, and administer dipyrone, 10 ml IV.

Acute Bacterial Pneumonia and Respiratory Distress in Foals Due to Etiologic Agents Other than *R. equi*

Common in neonatal foals (see p. 482) and rare in older foals. Fever and respiratory distress in a nursing foal and a radiographic cranioventral pattern of disease and/or pleural effusion are compatible with bacterial pneumonia. Age, tracheal wash, farm history, and so on, are important in ruling out *R. equi* in 2-week–4-months-old foals.

Diagnosis/Clinical Findings

- Auscultation of the chest varies; crackles and wheezes or a "consolidated bronchial tone sound" are frequently heard cranioventrally. Pleural effusion, occasionally quiet bronchial sounds heard ventrally on auscultation.
- Clinical pathology: The leukogram generally supports sepsis; toxic neutrophils with a left shift; and an elevated fibrinogen.
- Tracheal wash: Perform a transtracheal wash (TTW) and submit sputum for aerobic and anaerobic culture and a Gram stain. The most common organisms are gram-negative rods—e.g., *Pasteurella* spp., *Escherichia coli*, and occasionally anaerobic organisms.
- Thoracocentesis: *ONLY if* ultrasound indicates a pleural effusion *and* the fluid is believed contributing to respiratory distress, or when an etiologic agent is not isolated on TTW. Butorphanol, 0.025 mg/kg IM, or diazepam, 5 mg IV, can be administered before the procedure.
- Radiography: A chest radiograph may be needed to rule out *R. equi* and diffuse bronchointerstitial pneumonitis.
  □ Radiographic pattern suggesting abscessation and diffuse involvement of the lung is characteristic of *R. equi*. Multiple joint swellings, marked neutrophilia, and thrombocytosis indicate *R. equi*.

□ An acute interstitial pneumonia, viral or idiopathic, is ruled out by lower fibrinogen, less responsive leukogram, more diffuse disease pattern on clinical and radiographic examination, and absence of pathogenic bacteria on tracheal aspirate.

Treatment

- Broad-spectrum antibiotics:
  - □ Ticarcillin/clavulonic acid, 44–50 mg/kg IV q6h
    OR
  - □ Ceftiofur, 3–5 mg/kg IV q8–12h
  - □ Amikacin can be added for the synergistic benefit and improved gram-negative spectrum if renal function is normal and the foal is receiving IV fluids.
  - □ Metronidazole, 15 mg/kg PO q12–24h in foals <3 weeks of age and q8h in older foals, only if anaerobic organisms are seen on the TTW or if *E. coli* or *Enterobacter* spp. are cultured (which may indicate an anaerobic organism is present).
- Intranasal oxygen, 10–20 ml/kg/min
- Antiulcer prophylaxis:
  - □ Ranitidine, 6.6 mg/kg q8h PO or other H₂-blocker
  - □ Sucralfate, 1–2 gm q6–12h PO 60 minutes before ranitidine
- Remove pleural fluid using diazepam (Valium) for sedation and adequate restraint; use a teat cannula and 60-ml syringe with a three way stopcock. The fluid is often bright red.

Bronchointerstitial Pneumonia in Foals

A primary rule-out for *R. equi* infection affecting the same age or *older* foal and of unknown etiology. It causes severe respiratory distress with a high fever, *usually affecting one individual on a farm.* Consider this disease in *R. equi* suspects that are negative for *R. equi* on tracheal aspiration; the prognosis for these foals is fair with corticosteroid treatment. If not treated with corticosteroids, most of the affected individuals have respiratory distress for 3–5 days before dying. Some may survive. The cause of the syndrome is not known and may be toxic, immunologic, or nonbacterial infections.

Diagnosis

- Clinical presentation:
  - □ Respiratory distress—tachypnea and cyanosis
  - □ Frequently bright, alert, and nursing
  - □ High fever—102–107°F
  - □ No severe inflammatory changes on leukogram
  - □ Several weeks of age
  - □ *R. equi* negative
  - □ No intracellular bacteria on tracheal aspirate
- Radiograph findings:
  - □ Diffuse disease, with or without a nodular pattern
  - □ No abscesses

Treatment

- Corticosteroids: Dexamethasone, 0.4–0.8 mg/kg IV or IM q12h for 2 days, followed by a tapering dose (*only* if *R. equi* is believed unlikely based on age and no *R. equi* is found on TTW)
- Improvement should be seen within 48 hours after corticosteroids are started.
- Intranasal oxygen: 5 liters/min continuously. *CAUTION:* Small O_2 tanks may last for 1–2 hours only.
- Antibiotics: Ceftiofur, 3.0 mg/kg IV q12h
- Bronchodilators:
  □ Clenbuterol, 0.8–1.6 µg/kg PO q12h
  OR
  □ Albuterol, 0.016–0.032 mg/kg PO q12h
- DMSO, 1 gm/kg IV, diluted in 1 liter of an isotonic fluid and balanced polyionic fluids to maintain hydration. *Do not* administer sodium bicarbonate because this may increase respiratory rate and even lower blood pH if there are severe alveolar ventilation/perfusion abnormalities.
- Ulcer prophylaxis medication:
  □ Sucralfate, 1 to 2 gm PO q6–8h preferred,
  OR
  □ Ranitidine, 6.6 mg/kg PO q8h, or other H_2-proton pump blocker
- *Thermoregulatory control:*
  □ Alcohol or cold water bath and fan
  □ Dipyrone, 5–10 ml three to four times daily if needed

ACUTE RESPIRATORY DISTRESS IN FOALS AFTER ANTHELMINTIC TREATMENT

Although rare, nursing or weanling foals may develop respiratory distress 1–3 days after the administration of an anthelmintic. This is believed due to the death of a significant number of ascarid or strongyle larvae in the lungs.

Diagnosis

- History of receiving an anthelmintic, often for the first time
- Signs of respiratory distress within 48 hours after anthelmintic treatment
- Clinical signs:
  □ Labored breathing
  □ Tachypnea
  □ Coughing
  □ Nasal discharge
  □ Body temperature ranging from normal up to 102.5°
- Auscultation:
  □ Wheezes heard over lung fields bilaterally
- Transtracheal wash:
  □ Usually nonseptic
  □ Cellular reaction may be a mixture of neutrophils and eosinophils.

Treatment

- Corticosteroids, **single dose only**: Dexamethasone, 0.1 mg/kg; usually a significant improvement seen
- Antibiotics:
  - ☐ Trimethoprim-sulfa, 20 mg/kg PO q12h
    AND/OR
  - ☐ Procaine penicillin, 22,000 U/kg IM q12h
    OR
  - ☐ Ceftiofur alone, 3.0 mg/kg IV q12h

Prognosis

Good

PLEUROPNEUMONIA/SEPTIC PLEURITIS

- Although the disease process may be present for several days, *treat pleuropneumonia in the adult as an emergency!*
- Unlike the majority of foal pneumonias, adult pleuropneumonia is commonly complicated by anaerobic infections, which are associated with a greater risk for necrosis and infarction of the lung.
- *Pleuropneumonia is the most common cause of infectious pleural effusions in the horse.* See Table 33–1.

Clinical Signs

Usually most severe in the midventral right lung, and abnormal lung sounds are generally more prominent in this area. Other clinical signs include forelimb or sternal edema, *low grade colic*, pleurodynia, laminitis, fever, and anorexia.

Diagnosis

The sample odor obtained by transtracheal wash or thoracocentesis can be important in the management of the case! A fetid odor indicates the presence

TABLE 33–1. **Signs and Physical Findings of Pleuropneumonia**

	Clinical Signs	**Auscultation Findings**
Acute	Respiratory distress, cough (usually soft), red to dark brown exudate at nostril, severely depressed	Crackles and in some areas wheezes; increased bronchial sounds ventrally if effusion minimal
Subacute to Chronic	Weight loss, soft cough, poor performance, normal to increased respiratory rate	Pleural effusion, no lung sounds ventrally; normal to loud sounds dorsally; radiating heart sounds; normal to increased respiratory rate

of anaerobic bacteria, *worsens the prognosis and increases the cost of treatment.* Discuss this finding with the owner!

- Transtracheal aspirate (*preferred over bronchoalveolar lavage*). Use a BBL Vacutainer, Columbia broth with sodium polystyrene sulfonate (SPS) and increased cysteine (Becton-Dickinson, Cockeysville, MD). Submit for both aerobic and anaerobic culture.
- Thoracocentesis: Indicated if there is the suspicion of pleural effusion (decreased lung sounds ventrally and radiating heart sounds). Ultrasound confirms the presence of fluid.
    □ Quick method (for culture only). Requires: 18-gauge, 1.5-inch needle. Aerobic/anaerobic culture medium (BBL Vacutainer, Columbia broth with SPS and increased cysteine, Becton-Dickinson, Cockeysville, MD)
- Indwelling chest drain: Indicated if a large volume of fluid is present or if the effusion is flocculent and fetid (the same site as the thoracocentesis is preferred if the site is ventral enough to provide adequate drainage)
    □ Requires a blunt-tipped 24 F. trocar catheter (Deknatel, Howmedica, Inc., Floral Park, NY); oneway valve (a latex condom can be made into a oneway valve by opening the closed end and attaching the other end to the catheter with tape).

PROTOCOL

- Pass the blunt-tipped 24 F. trocar catheter 4–6 cm through the stab incision.
- Remove the trocar and manipulate the catheter to obtain the best flow rate.
- Attach the oneway valve to the catheter to prevent pneumothorax. Tape the condom over the end of the tube with the cut end distal and place a pursestring around the catheter to hold it in place.
- Determine the site for the thoracocatheter using ultrasound examination.

Treatment

- *Treat all cases of adult pleuropneumonia aggressively.*
- Start broad-spectrum antibiotics immediately.

OPTION 1

- Penicillin, 44,000 U/kg q6h IV *AND*
- Gentamicin,* once daily treatment with 6.6–8.8 mg/kg IV *AND*
- Metronidazole, 15 mg/kg PO q6–8h

OPTION 2

- If decreased renal function or if cost of option 1 is prohibitive:
    □ Ceftiofur, 3 mg/kg IV or IM q12h
    AND
    □ Metronidazole, 15 mg/kg PO q6–8h

---

*NOTE: Serum creatinine must be monitored during treatment. If azotemia is present, adminster fluids or use Option 2. Monitoring peak and trough gentamicin levels is the best method to prevent renal toxicity associated with aminoglycoside usage.

Supportive Treatment for Concurrent Toxemia

Adults with abnormal mucous membrane color, toxic-appearing neutrophils and/
or bands, and tachycardia:

- Fluid therapy IV, polyionic fluid
- Flunixin meglumine, 0.25 mg/kg q8h IV/IM
- J-5 hyperimmune plasma, 2 liters IV
- Prophylaxis for laminitis:
  □ Pentoxifylline, 8.4 mg/kg PO q12h
    AND/OR
  □ Aspirin, 11–20 mg/kg (90 grains/450 kg adult) PO q48h
  □ Intranasal oxygen, 10 to 20 ml/kg/min
  □ Nitroglycerine cream applied over digital arteries

Prognosis

Prognosis for life is generally good unless severe tachypnea, severe polypnea, toxemia, and hemorrhagic-fetid nasal exudate are present. These findings support pulmonary infarction and a poorer prognosis. In individuals with pulmonary infarctions, a rib resection may ultimately be required to improve recovery.

ASPIRATION PNEUMONIA

Occurs commonly in horses. Generally chronic, due to a mechanical or neurologic condition of the pharynx and/or larynx—not an emergency. Acute aspiration results from esophageal choke, iatrogenic causes, or meconium aspiration in foals. Rarely, horses spontaneously reflux gastric contents secondary to anterior enteritis, small bowel obstruction, or gastric dilatation.

Occasionally, individuals present with severe respiratory distress after aspirating a large volume of material. Those with severe respiratory distress are caused by misdirected stomach tubes and meconium aspiration in foals: *these are considered an emergency.*

Iatrogenic Aspiration Pneumonia

Diagnosis

- History of coughing and distress after tubing
- Auscultation of the trachea and lungs reveals a loud fluttering sound with crackles and wheezes hours later, with ingesta seen at the nostrils.
- Tracheal endoscopic examination
- Percutaneous transtracheal wash preferred over endoscopic aspirate to eliminate any possible confusion over contamination from the endoscope

Treatment

- Corticosteroids: Dexamethasone, 0.1–0.2 mg/kg q24h on day 1, and 0.05–0.1 mg/kg on day 2. NOTE: *Corticosteroids are for chemical aspiration only.*

- DMSO: 1 gm/kg diluted in 3 liters of saline and administered over 30–60 minutes.
- Antibiotics:
  □ Penicillin, 44,000 U/kg IV q6h
    AND
  □ Gentamicin, 6.6–8.8 mg/kg IV q24h. (**CAUTION**: Monitor renal function and/or provide IV fluids.)
    AND
  □ Metronidazole, 15–25 mg/kg PO q6–8h
    OR
  □ Ceftiofur, 3.0 mg/kg IV q12h
    AND
  □ Metronidazole, 15–25 mg/kg PO q6–8h

ADJUNCT SUPPORTIVE TREATMENT

- Intranasal oxygen: 10–20 ml/kg/min continuously. Place a soft rubber tube in the nasopharynx, suture to the false nostril, with humidified oxygen from a portable tank.
- Flunixin meglumine, 0.25–1.1 mg/kg, or phenylbutazone, 2.2–4.4 mg/kg IV or PO after discontinuing corticosteroid therapy
- Aspiration of the lower airway by infusing warm sterile saline followed by suction. If the suction is vigorous, via pump, simultaneously administer oxygen.

  NOTE: Rarely distress occurs associated with proper nasogastric tubing and administration of oral medication. These episodes of reflux esophageal spasm and/or esophageal or gastric irritation are alarming because the immediate concern is aspiration pneumonia or gastric rupture; however, within 30–60 minutes the affected individual is normal.

  NOTE: Almost all adults with choke have some aspiration pneumonia. Ultrasound examination of the chest 24–48 hours after the onset of choke generally reveals moderate to marked pleural abnormalities. In most cases, recovery is excellent regardless of these findings.

Meconium Aspiration in Foals

Diagnosis

Based primarily on the history; commonly seen with fetal (in utero) diarrhea and stress associated with a colicky mare. Typically, foals are born with brown stained amniotic fluid.

Foals with this history should be presumed to have aspirated meconium and generally show respiratory distress in the first few days of life.

Treatment

- Corticosteroids: Dexamethasone, 0.1–0.2 mg/kg IV q24h on day 1; 0.05–0.1 mg/kg on day 2. Use of corticosteroids is controversial, but in the newborn, a decreased pulmonary inflammatory response may be necessary to prevent hypoxia and reversion to fetal circulation via pulmonary hypertension.

- Broad-spectrum antibiotics:
  - ☐ Ticarcillin/clavulanate (Timentin), 44–50 mg/kg IV q6h
    OR
  - ☐ Ceftiofur, 3.0 mg/kg IV q12h as an alternative
- *If severe*, administer intranasal O_2 at 5 liters/hour (see p. 40), and DMSO, 1 gm/kg diluted in saline.
- Perform tracheal suction if a fluttering sound is heard on auscultation of the trachea: pass a catheter down the trachea, infuse 10 ml of saline and aspirate using a 60-ml syringe. Repeat several times if aspirated material is retrieved. Oxygen should be administered simultaneously, and aspiration brief to prevent further oxygen debt.

ADDITIONAL CAUSES OF RESPIRATORY DISTRESS

1. Diaphragmatic hernia (see p. 183)
2. Botulism (see p. 348)
3. Fractured ribs (foals) (see p. 293)
4. Internal respiratory failure caused by hemolysis or intoxication (see p. 294).

EPISTAXIS

Epistaxis caused by head trauma rarely requires emergency treatment unless the nares are obstructed. A tracheotomy is then required. Other conditions causing epistaxis that can be life threatening and require emergency evaluation and therapy:

- Guttural pouch mycosis
- Thrombocytopenia
- Rupture of the longus capitis muscle

Guttural Pouch Mycosis

Bleeding may be the only clinical sign in adults with guttural pouch mycosis; bleeding and neurologic signs rarely occur simultaneously. In some cases, a yellow exudate is seen at the nostril before bleeding. Middle-aged or older pastured individuals are most commonly affected. Owners report finding blood on the stall wall or on the nose before a major bleed. The bleeding is generally unilateral unless major bleeding occurs.

Diagnosis

- A tentative diagnosis is based on history; endoscopic examination is required for a definitive diagnosis.
- Endoscopic examination: Unless there is evidence of hypotension, elevated heart rate, pale mucous membranes, or slow capillary refill time, sedation facilitates the passage of the endoscope. Using a guide wire passed through the biopsy channel assists in entering the pouch or, alternatively, a Chambers catheter is passed on the opposite side of the

endoscope to elevate the guttural pouch flap. The lesion, often yellow to green, diphtheritic membrane, is most commonly found dorsally in the medial or lateral compartment.

Treatment

Once the diagnosis is confirmed, surgery is needed as soon as possible.

- If blood loss is severe, a blood transfusion (see p. 293) and polyionic fluids are needed to stabilize the patient. Generally, hypertonic saline is not administered unless hypovolemic shock is clinically evident.
- If sedation is required to transport the patient, use diazepam, 0.05 mg/kg IV.
- If the bleeding is uncontrollable and life threatening, ligation of the common carotid artery on the affected side is helpful even though bleeding continues. *NOTE:* Ligation of the common carotid artery can result in severe neurologic signs and blindness.

Epistaxis Due to Thrombocytopenia

Can be a severe problem and require emergency treatment.

Rupture of the Longus Capitis Muscle

Can mimic severe guttural pouch hemorrhage but is differentiated on endoscopic examination. Treatment is symptomatic: Keep the affected individual quiet; administer fluids, blood transfusion, and maintain a patent airway.

Ethmoid Hematoma

The initial clinical sign is usually a unilateral blood-tinged nasal discharge. With progression of the hematoma, respiratory noise from partial airway obstruction develops.

Diagnosis

Endoscopic examination usually reveals a dark red/black or even greenish discolored mass in the ethmoid turbinate region. Radiographs are helpful in identifying masses in the paranasal sinus(es).

Treatment

Laser or cryosurgery is generally recommended, although intralesion injections with formalin are also successful. Large ethmoid hematomas require excision of the mass via paranasal sinus surgery.

Exercise-Induced Pulmonary Hemorrhage

Rarely is the bleeding so severe that it results in respiratory distress and death. In some cases of acute death, bleeding is within the thoracic cavity.

Nasal Masses

Rarely are nasal masses (e.g., tumor, granuloma) a cause for emergency treatment; however, they are some of the most common causes of epistaxis and upper respiratory noise/obstruction.

SUGGESTED REFERENCES

Respiratory Distress with Noise

Altmaier K, Morris EA. Dorsal displacement of the soft palate in neonatal foals. Equine Vet J 1993;25(4):329–332.

Mair TS, Lane JG. The differential diagnoses of sudden-onset respiratory distress. Equine Vet Educ 1996;8:131–136.

Traub-Dargatz JL, Ingram JT, Stashak TS, et al. Respiratory stridor associated with polymyopathy suspected to be periodic paralysis in four Quarterhorse foals. J Am Vet Med Assoc 1992;201:83–85.

Bronchointerstitial Pneumonia in Foals

Lakritz J, Wilson D, Berry CR, et al. Bronchointerstitial pneumonia and respiratory distress in young horses: Clinical, clinicopathologic, radiographic, and pathologic findings in 23 cases (1984–1989). J Vet Intern Med 1993;7(5):277–288.

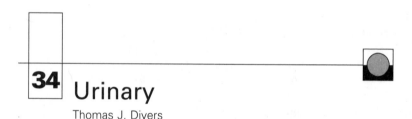

34 Urinary

Thomas J. Divers

Primary urinary tract emergencies in the horse are uncommon; however, when they do occur the disease progress can be fatal if not properly diagnosed and treated. The most common urinary system emergencies are: acute renal failure, discolored urine, lower urinary tract obstruction, and ruptured bladder in the foal and occasionally in the adult.

ACUTE RENAL FAILURE

Acute renal failure (ARF) usually results from nephrotoxic causes or vasomotor nephropathy (e.g., ischemic causes). The most common pathologic finding is acute tubular necrosis.

Nephrotoxic Causes

- Consider aminoglycoside nephrotoxicity if a patient becomes *depressed* while being treated with aminoglycosides or a few days after therapy is discontinued.
- Aminoglycoside-induced renal failure *usually* results in polyuric renal failure and is typically responsive to treatment if diagnosed early.

- Tetracycline-induced renal failure may occur if 20 mg/kg/day or greater is administered (foals appear more resistant to toxic effects).

DIAGNOSIS

History, physical examination, laboratory findings:

Laboratory Findings
- Azotemia, isosthenuria, hyponatremia, hypochloremia
- Azotemia in the horse is best determined by measuring serum creatinine.
  - □ In some cases of ARF, especially those with diarrhea, BUN may remain normal or mildly elevated, but the creatinine level is markedly elevated.
  - □ Prerenal azotemia is best determined by clinical examination, urinalysis and time required for serum creatinine to return to normal after fluid therapy is started (most prerenal azotemia is corrected within 36 hours after initiating fluid therapy). The upper range for creatinine from *prerenal azotemia* is generally *7–8 mg/dl.*
  - □ Suspect renal azotemia if the BUN:creatinine ratio is 10 or less, serum potassium is elevated, urine specific gravity is >1.006 in spite of large volumes of IV fluid therapy, and creatinine does not decline or declines slowly over several days after fluid therapy is started.
  - □ Newborn foals sporadically may have serum creatinine in the 5–8 mg/dl (and sometimes higher) range without other evidence of renal dysfunction. This is most common in foals born to mares with placental dysfunction. The creatinine generally returns to normal in these individuals within 2 days.

Serum potassium and calcium are typically normal or low with ARF, but potassium may be high if the renal failure is oliguric. The finding of hyperkalemia in an individual with acute renal failure suggests a guarded prognosis because it indicates oliguric/anuric renal failure.

TREATMENT

- **General treatment** (see p. 464)
- Specific treatment: Peritoneal or pleural dialysis may be useful in reducing toxic agents although results are variable, and is *rarely* needed.
- Dialysis protocol:
  - □ Monitor electrolyte status.
  - □ Warm lactated Ringer's solution with 1.5% dextrose for peritoneal dialysis
  - □ If no cardiopulmonary abnormalities are detected, dialysis may be administered at 40 ml/kg. After 30–60 minutes, drain fluid. At least 70% of fluid should be recovered.
  - □ In foals, the omentum often interferes with this procedure, making peritoneal dialysis difficult.

Nephropathy

PIGMENT NEPHROPATHY

- Most common after a severe tying-up episode or several milder episodes
- Grossly discolored urine is not a prerequisite for myositis-induced acute renal failure.

- Hemolysis is less likely to result in renal failure than myopathy, although individuals with hemolysis and disseminated intravascular coagulation are at risk for ARF.
- Depression caused by uremia occurs 3–7 days after the tying-up episode or hemolytic crisis.
- Aspartate aminotransferase (AST) measurement helps confirm previous myopathy.

VASOMOTOR NEPHROPATHY

- Any condition predisposing to hypotension and/or release of endogenous pressor agents potentiates hemodynamic-mediated acute renal failure.
- Causes:
  - ☐ Acute blood loss, severe intravascular volume deficits, septic shock, thrombotic episodes, coagulopathies, acute heart failure
- Vasomotor nephropathies may cause severe renal failure with accompanying histologic findings. A diffuse renal cortical or medullary necrosis occasionally occurs.

DIAGNOSIS

- History, physical examination, clinical signs
- Laboratory findings:
  - ☐ Elevated serum creatinine with concurrent low urine specific gravity (<1.020), hematuria, hypochloremia, hyponatremia
  - ☐ Hyperkalemia suggests primary intrinsic renal failure as opposed to prerenal azotemia.

General Treatment Principles for Acute Renal Failure

- Fluid replacement for volume deficits and electrolyte and acid-base correction. 0.9% NaCl is the preferred initial fluid therapy in most cases. Potassium (20 mEq/L) is added after it is apparent that the affected individual is polyuric.
- Monitor serum sodium, chloride, potassium, bicarbonate and correct any abnormalities.
- Assess character of ARF (polyuric [excessive secretion of urine] vs. oliguric [diminished urine secretion]).
  - ☐ Monitor blood pressure (BP) to assess adequacy of volume replacement. If BP remains low despite volume replacement, administer hypertonic saline and/or dobutamine, 5 μg/kg/min, to restore BP and assure adequate glomerular filtration.
  - ☐ *Determine whether patient has oliguric or polyuric renal failure.* If oliguric renal failure is suspected, monitor the packed cell volume (PCV), plasma protein concentration, and central venous pressure (CVP).
  - ☐ To measure CVP, insert a 20-cm Mylar catheter into the jugular vein and down the anterior vena cava. Use a manometer with a baseline at the level of the right atrium. Normal CVP is <8–10 cm H_2O.
- Once volume deficits are corrected and systemic BP restored, treat

the **oliguric** renal failure patient with **dopamine**, 3–7 μg/kg/min IV continuously, **dobutamine**, 2–5 μg/kg/min, and **furosemide**, 1 mg/kg q2h for four treatments. Blood pressure should not increase above normal values (mean 110–120 mm) during the infusion.

- □ Discontinue dopamine within 24–48 hours and furosemide immediately if therapy is successful in converting oliguria to polyuria.
- □ Continue to monitor urine output. If oliguria occurs again, repeat dopamine and furosemide.
- □ Furosemide therapy alone is contraindicated in rhabdomyolysis-induced renal failure.
- □ Aminophylline is administered, 0.5 mg/kg, to improve glomerular filtration rate (GFR) in premature or septic foals with respiratory distress and renal failure.

- **Polyuric** acute renal failure:
  - □ Administer 40–80 ml/kg/day of polyionic fluids (usually 0.9% NaCl with 20 mEq/L KCl) IV until a precipitous drop in serum creatinine occurs.
  - □ Continue with IV fluids at 40–80 ml/kg/day for the next several days until creatinine has returned to normal.
  - □ Furosemide and dopamine are not required in polyuric states.
  - □ If sedation is required, use small doses of xylazine, because it may increase urine production.
  - □ If the patient is anorexic, 50–100 gm of dextrose/liter is added to the IV fluids for calories.

ACUTE SEPTIC NEPHRITIS

Rare in horses other than from *Actinobacillus equuli* nephritis in foals. These foals are usually less than 7 days of age (most are 2 to 4 days old), and many are found dead in the pasture without obvious clinical signs. Overwhelming bacteremia and endotoxemia are the primary concerns with *A. equuli* rather than renal failure. Most infected foals have a low serum IgG concentration.

Leptospira interrogans serogroup *pomona* may cause acute renal failure and/or hematuria in an individual. Fever, leukocytosis, and pyuria without microscopically detectable bacteriuria should raise the index of suspicion for *L. pomona*. Serum titers are very high for *L. pomona* and the other serotypes. Treatment includes IV fluids as recommended for other causes of ARF. Additionally, administer penicillin, 22,000 U/kg IV q6h.

DISCOLORED URINE

This results from bilirubinuria (see pp. 274, 275), hemoglobinuria (see p. 274), myoglobinuria (see p. 356), pyuria, or hematuria (Table 34–1). *The color and consistency of normal adult urine varies greatly because of the amount of mucus in the urine.* The urine of some horses normally contain pigments that cause a red-brown discoloration best seen in urine stained snow.

TABLE 34–1. **Differential Diagnosis of Discolored Urine**

	Hematuria	Hemoglobinuria	Drugs	Bilirubinuria	Myoglobinuria
*Urine Color**	Red—bright or dark	Pink (also red or dark red)	Any color, e.g., orange—rifampin	Dark brown (green foam when shaken in a tube)	Brown to red to black
Consistency	Occasional clumps of blood are seen, and the discoloration is not uniform	Consistent discoloration	Consistent discoloration	Consistent discoloration	Consistent discoloration
Plasma Color	Normal	Usually pink	Variable	Icteric	Usually normal unless anuric
Urine Dipstick—Blood	Almost always positive for both hemolyzed and nonhemolyzed blood	Uniformly strongly positive for hemolyzed blood	Negative	Negative unless secondary renal disease with hemolysis or hematuria	Uniformly strongly positive for hemolyzed blood
Sediment and Cytology of Urine	RBCs and ghost cells	Pigment casts and some secondary RBCs due to tubular disease	Normal	Normal to few RBCs if renal disease	Pigment casts, RBCs due to tubular disease
Laboratory Tests	Variable PCV and protein; MCV may be increased; creatinine is increased if both kidneys sufficiently diseased	Low PCV; normal to high protein; MCV may be increased; increased unconjugated bilirubin	No change	Increased liver enzymes and bilirubin (both conjugated and unconjugated)	Increased creatine kinase; any increase in serum creatinine is a reflection of GFR

*Never use this alone for diagnosis.

Hematuria

Recognized blood clots or a uniform red discolored urine without blood clots. Most frequent causes:

- Urethral hemorrhage—habronemiasis, calculi, idiopathic (male proximal dorsal urethral hemorrhage), urethritis, neoplasia (squamous cell carcinoma most common)
- Bladder—calculi, cystitis, neoplasia, amorphous debris, bleeding diathesis (warfarin toxicity), blister beetle toxicity
- Kidney—calculi, trauma, nephritis, vascular anomaly, parasite migration, neoplasia, glomerulopathy, papillary necrosis, blister beetle, and leptospirosis

Diagnosis

- Signalment, age, duration of hematuria, and the time during urination when hematuria is most pronounced are helpful. Examples:
  - Hematuria after exercise—suspect cystic calculi.
  - Hematuria only at the beginning of urination indicates a urethral lesion.
  - Hematuria observed uniformly throughout urination implicates the bladder or more likely bleeding from the kidney.
  - Hematuria seen only at the end of urination suggests bladder hemorrhage or proximal urethral syndrome in adult males.
- If discolored urine is recognized but clots are not seen, hemoglobinuria, bilirubinuria, or myoglobinuria must be rule-outs.
  - Differentiate using urine dipstick evaluation, PCV, plasma protein, color of plasma, color of mucous membranes, serum chemistries (e.g., CK, AST, gamma-glutamyl transferase [GGT]), and urine sediment examination (presence of RBCs). A few individuals with normal urine produce red/brown spots in snow after urination. This is believed a result of a metabolized plant pigment that does not discolor urine but discolors the snow.
  - Confirm origin of hematuria by physical examination: examine urethra (after tranquilization in males); palpate urethra, bladder, ureters, left kidney. Endoscopy and/or ultrasonography is required. A 1-meter scope is usually sufficient to examine the bladder even in some males. After the instrument is disinfected, the patient is tranquilized for penile relaxation, and the scope is gently passed up the urethra after *lightly* lubricating the *outside* of the scope with sterile K-Y jelly. The mucous membrane of the urethra is generally pale white to pink, although a few small red foci are normal. *Minimal* dilation with air is needed in some cases to move the mucosa away from the tip of the scope. Excessive air causes the individual to strain and the urethral mucosa becomes hyperemic. Hyperemia and tortuous vessels in the urethra near the opening of the accessory sex glands is nearly diagnostic for idiopathic urethral hemorrhage in adult males. Hyperemia throughout the urethra is more consistent with urethritis. Once the endoscope is in the bladder, the ureteral openings can be seen.

Treatment

Emergency treatment is rarely required unless clots are causing urinary obstruction, or rupture of the kidney has occurred, resulting in life-threatening hemorrhage and/or colic. Treatment for life-threatening hemoglobinuria, myoglobinuria, and bilirubinuria are discussed under hemolytic anemia (see p. 284), rhabdomyolysis (see p. 356), and liver failure (see p. 275).

OBSTRUCTION OF THE LOWER URINARY TRACT

Clinical Signs

Hematuria, pollakiuria (frequent urination), dysuria (painful or difficult urination), and tenesmus (ineffectual and painful straining in urinating) are frequently seen. Dribbling of small amounts of urine and signs of colic, agitation, and sweating also occur. Stranguria (slow and painful discharge of urine) is most commonly a result of lower urinary tract obstruction and may occur from acute lower urinary tract infections or neurologic disorders, e.g., herpes myelitis.

General Information on Urinary Obstruction

- Usually caused by urethral calculi or calculi at the trigone of the bladder preventing normal urine voiding
- Rarely caused by blood clots
- Urethral obstruction is more common in males and rarely occurs in individuals less than 1 year of age.
- Urethral obstruction can occur from severe preputial trauma and/or cellulitis (see p. 408).

Diagnosis

- Rectal examination
  - □ Enlarged bladder (individuals with abdominal/intestinal pain may also have bladder distention)
  - □ Cystic calculi can be palpated during rectal examination.
  - □ In males, urethral calculi are frequently palpated percutaneously a few inches below the anus in the perineum.
  - □ In males, the urethra seems painful to palpation, and pulsations and/or swelling of the urethra is detected.
- Passing a urethral catheter (stallion catheter) after tranquilization is helpful.
- Ultrasonography of the perineal region and urethra with a 7.5-MHz scanner can detect calculi and urethral swelling.
- Urethral endoscopy is used although generally not necessary.

Laboratory Tests

Unless bladder rupture is suspected, laboratory tests are typically unnecessary (see next section).

Treatment

- Surgical removal of the stone
- In some cases, the stone is pushed back into the bladder by a urethral catheter during general anesthesia.
- Follow-up examination of the urinary tract is important to determine bladder function (via rectal examination), presence of other stones (ultrasound examination of the urinary tract), urinary tract infection (culture and urinalysis), and renal function (serum creatinine).

RUPTURED BLADDER

Most cases occur in young male foals within the first few days of life (average, 4 days), although it can occur in adults as a result of urinary calculi. Rupture of the bladder or urachus causing uroperitoneum occurs in older foals with urachal abscess, ischemia of the apex of the bladder, prolonged recumbency (e.g., premature foals, botulism, central nervous system disturbances), or from abdominal trauma.

If the urachus ruptures, a significant accumulation of subcutaneous urine causes severe stranguria, subcutaneous swelling, colic, and distress. Differentiate the subcutaneous swelling from a hematoma or septic cellulitis by aspiration and cytology. If urine is found, prompt surgical removal of the urachus is required.

Ruptured Bladder in Foals

Clinical Signs

- Usually seen within the first 2–3 days of life and most common in males
- Stranguria, dysuria, depression, bilaterally symmetric ventral abdominal distention
  - □ Stranguria and dysuria are often misinterpreted as rectal tenesmus. With tenesmus, the rear limbs are positioned further under the body than with stranguria/dysuria.

Diagnosis

- History—generally young males and can occur in females
- Clinical signs
- Laboratory findings
  - □ *Hyponatremia, hypochloremia, hyperkalemia, azotemia*
  - □ Ratio of peritoneal fluid creatinine concentration to serum creatinine is diagnostic of uroperitoneum (> 2:1). With large amounts of peritoneal fluid, e.g., uroperitoneum, it is preferable to perform the abdominocentesis using an 18-gauge needle. A teat cannula creates a large defect in the abdominal wall, and if surgery is not performed within a few hours, urine leaks through the abdominal wall defect into the subcutaneous tissues.

Treatment

- Stabilize acid-base and electrolyte abnormalities before surgery.
  - □ Administer 0.9% NaCl with 5% glucose IV.

☐ Avoid exogenous insulin therapy (to drive potassium into cells) for the hyperkalemia. If significant ECG abnormalities (QRS complexes without P waves) are found, administer 100 ml of 50% dextrose with 0.5 gm calcium borogluconate to raise the endogenous insulin and protect the myocardium.

☐ If severe hyperkalemia and abdominal distention are present, removal of abdominal fluid is beneficial before anesthesia. If the drainage is performed several hours before surgery, subcutaneous leakage of abdominal fluid results if the intraperitoneal catheter is removed.

Surgery

- Usually successful if performed within the first 5 days of life. The surgery is usually not an immediate emergency; electrolyte abnormalities are corrected and in some cases, e.g., severe distention and/or hyperkalemia, the abdominal fluid removed before surgery.
- Induction of anesthesia is best performed by mask induction with isoflurane.
- A second surgery is sometimes required if continued urine leakage from the bladder occurs.
  ☐ It is occasionally beneficial to place an indwelling urethral catheter at surgery for the first 24 hours postoperatively particularly in foals that have more chronic bladder distention before rupture due to other problems (e.g., maladjustment syndrome, prematurity, and so on).

BLADDER RUPTURE IN OLDER NURSING FOALS

This occurs without warning in 4–10-week-old foals. The apex of the bladder is necrotic, resulting in rupture. Affected foals are depressed, have abdominal distention, and may or may *not* have the classic electrolyte abnormalities, hyponatremia, hypochloremia, hyperkalemia seen in younger individuals. Diagnosis is by ultrasound examination and comparison of urine to blood creatinine. Treatment is similar to that for younger individuals, except the urachus and apex of the bladder are removed.

Ruptured Bladder in Adults

- Unusual in the adult for reasons other than urethral calculi.
  ☐ May occur after foaling

Clinical Signs

Difficult to diagnose from clinical signs alone. Depression and anorexia 2 days after the rupture may be the only signs observed. Stranguria may be present.

Diagnosis

- Peripheral blood sample:
  ☐ Azotemia
  ☐ Hyponatremia
  ☐ Hypochloremia
- Abdominal ultrasonography—large volume of slightly echogenic fluid
- Abdominocentesis:

□ Peritoneal fluid creatinine–plasma creatinine ratio (>2:1)
□ Identification of calcium carbonate crystals
- Endoscopy of the bladder is indicated to determine the extent of the tear.

Treatment

- Surgical repair—not needed immediately
  □ Small dorsal tears may not need surgery.
- Drainage of peritoneal fluid. Use indwelling mushroom catheter:
  □ Place at ventralmost aspect of midline.
  □ Clip and aseptically prepare area after local anesthesia.
  □ Make stab incision with No. 20 blade through skin into linea alba.
  □ Introduce 4-inch cannula—confirm presence of fluid.
  □ Use bitch catheter to help direct mushroom catheter into opening created by cannula.
  □ Suture the skin around mushroom catheter after removing bitch catheter. Apply antiseptic cream and keep catheter end clean when not draining; use a small syringe to prevent ascending contamination.
- IV fluids—polyionic fluids at maintenance or slightly greater rate
- Antimicrobial therapy: Trimethoprim/sulfamethoxazole, 20 mg/kg PO q12h.
- Heparin: 100 IU/kg SQ q12h to reduce abdominal adhesions.

PROLAPSE OF THE BLADDER

This may occur as eversion of the bladder or in association with prolapsed vagina. Eversion of the bladder through the urethra occurs in females with severe straining. The mucosal surface of the bladder is obvious, and the ureteral opening may be seen. The ureters may still be patent.

Treatment

- Epidural anesthesia is performed. For a 450-kg mare, 5–7 ml of 2% lidocaine or 80 mg of xylazine diluted with 8 ml of sterile saline is administered with an 18-gauge, 1.5-inch needle.
- Clean the bladder with sterile saline and examine to rule out the possibility of intestinal involvement in the herniated bladder. If part of the bladder is necrotic, remove and suture it.
- Gentle uniform pressure on the bladder is attempted to return the bladder into the abdomen either with or without a sphincterotomy. This is generally difficult because of bladder swelling; general anesthesia and abdominal laparotomy may be required. The bladder is returned to its normal position with a sphincterotomy and laparotomy, using the ligaments of the bladder as a guide for inverting the bladder through the urethra. One liter of warm saline is infused into the bladder to insure repositioning and to check for tears. A Foley catheter with the cuff distended with saline is left in the bladder for 24 hours and prophylactic antibiotics administered.

ACUTE URINARY INCONTINENCE ASSOCIATED WITH FOALING

This occurs because of damage to the bladder muscle, or more commonly from damage to the urethral spincter. If the urethral spincter is lacerated, it is sutured after a Foley catheter is placed in the bladder. If the sphincter is injured but not lacerated, treatment includes:

- Phenylpropanolamine, 1–2 mg/kg PO q12h
- Systemic antimicrobials, e.g., trimethoprim/sulfa

  If the bladder wall (detrusor muscle) is damaged and the bladder is enlarged with no physical obstruction of the urethra, treat the mare with:

  ☐ Bethanechol, 0.03–0.05 mg/kg SQ q8h, or 0.16 mg/kg PO q8h
  ☐ Phenyoxybenzamine, 0.4 mg/kg PO q6h

35 Neonatology; Foal Cardiopulmonary Resuscitation

NEONATOLOGY

Wendy E. Vaala

PHYSICAL EXAMINATION OF THE NEWBORN FOAL

Healthy, full-term foals are precocious neonates that can stand and nurse from the udder within 2 hours of delivery. Vital signs change dramatically within the first 24 hours of life (Table 35–1).

- At 20 minutes of age a normal, healthy foal has an effective suckle reflex, can sit sternal without assistance, and makes attempts to rise.
- A finger inserted in the ear or nostril results in a head shake and grimace reflex.
- A thoracolumbar stimulus performed by briskly running the thumb and forefingers down either side of the foal's thoracolumbar spine elicits gallant attempts to rise, characterized by throwing the front legs forward, lifting the head and neck skyward, and trying to push off with the hindlimbs.
- The foal's heart rate at this age approaches 100 beats/min, and the respiratory rate averages between 40 and 60 breaths/min.
- A newborn foal that displays generalized hypotonia, and an inability to rise, sit sternal, or suckle may be suffering from peripartum asphyxia, in utero acquired septicemia, or prematurity/dysmaturity. A thorough history

TABLE 35–1. **Neonatal Vital Signs During the First 24 Hours**

	Age		
Parameter	<10 Minutes	≤12 Hours	24 Hours
Heart rate (beats/min)	<60	100–120	80–100
Respiratory rate (breaths/min)	40–60	20–40	20–40
Body temperature (°F/°C)	99–102/37–39	99–102/37–39	99–102/37–39

of peripartum events and careful examination of the foal and placenta help distinguish among these differentials.

Placenta. A history of premature separation of placental membranes, prolonged delivery/dystocia, or meconium staining of the foal are periparturient events frequently associated with neonatal asphyxia. A maternal history of prepartum purulent vaginal discharge, precocious udder development and lactation, or evidence of abnormal discoloration of the placenta, particularly in the area of the cervical star, increases the index of suspicion for placentitis and in utero septicemia. A normal placenta should weigh 10%–11% of the foal's birth weight. Examine grossly unusually heavy or light placentas and submit samples for histopathology. Peracute cases of placentitis may produce only generalized edema without grossly obvious areas of infection. Small placentas with large areas of abnormal villi formation have been associated with neonatal dysmaturity. Therefore, histopathologic examination of the placenta is strongly recommended if a neonate shows early signs of compromise.

Prematurity. Foals from abnormally long gestations can show signs of prematurity, although we often use the term "dysmaturity" rather than prematurity. Unusually short (≤320 days') or abnormally long (≥360 days') gestation has been associated with the birth of foals showing signs of prematurity, including:

- Small body size
- Fine, silky hair coat
- Generalized weakness
- Increased passive range of limb motion
- Flexor tendon and periarticular ligament laxity
- Incomplete cuboidal bone ossification
- Domed forehead
- Floppy ears
- Inability to regulate body temperature

Mucous Membranes and Sclera

A healthy neonate's **mucous membranes** are pale pink with a capillary refill time of ≤2 seconds. Pale mucous membranes suggest anemia.

Gray or slightly blue mucous membranes indicate shock, poor peripheral perfusion, and/or hypoxia. Cyanosis appears only after $PaO_2 < 35$–40 mm Hg; tissue damage begins when $PaO_2 < 60$ mm Hg. Do not rely on mucous membrane color to diagnose hypoxemia.

Increased respiratory rate and effort are clinical signs of pulmonary disease. Of these two signs, increased effort is the most reliable, since foals suffering from central respiratory depression secondary to hypoxia, hypothermia, hypoglycemia, or hypocalcemia may not increase their respiratory rate appropriately in response to lung pathology.

Hyperemic, injected mucous membranes and hyperemic coronary bands indicate septicemia/endotoxemia. Petechiae on oral mucous membranes or inside the pinnae are associated with sepsis. Icteric mucous membranes are observed with hemolysis, septicemia, equine herpesvirus infection (EHV-1), and liver disease.

The **sclera** should be white with only faint vessels apparent. Marked injection is indicative of septicemia. Prominent scleral hemorrhages are observed following birth trauma.

Cardiovascular System

A neonate's **cardiac rhythm** should be regular. However, a sinus arrhythmia may be present for a few hours postpartum. **Heart rate** averages between 70 and 100 beats/min during the first week of life.

Bradycardia. Associated with severe

- Hypoglycemia—use rapid blood glucose strips to diagnose
- Hypothermia—apply heat, concentrating on the thorax
- Hyperkalemia—most common with anuric renal failure or ruptured bladder (see pp. 462 and 469)
- Asphyxia—hypertonic dextrose is not indicated in asphyxiated foals unless hypoglycemia is documented because hyperglycemia further increases cerebral acidosis.

Tachycardia. Observed with

- Sepsis—fever often absent at the time of examination
- Pain—abdominal or musculoskeletal in origin
- Stress
- Hypocalcemia—can be seen with severe asphyxia

Murmurs. Those associated with a patent ductus arteriosus (PDA) may persist for several days after birth. The typical PDA murmur is a continuous machinery murmur or a holosystolic murmur heard loudest over left side of the heart base. Soft, blowing murmurs are usually associated with blood flow and are exacerbated by anemia. **Persistent murmurs** that fail to improve with time or are associated with exercise intolerance and hypoxemia may be due to a persistent PDA, patent foramen ovale, ventral septal defect, or other congenital heart disease. Such foals are candidates for an echocardiogram.

Peripheral Pulses. Should be easy to palpate. The great metatarsal artery is the easiest site to use. Bounding, hyperkinetic pulses are associated with early stages of compensated sepsis. Weak, thready pulses herald cardiovascular collapse and shock.

Respiratory System

A newborn foal's resting **respiratory rate** averages between 20 and 40 breaths/min. Because of the foal's thin chest wall and relatively rapid respiratory rate, thoracic auscultation often reveals air movement throughout the chest even when there is lung pathology, especially diffuse interstitial disease. Moist end-expiratory crackles are commonly heard after birth as the foal expands its lungs. Unusually quiet lung sounds immediately after birth are compatible with incomplete alveolar inflation and lung atelectasis. Marked areas of ventral dullness on auscultation and percussion indicate areas of consolidation, atelectasis, or pleural effusion. Breathing effort should be minimal once the lung liquid has been reabsorbed.

Respiratory distress. Exacerbated by recumbency and characterized by

- Nostril flare
- Expiratory grunting
- Rib retractions
- Increased abdominal effort
- Paradoxic respiration (chest wall collapses during inspiration)

Apnea. Apnea and unusually slow or irregular respirations are abnormal and have been associated with

- Electrolyte disturbances, most frequently hypocalcemia
- Hypoglycemia
- Hypothermia
- Central respiratory depression secondary to asphyxia
- Prematurity

Thoracic radiography and **ultrasonography** help identify pulmonary consolidation and abscessation and pleural effusion. **Arterial blood gas** analysis provides the most accurate assessment of pulmonary function. These samples are most easily collected from the metatarsal artery. The artery can be used for repeated sampling. A small subcutaneous intradermal bleb of 2% lidocaine without epinephrine makes collection easier in foals hypersensitive to arteriopuncture.

Abdominal Examination

Abdominal Auscultation. Should reveal borborygmi bilaterally. Ingestion of colostrum and the act of suckling itself enhance gastrointestinal motility and meconium/manure passage.

Meconium. The first manure a foal passes, meconium, is composed of cellular debris, intestinal secretions, and amniotic fluid ingested by the fetus. It is dark, black-brown, or gray and is firm, pellet-like, or pasty in consistency. All meconium should be passed within 24 hours of birth and is followed by softer, tan "milk feces." Absence of manure passage can be associated with

- atresia coli
- meconium impaction
- ileus
- intestinal obstruction

Due to the foal's thin body wall, distention of small and/or large intestine results in visible, generalized abdominal enlargement. Simultaneous auscultation/percussion of tympany identifies a gas-distended viscus. Tight, tympanic, dorsally distributed distention is compatible with gas accumulation. Turgid, ventrally distributed, pendulous distention can be seen with uroperitoneum and peritoneal effusion.

Causes of Colic (With or Without Abdominal Distention)

- Meconium/fecal impaction—digital examination usually detects the impaction, although radiographs are needed to diagnose more proximal impactions.

- Enteritis (see p. 217)
- Ileus (see p. 156)
- Intussusception (see p. 175)—may be seen with ultrasound
- Gastroduodenal ulceration—classic signs include rolling onto back, sialorrhea, and odontoprisis (grinding teeth)
- Peritonitis—differentials include ruptured duodenal ulcer, enteritis, urachal abscess
- Intestinal volvulus—severe pain that may progress to depression
- Uroperitoneum—large amount of free fluid on sonogram, peritoneal creatinine at least two times serum creatinine (see p. 469)

Diagnostic Aids

Nasogastric Tube Intubation. Performed to check for reflux. **Reflux** is associated with ileus due to ischemic hypoxic gut damage, peritonitis, or enteritis or obstruction due to intussusception, impaction, volvulus, or duodenal stricture. Occult blood-positive reflux is associated with hypoxic gut damage and enteritis due to *Clostridia* sp. and occasionally *Salmonella* sp. If severe gastric distention is present, passage of the tube through the cardia may be impeded. Lidocaine applied to the nasogastric tube or injected down the tube may help relax the esophagus and facilitate entry into the stomach.

Abdominal Radiography. Can determine the location, but not necessarily the cause, of gas or fluid distention. Gaseous distention of the small intestine characterized by gas/fluid interfaces within the lumen can be observed in foals with ileus due to enteritis, peritonitis, hypoxic gut damage, and small intestinal obstruction (see p. 225). Concurrent large bowel distention is frequently associated with ileus due to hypoxia or enteritis. Primary large bowel distention occurs with obstruction due to meconium retention, volvulus, and/or displacement.

Radiograph settings using a portable machine and DuPont-Quanta 3 Screen:

- Setting for neonate: 20 MA/12–16 MAS/80 KVP

Stationary machine: using DuPont-Quanta 3 screen with 5:1 grid:

- Setting for neonate: 1000 MA/25 MAS/80 KVP
- Setting for 2-month-old: 1000 MA/20 MAS/80 KVP

Contrast Studies. Using barium enemas (1 liter barium mixed with warm water and administered through a cuffed Foley catheter inserted in the rectum), these studies help identify meconium impactions. Upper GI contrast radiography is used to document delayed gastric emptying and prolonged transit times observed with ileus and obstructions and to identify small intestinal stricture formation associated with gastroduodenal ulcer disease.

Contrast radiography of the upper gastrointestinal tract is performed by administering **5 ml/kg barium sulfate suspension** via nasogastric tube followed by serial radiographs obtained at 1, 15, and 30 minutes and 2-hour intervals. Contrast radiography is used to demonstrate gastrointestinal obstruction and/or ulceration. Normal findings:

- Barium begins leaving the stomach immediately and is gone after 1.5–2 hours.

- The cecum fills by 2 hours.
- The transverse colon fills by 3 hours.

Transabdominal Ultrasonography. Permits evaluation of

- Small intestinal motility
- Bowel wall thickness
- Degree of gastric or small or large intestinal distention
- Volume and character of peritoneal fluid

Healthy foals have flaccid, motile, fluid-filled loops of small intestine, with wall thickness ≤ 0.4 mm and neglible amounts of peritoneal fluid. Round, fluid-distended loops of bowel can be seen with ileus, enteritis, and small bowel obstructive disease. Enteritis results in a generalized increase in bowel wall thickness and edema. Severe hypoxic-ischemic bowel disease can produce focal increases in bowel wall thickness with or without intramural gas accumulation (i.e., intestinalis pneumatosis). Small intestinal intussusceptions appear as dough-nut-shaped patterns caused by the telescoping of one segment of bowel into another. An excessive volume of clear, nonechogenic peritoneal fluid is compatible with uroperitoneum. An increase in peritoneal fluid echogenicity is associated with increased cellularity as seen with peritonitis or ruptured abdominal viscus.

Abdominocentesis. Used to obtain peritoneal fluid for analysis and cytology. The procedure is best performed with ultrasound guidance using an 18-gauge needle or a teat cannula. Peritoneal fluid with an increased nucleated cell count and protein concentration is consistent with peritonitis. Peritoneal fluid with a creatinine concentration greater than twice serum creatinine concentration is diagnostic for uroperitoneum. If there is distended small intestine, abdominocentesis may result in bowel perforation and peritonitis.

Gastroscopy. Documents gastroduodenal ulceration. The foal should be fasted for a minimum of 3–6 hours before gastroscopy to ensure adequate gastric emptying.

Urogenital System

Urination

Time to first urination is approximately 8 hours, with fillies taking slightly longer than colts to void for the first time. Due to a persistent frenulum, some colts do not drop their penis to urinate for the first week following birth. Observe urination closely to be certain the foal does not have a **patent urachus,** in which case urine drips from the umbilicus.

Healthy, well-hydrated foals urinate frequently, often after nursing. The **urine specific gravity** is low in nursing foals (1.001–1.025) due to the high-volume liquid diet and relative renal immaturity. Foals suffering from peripartum asphyxia may exhibit oliguria due to decreased renal blood flow and urine production. Dysuria can be observed with uroperitoneum, urachitis, patent urachus, or urachal diverticulum.

A ruptured bladder can occur during birth owing to trauma or postpartum associated with cystitis, umbilical remnant infection, or frequent lifting of recumbent foals. Signs include:

- Decreased urination
- Straining to urinate
- Pendulous, fluid-filled abdominal distention
- Mild abdominal malaise and depression

Large amounts of free fluid on sonogram, peritoneal fluid creatinine at least two times serum creatinine. Ruptured ureter(s) or urachus (subcutaneous or intra-abdominal) causes a postrenal azotemia.

Umbilicus

Examine the **umbilical stump** for signs of infection characterized by thickening or abnormal discharge. Transabdominal ultrasound is used to measure internal umbilical remnants. Normal diameter measurements:

- Umbilical vein at external stump ≤ 1 cm
- Umbilical vein at liver ≤ 1 cm
- Umbilical artery at bladder ≤ 1 cm
- Umbilical arteries and urachus < 2.5 cm

Palpate the umbilicus, inguinal region, and scrotum (in colts) for congenital hernias. The testes may not be descended at birth.

Ophthalmic Examination

- **A pupillary light response** is present and is more sluggish than in the adult.
- Often, a consistent menace response is not present until 2–3 weeks of age.
- Ventral medial strabismus is common.
- Examine the foal's eyes for corneal cloudiness, congenital cataracts, or entropion.
- Ophthalmic examination may reveal a persistent hyaloid artery remnant coursing from the optic disc to spread on the posterior lens capsule, often resembling a spider's web. Suture lines frequently can be seen in the center of the lens.
- Examine the retina for signs of detachment and hemorrhage. Scleral hemorrhage is associated with birth trauma.

Neurologic Evaluation

Healthy foals are bright, alert, and very responsive to touch and sound. While being restrained in a standing position, foals often alternate between periods of hyperactivity and struggling and episodes of sudden, complete relaxation (flopping). Foals should stand with an erect, angular head and neck carriage and a basewide stance in front. Their gait is exaggerated. **Limb reflexes** are increased. When recumbent, foals have strong resting extensor tone and a crossed extensor reflex that exists for up to 1 month of age. Foals normally spend about 50% of their time sleeping. When sound asleep, normal foals may be extremely difficult to arouse and may exhibit rapid eye movement, limb twitching, and irregular breathing patterns.

Neurologic Disease

The most common cause of neurologic disease in the newborn foal is peripartum hypoxic damage. Cerebral and brain stem edema from **hypoxic-ischemic encephalopathy** can produce

- Loss of menace response; central blindness
- Fixed, dilated pupils
- Nystagmus
- Jittery behavior
- Seizure activity ranging from grand mal clonic seizures to tonic posturing, extensor rigidity, and focal seizures
- Stuporous attitude, hypotonia
- Coma

Causes of Neonatal Seizures

- Hepatoencephalopathy—unusual
- Congenital malformations
- Head trauma—cerebrospinal fluid (CSF) aspirate may be indicated. Treatment with mannitol unless there is severe bleeding as suggested by CSF fluid. Dexamethasone, 2–4 mg/kg, may be helpful early in the course of the cerebral ischemia. Administer dimethyl sulfoxide (DMSO), 1 gm/kg IV, diluted in 1 liter of lactated Ringer's solution q12 or 24h.
- Hypoxia—ischemic encephalopathy—do not administer hypertonic dextrose or calcium. Hypertonic dextrose may increase cellular lactic acidosis and calcium may increase arterial tone and decrease cerebral perfusion and/or cause enhanced cell toxicity. Administer oxygen and improve cardiac function, polyionic crystalloids, colloids (plasma), and positive inotropes, e.g., dobutamine, 2–10 μg/kg/min, to normalize arterial pressure with hypoxia, and/or head trauma. Ventilation may be needed to maintain $PaCO_2$ low normal to low to decrease cerebral venous dilatation.
- Meningitis—In addition to antibiotics and other supportive therapy, pentoxifylline, 8.4 mg/kg q12h, and a single dose of dexamethasone, 1–4 mg/kg IV, may be beneficial.
- Hypoglycemia—see p. 488
- Hypocalcemia—administer 1–2 ml/kg of 10% calcium gluconate, 9–18 mg Ca^{++}/kg, slowly IV over 5–10 minutes. Slow or stop infusion if bradycardia develops. Follow with a maintenance infusion of calcium: 5 ml/kg/day of 10% calcium gluconate.
- Hyponatremia—hypertonic saline 1 mg/kg repeated dose administration every 15 minutes until serum Na^+ is >125 mEq/L **but** <135 mEq/L.
- Toxins—e.g., aminophylline

Musculoskeletal System

Examine the foal's **musculoskeletal system**, including mandible, limbs, and ribs, for fractures due to birth trauma. Fractured ribs are often difficult to detect but frequently produce a clicking sound on auscultation, heard in synchrony with respiration. Keep foals with fractured ribs quiet, with the affected side down. Foals normally have a mild carpal and fetlock valgus conformation in front. Examine limbs for more severe angular and flexural deformities. Palpate joints and physes for signs of swelling and heat (see p. 334).

Dysmaturity/Prematurity. Musculoskeletal signs:

- Increased passive range of joint motion
- Periarticular ligament and flexor tendon laxity
- Incomplete cuboidal bone ossification (detectable only on radiographs) of carpus and tarsus. If severe, restrict exercise and apply a cylinder cast to protect the incompletely ossified bones.

Severe Flexor Tendon Laxity. Treatment includes:

- Controlled exercise
- Shoes with heel extension
- Light protective wraps if weight bearing results in trauma to heel bulbs and fetlock
- If incomplete cuboidal bone ossification is severe, the foal may require rigid support using sleeve casts in addition to stall confinement and corrective shoeing.

Septic Arthritis Signs
- Lameness
- Fever
- Painful, warm joint effusion accompanied by marked leukocytosis and hyperfibrinogenemia
- Treat with joint lavage using balanced electrolyte solution with 10–20 gm DMSO added to one liter, systemic antibiotics, low-dose flunixin meglumine (Banamine) 0.25 mg/kg IV q8h or carprofen, 1.4 mg/kg PO q24h.

Septic Osteomyelitis
- Variable lameness
- Fever
- Painful swelling over physis or epiphysis proximal to joint, with or without sympathetic joint effusion
- Radiographic evidence of periosteal osteolytic and proliferative changes
- Leukocytosis and hyperfibrinogenemia usually accompany the condition.
- Treat with long-term antibiotic therapy; aspirate physis for culture and sensitivity; conservative use of nonsteroidal drugs to provide analgesia and decrease inflammation. Support unaffected limbs.

Limb Contracture. Can involve proximal (carpus, tarsus) or more distal (fetlocks, pasterns) joints. Tendon contracture has been associated with in utero malpositioning, toxins, and neonatal hypothyroidism. Therapy for **contracted tendons** includes physical therapy, systemic analgesics, splinting, casting, controlled exercise to prevent extensor tendon rupture, and IV oxytetracycline, 1–3 gm IV q24–36h for maximum of three doses. Evaluate serum creatinine pre/post treatment.

Nursing Behavior

A healthy foal **consumes between 15% and 30% of its body weight in milk daily**, with an average weight gain of 1–2 pounds per day. Foals nurse at least several times an hour. Udder distention in the mare is one of the earliest signs of a "fading foal" that is no longer nursing effectively. Milk seen dripping from the nose following nursing may be due to

- Cleft palate
- Subepiglottic cyst
- Dorsal displacement of the soft palate
- Generalized weakness due to sepsis; dysmaturity, peripartum hypoxia
- Dysphagia associated with dysmaturity, peripartum hypoxia
- White muscle disease

Catheterization and Blood Sampling

The jugular vein is the most common site for venipuncture in the awake, active foal. In more depressed foals the saphenous and cephalic veins can be used. Sites for arterial blood gas sampling include the great metatarsal (first choice), brachial, femoral, and facial arteries.

GENERALIZED WEAKNESS, LOSS OF SUCKLE

The most common causes of weakness and reluctance to suckle in newborn foals are

- Septicemia
- Peripartum asphyxia
- Prematurity/dysmaturity

Septicemia

The leading cause of neonatal foal morbidity and mortality; most commonly associated with gram-negative bacterial infection and endotoxemia. Sepsis is the result of overactivation of the immune system following exposure to microbial toxins. During septicemia an uncontrolled release of endogenous mediators (e.g., endotoxin, tumor necrosis factor) precipitates a cascade of metabolic and hemodynamic changes that culminate in multiple organ system failure. As septic shock advances, the patient dies from a combination of cardiopulmonary failure, generalized coagulopathies, complete disruption of metabolic pathways, and loss of vascular endothelial integrity throughout the body.

The organisms most commonly associated with foal septicemia include *Escherichia coli, Actinobacillus, Pasteurella, Klebsiella, Salmonella,* and *Streptococci.* Anaerobic infections with *Clostridia* sp. occur less frequently and are usually associated with colic and severe, often hemorrhagic, diarrhea or reflux within the first week of life.

Clinical Signs/Diagnosis

The spectrum of clinical signs observed during sepsis depends on the integrity of the host's immune system, the duration of illness, and severity of the infection.

SIGNS DURING EARLY HYPERDYNAMIC PHASES OF SEPSIS

- Lethargy
- Loss of suckle

- Hyperemic, injected mucous membranes and sclera
- Hyperemic coronary bands
- Petechiae inside pinnae and on oral mucosa
- Decreased capillary refill time
- Tachycardia, increased cardiac output, hyperkinetic bounding pulses
- Tachypnea
- Variable body temperature
- Extremities often still warm
- Foal still responsive

SIGNS OBSERVED DURING ADVANCED UNCOMPENSATED SEPTIC SHOCK

- Depression
- Profound weakness; recumbency
- Dehydration
- Severe moribund hypotension
- Decreased cardiac output, tachycardia, cold extremities, thready peripheral pulses
- Prolonged capillary refill time
- Oliguria
- Hypothermia
- Respiratory compromise: tachypnea, dyspnea, hypoxemia, cyanosis

LOCALIZED SITES OF INFECTION: SPECIFIC SIGNS

- **Pneumonia, pleuritis:** Tachypnea, dyspnea, fever, abnormal lung sounds, ventral dullness, and friction rubs with pleural effusion
- **Meningitis:** Seizures, stupor, opisthotonos
- **Hepatitis:** Icterus
- **Nephritis:** Variable urine production, proteinuria
- **Peritonitis/enteritis:** Colic, ileus, diarrhea, abdominal distention
- **Synovitis:** Painful, warm joint distention, lameness, fever
- **Physeal/epiphyseal osteomyelitis:** Variable joint distention, localized pain over epiphysis/physis, lameness, fever
- **Uveitis:** Blepharospasm, miosis, hypopyon, epiphora
- **Omphalitis:** Variable enlargement of umbilical remnant, ± umbilical discharge, fever

Clinical Pathology

- **Leukopenia**, neutropenia (WBC ≤ 5000/μl, neutrophils ≤ 4000/μl), elevated band neutrophil count (bands ≥ 50-100/μl). Neutrophils show toxic changes (toxic granules; hyposegmentation).
- **Fibrinogen** concentration normal with acute sepsis. Fibrinogen increases in response to inflammation over 48–72 hours. Hyperfibrinogenemia in a newborn foal indicates chronicity and suggests in utero infection.
- **Hemoconcentration** due to poor nursing
- **Hypoglycemia** (glucose < 60 mg/dl) due to anorexia and acute bacteremia
- **Hypogammaglobulinemia** due to failure to absorb colostral antibodies and/or increased protein catabolism due to sepsis. Normal foals have

serum [IgG] > 800 mg/dl. Partial failure of passive transfer (FPT): IgG between 200 and 800 mg/dl. Complete FPT: IgG < 200 mg/dl

- **Hyperbilirubinemia** due to a combination of sepsis, induced hemolysis, and decreased hepatic function
- **Lipemia** resulting in opalescent serum due to impaired lipid clearance
- **Azotemia**—Creatinine > 3.0–3.5 mg/dl associated with dehydration, renal ischemia, and direct renal damage
- **Hypoxemia**—PaO_2 ≤ 60 mm Hg, associated with ventilation/perfusion mismatching, pulmonary hypertension, and decreasing cardiac output
- **Acidosis**—arterial pH < 7.35, HCO_3 ≤ 23 mEq/L due to poor peripheral perfusion and anaerobic metabolism

Other Diagnostic Aids

Culture. Blood, synovial fluid, cerebrospinal fluid, peritoneal fluid, urine. Tracheal aspirates, although useful in foals with pneumonia, are often too stressful to perform in septic neonates with severe respiratory distress.

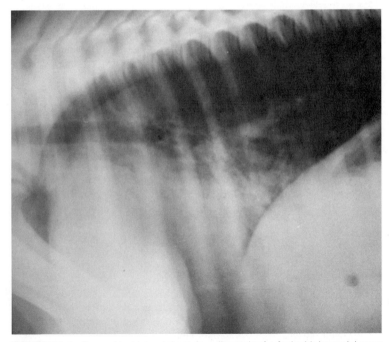

FIGURE 35–1. Recumbent lateral thoracic radiograph of a foal with bacterial pneumonia. The radiograph demonstrates a marked alveolar infiltrate involving the caudal and ventral lung fields, compatible with consolidation secondary to bronchopneumonia.

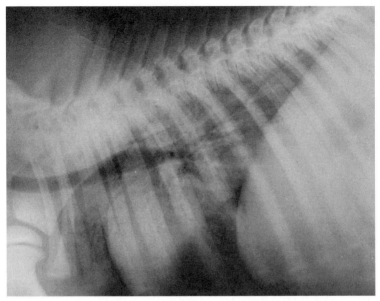

FIGURE 35–2. Recumbent lateral thoracic radiograph of a 24-hour-old foal that was the result of a pregnancy complicated by severe bacterial placentitis. The radiograph demonstrates an interstitial pattern most pronounced in the caudodorsal lung fields.

Radiographs

Take thoracic radiographs with the foal in lateral recumbency and the forelegs pulled forward to improve evaluation of the cranioventral lung fields.

- **Bacterial bronchopneumonia** is associated commonly with an alveolar pattern and air bronchograms observed in the cranioventral lung fields (Fig. 35–1). Acute bacterial pneumonia can also present as diffuse interstitial disease.
- Viral pneumonia is characterized by a diffuse interstitial pattern (Fig. 35–2).
- Aspiration pneumonia is associated with caudoventral and cranioventral infiltrates.
- Surfactant deficiency and **hyaline membrane** formation produce a diffuse, ground-glass appearance to the lung, with prominent air bronchograms (Fig. 35–3).

Serial **radiographs of swollen joints or painful physes** at a minimum of 5-day intervals are recommended to detect signs of articular damage and osteomyelitis.

Plain **abdominal radiographs** can help identify the location of gas distention. Ileus associated with **enteritis** or **peritonitis** is associated with generalized, mild to moderate distention of small and large intestine.

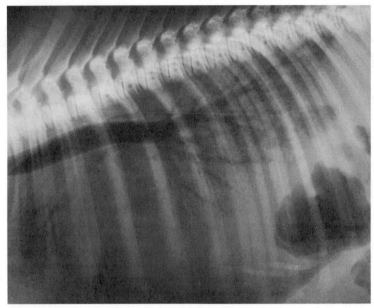

FIGURE 35–3. Recumbent lateral thoracic radiograph of a premature foal that was the result of a cesarean section and 322-day gestation. A diffuse alveolar pattern is seen in all lung fields, compatible with diffuse pulmonary atelectasis.

OTHER DIFFERENTIAL RULE-OUTS FOR GENERALIZED WEAKNESS

- **Neonatal maladjustment syndrome:** Behavior changes, loss of suckle and dam recognition, seizures
- **Neonatal isoerythrolysis:** Icterus, hemolysis, anemia, hemoglobinuria
- **Ruptured bladder:** Abdominal distention, dysuria, hyponatremia, hypochloremia, hyperkalemia, azotemia
- **Meconium impaction:** Colic, straining to defecate, tail flagging
- **Prematurity/dysmaturity:** Small body size, silky hair coat, tendon and joint laxity, domed forehead, floppy ears
- **Tyzzer disease:** Icterus, markedly elevated concentration of hepatocellular enzymes

General Therapy for Septicemia

CARDIOVASCULAR SUPPORT

Fluid Therapy

- Crystalloids—20–40 ml/kg/h to treat severe hypovolemia/hypotension. Balanced electrolyte solutions are optimal for rapid rehydration. Avoid dextrose-containing fluids as the primary rehydrating fluid to avoid severe hyperglycemia.

- 5–8 ml/kg/h maintenance rate. Balanced electrolyte solutions with or without 2.5–5.0% dextrose can be used for maintenance fluid therapy.
- Monitor BP (goal, > 70 mm Hg), central venous pressure (CVP) (goal, 2–6 cm H_2O), urine output, heart rate (HR), peripheral pulses, and respiratory function.
- Plasma may be required to maintain oncotic pressure and intravascular fluid volume. Minimum volume to administer is 20 ml/kg over 60 minutes.
- Volume expansion alone may be sufficient to correct mild to moderate metabolic acidosis. Severe acidosis requires bicarbonate supplementation. Prefer isotonic (1.3%) solutions (150 mEq $NaHCO_3$/L). Ensure adequate ventilation before administering bicarbonate. Rapid infusions may induce respiratory or CNS acidosis.

Sepsis-induced hypotension can be difficult to reverse, because foals appear to be less responsive to adrenergic drugs. **Treatment** recommendations in suggested order of use:

1. Isotonic fluids as indicated above
2. **Dopamine:** 2–10 μg/kg/min continuous infusion; low doses stimulate dopaminergic receptors and improve renal blood flow. Moderate doses stimulate β-adrenergic receptors and support cardiac function. High doses (>10–12 μg/kg/min) produce α- and β-adrenergic effects with tachycardia (if HR increases >50%, therapy should be slowed), increased blood pressure, and reduced splanchnic perfusion and urine output. Titrate dose for each patient.
3. **Dobutamine:** 2–15 μg/kg/min continuous infusion; used in patients with adequate volume expansion as a β-adrenergic, inotropic agent to improve cardiac output and O_2 delivery. Titrate dose to effect. Discontinue if severe tachycardia (>50% increase) or hypertension develops.
4. For unresponsive, severe hypotension:

   □ **Norepinephrine:** 0.1–3.0 mg/kg/min
   □ **Epinephrine:** 0.1–1.0 mg/kg/min
   □ **Phenylephrine:** 9–20 mg/kg/min
   □ **New methylene blue:** 2 mg/kg IV bolus

RESPIRATORY SUPPORT

The aim of therapy is to minimize ventilation/perfusion mismatching.

- **Cautious fluid therapy** to maintain adequate left ventricular and atrial pressure to promote more uniform lung perfusion
- **Frequent repositioning** of foal's thorax to reduce dependent lung atelectasis and development of pulmonary edema. Encourage sternal recumbency and stimulate periodic deep breathing. "Coupage" the thorax with cupped hands to stimulate a cough.
- **Intranasal (IN) humidified O_2 therapy** to treat hypoxemia (PaO_2 ≤ 70 mm Hg) if ventilation is adequate. Use O_2 flows of 2–10 L/min (3 L/min provides approximately 30% FIO_2; 10 L/min provides approximately 50% FIO_2). Administered via an oxygen cannula positioned in the nasal passage, with the end of the cannula at the level of the medial

canthus of the foal's eye. Tape or suture nasal cannula in place. Oxygen tubes in both nostrils may be used to increase positive airway pressure.

- **Mechanical positive-pressure ventilation** (PPV) to prevent alveolar collapse, reduce respiratory muscle fatigue, and address increased O_2 consumption associated with sepsis. Positive end-expiratory pressure (**PEEP**) (8–15 cm H_2O) is required to counteract the increased tissue pressure of interstitial edema compressing respiratory bronchioles. **PPV** is indicated if intranasal (IN) oxygen therapy alone fails to correct hypoxemia and/or $PaCO_2 \geq 65$ mm Hg. Peak airway pressure should be kept at a minimum level and <30 cm H_2O to prevent barotrauma even if $PaCO_2$ remains elevated (permissive hypercapnia). Oxygen concentration should be reduced to $<50\%$ by day 2. Prolonged oxygen at $>50\%$ may result in oxygen toxicity and/or *collapse of poorly ventilated alveoli.*
- **Caffeine** administration to treat abnormally slow respiratory rate and respiratory acidosis secondary to central respiratory center depression. Administer 10 mg/kg PO as a loading dose, followed by 2.5–3 mg/kg PO once daily as a maintenance dose. Therapeutic trough serum concentration is 5–25 μg/ml. Toxicity is associated with concentrations greater than 40–50 μg/ml.

NUTRITIONAL SUPPORT

- **Hypoglycemia** is treated initially with a glucose infusion best administered as a constant infusion using a 5% or 10% solution at a rate of 4–8 mg/kg/min. Using this rate, a 50-kg foal would receive 120–240 ml of 10% dextrose/hour. Once hypoglycemia is corrected, a decision must be made regarding long-term nutritional support.
- **Caloric requirements:** A healthy foal consumes 15%–25% of its body weight (BW) daily in milk, which equals 100–120 kcal/kg/day. Sepsis and fever may increase caloric requirements to 150 kcal/kg/day.
- **Enteral feeding:** Use mare's milk, foal milk replacer, or goat's milk. The goal is **15%–25% of BW/day in milk administered in small volumes every 2–3 hours.** If GI function is questionable, begin enteral feedings cautiously at 5%–10% of foal's BW/day. Supplement with parenteral nutrition if $< 10\%$ of BW in milk is fed daily for ≥ 2 consecutive days. (**Do not feed foals that are generally hypotensive or hypothermic.**)
- **Parenteral nutrition:** Solutions are hypertonic and must be administered continuously, using large peripheral veins and long catheters (≥ 5 inches long) at precise flow rates. Use infusion pumps, dial-a-flow regulators, or buretrols/solution sets to administer total parenteral nutrition (TPN). Monitor blood for hyper/hypoglycemia and check urine for glucosuria to help regulate amount of glucose delivered. Monitor serum for lipemia. Monitor PCV/total protein (TP) for signs of dehydration.

Components of Parenteral Nutrition

- **50% dextrose**
- **8.5 or 10% amino acids**
- **10 or 20% lipids**

Daily caloric requirements should be met primarily by lipids and glucose.

Lipids should contribute ≤ 50% nonprotein calories. To ensure the amino acids are used for structural protein and not catabolized for energy, the ratio of non protein calories: grams of nitrogen should be maintained between 100 and 200.

Caloric Density

- Lipids = 9–11 kcal/gm
- Carbohydrate (glucose) = 3.4 kcal/gm
- Protein (amino acids) = 4.0 kcal/gm

Starting formula for parenteral nutrition:

- 10 gm/kg/day of dextrose
- 2 gm/kg/day of amino acids
- 1 gm/kg/day of lipids
- 5–10 ml/day of multivitamins
- Add trace minerals if foal requires prolonged parenteral nutritional support.
- Potassium chloride can also be added to the parenteral formula.

When first starting TPN, begin at one third of the desired flow rate. Check blood for lipemia and blood/urine for hyperglycemia (blood glucose > 180 mg/dl) at 3–4 hour intervals and increase flow rate by one third until final rate is achieved. **Sample calculation for 50-kg foal:**

- **Dextrose** = 10 gm/kg/day = 500 gm = 1 L of 50% dextrose
- **Amino acids** = 2 gm/kg/day = 100 gm = 1 L of 10% amino acids
- **Lipids** = 1 gm/kg/day = 50 gm = 0.5 L of 10% lipids
- **Total volume** = 2.5 L of TPN administered over 24 hours at 140 ml/h.

Begin TPN at 45 ml/h. Slowly increase rate every 3–4 hours by 45–50 ml until 140 ml/h is reached. Increase TPN flow to target rate provided blood glucose concentration is ≤ 180 mg/dl and serum is not lipemic.

Antibiotic Therapy. Broad-spectrum, bactericidal antibiotics are indicated. Administer for a minimum of 10–14 days provided no localized areas of infection develop. Specific sites of infection (e.g., pneumonia, meningitis, arthritis/osteomyelitis) require prolonged antibiotic therapy. Penicillin and aminoglycoside are a popular combination that provides coverage against gram-positive and gram-negative aerobes and anaerobes. Antibiotic dosages:

- Penicillin: 15,000–30,000 U/kg IV q6h
- Amikacin: 6.6 mg/kg IV/IM q8h, or 25–30 mg/kg IV q24h (preferred)
- Gentamicin: 1–2 mg/kg IV/IM q6–8h, or 6.6 mg/kg IV q24h (preferred). More nephrotoxic than amikacin in very young foals, use cautiously only in well-hydrated foals. Many gram-negative organisms may be resistant to gentamicin; therefore, it is not considered first-line treatment in septicemia.
- Ceftiofur: 2–10 mg/kg IV q6–8h; less nephrotoxic; must be administered frequently if IV route is used: 2–5 mg/kg IM q12h
- Ticarcillin/clavulanic acid: 50–75 mg/kg IV q6h; less nephrotoxic
- Trimethoprim/sulfa: 25–35 mg/kg PO q12h; do not use with uncertain GI function. Many gram-negative organisms may be resistant.
- Third-generation cephalosporins if meningitis is suspected: Cefotaxime, 50 mg/kg IV q6–8h

- Imipenem—cilastatin sodium—broadest spectrum beta-lactam bactericidal antibiotic. A recommended dose is 15 mg/kg slowly IV q6h (NOTE: expensive).
- Fluconazole for fungal infections: 8.8 mg/kg PO q24h loading dose; 4.4 mg/kg PO q24h maintenance dose

IMMUNE SYSTEM SUPPORT: COLOSTRUM ADMINISTRATION

- Feed only those foals with normal BP and body temperature.
- Ideally, foals should receive ≥1 liter of colostrum with a specific gravity ≥1.060, administered in three to four feedings during the first 8–10 hours of life. This dose is equivalent to 1 gm IgG/kg BW.

PLASMA TRANSFUSION

- Use plasma to treat FPT (failure of passive transfer) to provide opsonins, to improve immune response, and to support oncotic pressure and defend intravascular fluid volume.
- Administer hyperimmune plasma from donors negative for A and Q antigens and antibodies.
- If orally administered, serum-derived commercial IgG products are used, they should be mixed with colostrum to improve absorption. The same dose of 1 gm IgG/kg BW is recommended.
- Foals ≥18 hours of age or foals with gut dysfunction may be unable to absorb sufficient colostral antibodies and require plasma transfusion.
- **Minimum plasma volume** to administer: **20 ml/kg.** The volume of plasma required to treat FPT depends on the IgG concentrations in recipient's blood and donor's plasma. Due to sepsis-induced protein catabolism, septic foals require a larger volume of plasma than healthy foals to increase serum [IgG] to the same level. Administer sufficient plasma to raise serum [IgG] above 800 mg/dl for septicemia.

Sources of Commercial Plasma: IgG > 2500 mg/dl

HiGamm Equi: [IgG] = 2500 mg/dl
Lake Immunogenics
348 Berg Road
Ontario, NY 14519
(800) 648 9990

Polymune Plus: [IgG] = 2500 mg/dl
Veterinary Dynamics, Inc.
P.O. Box 2406
Chino, CA 91708-2406
(800) 654 9743

General Nursing Care

- **Provide warmth**, using heating pads, warm fluids, radiant warmers, forced hot air blankets, and fluid jacket warmers (Intratherm, a warm IV fluid pouch, and Safe and Warm reusable instant heat measuring 7″ × 9″, from Safe and Warm Inc., Boulder City, NV 89005; [800] 421 3237).
- **Maintain sternal recumbency** as much as possible. Frequent repositioning helps prevent decubital sores and dependent lung atelectasis.
- Apply **sterile ocular lubricant** to eyes of foals that spend majority of time in lateral recumbency to prevent exposure keratitis/ulceration.
- Administer **antiulcer medication** to reduce the risk of gastroduodenal ulcers associated with stress and GI hypoperfusion:

□ **Ranitidine**, 6.6 mg/kg PO q8h; 1.5 mg/kg IV q8h, and/or
□ **Sucralfate**, 1–2 gm/45 kg PO q6h

Peripartum Asphyxia (Neonatal Maladjustment Syndrome)

Asphyxia can result from any periparturient event that impairs or disrupts uteroplacental perfusion or umbilical blood flow. Asphyxia produces multiorgan system damage in addition to the more commonly recognized behavioral and neurologic deficits.

Periparturient events associated with fetal/neonatal asphyxia:

- Dystocia—supply more O_2 via nasotracheal tube for mare to help reduce fetal hypoxia.
- Induced delivery—cervical dilatation is a prerequisite for induction to reduce risk of dystocia.
- Cesarean section
- Premature placental separation
- Placentitis—fetal membranes greater than 11% of foal's body weight (BW)
- Severe placental edema—uteroplacental thickness greater than 2.0 cm
- In utero meconium passage with or without postpartum meconium aspiration
- Twinning
- Severe maternal illness—especially with hypoxia
- Abnormally prolonged gestation
- Pregnancy complicated by reduced fetal fluid volume increases risk of umbilical cord compression during labor and suggests the presence of chronic placental dysfunction.

Diagnosis

Peripartum asphyxia produces a wide range of clinical signs. Asphyxia induces a critical **redistribution of cardiac output** resulting in preferential blood flow to heart, brain, and adrenal glands and decreased perfusion of lungs, gut, spleen liver, kidneys, skin, and muscles. Diagnosis is based primarily on clinical signs. Placental dysfunction causes increased creatinine (>3.0 mg/dl) in the newborn foal.

SIGNS ASSOCIATED WITH SPECIFIC ORGAN INJURY

- **CNS hemorrhage/edema/necrosis (hypoxic ischemic encephalopathy):** Loss of suckle, loss of dam recognition, apnea, hypotonia, anisocoria, sluggish pupillary light reflex (PLR), dilated pupils, depression, and tonic posturing: preference to lie in extensor posture with occasional pedaling limb movements, hyperesthesia, focal or grand mal seizures, and coma
- **Renal tubular necrosis:** Oliguria, anuria, generalized edema
- **Ischemic enterocolitis:** Colic, ileus, abdominal distention, gastric reflux, diarrhea (± bloody)
- **Meconium aspiration, pulmonary hypertension, and/or surfactant dysfunction:** Respiratory distress, tachypnea, dyspnea, rib retractions, apnea

- **Cardiac dysfunction due to myocardial infarcts and persistent fetal circulation (PFC):** Arrhythmia, tachycardia, murmurs, generalized edema, hypotension
- **Hepatocellular necrosis, biliary stasis:** Icterus
- **Adrenal gland necrosis:** Weakness, hypotension
- **Parathyroid necrosis:** Lipemia, seizures

BIOCHEMICAL ABNORMALITIES

Vary greatly depending on the severity of specific organ injury.

- **CNS:** Increased blood/brain barrier permeability, ± increased intracranial pressure, elevated CSF protein
- **Renal:** Proteinuria, increased urinary gamma-glutamyltransferase (GGT), azotemia, hyponatremia, hypochloremia
- **Gastrointestinal:** Occult blood–positive reflux/diarrhea
- **Respiratory:** Hypoxemia, hypercapnia, respiratory acidosis
- **Cardiac:** Hypoxemia, elevated myocardial enzymes, tachycardia or bradycardia
- **Hepatic:** Elevated hepatocellular and biliary enzymes, hyperbilirubinemia
- **Endocrine:** Hypocortisolemia, hypocalcemia

OTHER DIAGNOSTIC AIDS

- **Abdominal ultrasound or radiography** (recommended technique: 85 KVP/20 MAS) to assess for intramural gas accumulation, generalized intestinal distention, thickening of bowel wall; associated with necrotizing enterocolitis
- **Thoracic radiographs** (65–75 KVP/5–8 MAS) to detect diffuse lung atelectasis due to surfactant dysfunction associated with meconium aspiration and/or hypoxia; decreased pulmonary vascular pattern secondary to pulmonary hypertension and persistent fetal circulation (PFC). Normal thoracic radiographs do not rule out respiratory distress syndrome.
- **Echocardiography** to assess for patent foramen ovale, patient ductus arteriosus, and pulmonary hypertension associated with persistent fetal circulation

Therapy

CNS DISTURBANCES

- Administer **diazepam**, 0.11–0.44 mg/kg IV, for immediate seizure control; effect is short lived; repetitive doses contribute to respiratory depression. For severe or persistent seizure activity, use **phenobarbital**, 2–10 mg/kg IV q8–12h; monitor serum levels (15–40 μg/ml). Higher doses can produce respiratory depression and hypotension.
- **Avoid xylazine** for sedation unless it is the only drug available, since it causes transient hypertension, exacerbates existing CNS hemorrhage, and contributes to respiratory depression and reduced GI motility.
- **Avoid acepromazine**, since it lowers seizure threshold and produces hypotension.

- **To reduce cerebral edema:** administer **DMSO**, 0.5–1.0 gm/kg slowly as 10%–20% solution over 1 hour; stabilizes membranes, prevents platelet aggregation, maintains vascular integrity, scavenges free radicals during reperfusion. Administer IV **mannitol**, 0.25–1.0 mg/kg, as 20% solution over 10–20 min; osmotic diuretic; may exacerbate cerebral hemorrhage.
- **Protect from self-trauma.** Wrap legs, apply soft head helmet (Velcro foam leg wraps and helmet; (702) 851 1217); pad walls and provide soft bedding. Apply ocular lubricant to reduce risk of traumatic corneal ulceration.
- Head low during resuscitation
- Head elevated 30° when in lateral recumbency if suspect cerebral injury and/or after successful resuscitation
- Keep $PaCO_2$ normal or low if cerebral edema suspected.
- Do not overhydrate (maintain CVP at low normal value).

RENAL FAILURE

- **Monitor fluid in/urine out** to evaluate renal function and avoid overhydration.
- **Dopamine infusion**: 2–10 μg/kg/min. Lower doses stimulate dopaminergic receptors and enhance renal blood flow. Medium doses recruit β-receptors and support cardiac function, which may further improve renal perfusion. Higher doses stimulate α-receptors and result in decreased splanchnic blood flow, renal blood flow, and urine production. Titrate dose to individual patient. Recommend **catheterizing bladder** to allow accurate assessment of urine production.
- **Furosemide:** Administer small amounts (0.25–0.5 mg/kg q30–60 min) during dopamine infusion to enhance diuresis, or begin continuous infusion (0.25–2.0 mg/kg/h). If administering through same IV line as dopamine, avoid prolonged mixing of solutions in IV line by administering either dopamine or furosemide solution as close to catheter port as possible. Protect furosemide solution from light by wrapping line in paper or foil.
- **Mannitol**: 0.5–1.0 mg/kg administered IV as 20% solution over 15 min; osmotic diuretic.
- **Dobutamine:** (2–15 μg/kg/min). Use if cardiac dysfunction and secondary hypotension are contributing to poor renal perfusion; discontinue or reduce dosage if tachycardia develops.
- **Colic, reflux, abdominal distention: Nasogastric decompression** to check for reflux. Discontinue or reduce the volume/frequency of enteral feeding if reflux is present. **Percutaneous large bowel trocarization** if abdominal distention is severe causing respiratory compromise and continuous colic. Use 16-gauge, 3.5-inch catheter-over-stylet attached to 30-inch extension set. Sedate foal if necessary to keep quiet in lateral recumbency; clip and surgically prepare a site over one or both paralumbar fossae at point of maximal bowel distention. Infuse small bleb of lidocaine at puncture site. Using sterile technique, advance catheter/stylet through skin and body wall into distended viscus. Remove stylet and connect extension set. Place free end of extension set into a small beaker of sterile water to monitor gas/bubble production. Once bubbling stops, a small volume of antibiotic (e.g., amikacin diluted 50:50 with sterile water) can be infused as the catheter is withdrawn. Broad-spectrum

systemic antibiotic therapy is recommended for 3–5 days following trocarization.

- **Prokinetic drugs** for gastrointestinal dysmotility:
  - □ **Erythromycin**, 1–2 mg/kg PO, or as slow IV infusion q6h; observe for colic/diarrhea/intussusception; stimulates small and large intestinal motility
  - □ **Metoclopramide**, 0.25–0.5 mg/kg, as slow IV infusion, or per rectum, q6h; observe for excitement; stimulates gastroduodenal motility
  - □ **Cisapride**, 0.2–0.4 mg/kg q4-8h PO; stimulates small and large intestinal motility
  - □ **Lidocaine**, 1–2 mg/kg slowly IV followed by 0.05 mg/kg/min
- Antiulcer medication: Foals with hypoxic/ischemic gastrointestinal damage are at increased risk for GI ulcers.
  - □ **Ranitidine**, 6.6 mg/kg PO q8h, 1.5 mg/kg IV q8h, to increase gastric pH
  - □ **Sucralfate**, 20–40 mg/kg PO q6h, as cytoprotective agent
  - □ **Antacids**: Maalox; Di-Gel: 30–60 ml q3–4h; most antacids have a very short half-life, produce minimal change in gastric pH and may provide transient pain relief.
- **Broad-spectrum, bactericidal antibiotics** to reduce the risk of septicemia/endotoxemia secondary to invasion of luminal bacteria across compromised gastrointestinal mucosa
- **Parenteral nutrition:** With mild GI compromise, reduce volume/frequency of enteral feeding and support foal with partial parenteral nutrition. In cases of severe asphyxia accompanied by hypothermia, hypotension, shock, and/or advanced prematurity, recommend delaying all enteral feeds and providing TPN.

PERSISTENT FETAL CIRCULATION (PFC) PULMONARY VASOCONSTRICTION

- Treat **hypoxemia**, since it is a consistent stimulus for pulmonary vasoconstriction; provide high concentrations of O_2, up to 100% if necessary. 100% *intranasal* O_2 at 10 L/min results in only approximately 50% O_2 delivery.
  - □ Intranasal (IN):O_2 5–10 L/min
  - □ Positive-pressure ventilation can deliver 100% O_2.
- Acidosis accentuates hypoxic pulmonary vasoconstriction. Correct any *existing acid-base imbalance.* Attempt to achieve pH of 7.4
- Pulmonary vasospasm may be relieved by creating metabolic and respiratory alkalosis. *Hyperventilate* to drive pCO_2 below 20 mm Hg.
- Consider pulmonary vasodilators if other techniques fail:
  - □ **Tolazoline:** Infant dose: 1–2 mg/kg IV over 10 min; if response is positive with increase in PaO_2, then follow with IV infusion at 0.2 mg/kg/h for each 1 mg/kg pulse-dose administered. Causes adrenergic blockade, peripheral vasodilatation, GI stimulation, and cardiac stimulation
  - □ **Nitric oxide (NO):** NO is an important modulator of vascular tone in the perinatal pulmonary circulation. Acetylcholine mediates pulmonary vasodilatation in the newborn foal in an NO-dependent manner. Ventilation with NO reduces pulmonary vascular resistance. Inhalation of

20–80 ppm NO has been effective in reversing hypoxic pulmonary vasoconstriction.
- **Monitor blood pressure.** Support cardiac function with dopamine and dobutamine if indicated.
- Correct hyperthermia if present—remove covers, heating pads, and so on.

RESPIRATORY COMPROMISE

- **Mild hypoxemia** (PaO_2 between 60 and 80 mm Hg): Increase periods of time foal spends in sternal or standing position; turn q2h if recumbent; stimulate periodic deep breathing to reinflate atelectatic lungs; administer humidified IN oxygen, 2–10 L/min.
- **Moderate-severe hypoxemia** (PaO_2 < 60 mm Hg) accompanied by **hypercapnia** ($PaCO_2$ > 70 mm Hg): Provide **positive-pressure ventilation** (PPV). Intubate nasotracheally, using a 7–10-mm-diameter, 55-cm-long, cuffed, silicone nasotracheal tube (Bivona Inc., Gary IN; [800] 348 6064).
- Begin PPV with initial **tidal volume of 12–15 ml/kg** and **positive end-expiratory pressure (PEEP) of at least 4–6 cm H_2O.**
- Use inspired oxygen concentration of 60%–80% and re-evaluate arterial blood gas values within 30 min of initiating PPV. Adjust inspired O_2 concentration accordingly, with the goal of reducing F_1O_2 to < 50% as soon as possible to minimize risk of O_2 toxicity.
- Attempt to maintain airway pressures below 30–40 cm H_2O to reduce barotrauma.
- Respiratory rate is determined by $PaCO_2$ and foal's initial breathing rate (some elevation in $PaCO_2$ is permissible and may be necessary to prevent barotrauma).
- If **meconium aspiration** has occurred, suction upper airway and attempt to treat with IN O_2 alone. PPV can predispose to alveolar rupture/pneumothorax in these cases. Do not perform prolonged suction without O_2 administration.
- **Intratracheal surfactant** instillation may be beneficial if surfactant dysfunction is suspected secondary to severe asphyxia, pulmonary hypoperfusion, and/or meconium aspiration (may be nebulized).
- **Apnea and irregular respiration:** May be due to hypoxic-ischemic damage to central respiratory center, hypocalcemia, hypoglycemia, or hypothermia. Check body temperature and correct hypothermia if present. Correct hypoglycemia or hypocalcemia. If central respiratory depression is suspected, consider respiratory stimulants:
  - **Theophylline:** Loading dose of 5–6 mg/kg administered slowly IV q12h
    - Therapeutic levels, 6–12 mg/L
    - Signs of toxicity: Seizures, colic, hyperesthesia, tachycardia occur at levels > 20 mg/L.
    - Aminophylline, a precursor of theophylline, can be substituted; 1 mg aminophylline = 0.8 mg theophylline.
  - **Caffeine:** Loading dose of 10 mg/kg PO initially; maintenance dose of 2.5–3 mg/kg PO q24h
    - Therapeutic range, 5–20 mg/L; toxic levels ≥ 40 mg/L
  - If apnea persists, **CPAP** (continuous positive airway pressure) can be

tried requiring nasotracheal intubation, or else a high flow rate via two intranasal catheters. If CPAP is ineffective, **PPV** is required.

☐ **If PaO$_2$ does not have a 3–5 fold increase with 100% 0$_2$, suspect shunt(s), which is a poor prognostic indicator.**

SECONDARY INFECTION

Evaluate serum [IgG]. If IgG is less than 800 mg/dl and foal is $\geq$ 18 hours of age and has a functional GI tract, administer good-quality **colostrum** (specific gravity > 1.060) enterally, and/or administer plasma transfusion. If foal is $\leq$ 18 hours of age or has compromised gut function, administer **plasma**. Serum [IgG] should remain above 800 mg/dl. Maintain foal on broad-spectrum, bactericidal antibiotics if GI compromise is suspected, or if foal shows signs of sepsis, and/or serum [IgG] is less than 800 mg/dl.

Prognosis

60%–80% of foals suffering from peripartum asphyxia recover fully and mature into neurologically normal adults. A poor outcome is associated with severe, recurrent seizures that persist for more than 5 days postpartum, severe hypotonia that progresses to coma, severe multiorgan system damage and includes unresponsive renal failure and/or hypotension, and the development of concurrent septicemia. **Dysmature** and **premature foals** exposed to **severe peripartum asphyxia** have a poorer outcome than term foals.

Prematurity/Dysmaturity

Prematurity describes foals that are the product of a gestation length less than 320 days.

Dysmaturity describes foals that are the product of a normal or prolonged gestation length and show signs of underdevelopment. Dysmaturity is associated with abnormal uteroplacental function that can result in delayed fetal growth and maturation when chronic and varying degrees of fetal asphyxia when acute.

Clinical Signs

In addition to **generalized weakness** and **hypotonia**, the following signs are also characteristic of dysmaturity/prematurity:

- Low birth weight; thin body condition
- Short, silky hair coat
- Floppy ears, soft muzzle, flexor tendon laxity, periarticular laxity
- Increased range of passive limb motion
- Domed forehead
- Absent or diminished suckle reflex; ineffective swallow reflex
- Time to nurse and stand delayed more than 3–4 hours post partum
- Hypothermia due to poor thermoregulation
- Intolerance to enteral feeds; colic, abdominal distention, diarrhea, reflux
- Respiratory distress due to lung immaturity or surfactant dysfunction
- Visceral wasting—"gaunt" abdomen

Laboratory Findings:

- **Leukopenia:** WBC $< 6.0 \times 10^9$/ml; neutropenia with neutrophil:lymphocyte ratio < 1.0
- **Hypoglycemia** due to insulin response contributing to abnormal glucose homeostasis
- **Hypocortisolemia** and poor cortisol response to stress and exogenous ACTH
- **Hypoxemia,** variable hypercapnia, and lower pH values due to lung immaturity
- **Hyponatremia** and hypochloremia associated with renal immaturity

Therapy

Try to establish cause of prematurity/dysmaturity. **Examine placenta.** If evidence of placentitis, initiate broad-spectrum, bactericidal antibiotic therapy.

Observe closely for signs of **respiratory distress** and progressive respiratory fatigue. Therapy depends on degree of respiratory dysfunction:

- $PaO_2 < 60$ mm Hg, $PaCO_2 < 60$ mm Hg: Try intranasal O_2 therapy, 3–10 L/min; increase time spent in sternal recumbency; monitor arterial blood gases.
- $PaO_2 < 60$ mm Hg, $PaCO_2 > 65$–70 mm Hg: Begin positive-pressure ventilation (PPV) with positive end-expiratory pressure (PEEP). Use PPV with tidal volumes of 12–15 ml/kg. Attempt to keep peak airway pressures < 30–40 cm H_2O, and inspired O_2 concentrations $\leq 50\%$ to reduce risk of barotrauma and O_2 toxicity; PEEP at 4–10 cm H_2O. Excessive PEEP reduces cardiac output, requiring dobutamine drip. Insufficient PEEP may not increase functional residual volume as desired.
- If foal shows signs of advanced prematurity and signs of severe respiratory distress immediately postpartum, consider intratracheal instillation of surfactant in addition to PPV.

Hypothermia. Maintain carefully controlled environmental temperature if foal shows poor thermoregulation. Provide external warmth using warm water pads, radiant heaters, forced warm air blankets, warmed IV fluids, and insulated fluid jacket warmers.

Self-Trauma. Reduce risk of decubital sores by providing soft bedding (e.g., synthetic sheep skin) for recumbent foals.

Metabolic Disturbances. Monitor serum electrolyte concentrations. Hyponatremia and hypochloremia are the most common disturbances associated with renal and endocrine immaturity.

Nutrition. Ideally, foals should receive approximately 20%–25% of their BW in milk per day. Begin enteral feedings cautiously at a rate of 10% BW in milk divided into 10–12 feedings per day. If foal cannot tolerate sufficient enteral nutritional support, supply additional calories using partial or complete parenteral nutrition.

Incomplete Cuboidal Bone Ossification. Most premature and dysmature foals suffer varying degrees of incomplete cuboidal bone ossification. Radiograph one carpus (AP view) and tarsus (lateral view) to evaluate degree of ossification. If foal is active but has minimal cuboidal bone ossification, apply

sleeve casts for support and/or **restrict exercise** (i.e., stall confinement). If only mild incomplete ossification exists, restrict exercise and use **corrective shoeing/foot trimming** as needed to maintain proper weight-bearing axis (see p. 334).

Evaluate Serum [IgG]. Do this within 12 hours of birth. If [IgG] < 800 mg/dl, administer colostrum supplementation and/or plasma transfusion.

Secondary Bacterial Infections. Premature/dysmature foals are at increased risk. Consider broad-spectrum, bactericidal antibiotic therapy until foal is up and nursing normally.

COLIC

Signs of colic in newborn foals:

- Poor nursing behavior
- Rolling, treading
- Abdominal distention
- Teeth grinding
- Tachycardia, tachypnea

Common Causes

- **Meconium impaction**—can generally be palpated on digital examination and may require abdominal radiographs. Overzealous treatment for meconium impaction can result in colic.
- **Ileus** associated with gastrointestinal ischemia secondary to severe peripartum asphyxia or septic shock
- **Intussusception**—can be seen with ultrasound
- **Enteritis/peritonitis**—frequently *Clostridium* spp. and accompanying bacteremia
- **Gastroduodenal ulceration**
- **Intestinal volvulus**

Meconium Impaction

Meconium impaction is **more common in colts** than in fillies. In addition to colic, abdominal distention, and poor nursing behavior, affected foals may show **tenesmus, tail flagging**, and an **arched-back posture**. If obstruction is complete, abdominal distention can develop rapidly.

Diagnosis

- Palpation of firm meconium within the rectum/pelvic canal on **digital examination**
- A history of unsuccessful **straining to defecate**
- Demonstration of firm fecal material within the pelvic inlet, using plain radiography or contrast radiography following a barium enema
- Sonographic detection of echogenic material within the distal colon, rectum

Therapy

Warm, Soapy (Ivory Soap), Water Gravity Enemas. Use a soft, urinary catheter or small feeding tube and enema bucket with 75–180 ml of the solutions. If repetitive enemas are required, alternate soapy water with warm water or water mixed with J-lube or rectal lubricant to minimize excessive mucosal irritation. Avoid dioctyl sodium sulfosuccinate (DSS) enemas because of irritation. Repeated enemas may lead to pathologic tenesmus.

Retention Enemas. Use Mucomyst or powdered *N*-acetyl-L-cysteine. If Mucomyst, add 40 ml of 20% solution to 160 ml water to make a 4% solution. If using the powder, add 8 gm of powder and 1.5 tablespoon of sodium bicarbonate (baking soda) to 200 ml of water. Insert a lubricated Foley urinary catheter with a balloon tip approximately 2–4 inches into the rectum and inflate balloon. Slowly infuse 4–6 oz (120–180 ml) of acetylcysteine solution into rectum. Occlude catheter end for at least 15 minutes. Deflate balloon and remove catheter. The retention enema can be repeated several times.

Oral Laxatives. Proximal (high) impactions require oral laxatives in addition to enemas. The safest, least irritating laxative is **mineral oil** (120–160 oz), administered via nasogastric tube. Mineral oil lubricates around the impaction and reduces the risk of complete obstruction, which can rapidly result in severe and painful gas accumulations and abdominal distention.

Milk of Magnesia (60–120 ml) is another oral laxative that should be used conservatively. Castor oil or DSS orally is not recommended due to excessive mucosal irritation and increased risk of severe diarrhea and colic.

Intravenous Fluid Therapy. Useful in cases of refractory impactions. Dextrose supplementation is recommended if nursing behavior is curtailed due to increasing abdominal distention and colic. Maintenance IV fluid rate: 4–6 ml/kg/h for newborn foal.

Percutaneous Bowel Trocarization. If severe abdominal distention develops before the impaction can be resolved consider this (technique described under Peripartum Asphyxia, p. 491). Trocarization often provides immediate pain relief without excessive medication and allows time for medical therapies to work.

Analgesics and Sedatives. May be required to prevent self-trauma in foals that are down and rolling.

- **Dipyrone:** 11–22 mg/kg IV/IM, effective in mild cases; can be repeated several times as needed (no longer marketed in the USA).
- **Flunixin meglumine**, 0.5–1.0 mg/kg IV q24–36h; avoid repetitive doses owing to its ulcerogenic potential.
- **Butorphanol**, 0.01–0.04 mg/kg IV
- **Xylazine**, 0.1–0.5 mg/kg IV; use sparingly due to adverse effect on GI motility; some debilitated neonatal foals experience marked ileus and/or respiratory compromise following its use. Administering butorphanol and xylazine together allows a smaller dose of xylazine to be used.

Ileus

Decreased gastrointestinal motility is associated with ischemic/hypoxic bowel damage secondary to septic shock and/or peripartum hypoxia. Beware that intussusceptions may develop as a result of the ileus and/or prokinetic drugs used to promote motility.

Clinical Signs

- Decreased or absent borborygmi
- Tympanitic abdominal distention
- Colic
- Gastric reflux ($\pm$ blood)
- Diarrhea/constipation

Diagnosis

Based on physical examination and supported by several diagnostic techniques:

- **Transabdominal ultrasound** reveals distended bowel, lack of propulsive motility. If **necrotizing enterocolitis** is present, ultrasound reveals gas echoes within bowel walls.
- **Abdominal radiographs** demonstrate generalized small and large bowel distention. **Pneumatosis intestinalis,** gas formation within bowel wall, is observed with severe necrotizing enterocolitis.

Therapy

Depends on the underlying cause. Treatment for **severe hypoxic/ischemic gut damage with severe gastric reflux, bloody diarrhea:**

- **Gut rest**, discontinue all enteral feeding until reflux and diarrhea abate and borborygmi return. Severe cases may require ≥7 days of **complete** gut rest. Small amounts of enteral food (milk or commercial isotonic, easily digested products) supports enterocyte and enzyme production.
- **Parenteral alimentation** (see p. 488)
- **Broad-spectrum, bactericidal antibiotics** recommended (see p. 489)
- **Antiulcer medication: Sucralfate**, 20–40 mg/kg PO q6h and/or **ranitidine**, 6.6 mg/kg PO q8h; 1.5 mg/kg IV q8h.
- If foal show signs of endotoxemia, consider administering **1 liter of hyperimmune plasma** to provide opsonins and immunoglobulins to support immune system.
- **Cautious use of prokinetic agents** after periods of gut rest:
  - **Metoclopramide:** 0.25–0.50 mg/kg IV as 1-hour infusion q4–8h; 0.6 mg/kg PO, or per rectum q4–6h
  - **Cisapride:** 0.2–0.4 mg/kg PO q4–8h—preferred treatment
  - **Erythromycin:** 1.0–2.0 mg/kg IV q6h, administer as 1-hour infusion, or PO q6h
- Slowly reintroduce enteral feeds, beginning with small volumes of colostrum or dilute mare's milk.
- **Complications** associated with necrotizing enterocolitis include septicemia, intussusception, peritonitis, and stricture formation.
- Rule out *Clostridium perfringens* or *difficile* (see p. 225).

Treatment of **mild to moderate ileus, mild colic associated with feeding, variable amounts of reflux, and variable manure production:**

- **Conservative use of** prokinetics, described above. Begin erythromycin or metoclopramide infusion 15–20 min before feedings.

- **Decrease volume of enteral feedings** temporarily and support with partial parenteral nutrition.
- **Controlled exercise**
- If **constipation** develops, treat with enemas, oral laxatives (mineral oil), psyllium in small amounts, and maintain hydration with PO or IV fluids.
- **Oral probiotic agents:** Commercial products or 2–3 oz of active culture yogurt PO q12–24h

Intussusception

Colic due to intussusception may be mild to severe, depending on location and duration of obstruction. **Abdominal distention** and **reflux** usually develop.

Diagnosis is often made with **transabdominal ultrasound**. Sonography demonstrates "bull's eye" target lesions that represent cross-section view of intussuscepted bowel. Contrast radiography may help identify location of obstruction.

Surgical resection is the only definitive treatment. Prognosis for survival is guarded to grave if multiple intussusceptions are found, if there are large sections of compromised bowel, and/or if peritonitis is severe. **Postoperative complications** include recurrent intussusception, stricture formation, intra-abdominal adhesions.

Enteritis (With or Without Peritonitis)

May be due to a primary GI disorder or secondary to other systemic conditions, such as septicemia and peripartum hypoxia (also see pp. 482 and 491).

Clinical Signs

- Colic
- Abdominal distention, reduced or absent borborygmi, tympany
- Diarrhea (± blood, mucus)
- Variable temperature
- Injected sclera, hyperemic mucous membranes if enteritis is associated with endotoxemia
- Prolonged capillary refill time, dehydration
- Tachycardia

Possible Infectious Causes of Enteritis in Neonatal Foals

BACTERIAL

- *Salmonella* sp. can cause acute to peracute diarrhea accompanied by peritonitis and endotoxemia. Affected foals are often bacteremic, with increased risk of developing septic osteomyelitis/arthritis.
- *E. coli* septicemia: the *E. coli* isolates recovered from the blood of foals with diarrhea have **not** been shown definitively to be enteric pathogens; many foals with *E. coli* bacteremia also have enteritis.

- *Clostridium* spp. (*C. perfringens, C. sordellii, C. welchii, C. difficile*) can produce fetid diarrhea that is often bloody, particularly *C. perfringens.* Affected foals are often septicemic.
- *Rhodococcus equi* is associated with chronic diarrhea, weight loss, and peritonitis in older foals (1–4 months of age) affected with the more common respiratory form of this disease.

VIRAL

Although corona virus, adenovirus, and parvovirus have been isolated from foals with diarrhea, **rotavirus** is the most common cause of viral diarrhea in neonatal foals. Rotavirus produces a nonfetid, watery diarrhea that may be accompanied by fever and anorexia. There has also been an increased incidence of gastroduodenal ulcer disease during some rotavirus endemics.

PARASITIC

Strongyloides westeri nematode larvae have been associated with mild neonatal foal enteritis.

NUTRITIONAL

Overfeeding can produce gastric distention, ileus, and diarrhea. If the gastric digestive/absorptive capacities are overwhelmed, a large, rapidly fermentable carbohydrate load reaches the colon, resulting in diarrhea.

Sudden diet changes (e.g., changes from mare's milk to artificial replacer) can result in diarrhea.

OTHER

Enterocolitis associated with hypoxic/ischemic gut damage (e.g., necrotizing enterocolitis). See section on Peripartum Asphyxia, p. 491.

Foal heat diarrhea is due to physiologic changes occurring in the foal's gastrointestinal tract and usually results in a self-limiting diarrhea that occurs between 5 and 14 days of age and lasts less than 5–7 days.

Diagnosis

- **Blood culture** if septicemia is suspected (e.g., *Salmonella, E. coli, Clostridium*)
- **Fecal culture** for *Salmonella* sp., *Clostridium* spp.—polymerase chain reaction (PCR) can be used for Salmonella (see p. 229), and toxin assays should be performed on *Clostridium* spp. (see p. 225).
- **Fecal flotation, direct smear**
- **Rotavirus** test: Rotazyme (ELISA), Abbott Laboratories, North Chicago, IL; Rota test (latex agglutination), Wampole Laboratories, Carter Wallace Inc., Cranbury, NJ.
- **Abdominal radiography:** Enteritis, especially during the early stages, is often associated with varying degrees of ileus and generalized gas/fluid accumulation within the bowel lumen. Intramural gas accumulation *(pneumatosis intestinalis)* is observed with severe necrotizing enterocolitis. **Pneumoperitoneum** is seen with bowel rupture.
- **Transabdominal ultrasonography:** An increased volume of intraluminal fluid and bowel wall edema are seen with enteritis. Peritonitis is associ-

ated with an increased volume of echogenic peritoneal fluid with or without fibrin tags. Intramural gas accumulation casts bright white echoes and is associated with hypoxic gut damage.

- **Hematology/chemistry: Leukopenia, neutropenia** are associated with endotoxemia. Secretory diarrhea usually results in **hypochloremia, hyponatremia,** varying degrees of metabolic acidosis, hemoconcentration, and variable potassium concentrations.
- **Abdominocentesis** if peritonitis is suspected. Peritoneal fluid contains increased protein concentration and nucleated cell count.

Therapy

- **Maintain hydration**, using polyionic fluids. Monitor serum concentrations of electrolytes, glucose and creatinine, acid/base balance, and PCV/TP. If foal is anorexic, parenteral alimentation is required.
- **Broad-spectrum, bactericidal, parenteral antibiotic therapy** is recommended for foals with severe diarrhea and toxic mucous membranes, because of the increased risk of gram-negative septicemia.
- **Intestinal protectants: Bismuth subsalicylate** (Corrective Suspension, Phoenix Pharmaceutical Inc., St. Joseph, MO 64506): 0.5–1 ml/kg PO q4–6h; **kaolin and pectin:** 4–8 ml/kg PO q12h
- **Nonsteroidal anti-inflammatory drug therapy** is recommended if foal shows signs of endotoxemia. A "low-dose" of flunixin meglumine, 0.25 mg/kg IV q8–12h, is preferred. *Conservative use of this drug is advised owing to its ulcerogenic potential.*
- **Plasma** administration benefits foals showing signs of endotoxemia and foals suffering from FPT and/or hypoproteinemia 20 ml/kg.
- Consider **Antiulcer medication:**
  □ **Ranitidine**, 6.6 mg/kg PO q6–8h; 1.5 mg/kg IV q6–8h
  □ **Sucralfate**, 20–40 mg/kg PO q6h
- **Loperamide:** 4–16 mg PO q6h beginning with low dose and increasing by 2-mg increments every 2–3 doses. Because loperamide increases segmentation rate and slows transit time, it may enhance toxin absorption in cases of acute, infectious enteritis. Therefore, its use should be reserved for foals that do not show signs of severe endotoxemia.

FOAL CARDIOPULMONARY RESUSCITATION

Jonathan E. Palmer

OVERVIEW/IMPORTANT FACTS

- Cardiopulmonary failure in foals is secondary to other systemic conditions.
  □ Shock and respiratory failure, which are progressive and in early stages treatable, lead to bradycardia, which then deteriorates to asystole.
  □ Unlike in people, in whom the principal cause of cardiopulmonary failure is coronary artery disease, ventricular fibrillation is not a common presenting arrhythmia.

- **The key to successful treatment is early recognition and treatment of the predisposing conditions.**
- A high-risk period is during birth because neonates may fail the transition from fetal to neonatal physiology. Prompt intervention is vital in these cases.

Thorough preparation is as important as early intervention. *At the moment of crisis, there is no time to formulate a plan. Rather, one of several well-thought-out plans must be initiated once the nature of the crisis is recognized.*

It is most convenient to store airway equipment and emergency drugs in one or two grips that can easily be transported stallside (see Tables 35–2 and 35–3.) Also include resuscitation flow sheets with drug doses shown in milliliters needed for the typical foal, as demonstrated later (see Table 35–4). Code drug vials with colored tape so that you can easily direct bystanders to retrieve the appropriate drugs.

In general, people are much more knowledgeable about proper CPR techniques than in the past, partly due to the efforts of the American Heart Association to teach basic life support and partly due to the portrayal of realistic CPR

TABLE 35–2. **Equipment Required for Resuscitation**

1. **Self-inflating Bag-valve Device**
Adult size–1600 ml with O_2 reservoir bag–2600 ml
Laerdal silicone resuscitator
Laerdal Medical Corp.
1 Labriola Court
Armonk, NY 10504
800 431 1055

2. **Silicone Cuffed Endotracheal Tubes**
Sizes 7 mm, 9 mm, 10 or 12 mm–55 cm long
Several suppliers, such as:
Air Vet(Bivona) Inc
5425 Raines Rd, Suite 3
Memphis, TN 38115
800 343 6237

Cook Veterinary Products
PO Box 489
Bloomingham, Indiana 47402
800 826 2380

Rusch Inc.
53 West 23rd St.
New York, NY 10010
212 675 5556

3. **Bubble-Jet Humidifier**
Puritan Bennett Corp.
9410 Indian Creek PKY#300
Shawnee Mission, KS 66225-5905
913 661 0444

4. **Intranasal O_2 Tubing**
A number of options; one suggestion:
16 F Levin 127 cm tubing
Davol, Inc
100 Sockanosset Crossroad
Cranston, RI 02920
401 463 7000

5. **O_2 Line**
A number of options; one suggestion:
Clear vinyl tubing 3/8" ID, 1/2" OD (1/16" thick)
VWR Scientific
200 Center Square Rd.
Bridgeport, NJ 08014
609 467 3333

6. **O_2 Flow Meters**
1–15 L range
Any local medical supply co.

O_2 Tank
With regular adapted for humidifier/flow meter
Small "E" tank (655L)-local medical gas company

TABLE 35–3. **Useful Equipment for Resuscitation**

1. **Compact Suction Unit**
   Laerdal Medical Corp.
   1 Labriola Court
   Armonk, NY 10504
   800 431 1055

2. **Dextrometer**
   ACCU-CHEK III-Chemstrip bG
   Boehringer Mannhein
   9115 Hauge Rd.
   Indianapolis, IN 46250
   800 858 8072

3. **Noninvasive Blood Pressure Monitor**
   Critikon, Inc.
   5820 West Cypress
   Suite B
   Tampa, FL 33634
   813 887 2000

   Datascope Corp.
   580 Winters Ave.
   Paramus, NJ 07632
   800 288 2121

4. **IV Pumps**
   Gemini PC-1
   IMED Corp.
   9775 Businesspark Ave.
   San Diego, CA 92131-1192
   800 854 2033

5. **IV Catheters**
   Arrow International, Inc.
   P.Q. Box 12888
   3000 Bemville Rd.
   Reading, PA 19612
   610 378 0131

6. **HME filter (Heat-Moisture Exchange Filter)**
   Provides heat and moisture to airway and filters bacteria/viruses
   Pall Biomedical Products Corporation
   Glen Cove, NY 11542
   800 645 6578

7. **Blood Gas Analyzer**
   StatPal II-PPG Industries
   Biomedical Systems Division
   11077 Torrey Pines Rd.
   La Jolla, CA 92037
   800 369 3457

8. **Defibrillator with ECG**
   Life Pak-10
   Physiocontrol Corp.
   Box 97006
   Redmond, WA 98073-9706

   Automated External Defibrillator
   Currently being developed by a
   number of companies

9. **ECG**
   Datascope Corp.
   580 Winters Ave.
   Paramus, NJ 07632
   800 288 2121

scenes in popular television series. This is important in resuscitation because with minimal prompting bystanders can be enlisted to help.

Here techniques ranging from basic to advanced life support are outlined in an effort to prepare the clinician to meet the challenge of the moment of crisis with equipment that results in a successful outcome.

Humane Aspects of CPR

- Often it is mechanically possible to successfully resuscitate a foal but not humanely appropriate to do so.

- Most arrests in foals are secondary to progressive systemic disease.
  - ☐ If the underlying disease is incurable (relative to available facilities, technology, and skill), it is not in the best interest of the foal to attempt resuscitation.
  - ☐ If the likely outcome is not as predictable, initiation of resuscitation efforts becomes a value judgment.
- Whether or not resuscitation is appropriate should be discussed before the crisis develops.

GENERAL CARDIOPULMONARY RESUSCITATION

Reasons for Cardiopulmonary Failure

Primary cardiac failure (unusual). Possible causes:

- Hypoxic-ischemic myocardial damage
- Congenital cardiac defects
- Myocarditis
- Endocarditis with coronary artery embolism

Ventricular tachycardia or fibrillation, the expected consequences of primary cardiac failure, occurs as the initial arrhythmia in only about 10% of pediatric cases of cardiopulmonary arrest.

Cardiopulmonary failure in foals usually occurs secondary to systemic disease, which may cause respiratory or cardiac failure leading to hypoxic acidosis. The hypoxic acidosis, in turn, causes respiratory arrest, followed by development of a nonperfusing bradycardia and finally, asystole. If resuscitation is begun before a nonperfusing cardiac rhythm develops, the likelihood of revival is good (survival rate as high as 50%). However, if resuscitation efforts are delayed until after development of asystole, expect less than 10% survival rate. Since the cause of arrest in most cases is systemic disease and the onset of arrest follows progressive respiratory and circulatory failure, with careful attention to development of signs, resuscitation can be begun before complete failure.

Common causes of cardiopulmonary arrest:

- Perinatal hypoxia leading to central respiratory center damage, resulting in hypoventilation
- Primary lung disease leading to hypoventilation and hypoxia
- Septic shock
- Hypovolemia
- Metabolic acidosis
- Hyperkalemia (e.g., ruptured bladder)
- Vasovagal reflex
- Hypothermia

To revive the patient successfully, the underlying cause of the arrest must be recognized and treated.

Recognition of Impending Failure

- Respiratory failure is marked by hypercapnia and hypoxia caused by inadequate ventilation.

- Foals with failure due to respiratory center damage secondary to peripartum asphyxia:
  - Do not sense the hypoxia/hypercapnia.
  - Have an inadequate respiratory effort.
  - Have periods of apnea.
  - Have apparently normal respiratory rate and minimal effort.
- **If there is a lack of responsiveness or loss of consciousness, respiratory failure should be assumed until disproved.**
- Failure secondary to intrinsic lung disease or airway obstruction results in progressive respiratory failure.
  - Signs of respiratory compensation:
  - Increased respiratory rate (tachypnea)
  - Increased respiratory depth (hyperpnea)
  - Increased work of breathing
  - Nostril flare
  - Use of accessory respiratory muscles
  - Sinus tachycardia
  - Respiratory compensation followed by what appears to be rapid improvement may, in fact, be fatigue or toxic effects of extreme hypercapnia and prolonged hypoxia preceding respiratory arrest.
- Uncontrolled shock (inadequate delivery of O_2 and metabolic substrates to tissues) leads to cardiopulmonary arrest.
  - Shock can occur with normal, decreased, or increased cardiac output and blood pressure.
  - Respiratory failure and shock may begin as distinct problems and progress in concert to cardiopulmonary failure.
  - There is a dynamic balance between oxygen content of blood and cardiac output.
    If either falls, the other must increase to insure adequate oxygen delivery to the tissues.
    Oxygen content can increase only marginally when breathing room air. Any significant decrease in cardiac output results in decreased oxygen delivery unless oxygen content is increased by increasing the concentration of inspired oxygen with intranasal oxygen.

  Cardiopulmonary failure leads inevitably to cardiopulmonary arrest.

- Signs of cardiopulmonary failure:
  - Tachycardia
  - Depression (nonresponsiveness)
  - Oliguria
  - Hypotonia
  - Weak proximal pulse with weak or absent peripheral pulse
  - Prolonged capillary refill time
- Late ominous signs:
  - Bradycardia
  - Hypotension
  - Irregular respiratory pattern

Clinical Approach to CPR

(See Diagram 35–1 and Diagram 35–2.)

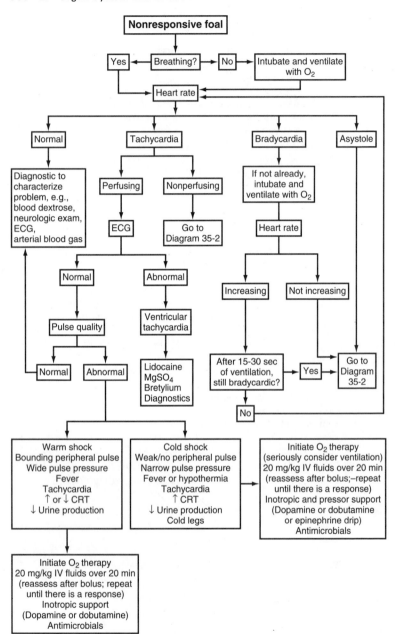

DIAGRAM 35–1. Nonresponsive foal algorithm.

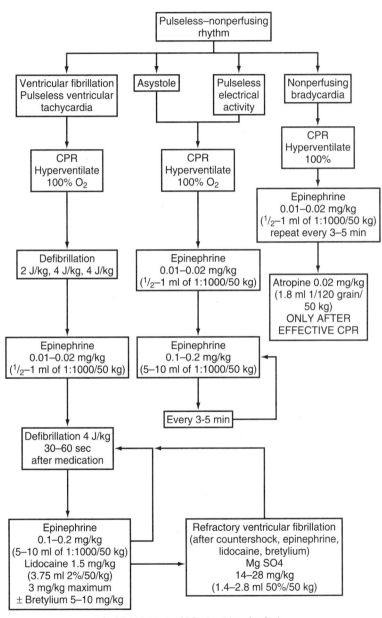

DIAGRAM 35–2. CPR algorithm for foals.

- Establish an airway.
- Begin ventilation.
- Begin chest compressions.
- Administer epinephrine.
- Determine cardiac arrhythmia and treat accordingly.

The initial intent of resuscitation is to establish oxygen and blood flow to the brain and heart.

Establishing an Airway

MOUTH-TO-NOSE VENTILATION

(Fig. 35–4)

- Use when an endotracheal tube is not available.
- Can be very effective because foals are obligate nasal breathers
- Technique:
  - □ Place the fingers of one hand just behind the chin with the palm and thumb occluding the down nostril.
  - □ Place the other hand on the poll so that the head can be maximally dorsiflexed straightening the airway, decreasing the possibility of aerophagia.
  - □ Alternatively, the head can be turned so that the poll is on the ground, resulting in maximal dorsiflexion, and allowing the free hand to place pressure on the cricoid to insure occlusion of the esophagus.
  - □ **The head should not be elevated** (could further compromise cerebral circulation).
- Place an endotracheal tube without delay, since the fractional inspired O_2 content (i.e., percent inspired) is no greater than 16%–18%.

ENDOTRACHEAL TUBE PLACEMENT

- Internal diameter: 9-mm endotracheal tube for the average Thoroughbred or Standardbred foal. Small foals (e.g., Arabians), 7-mm tube; large foals, 10–12-mm tube.
- Length: 55 cm so that full nasotracheal tube insertion places the cuff in the midtrachea.
- Use sterile technique whenever possible, to avoid introduction of nosocomial pathogens, and because time is of the essence, the first priority is rapid intubation and initiation of resuscitation.

Intubation Technique

- Nasotracheal intubation can be performed without assistance in cardiopulmonary failure, allowing others to begin cardiac compressions, establish IV access, prepare appropriate drug dosages, or attach monitoring equipment.
- Place foal in lateral recumbency so that cardiac compression can begin without delay.

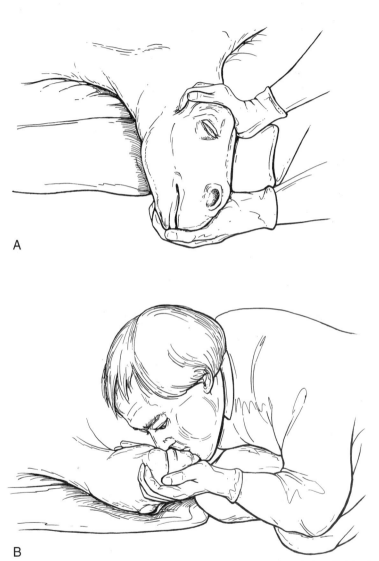

A

B

FIGURE 35–4. *A,* Position of foal's head for mouth-to-nose ventilation. *B,* Mouth-to-nose ventilation.

- **Do not elevate the foal's head** (further compromises cerebral blood flow).
- Dorsiflex the head to straighten the airway (Fig. 35–5).
  - □ If an assistant is available: place one hand under the chin, extending the head and neck, with the other pushing down on the poll, achieving dorsiflexion.
- Pass endotracheal tube through the nasal passage.
- Use the largest diameter tube that passes through the nasal passage.
- Once the tube reaches the level of the arytenoids, a twisting motion facilitates passage by allowing the beveled end to spread the arytenoids.
- *Palpate the esophagus to insure proper placement.* Inadvertent inflation of the stomach is contraindicated.
- Advance the endotracheal tube until only the adapter is visible at the nostril, to minimize dead space.
- Secure with ties to a halter or around the poll.
- Inflate the cuff to insure a tight seal (fill cuff until no air leak is heard during positive-pressure ventilation).

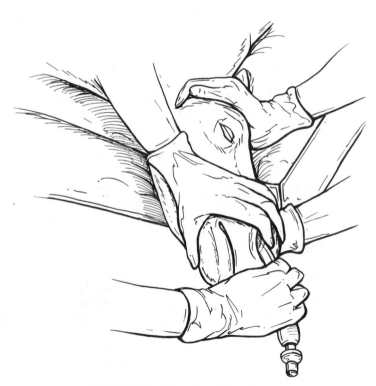

FIGURE 35–5. Nasotracheal tube placement.

Ventilatory Aids

ANESTHESIA BAG

- Consists of a reservoir bag, an overflow port with pop-off valve, and a gas inflow port attached to an O_2 supply
- Proper use of an anesthesia bag requires extensive training.

DEMAND VALVE

- Requires a pressurized O_2 supply
- Simple to use
- **Very prone to inducing barotrauma** when the operator is not trained or becomes distracted

SELF-INFLATING BAG-VALVE DEVICE (AMBU BAG)

- Of the three, this is easiest to use, most versatile, and safest.
- Use a bag designed for human adult resuscitation (1600-ml, with a 2600-ml O_2 reservoir bag).
- Operation:
  □ The bag fills via recoil, drawing from the gas intake valve, O_2 input line, or O_2 reservoir.
  □ When the bag is compressed, the intake valve closes and the patient outlet valve connected to the endotracheal tube opens, allowing gas to flow to the patient.
  □ During exhalation, the patient outlet valve closes (to prevent rebreathing of exhaled gas on the next breath), and the exhalation valve near the patient connection opens.
  □ The bag's recoil draws gas into it for the next breath.
- An O_2 source is not needed.
  □ The bag draws room air if no other gas source is available.
  □ It is preferable to use a high concentration of O_2 during resuscitation; resuscitation using room air can be very effective.
- With an O_2 line attached:
  □ The delivered O_2 concentration is between 30% and 80%.
  □ With an O_2 reservoir bag and high flows (> 15 Lpm), O_2 concentrations of 60%–95% can be maintained. *Keep the reservoir full to maintain these high concentrations. The flow needed to maintain the reservoir depends on the minute volume being delivered.*
- If the self-inflating bag has a pop-off valve (usually set to 35–45 cm H_2O to avoid barotrauma during normal ventilation), it needs to be easily occluded when low lung compliance, high airway resistance, an endotracheal tube obstructed by secretions or kinks, or the presence of pneumothorax makes high airway pressures a necessary risk.

Ventilation During Resuscitation

- Rate: Hyperventilate (40–60 breaths per minute)
- Tidal volume: Estimated at 10 ml/kg
  □ Best gauged by careful observation of chest excursion to insure proper ventilation.

- Auscultation of the lung fields after endotracheal placement to ensure even air flow is helpful (occlusion of the main stem bronchi from overinsertion of the endotracheal tube is uncommon but possible).

Cardiovascular Support—Establishing Circulation

> **Initiate chest compressions immediately if a nonperfusing cardiac rhythm is present. Do not delay until cardiac contractions stop.**

How blood flow occurs during chest compression is not clear. The *cardiac pump theory* suggests that chest pressure causes direct cardiac compression propelling the blood, the cardiac valves directing the blood flow forward. The *thoracic pump theory* suggests that the increased thoracic pressure caused by the compression propels the blood, and the venous valves direct it forward, whereas noncompliant cardiac valves (as a result of myocardial rigor) make the cardiac contribution to blood flow minimal. There is evidence for both explanations.

Cardiac Compression
(Fig. 35–6)

- Place the foal on a firm surface by removing any bedding.
- Position the foal with its withers against a wall so that it does not move during forceful compressions.
  - □ There is no difference in effectiveness of chest compressions from one side to the other.
  - □ Time is of the essence—do not waste it by repositioning the foal.

COMPRESSION TECHNIQUE

- Place the palm of the hand with the fist closed over the heart.
- Place the other hand to reinforce the compressing hand.
- Elbows remain straight, and the motion for compression originates from the waist (the upper body weight powering the compression results in increased endurance).
- Closed chest compression results in no more than 15%–20% of normal cardiac output.
- To maximize cardiac output, make half the duty cycle compression and half relaxation.
  - □ Easiest to achieve with a rapid compression rate of 100–120 per minute.
  - □ Do not be overly ambitious in setting a rate. Too rapid a rate results in early operator fatigue.
- If an airway is secured, coordination between ventilation and chest compression is not needed.
  - □ Cardiac output is enhanced by ventilation superimposed on chest compression.

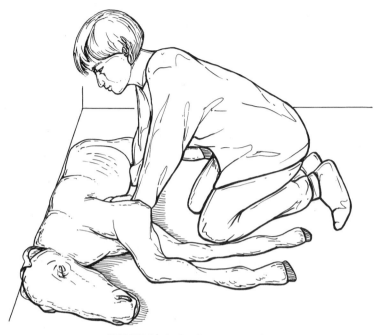

FIGURE 35–6. Cardiac compression.

□ **Routine superimposition of chest compression and ventilation** results in increased cerebral pressure, which is clearly contraindicated in cases with hypoxic-ischemic encephalopathy and **should be avoided** in neonatal foals with possible perinatal hypoxia.

Methods for measuring effectiveness of cardiac output:

- Feel a central arterial pulse.
- Monitor pupil size (becomes less dilated).
- Measure end-tidal CO_2 (begins to increase).

Central Arterial Pulse

- Traditional assessment of effectiveness of the chest compressions
- Carotid or femoral artery
- Can be difficult for several reasons:
  □ Motion caused by chest compressions makes rapid location of the pulse difficult.
  □ Skill and practice at locating central artery pulse are needed to make the judgment of an adequate pulse within seconds.

☐ If an individual talented enough to detect efficiently the presence of a pulse is available, it is likely that his or her talent is better utilized performing other vital tasks, such as establishing a central IV line.

Pupil Size

- Preferable method—an indirect indication of adequate cerebral perfusion:
  ☐ When perfusion of the head becomes inadequate (e.g., cardiac arrest) the pupils dilate widely.
  ☐ When chest compression results in adequate perfusion to the head, the pupils assume a more neutral size.
- Pupil size can be monitored by the same person who is performing the chest compression.
- Adjust chest compression technique as indicated by pupil size.

End-Tidal CO_2 (P_{ETCO_2})

The most effective measurement of cardiac output, best measured using a capnograph. When there is no cardiac output to the lungs, the P_{ETCO_2} is 0 (alveoli are ventilated but not perfused). If chest compression results in effective cardiac output and lung perfusion occurs, the P_{ETCO_2} increases.

- The more effective the chest compression in producing cardiac output, the higher the P_{ETCO_2}.
- Effective compressions result in a P_{ETCO_2} of 12–18 torr.
- Manipulations during CPR that cause a change in P_{ETCO_2} independent of cardiac output:
  ☐ High-dose epinephrine therapy causes a decrease in P_{ETCO_2}.
  ☐ Treatment with bicarbonate increases P_{ETCO_2} (buffering of acid in the central venous system results in a higher concentration of CO_2 in the blood delivered to the lungs).
- Capnography results in immediate feedback to the resuscitator, allowing for beat-to-beat modification of technique, ensuring that the most effective cardiac output is achieved.

Complications of Chest Compression

Rib fractures, which can result in:

- Hemorrhage and possible hemothorax
- Lung and myocardial lacerations
- Flail chest
- **Chest compression must be applied above the costochondral junction in order to produce effective cardiac output,** increasing the possibility of rib fractures. (The compliant nature of the ribs in neonatal foals makes fractures less likely.)
- Pulmonary and myocardial contusions

Vascular Access

Establishing vascular access is essential if the neonate does not respond immediately to ventilation and chest compression. Because cardiopulmonary failure in neonates is usually secondary to other serious systemic disease, cases may already have an intravenous catheter. For those that do not, catheterize the jugular vein using whatever available materials the resuscitator believes results in the most rapid vascular access.

NOTE: **Administering drugs via the intracardiac route is contraindicated!** The delivery of drugs is no more rapid than by the intravenous or intratracheal access route.

COMPLICATIONS OF INTRACARDIAC INJECTIONS

- Interruption of chest compressions
- Coronary artery laceration
- Cardiac tamponade
- Pneumothorax

DRUGS THAT CAN BE ADMINISTERED BY INTRATRACHEAL ROUTE

Some low-volume drugs can be administered by the intratracheal route before vascular access is secured:

- Epinephrine (use high dose)
- Lidocaine
- Atropine
- Naloxone

To be absorbed, **the drug must be delivered beyond the endotracheal tube into the bronchial tree,** by passing infusion tubing down the endotracheal tube and chasing the drug with fluids. However, this requires interruption of ventilation. An equally effective and more expedient method involves **transtracheal injection** of the drugs:

- Palpate the trachea to identify the level of the inflated cuff.
- Estimate where the end of the endotracheal tube is.
- Inject the drug transtracheally below the tube (usually close to the thoracic inlet).
- Follow the injection with several large breaths.

Drug Therapy During Resuscitation (Table 35–4)

EPINEPHRINE

Key points: Epinephrine is an endogenous catecholamine with both α- and β-adrenergic effects.

- α-Adrenergic effects:
  - Increase systemic vascular resistance
  - Elevate systolic and diastolic blood pressure
  - Decrease perfusion of splanchnic, renal, mucosal, and dermal circulation
- β-Adrenergic effects:
  - Increase myocardial contractility
  - Increase heart rate
  - Relax smooth muscle in bronchi
  - Relax skeletal muscle vasculature

TABLE 35-4. Dosage (ml/kg) of Drugs Commonly Used in CPR

Drug	Supplied	Dose/kg	ml/kg	ml/20 kg	ml/30 kg	ml/40 kg	ml/50 kg	ml/60 kg	ml/70 kg
Epinephrine low dose	1 mg/ml	0.01–0.02 mg	0.01–0.02	0.02–0.4 3–5 min	0.3–0.6 3–5 min	0.4–0.8 3–5 min	0.5–1 3–5 min	0.6–1.2 3–5 min	0.7–14 3–5 min
Epinephrine high dose	1 mg/ml	0.1 mg	0.1	2 3–5 min	3 3–5 min	4 3–5 min	5 3–5 min	6 3–5 min	7 3–5 min
Lidocaine	2% 20 mg/ml	1.5 mg	0.075	1.6	2.25	3	3.75	4.5	5.25
				every 5 minutes max. 3 mg/kg					
Bretylium	50 mg/ml	5–10 mg max. 30–35 mg/kg	0.1–0.2	2–4 10 min	3–6 10 min	4–8 10 min	5–10 10 min	6–12 10 min	7–14 10 min
Atropine	0.54 mg/ml	0.02 mg	0.037	0.8 max. 2X	1.1 max. 2X	1.5 max. 2X	1.8 max. 2X	2.2 max. 2X	2.6 max. 2X
Ca Cl	10% CaCl	20 mg(CaCl)	0.2	4	6	8	10	12	14
Na HCO₃	1 mEq/ml	0.5–1 mEq/kg	0.5–1	10–20	15–30	20–40	25–50	30–60	35–70
Mg SO₄	50% 500 mg/ml	14–28 mg/kg	0.028–0.056	0.6–1.1	0.8–1.7	1.1–2.2	1.4–2.8	1.7–3.4	2–4

The most important advance in the understanding of the mechanism of drug activity in CPR in the past 15 years is the insight into the importance of epinephrine in improving coronary perfusion pressure during cardiac arrest. During chest compression, coronary blood flow is restricted to the diastolic period. *Diastolic aortic pressure determines coronary perfusion*, because during cardiac arrest there is no coronary capillary resistance, and central venous pressure is low due to minimal venous return. Epinephrine increases diastolic aortic pressure by simultaneously preventing run-off into peripheral tissues (by peripheral arterial constriction) and by increasing aortic tone. The combination of effective chest compression and the action of epinephrine results in a return of coronary perfusion, which is the most important step in resolving cardiac arrest no matter what the cause. **Without coronary perfusion there is no hope of return to a normal cardiac rhythm.**

Indications for Epinephrine

- Cardiac arrest regardless of underlying cause
  □ Asystole
  □ Idioventricular rhythms
  □ Pulseless electrical activity
  □ Symptomatic bradycardia (nonresponsive to ventilation with oxygen)
- Hypotension not related to volume depletion

Epinephrine Dose for Pulseless Cardiac Arrest
- Initial IV dose: 0.01–0.02 mg/kg (0.5–1.0 ml/50 kg of 1:1000 epinephrine)
- Subsequent IV doses and all intratracheal doses: 0.1 mg/kg
- Dosing interval: Repeat every 3–5 minutes

Complications/Precautions
- Postresuscitation hypertension/tachyarrhythmias
- ↑ Cardiac oxygen demand/myocardial necrosis
- *Inactivated when mixed with bicarbonate*

FLUIDS

Key points:

- Large volumes of fluids are important in treating hypovolemic/septic shock that frequently leads to cardiac arrest.
- After cardiac arrest, **overzealous fluid administration is contraindicated**.
  □ When hypovolemia leads to cardiac arrest, a nonperfusing rhythm develops and the situation resembles congestive heart failure, with ineffective cardiac output.
  □ With effective chest compressions, the cardiac output is only 15%–20% of normal.
  □ If fluids are administered rapidly the venous pressure rises, impeding coronary perfusion and return of a normal cardiac rhythm, despite effective chest compressions and high doses of epinephrine.

☐ *If volume replacement is indicated because of severe dehydration, bolus administration is preferred rather than a continuous high flow rate.*

☐ Use moderate fluid rate ideally with crystalloid containing magnesium (which may help abolish post arrest cerebral hypoperfusion) until spontaneous cardiac rhythm returns.

- Once a perfusing rhythm returns, increased fluid rates may be needed to help maintain cardiac output.
- Severe hypoglycemia can lead to cardiac arrest; however, **avoid glucose-containing fluids during resuscitation** unless a patient-side glucose determination indicates severe hypoglycemia.

☐ Hyperglycemia and hyperosmolality secondary to rapid glucose infusion during resuscitation is associated with poor neurologic outcome in humans.

SODIUM BICARBONATE

Key points:

The use of bicarbonate during cardiac arrest remains controversial. Theoretical contraindications:

- Sodium bicarbonate buffers acid by forming CO_2, eliminated by ventilation.
- During resuscitation, CO_2 is not eliminated efficiently.
- CO_2 is very soluble and moves across cell membranes rapidly.

☐ Organic acids tend to accumulate in the blood during prolonged cardiac arrest.

☐ Intracellular acidosis increases when bicarbonate buffers these organic acids, producing CO_2 that re-enters cells since, because of capillary blood stasis, it is not carried away.

- During CPR, a venoarterial paradox develops.

☐ Slow venous return produces a severe venous hypercapnic acidemia.

☐ The blood passing through the lungs is overventilated, resulting in arterial hypocapnic alkalemia.

☐ The poorer the cardiac output, the more extreme the venoarterial difference.

☐ When there is a large venoarterial difference, the administration of bicarbonate may exacerbate the acidosis.

☐ Myocardial acidosis is more marked than acidosis in other tissues. Increased intracellular acidosis results in significant cardiac depression.

- **With poor cardiac output and coronary perfusion, the use of bicarbonate therapy is contraindicated.**
- Once efficient cardiac output is achieved, administration of bicarbonate may be helpful in returning the heart to a spontaneous perfusing rhythm.

☐ If bicarbonate is administered to a patient being hyperventilated with 100% O_2 and who has effective cardiac output, it helps reverse acidosis-induced cardiac depression.

☐ It also increases the effectiveness of epinephrine; *do not mix in the same IV line.*

☐ The combination of epinephrine and bicarbonate therapy under these circumstances can significantly improve recovery.

☐ *Maintaining a good cardiac output is crucial for this effect.*

Indications for Bicarbonate Administration

Absolute indication:

- Hyperkalemia (as secondary to ruptured bladder)

Probable indications:

- Pre-existing metabolic acidosis leading to arrest
- Phenobarbital overdose

Controversial indications:

- In prolonged, nonresponsive arrests
- After return to spontaneous circulation

Contraindication:

- Hypoxic lactic acidosis

Sodium Bicarbonate Dosage

- 0.5–1 mEq/kg over 1–2 minutes
- Repeat once in 5–10 minutes if indicated

Potential Complications

- Significant cardiac depression secondary to increased intracellular CO_2
- Hypernatremia with secondary cerebral hemorrhages
- Hyperosmolality with secondary cerebral hemorrhages
- Left shift of oxyhemoglobin saturation curve (less O_2 to tissues)
- **Bicarbonate and epinephrine cannot be administered through the same IV line, because epinephrine is inactivated.**

ATROPINE

Key point: Atropine is a parasympatholytic drug that accelerates sinus or atrial pacemakers and atrioventricular conduction.

Indications
Major indication: vagally mediated bradycardia

- High vagal tone (except secondary to hypoxia) is an uncommon cause of bradycardia in neonatal foals.
- *Neonatal bradycardia is generally caused by hypoxia and is treated by hyperventilation with 100% O_2 **and** epinephrine.*
    □ Early treatment with atropine may exacerbate the hypoxic insult by increasing the heart rate, resulting in a higher oxygen demand of cardiac muscle in the face of inadequate oxygen delivery.
- Hypoxemia and hypercapnia result in stimulation of the carotid body, increasing vagal tone with secondary bradycardia.
    □ Hyperventilation corrects this form of vagally mediated bradycardia, because lung inflation stimulates pulmonary receptors that override the carotid body stimulus.
    □ If hyperventilation and epinephrine treatment do not reverse the bradycardia, atropine therapy is indicated.

- Excessive vagal tone can be associated with GI disease.
  - ☐ Extreme intestinal distention secondary to meconium impactions, necrotizing enterocolitis, and bacterial enteritis (clostridiosis, salmonellosis)
  - ☐ Hypoglycemia often complicates this condition.
  - ☐ If hyperventilation with 100% O_2, effective chest compressions, and repeated treatment with epinephrine do not resolve the bradycardia, atropine is indicated.
- **In all cases of bradycardia, atropine should not be administered before hyperventilation with 100% O_2.**

Atropine Dosage

- 0.02 mg/kg IV
- 0.04–0.06 mg/kg intratracheally
- Repeat once in 5 minutes if indicated

Potential Complications

- Tachycardia
- Exacerbation of hypoxic insult by increasing the oxygen demand of cardiac muscle

CALCIUM

Key points:

- Calcium is essential for cardiac contraction.
  - ☐ Calcium entry into myocardial cells induces actin-myosin coupling.
  - ☐ Contraction is terminated when calcium is pumped out of the cell.
- Myocardial contractility is increased when calcium is infused in normal patients.
- Calcium therapy during cardiac arrest may hasten cell death.
  - ☐ During cardiac arrest, calcium entry into the cell cytoplasm is believed to be the final common pathway of cell death.
  - ☐ Calcium channel blockers are protective during cardiopulmonary bypass.
- **Calcium is not recommended for treatment of asystole or pulseless electrical activity.** Epinephrine is more useful.

Indications

- Hyperkalemia (secondary to ruptured bladder)
- Hypocalcemia
- Hypermagnesemia

CaCl Dosage

- 5–7 mg/kg (elemental calcium)
  - ☐ 10% CaCl—0.2–0.25 ml/kg
  - ☐ 10% Ca gluconate—0.6–0.75 ml/kg

Potential Complications

- Can result in more rapid cell death in presence of hypoxic damage
- Rapid infusion results in bradycardia or cardiac standstill.

LIDOCAINE

Key points:

- Lidocaine suppresses ventricular arrhythmias by decreasing automaticity.
  - □ Its local anesthetic properties suppress ventricular ectopy after myocardial infarction.
  - □ It decreases conduction of reentrant pathways.
  - □ It reduces the disparity in action potential duration between ischemic and normal tissue.
  - □ It prolongs conduction and refractoriness in ischemic tissue.
- There is no experimental support for a major antifibrillatory effect, but it may prevent recurrence once converted.

Indications

- Ventricular fibrillation
- Ventricular tachycardia

Lidocaine Dosage

- Bolus dosage
  - □ Initial dose: 1.5 mg/kg IV
  - □ Repeat once in 5 minutes
  - □ Then 8–10 minutes later with 0.5 mg/kg
  - □ Use in conjunction with defibrillation
- IV infusion
  - □ 1 mg/kg loading dose
  - □ 20–50 μg/kg/min (6 × body weight in kg = mg of lidocaine added to 100 ml fluids; 20–50 ml/h results in a dose of 20–50 μg/kg/min)

Precautions

- Toxic effects
- Neurologic signs
  - □ Depression
  - □ Paresthesia
  - □ Muscle twitching
  - □ Seizures
- Myocardial depression
- Circulatory depression

BRETYLIUM TOSYLATE

Key points:

- Prevent recurrence of ventricular fibrillation or ventricular tachycardia and wide-complex tachycardia (which is usually ventricular)

- Bretylium is an adrenergic neuronal blocker.
- Increases fibrillation threshold
- Synergistic with lidocaine
- Has direct myocardial effects
- Has biphasic adrenergic effects causing hypertension followed by hypotension (in normal individuals)
  - ☐ Initially, bretylium releases norepinephrine from adrenergic nerve endings for about 20 minutes.
  - ☐ Subsequently, it produces an adrenergic blockade that peaks at 45–60 minutes.
- Antiarrhythmic action is poorly understood.
- Increases action potential duration and effective refractory period

Indications (After Countershock, Epinephrine, Lidocaine)

- Ventricular fibrillation
- Ventricular tachycardia

Bretylium Tosylate Dosage

- 5 mg/kg undiluted IV rapidly, followed in 30–60 seconds by defibrillation
- If ventricular fibrillation persists, repeat with 10 mg/kg boluses
- Do not administer more than a total of 35 mg/kg

Precautions

- Toxic effects:
  - ☐ Hypotension
  - ☐ Hypertension
  - ☐ Tachycardia

MAGNESIUM SULFATE ($MgSO_4$)

Key point: Use in refractory fibrillation when countershock, epinephrine, lidocaine, and bretylium have failed.

Indications
- Refractory ventricular fibrillation
- Hypomagnesemia
- Torsades de pointes (see p. 115)

$MgSO_4$ Dosage

- 14–28 mg/kg diluted to 10 ml in 5% dextrose in water, IV push

---

Precautions

- Hypotension
- Use caution with renal failure

DEFIBRILLATION

Key points:

- The definitive treatment for ventricular fibrillation and pulseless ventricular tachycardia
- **Do not use to treat asystole or bradyarrhythmias.**
- Continue ventilation with 100% O_2 and chest compressions until the moment of defibrillation.
- Defibrillation results in depolarization of a critical mass of myocardial cells to allow spontaneous organized myocardial depolarization to resume.
  □ Defibrillation requires electrical current to pass through the heart.
  □ The amount of current delivered to the heart depends on the energy delivered from the paddles and the transthoracic resistance.
  □ There are numerous determinants of current flow through the heart.

Indications

- Ventricular fibrillation
- Pulseless ventricular tachycardia

Defibrillation Dose

- Initial series of up to 3 rapid charges: 2 J/kg, 4 J/kg, 4 J/kg
- Subsequent defibrillations—4 J/kg 30–60 seconds after treatment with epinephrine, lidocaine, or bretylium

---

Complications

- Potentially dangerous to the operator and other personnel
  □ No one should attempt defibrillation until trained both in the technique and on the defibrillator being used.
  □ Improper placement of the paddles can cause serious burns.
- *Use of alcohol before defibrillation is a fire hazard.*

POSTRESUSCITATION TREATMENT

Goals

- To prevent secondary organ failure
- To allow transportation to a facility where intensive care can be delivered

Continued evaluation of cardiopulmonary function is vital, even if the foal is easily resuscitated and its condition initially appears stable. Foals often suffer recurrent episodes of hypoxia, hypercapnia, or cardiovascular instability. The underlying cause of cardiopulmonary failure must be recognized and treated. Whatever the original etiology, if periods of hypoxia and hypotension go unrecognized and untreated, a fatal outcome is almost certain.

Guidelines for Postresuscitation Treatment

- Search for and treat the underlying cause of cardiopulmonary failure.
- Frequently assess cardiopulmonary function:

- Signs of inadequate pulmonary function:
  - □ Minimal and uneven chest excursions
  - □ Inadequate or unequal breath sounds
  - □ Increased respiratory effort (nasal flare, rib retraction)
  - □ Paradoxic ventilation (increased diaphragmatic efforts drawing chest wall in on inspiration)
- Periodic arterial and venous (VO_2 gives best measurment of O_2 uptake) blood gas analysis
- Continuous ECG to monitor heart rate and rhythm
- Evaluate peripheral circulation and end-organ perfusion:
  - □ Skin temperature
  - □ Capillary refill time
  - □ Quality of distal pulses
  - □ CNS responsiveness
  - □ Urine output
  - □ Serial indirect blood pressure determinations
- Place on humidified intranasal oxygen insufflation at 6–10 L/min.
- Treat hypothermia and maintain core temperature (if transporting, place in heated cab and not in cold van).
- Continued intravenous fluid therapy:
  - □ If in septic shock, once spontaneous circulation returns initiate aggressive fluid therapy—20-ml/kg boluses over 20 minutes with reassessment and monitoring of CVP after completing each bolus administration.
  - □ Continue maintenance fluids after successful fluid resuscitation.
- Pressor and inotropic support as needed (*must use IV infusion pump*): (see Table 35–5)
  - □ Dopamine, 3–6 μg/kg/min initially, titrate to effect up to 20 μg/kg/min
  - □ Dobutamine, 3–6 μg/kg/min initially, titrate to effect up to 25 μg/kg/min or higher

> To prepare dopamine or dobutamine infusion:
> 6 × body weight in kg = mg of drug added to 100 ml of fluids
> 1 ml/h equals a dose of 1 μg/kg/min

  - □ Epinephrine, 0.1 μg/kg/min initially, titrate to effect up to 1 μg/kg/min or higher

> To prepare epinephrine infusion:
> 0.6 × body weight in kg = mg of epinephrine added to 100 ml of fluids
> 1 ml/h equals a dose of 0.1 μg/kg/minute

  - □ If no response to traditional pressors, methylene blue therapy (0.5–2 mg/kg) may be helpful. It blocks the action of nitric oxide, which is the local messenger causing active vasodilation. Limited experience indicates this is a very effective pressor when used in foals in endotoxic shock. **CAUTION:** *Do not overdo pressor response with this drug.*

TABLE 35–5. **Relative Potency of Inotropes and Pressors**

Drug	Infusion Rate*	α Effect (Pressor)	β Effect (Inotropic)	Use
Dopamine	1–5 μg/kg/min (dopaminergic effect)	+	+	1st line choice, good
	5–15 μg/kg/min	+ +	+ +	mixed α
	10–20 μg/kg/min	+ + +	+ +	and β response
Dobutamine	2–20 μg/kg/min (high doses)	+ (+ +)	+ + +	Good β effects; add to dopamine for additional inotropic effect (limiting tachycardia)
Epinephrine	0.1–1 μg/kg/min (max 3 μg/kg/min)	+ + +	+ + +	Use if not responding to dopamine; good mixed α and β response
Norepinephrine	0.05–1 μg/kg/min (max 2 μg/kg/min)	+ + +	+	Primarily α effect; should be combined with a β drug
Phenylephrine	0.1–1 μg/kg/min	+ + +	0	Primarily α effect; should be combined with a β drug

*These rates serve as guidelines for treatment. The pharmacokinetics of these drugs are not consistent between individuals and within the same foal over time. Therefore, the dosage must be titrated for the individual and adjusted over time.

□ Naloxone may be useful in blocking endorphin-mediated hypotension (hemorrhagic and septic shock). It also enhances myocardial sensitivity to β-adrenergics.
■ **Remember: The goal of pressor therapy is not to increase blood pressure but to increase and direct perfusion of tissues and maintain cardiac perfusion by maintaining diastolic pressure.** As blood pressure increases, afterload increases and cardiac output drops. It is *counterpro-*

ductive to increase blood pressure at the expense of cardiac output. As blood pressure increases, more inotropic support of the heart is needed concurrently to support the cardiac output. This is the reason mixed α- and β-support (dopamine, dobutamine, epinephrine) is useful.

- When adequately oxygenated, begin 4–8 mg/kg/min glucose to help clear metabolic acidosis. This is important because myocardial glycogen is generally depleted and helps prevent postasphyxia hypoglycemia. Monitoring blood glucose levels (every 30 minutes until stable using a stallside test, e.g., a glucometer) is necessary because the glucose infusion rate frequently needs to be adjusted to prevent hyperglycemia or hypoglycemia. Occasionally the infusion rate needs to be greater than 8 mg/kg/min to satisfy glucose demands.

BIRTH RESUSCITATION

Although most newborns make the transition from fetal life without incident, rapid recognition of the need to intervene is vital in achieving a successful outcome in those that do not (see Diagram 35–3). The cause of cardiopulmonary failure at birth is readily evident. The lack of anticipation, however, may catch the attending clinician off guard. In a few cases the risk to the foal may be clear (e.g., with dystocia or peripartum maternal disease). In others it is not. Even when attending what is expected to be a normal birth, the clinician must monitor the progress of the foal's transition and be prepared to intervene when indicated. *Birth resuscitation represents a special case of general resuscitation requiring some modification in approach.*

Fetal/Neonatal Transition

The fetus depends on the placenta for gas exchange. When compared with the newborn foal, the fetus is hypoxemic, with a Pa_{O_2} of 40 torr in the umbilical vein. This does not imply tissue hypoxia, since compensatory mechanisms allow for adequate delivery of O_2 to tissues. Hypoxemia is largely responsible for the pulmonary hypertension that insures proper fetal blood flow.

Fetal Circulation

- Oxygen-rich blood, returning from the placenta by way of the umbilical vein, is directed to the heart and brain:
  - □ It bypasses the liver through the ductus venosus (which closes 30 days before birth in foals).
  - □ It travels to the right side of the heart via the posterior vena cava.
  - □ It enters the right atrium directly across from the foramen ovale. This blood tends to stream, flowing directly across the right atrium, through the foramen ovale. Oxygen-rich blood fills the left atrium.
  - □ Oxygen-rich blood is pumped by the left ventricle into the ascending aorta, which feeds the coronary arteries and the brachiocephalic artery, ensuring that the heart and brain receive the most oxygen-rich blood.
- Blood returning from the head and trunk is directed to the lower body and back to the placenta.

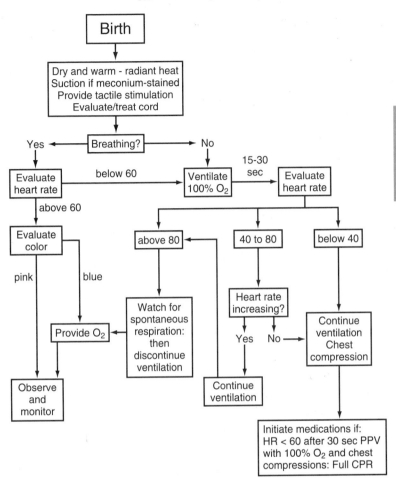

DIAGRAM 35–3. Overview of resuscitation of the foal at birth.

- □ Blood from the anterior vena cava fills the right ventricle.
- □ Because it enters the heart perpendicular to the foramen ovale and across from the tricuspid valve, it flows into the right ventricle.
- □ This blood is pumped into the pulmonary artery and is shunted through the ductus arteriosus to the descending aorta. Hypoxemia-induced pulmonary hypertension insures little pulmonary artery flow. Relative systemic hypotension (due to the placental circulation accommodating 40% of the cardiac output) allows right-to-left shunting of the blood.
- □ The descending aorta sends the blood to the lower body or back to the placenta.
- □ Blood returning to the placenta has a Pa_{O_2} of 15–25 torr.

During Labor

Mild asphyxia (exacerbated hypoxemia plus hypercapnia) **occurs in all neonates.**

- Uterine contractions prevent effective placental perfusion, resulting in
  - Mild tissue hypoxia
  - Secondary mild metabolic acidosis
  - Respiratory acidosis
- Between contractions, there is partial but not complete recovery.
- Uterine contractions also help empty the blood from the placenta.

At Birth

- Removal of the placental vascular space results in an increase in systemic blood pressure.
- Vigorous breathing efforts at birth originate from central and peripheral chemoreceptors stimulated by
  - The increase in systemic blood pressure
  - External stimuli
  - Progressive asphyxia
- There is a rapid drop in pulmonary blood pressure with the first breath.
  - The first breath is accompanied by a forceful expiration against a partially closed glottis, resulting in effective distribution of air in alveoli.
  - An adequate functional residual capacity is rapidly established.
  - Initial expansion of the lungs stimulates surfactant release, which allows further lung expansion
  - Lung expansion is responsible for an initial drop in pulmonary hypertension.
  - Ventilation with air results in a fall in PCO_2 and a rise in pH and PO_2 in the lungs, resulting in a dramatic drop in pulmonary vascular resistance.
- The reversal of the relative pulmonary and systemic pressures results in a closing of the foramen ovale and a reversal of the shunting of blood through the ductus arteriosus.
  - The increase in O_2 flowing through the ductus arteriosus stimulates its closure.

Unsuccessful Transition

If more than mild asphyxia occurs, the transition may be unsuccessful.

- Moderate to severe asphyxia may result from
  - Maternal systemic disease (colic, endotoxemia, hypotension, general anesthesia)
  - Placental disease (placentitis, premature placental separation)
  - Fetal disease (fetal infections, cord compression)
  - Intrapartum problems (dystocia, uterine inertia, premature placental separation)

- The fetus responds to asphyxia by reinforcing the fetal circulatory pattern. The neonate responds by reverting to the fetal pattern.
  □ Increased hypoxemia and acidemia increases pulmonary vascular vasoconstriction, resulting in the following chain of events: Decrease in pulmonary blood flow→ Decreasing left atrial return→ Resulting in a drop in left atrial pressure→ Resulting in increasing right-to-left shunting through the foramen ovale.
  □ In the fetus this may be appropriate because it would increase the amount of well-oxygenated blood (returning from the placenta) diverted to the heart and brain.
  □ In the neonate without placental function, it makes things worse, because the blood completely bypasses the lungs.

Development of Primary and Secondary Apnea

- Early, severe asphyxia results in stimulation of the fetus to breathe while still in utero.
- If the resulting gasping activity does not correct the asphyxia, this activity stops, resulting in a period known as *primary apnea.*
- Within minutes a second series of gasping activity (more irregular) occurs.
- If this second attempt to establish normal ventilation fails, the foal enters into a period of *secondary apnea.* **Secondary apnea is irreversible unless resuscitation is initiated.**
  □ It is very difficult to determine how far the asphyxia has progressed at the time of delivery.
  □ **Assume that foals that do not breathe at birth are in secondary apnea and treat accordingly.**

Birth Resuscitation Steps

(See Diagram 35–3)

Assessment

- *Initial assessment of the neonate begins during presentation.*
  □ Make a rapid evaluation of the peripheral pulse when the vaginal positioning of the foal is checked.
  □ Relative pulse rate and strength form a basis for monitoring the expected changes during this dynamic period.
  □ This assessment takes only 5–10 seconds.
  □ Calculating an accurate pulse rate is unnecessary and counterproductive with the rapid changes occurring.
  □ Assess the apical pulse as soon as the chest clears the birth canal.
- Bradycardia (heart rate of 40 or below) is expected during forceful contractions while passing through the birth canal.
- A transient, marked sinus arrhythmia commonly occurs when the first breaths are taken.
- Once the chest clears the birth canal, the heart rate rapidly increases.
- **Persistent bradycardia is an indication for rapid intervention.**

- Calculating a modified Apgar score (see Table 35–6)
  - □ Helps direct the urgency and extent of intervention needed.
  - □ Waiting for the traditional 1-minute and 5-minute scores is inappropriate if severe in utero asphyxia has occurred. *Initiate resuscitation before the 1-minute score is calculated in severely compromised neonates.*

Clear the Airway

- Remove the membranes from the nostrils as soon as the nose is seen.
- If meconium staining is present and the foal is not yet active:
  - □ Suction the nasal passages and nasopharynx. (Meconium is very difficult to suction because of its consistency.)
  - □ If this is rewarding and the foal is severely asphyxiated, suction the trachea.
- Avoid overzealous suctioning, which causes bradycardia and prolonged apnea.
- Since suctioning removes the air in the lung, limit suctioning episodes to 10–15 seconds at a time, with high flows of O_2 before and after each attempt.
- If the foal is vigorous and responsive, suctioning attempts are not beneficial.

Tactile Stimulation

- If spontaneous respiration and movement do not begin within seconds of birth, tactile stimulation is useful.
  - □ Rub the chest and head with a dry towel.
  - □ Stimulate the ear canal or nasal canal.
  - □ Gently compress the chest wall.
- **If spontaneous breathing efforts are not stimulated, intubate and ventilate immediately.**

TABLE 35–6. **Apgar Score Modified for the Foal**

Score	0	1	2
Heart rate	Absent	< 60 irregular	> 60 regular
Respiratory rate	Absent	Irregular	Regular
Muscle tone	Limp, lateral	Some flexion	Active, sternal
Reflex, nasal stimulation, ear tickle	No response	Grimace, weak ear flick	Sneeze/cough; ear flick/head shake

Score 7–8 = Normal
Score 4–6 = Mild to moderate asphyxia—stimulate, intranasal O_2, ventilate
Score 0–3 = Severe asphyxia—begin CPR

Respiratory Support

Apneic foals who have an irregular, gasping respiratory pattern or remain bradycardic (< 60 beats/min), need respiratory support.

- If spontaneous respiratory efforts are present, administer free-flow intranasal oxygen at a rate to 8–10 liters/min.
- If no spontaneous respiration is present, intubate and hyperventilate with 100% oxygen.
  - □ If oxygen is unavailable, use room air.

If ventilatory equipment is unavailable, use mouth-to-nose ventilation.

Hyperventilation with 100% oxygen is the most important step in birth resuscitation. GOAL: to reverse persistent fetal circulation by inflating the lungs, delivering high O_2 concentration, and producing respiratory alkalosis. **90% of foals requiring birth resuscitation respond when ventilated.**

- With the first delivered breath, give a prolonged inspiratory phase lasting about 5 seconds to insure lung expansion.
  - □ Give a delivered breath rate of 40–60/min.
  - □ Gauge the depth by chest excursions.
- Consistent volumes of lung fluid should be seen escaping from the nostril during both spontaneous and delivered ventilation.
- *If the asphyxia is mild and short lived,* after 30 seconds of ventilation with 100% oxygen the heart rate is above 60 and soon approaches 100 beats/min.
  - □ *Watch for spontaneous respiration.* Once present, extubate and place on free-flow intranasal oxygen.
- *If the asphyxia is advanced and myocardial damage is present,* bradycardia persists; initiate cardiovascular support.
  - □ The more advanced the asphyxia, the longer until spontaneous ventilation.

Cardiovascular Support

- Begin chest compressions immediately if
  - □ The foal remains bradycardic despite ventilation and develops a nonperfusing rhythm.
  - □ There is a nonperfusing rhythm or cardiac standstill at birth.
- If a perfusing, spontaneous cardiac rhythm does not develop within 30–60 sec of chest compressions, initiate drug therapy.

Thermal Management

- Birthing areas for foals are usually cold.
- The healthy foal has little trouble handling cold environmental temperatures.
- The foal with even mild asphyxia has difficulty with thermal control.
  - □ Towel-dry
  - □ Place on dry bedding

- □ Provide an external heat source: heat lamp, hot water bottles, warm water heating pads, hot air blanket.
- □ If the foal is depressed and remains hypothermic, move to a warm environment.

Drug Treatment

- As in all cases of cardiopulmonary failure, administer epinephrine early and often.
- **Epinephrine is the most useful drug to treat cardiac failure secondary to birth asphyxia.**
- Follow the guidelines described earlier for general CPR (see Diagram 35–2), except as indicated below:

ATROPINE

Do not use to treat bradycardia in newborn foals.

- The initial bradycardia stimulated by hypoxia is vagally mediated.
- Reasons not to use atropine:
  - □ The atropine-mediated reversal of early hypoxic bradycardia is purely symptomatic and does not treat the underlying cause (hypoxia).
  - □ If the heart rate increases and the hypoxia is not corrected, the myocardium goes further into oxygen debt.
  - □ This leads to a return of an atropine-nonresponsive bradycardia due to hypoxic myocardial damage.
  - □ Treating the underlying cause, hypoxia, through ventilation with 100% oxygen, chest compressions, and epinephrine reverses the bradycardia as rapidly as atropine therapy and prevents further damage.

DOXAPRAM

Do not use to treat apneic newborn foals.

- Doxapram stimulates respiration in primary apnea.
- In secondary apnea, the respiratory center is unresponsive to doxapram, and the drug increases the oxygen demand of the myocardium in the face of prolonged and severe hypoxia.
- Administering doxapram wastes valuable time.
- Ventilating (even if supplemental oxygen is not available) is as effective in reversing primary apnea and is the only effective therapy during secondary apnea.
- **At birth it is impossible to differentiate primary from secondary apnea.**

FLUID THERAPY

During the resuscitation of the newborn foal, administer fluids conservatively.

- The neonate is not volume depleted, unless bleeding has occurred (e.g., cord hemorrhage, fractured rib).
- Severe in utero asphyxia results in larger than normal vascular volume.
  - □ Fetal myocardial asphyxia causes decreased cardiac output, resulting in less flow to placenta.

□ With the aid of uterine contractions, the fetus still has adequate venous return from the placenta.

□ The result is a higher than normal vascular volume in neonates suffering from severe prepartum asphyxia.

□ The decreased blood pressure is from effects of asphyxia on myocardial function.

■ Fluid overloading can exacerbate a failing heart. High fluid rates decrease coronary perfusion.

■ Cases of hemorrhagic shock benefit from a bolus of 20 ml/kg of nonglucose-containing fluids, if initial resuscitation attempts are not successful.

■ Once spontaneous circulation is established and the foal is adequately oxygenated, then treatment with glucose-containing fluids at a rate of 4–8 mg/kg/min glucose is indicated.

□ To help clear metabolic acidosis.

□ To support cardiac output since myocardial glycogen stores are depleted.

□ To help prevent postasphyxia hypoglycemia.

Persistent Pulmonary Hypertension

■ Despite successful return of spontaneous circulation, some foals retain the fetal circulation pattern, with pulmonary hypertension and right-to-left shunting through the foramen ovale and patent ductus arteriosus.

■ These foals benefit from

□ Mechanical ventilation with 100% oxygen

□ Maintaining an arterial blood pH above 7.45–7.50 by a high respiratory rate to produce respiratory alkalosis. (**CAUTION:** Do not allow the Pa_{CO_2} to decrease below 30 torr.)

□ Bicarbonate administration to produce a metabolic alkalosis

□ Surfactant to reduce surface tension

■ **The most effective treatment for persistent pulmonary hypertension is inhalation therapy with 5–40 ppm of nitric oxide.**

□ Nitric oxide causes pulmonary vasodilation without affecting systemic blood pressure.

□ Limited clinical experience shows nitric oxide to be very effective in foals, even at low concentrations.

Neonatal Hypoxia

■ Many foals may remain hypoxemic ($PaO_2 < 60$ torr) after birth.

□ Hypoxic ischemic encephalopathy leading to general depression

□ Central respiratory center damage

□ Systemic hypoxic damage leading to hypotension

□ Hypoxic lung damage

□ Ventilation/perfusion mismatching

□ Primary lung disease

□ Sepsis

■ These foals are generally weak.

□ Encourage them to remain sternal

□ Turn from side to side (on the sternum) every 2 hours.

- Administer nasal insufflation of moist oxygen at a rate of 4–10 L/min.
  □ Monitor their PaO_2 by arterial blood gases every 4–6 hours.

Neonatal Hypercapnia

Many foals with peripartum asphyxia suffer from hypoxic-ischemic encephalopathy, resulting in depression of central respiratory receptors. Although these foals are good candidates for transient mechanical ventilation, some respond adequately to respiratory center stimulants such as caffeine.

CAFFEINE

- Oral loading dose of 10 mg/kg
- Oral maintenance dose of 2.5 mg/kg
- Serum half-life of caffeine in human neonates is variable, making the pharmacodynamics difficult to predict.
  □ Therapeutic trough serum concentrations in human neonates are between 5 and 25 μg/ml.
  □ Toxic reactions in human neonates occur with plasma levels above 40 μg/ml.
  □ Limited experience in foals indicates that trough blood levels range between 4 and 10 μg/ml.
- Treated foals have an elevated level of arousal and become more reactive to environmental stimuli.
- Adverse reactions:
  □ Restlessness
  □ Hyperactivity
  □ Tachycardia
- Caffeine therapy fails if the hypercapnia is compensation for metabolic alkalosis and the pH is not low.
  □ Critically ill neonatal foals commonly develop electrolyte imbalances that result in metabolic alkalosis, as explained by the strong ion difference theory.
  □ These foals have a secondary hypercapnia in an effort to counteract the alkalosis.
  □ Treat this physiologic response by correcting the electrolyte abnormalities and not by manipulating the respiratory system with drugs or mechanical ventilation.

Respiratory Support During Dystocia

- During a prolonged dystocia, foals die from asphyxia. This can be prevented if the foal's nose is accessible while it is in the birth canal.
- Place an endotracheal tube:
  □ Confirm that the endotracheal tube is in the trachea.
  □ Use a capnograph to verify endotracheal tube placement and obtain information concerning the effectiveness of cardiac output.
- Once the airway is secured and the foal is ventilated, much of the urgency to correct the dystocia is eliminated, allowing for a reassessment of the situation and more time for manipulation.

- If correction of the dystocia is further delayed and the tongue is accessible, use arterial blood gas samples from the lingual artery to assess the effectiveness of ventilation.

FURTHER READING

Fisher DE, Paton JB. Resuscitation of the newborn infant. *In* Klaus MH, Fanaroff AA (eds): Care of the High-Risk Neonate, 4th ed. Philadelphia, W.B. Saunders, 1993, pp 38–61.

Peckham GJ. Resuscitation of the Newborn. I. Holbrook, PR (ed). Textbook of Pediatric Critical Care. Philadelphia, W.B. Saunders, 1993, pp 61–70.

Chameides L, Hazinski MF (eds). Textbook of Pediatric Advanced Life Support. Dallas, American Heart Association, 1994.

Hazinski MF, Cummins RO (eds). 1996 Handbook of Emergency Cardiac Care for Healthcare Providers. Dallas, American Heart Association, 1996.

Guidelines for cardiopulmonary resuscitation and emergency cardiac care. V, VI, VII. JAMA 1992;268:2251–2281.

Bloom RS: Delivery room resuscitation of the newborn. *In* Fanaroff AA, Martin RJ (eds): Neonatal-Perinatal Medicine, Diseases of the Fetus and Infant, 5th ed. St. Louis, Mosby–Year Book, 1992, pp 301–324.

2

PART III

Shock and Temperature-Related Problems

36 Shock and Systemic Inflammatory Response Syndrome

Thomas J. Divers

Shock: *Inadequate tissue oxygenation*, most often caused by *decreased perfusion*

Septic shock: Most commonly a result of bacteremia or endotoxemia, which is responsible for triggering a cascade of mediators causing the cardiopulmonary and vascular changes found in shock

Systemic inflammatory response syndrome (SIRS): The systemic response associated with release of vasoactive and inflammatory mediators that cause shock. Initiated by:

- Bacteremia
- Endotoxemia
- Traumatic shock
- Hemolysis
- Anaphylactoid-like reactions

- Localized infections
- Hyperthermia
- Hypothermia
- Dehydration
- Hypotension

- And/or any organ injury that causes hypoxia and release of vasoactive and/or inflammatory mediators.

In both septic shock and SIRS, inadequate tissue perfusion and oxygenation are mostly a result of:

- Intravascular fluid volume loss
- Hypotension
- Heart failure

- Maldistribution of blood flow
- And/or diminished oxygenation of hemoglobin

Early in the course of septic shock/SIRS, the predominant cause of inadequate tissue perfusion-oxygenation is *maldistribution of blood flow*, frequently followed by systemic hypotension.

Early maldistribution of blood flow results from:

- Changes in arteriovenous tone caused by endogenous release of β-catecholamines and release of mediators such as nitric oxide, cytokines, and autocoids.

- *Leaky vessels*, which result from:
  - ☐ Arachidonic acid metabolism, prostanoids, leukotrienes
  - ☐ *Macrophage* procoagulant production
  - ☐ Neutrophil and platelet adherence to vessels, causing inflammatory mediator release, oxidative enzyme activity, proteases and other damaging enzymes
  - ☐ Release of autocoids (histamine, endorphorins, and so on)
  - ☐ Microthrombosis: Platelet aggregation, exposure of subendothelial collagen and release of tissue factor

Treatment is most successful during the early stage of shock/SIRS. This is frequently termed the hyperdynamic phase of shock, associated with left ventricular dilation, increased heart rate, increased cardiac output (mostly due to increased heart rate), and decreased vascular resistance. The mucous membranes are generally hyperemic during this phase.

- Later stages of shock are associated with:
  - ☐ Decreased cardiac index
  - ☐ Diminished β_1 and α response
- Further maldistribution of blood flow:
  - ☐ Shunts
  - ☐ Sludging in capillaries
  - ☐ Increased vascular permeability
  - ☐ Vascular obstruction
- Diminished cellular oxygenation and increased cellular acid production
- Free radical formation and cellular death
- Pulmonary dysfunction, organ failure, and death

At this stage,

- Extremities are cold.
- Peripheral pulse is weak.
- Mucous membranes are dark.
- Capillary refill is slow (> 3 sec).
- Mentality is altered.
- Petechiations may be seen.
- Urine production is diminished or absent.

As a result of the severe hypoxemia, the intestinal barrier is damaged, allowing systemic absorption of normal enteric endotoxin and/or bacterial translocation (from the gut to blood and organs). Diminished hepatic phagocytosis of endotoxin and bacteria further exacerbates the systemic demise.

In the horse, damage to the pulmonary and foot circulation are the most life-threatening injuries associated with septic shock/SIRS.

TREATMENT OF SEPTIC SHOCK/SIRS

Re-establish tissue blood flow to *above normal values!*

Volume Support

- Crystalloids: Hypertonic saline, balanced electrolyte fluid, or both. Hypertonic saline has the advantage of causing a rapid increase in cardiac output and systemic arterial pressure but a decrease in pulmonary arterial pressure and diminished vascular tone.

- Administer these fluids rapidly and *ideally* while measuring systemic arterial pressure and central venous pressure (see p. 464).
- Although more expensive, the ideal fluid therapy is a combination of crystalloids and *colloids*. Colloids are particularly important in treating septic shock/SIRS because of the leaky vessels that occur and the inability of crystalloids to remain in the intravascular bed longer than 1 hour.
- Either plasma or hetastarch are administered; *plasma is preferred* because it has
  - ☐ *Albumin*, comparable to synthetic colloids in maintaining oncotic pressure. Although synthetic colloids have a larger molecular weight, plasma has an advantage of being negatively charged and, therefore, maintains cations in the intravascular bed longer. Plasma also has a longer half-life in the horse than synthetic colloids.
  - ☐ *Antithrombin III*, an important inhibitor of the coagulation cascade; 100 units of heparin/kg body weight is added to the plasma at least 10 minutes before administration.
  - ☐ Fibronectin, enhances opsonization of endotoxin and prevents bacterial translocation
  - ☐ Proteins C and S, serve to inactivate clotting factors and enhance fibrinolysis
  - ☐ α_2-Macroglobulin, inhibits proteases
  - ☐ Antibody against lipopolysaccharide (LPS) or cytokines, of some benefit but not as important as the other plasma factors in treating septic/SIRS shock

Pump Support

If fluid therapy alone is unsuccessful in supporting normal or elevated blood pressure, cardiac output, and perfusion, or when central venous pressure (CVP) increases, use β_1-agonist therapy:

- Dobutamine*—2–15 μg/kg/min diluted in saline, for β_1-activity
- Dopamine*—2–15 μg/kg/min diluted in saline; *low dose* stimulates renal dopaminergic receptors and increases renal blood flow; *middle dose* also stimulates β_1-receptors; *high dose* causes β_1- and α-stimulation, which decreases renal perfusion.
- **Adequate** O_2—normal or *above normal.*
- Hemoglobin levels—maintain within normal range
  - ☐ Too low (< 3–7 gm/dl)* means transfusion.
  - ☐ Too high (variable) means additional fluids.

Oxygen Therapy

- For most patients—a single or double intranasal tubing with humidified oxygen

---

*Systolic blood pressure must be maintained at more than 70 mm Hg. Variable depending on blood volume and tissue oxygen uptake.

- For the septic foal with respiratory distress—positive-pressure ventilation with 50% or more O_2 concentration is required.
- NOTE: PaO_2 must be maintained at greater than 70 mm Hg, $PvO_2 > 45$ mm Hg and lactate* <4 mm/L.

Antimicrobial Support

Broad-spectrum coverage for gram-positive and gram-negative aerobes and anaerobes (e.g., ticarcillin/clavulanic acid, amikacin)

Surgical Treatment

Establish drainage, resect and debride necrotic tissue.

Prostanoid Inhibitors

- Flunixin meglumine 0.25 mg kg q8h
- Aspirin to inhibit platelet function: 60–90 gr/450-kg adult PO q2–3 days; may be administered per rectum, 120 gr/450-kg adult. Aspirin is reported not to inhibit in vitro endotoxin stimulated coagulation.

Additional Therapy

- Steroids: 0.25 mg/kg dexamethasone; most studies show little value; inhibits arachidonic acid metabolism and, therefore, commonly used.
- Pentoxifylline, 8.4 mg/kg PO q12h: commonly used to inhibit platelet aggregation and cytokines; improves deformability of RBCs
- Oxygen free radical inhibitors:
  □ Dimethyl sulfoxide (DMSO) commonly used, of questionable value
  □ Vitamin E
  □ Allopurinol—little indication for use in the horse
  □ Carolina rinse contains several antioxidants and cell protectants and has been used experimentally in abdominal surgery
  □ Antihistamines—rarely used in treating shock and unlikely beneficial once clinical signs are present
  □ Furosemide—used to decrease pulmonary arterial wedge pressure (pulmonary edema) and may cause systemic vasodilation and decreased cardiac output
  □ Glutamine per os—oral fluids with essential amino acids, including glutamine, provided when the GI tract is functional to support enterocyte function and decrease endotoxin absorption and bacterial translocation
  □ Sodium bicarbonate—used only when blood pH < 7.2—controversial. Do not use with respiratory acidosis (increased $PaCO_2$, hypocalcemia or hypokalemia)

*Estimated by measuring anion gap.

□ Nitroprusside—used topically, e.g., coronary band, if blood pressure normal and suspect hypoperfusion—vasodilation may cause hypotension

□ Additional therapy for persistent hypotension when fluids or pump drugs have been unsuccessful is methylene blue (0.5–2.0 mg/kg), to inhibit nitrous oxide; and naloxone (0.02 mg/kg), an opioid antagonist; and/or 50% glucose (1 g/kg, with insulin [0.5 IU/kg/h]) plus 40 mEq KCl/L.

Monitoring During Treatment of Septic Shock/SIRS

- Heart rate
- Arterial pressure—tail cuff or subjective digital pulse pressure (> 70 mm Hg, ideally 120–130 mm Hg systolic)
- Plasma protein → 4.2 gm/dl to maintain oncotic pressure and prevent edema formation
- Packed cell volume (PCV)—30%–45%
- PaO_2 → >100 mm Hg
- PvO_2 → >40 mm Hg. Lower values indicate abnormal oxygen delivery or increased O_2 extraction.
- CVP—5–15 cm H_2O. Too low is an indication for increased fluid rate; too high is an indication for decreased fluid rate, pump therapy, and treatment of renal failure.
- Blood pH—determine metabolic or respiratory component and treat accordingly.
- Anion gap—to detect increased unmeasured anions (assuming plasma protein normal) and treat appropriately. Most commonly, increased unmeasured anions are associated with lactic acidosis or renal failure/metabolic acidosis.
- Urine production—should be normal or increased after beginning IV fluids
- ECG—treat arrhythmias
- Platelet count, neutrophil count, and neutrophil morphology—as prognostic and therapeutic indicators
- Mucous membrane color—indicates perfusion quality and tissue oxygenation at that site

37 Temperature-Related Problems

Thomas J. Divers

HEAT STROKE

Usually seen in poorly conditioned athletes that are overworked in hot and humid climates. However, it can occur in individuals confined to poorly ventilated areas during hot and humid weather; this especially is a problem during transporting. May also infrequently occur in foals treated with erythromycin.

Diagnosis

Early diagnosis is important for effective treatment. The diagnosis is made on history and clinical signs.

Clinical Signs

- Poor sweating response
  - □ Hot, dry skin signals the early onset of heat stroke.
- Tachycardia (with or without arrhythmias)
- Tachypnea (with or without arrhythmias)
- Elevated rectal temperature (with or without arrhythmias) (106–110° F)
- Prolonged capillary refill time, muddy mucous membranes
- Depression
  - □ May progress to coma and death
- Weakness
  - □ May progress to collapse or ataxia
- Decreased appetite, refusal to work

Treatment

- Lower the body temperature:
  - □ Move the affected individual to a shaded, well-ventilated area (use fans if available).
  - □ Cold water hydrotherapy, applied to entire body. Use alcohol baths over neck, thorax, and abdomen if cold water unavailable.
  - □ Ice water enemas ONLY if the temperature is critically high. (Use with caution—overzealous treatment results in rectal tears.)
  - □ Antipyretic: Flunixin meglumine (also useful for antiendotoxin effect)—**many exhausted horses may be endotoxemic!**

- Restore blood volume.
  - □ Any (crystalloid) fluid is used, but 0.9% NaCl *with 20–40 mEq KCl/L* is recommended.
  - □ Use hypertonic saline if heart rate is very high and capillary refill time markedly increased (5 seconds or greater).
- Administer 2 liters of hyperimmune plasma (antibodies against endotoxin) for more severe cases.

ANHYDROSIS

Usually seen in exercising athletes; can be seen in stabled individuals subjected to hot and humid environments for long periods of time. The condition represents an *inability to sweat* in response to normal stimuli. The problem can develop acutely but generally develops over time.

Diagnosis

Clinical Signs

- Failure to sweat with appropriate stimuli (heat, exercise). NOTE: Some individuals have patches of sweating under the mane, in the pectoral or perineal region.
- Tachypnea (some pant); decreased exercise tolerance, rectal temperature higher than normal following exercise (>104°F/40°C)
- Respiratory rate higher than heart rate.

LESS COMMON CLINICAL SIGNS

Depression, anorexia, weight loss, alopecia

EPINEPHRINE/TERBUTALINE CHALLENGE

1:1000 and 1:10,000 Epinephrine—0.1 ml both concentrations intradermal. Affected individuals exhibit little or no response (local sweating) within 1 hour.
NOTE: Intravenous epinephrine worsens the problem in affected individuals and should be avoided.
Terbutaline—0.5 mg intradermal injection is also used.

Treatment

- Antipyretics, e.g., flunixin meglumine; cold water hydrotherapy; and shade, with a fan if possible
- The only proven prevention is to move the affected individual to a more temperate climate or to air-condition the stall.
- Provide electrolyte supplementation to all individuals exercising in hot weather (one AC, an electrolyte supplement is obtained from MPCO, LLC, Phoenix, AZ).
- Clip body hair

EXHAUSTIVE DISEASE SYNDROME

Multisystemic changes are seen in athletes subjected to either brief maximal or longer submaximal-intensity exercise, especially during hot and humid weather.

Problems develop in association with fluid and electrolyte losses, acid-base changes associated with exercise, and depletion of the body's energy stores.

Diagnosis

Clinical Signs

- Tachypnea* (>40 bpm after a 30-minute rest)
- Tachycardia* (>60 bpm after a 30-minute rest)
- Elevated rectal temperature (104–106° F/40–41.1°C)
- Dehydration (may have fluid deficits of 20–40 liters) (do not exhibit much interest in water or food despite the severe dehydration)
- Severe depression, decreased pulse pressure, decreased jugular distention, prolonged capillary refill time
- *Continued sweating* at reduced rate
- Cardiac irregularities (e.g., ventricular tachycardia)
- Muscle cramps or spasms
- Decreased or absent intestinal sounds (unless spasmodic colic develops)
- Lack of anal tone
- Synchronous diaphragmatic flutter—often ileus associated with it
- CNS signs.
- Loss of >7% body weight

Treatment

- Decrease body temperature
    - □ Move the affected individual to a shaded, well-ventilated area.
    - □ Cold water hydrotherapy, applied repetitively to entire body
    - □ Ice water enemas ONLY if the temperature is critically high. Use with caution—overzealous treatment results in rectal tears.
- *Fluid therapy* for exhausted patients is to replace volume, correct electrolyte abnormalities, and provide a source of calories. To facilitate more rapid rehydration, use two catheters or administer hypertonic saline, 4 ml/kg.
    - □ Lactated Ringer's solution + 20 mEq/L KCl, 10–20 L/h
    - □ 0.9% NaCl + 20 mEq/L KCL, 10–20 L/h; *WITH* 5% dextrose, 2 L/h

If urination does not occur after several liters of fluids, discontinue KCl. If urination is normal, KCl can be increased to 40 mEq/L.

- If synchronous diaphragmatic flutter (SDF) or intestinal atony is found on physical examination, administer 100–300 ml of 20% calcium borogluconate IV SLOWLY over 30 minutes. *Discontinue administration if cardiac irregularities develop or worsen.*
- If evidence of organ failure or severe metabolic acidosis (pH <7.1) is seen, administer bicarbonate solutions. NOTE: *Bicarbonate is contraindicated if SDF is present and is not routinely used in exhausted individuals.*

---

*May see a transient inversion—respiratory rate may be higher than the heart rate. This is more common in humid environments.

- Administer oral fluids as long as there is no intestinal dysfunction: 5–8 liters of electrolyte solution q30min as needed.
- Electrolyte solution:
  - 2 Tbsp NaCl
  - 1 Tbsp KCl (Morton's Lite salt)
  - 1 liter water
  - Amino acids, e.g., glutamine
- Discontinue if discomfort or gastric reflux develops.
- Do not use phenothiazine tranquilizers—these patients are at high risk for cardiovascular collapse and death.
- Flunixin meglumine, 1 mg/kg IV initially then 0.3 mg/kg q8h.
- Hyperimmune plasma with antibodies against endotoxin, 2 liters (exhausted individuals have increased potential to be endotoxic).

Prognosis

Generally good if appropriate therapy instituted early. However, multisystemic complications develop in some individuals 2–4 days after an episode of exhaustion. These manifestations include:

- Myopathy
- Rapidly progressive laminitis
- Renal dysfunction
- GI ulceration
- Elevation in liver-derived enzymes and elevated bilirubin

Administration of nonsteroidal anti-inflammatory drugs (NSAIDs) without appropriate fluid replacement is not recommended.

FROSTBITE

Rarely seen in horses but may occur in debilitated patients or foals exposed to extreme cold.

Diagnosis

Cold extremity with color change: white to deep purple (may be warm and red if recirculation has started).

Treatment

- Rewarm extremity.
  - Move affected individual to heated area or at least out of the wind.
  - Apply warm, damp towels (avoid rubbing, which damages frozen cells).
- Restore dermal microcirculation.
  - Antiprostaglandin: flunixin meglumine (Banamine) IV (not in foals)
  - Pentoxifylline, 8.4 mg/kg PO q12h
  - Vasodilator: Acepromazine
  - Platelet aggregation inhibitor: Aspirin
- Local treatment:
  - Topical aloe vera gel three to four times per day

　　□ Nitroglycerin ointment (2%). NOTE: Wear gloves when handling ointment.
- Antimicrobials if necrosis is anticipated

Prognosis

Influencing factors:

- Time of exposure
- Temperature
- Wind chill
- Moisture on skin
- Circulatory status of patient
- Effectiveness of treatment.

Some individuals slough skin and/or hooves in the affected limbs, whereas others have no further signs once the limb is rewarmed. Generally edema and failure to rewarm are indicators of poor prognosis for the limb.

In cases of septicemia, especially in foals, a similar syndrome occurs due to arterial thrombosis. It is probable that septic foals are more prone to frostbite due to compromised circulation.

Laboratory Tests

38. Cytology   550

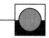

38 Cytology

Kent A. Humber

- Cytologic evaluation provides useful information rapidly.
- Answers are not always clear-cut.
  □ Samples may be nondiagnostic.
  □ Biopsy and histopathology may be necessary for definitive diagnosis.
- Proficiency requires practice.
  □ Duplicate slides can be kept and compared with the description and report from the cytopathologist.

MANAGEMENT OF CYTOLOGIC SPECIMENS

- Interpretation of specimen is limited by the quality of the sample.
- Maximizing the chance of achieving diagnostic samples depends on interrelated procedures:
  □ obtaining the specimen
  □ preparation of the glass slides
  □ staining
  □ microscopic evaluation and interpretation

Obtaining the Specimen

Techniques for collection of peritoneal, thoracic, synovial fluid, bronchoalveolar lavage (BAL), and transtracheal wash are discussed elsewhere (see pp. 36, 38, 50, 55, and 65).

Preparation of the Glass Slides

- Prepare as soon as practical after collection; cells are alive and continue to perform inherent "duties":
  □ Neutrophils phagocytize contaminant bacteria, simulating a septic condition.
  □ Macrophages phagocytize red blood cells, simulating previous hemorrhage.
- Use new, precleaned glass slides: do not wash slides and reuse.
  □ Residues alter cellular morphology and staining characteristics.

Staining

- Most common stains are Romanowsky-type (combinations of basic and acidic stains dissolved in methyl alcohol).
  □ Examples: Wright's stain, Giemsa stain, "quick" polychromatic stains

- Polychromatic stains (e.g., Diff-Quik, DipStat, Stat III) are widely used in veterinary practices.
  □ These stains do not undergo a metachromatic reaction, and some mast cell granules do not stain, resulting in misclassification of the cells as macrophages, leading to possible misdiagnosis of mast cell tumors.
- Staining protocols should follow those recommended by the manufacturer; however, make adaptations depending on the sample:
  □ Thin smears and samples with lower total protein content require less time in the stain.
  □ Thick smears and samples with higher protein content require more time in the stain.
- Slides can be restained if staining is insufficient in either the eosinophilic or basophilic tinctorial properties (skip the fixation step and immerse in the staining vat needed to correct the deficiency).
- These stains deteriorate with time and use.
  □ Staining quality gradually decreases indicating the need to replace the stain.
- The stains support bacterial and fungal growth; *consistent* presence of microorganisms indicates the need to change the stains, rather than true septic conditions.
- Bacterial and fungal elements stain basophilic in the Romanowsky-type stains; shape and morphology of the bacteria are discernible, but Gram stain is necessary for further classification.
- New methylene blue stain is a basic dye taken up readily by nuclei, nucleoli, and mast cells. Eosinophil granules do not take up the dye. Erythrocytes do not stain and appear as clear or pale blue circular areas.

Microscopic Evaluation

- Allow slide to dry in near-vertical position after staining.
- Film of stain on the back (bottom) of slide can be removed with an alcohol-moistened gauze sponge.
- Scan smear using 4–10× objective to evaluate staining quality and look for localized areas of increased cellularity or unique staining features.
- Look for large objects such as crystals, foreign bodies, parasites, and fungal hyphae.
- Detailed evaluation is made using oil-immersion objectives (50–100×) to study nuclear and cytoplasmic morphology, the presence of cellular inclusions, and presence and characteristics of microorganisms.

Interpretation

- A definitive diagnosis may not always be achieved; however, the general disease process (inflammation or neoplasia) is recognized quickly if a logical, methodical approach is utilized.
- A definitive diagnosis is not always necessary for immediate management of a case; preliminary findings are used to direct further diagnostic efforts as well as initial therapeutic regimens.

Inflammation

- In the equine patient, most cytologic evaluations performed on an emergency basis are approached with the goal of identifying or ruling out an inflammatory process; and, if an inflammatory process exists, can a causative microorganism be identified?
- Inflammation may accompany neoplastic processes; therefore, the presence of inflammation does not rule out concurrent neoplasia.
- Inflammation may cause morphologic changes in cell populations that mimic neoplasia, and it may not be possible to rule the presence of neoplasia out before the inflammation is controlled with therapy utilizing antimicrobial or anti-inflammatory agents.
- Inflammation is identified by increased numbers of inflammatory cells:
  □ Neutrophils
  □ Eosinophils
  □ Lymphocytes
  □ Plasma cells
  □ Macrophages
  □ Giant cells
  □ Mast cells
  □ Basophils

Mast cells and basophils are rare in horses.

- Inflammation is classified by terminology implying *duration* or the *type* of inflammation:

DURATION

- *Acute*: neutrophils > 70% of inflammatory cells
- *Subacute or Chronic Active*: 50–70% neutrophils, 30–50% macrophages
- *Chronic*: > 50% macrophages

TYPE OF INFLAMMATION

- *Suppurative:* neutrophils > 85%
  □ Septic or purulent: presence of intracellular bacteria
- *Mononuclear:* predominantly mononuclear cells without a significant suppurative component
- *Granulomatous*: numerous epithelioid macrophages or giant cells
- *Eosinophilic*: numerous eosinophils
- Inflammatory processes are not always "pure":
  □ *Pyogranulomatous*: suppurative or purulent process accompanied by granulomatous inflammation

SUBMISSION OF CYTOLOGIC PREPARATIONS AND SAMPLES FOR INTERPRETATION

- Provide adequate history!
  □ The cytopathologist who has a thorough understanding of the case is better able to provide meaningful information.
- Contact laboratory before submission regarding sample handling, fixa-

tion, number of slides, packing, and shipping methods to maximize chances of yielding useful information.

□ Generally, submit two to three air-dried, unfixed, unstained smears, along with two to three Romanowsky-stained smears (some tissues stain poorly when staining is delayed after preparation of the slides).

□ Submitting unstained smears allows the cytopathologists to stain the slides with their preferred stain in addition to providing slides for special stains.

□ Improperly packed slides often shatter during transport, slowing the diagnostic process or making diagnosis impossible.

□ Simple cardboard mailers do not provide sufficient protection to prevent slide breakage if mailed in unpadded envelopes: use bubble wrap, Styrofoam, or plastic slide boxes.

□ Mark slides with the name of the client, date collected, and sample site. Pencil works well on the frosted area of slides; use alcohol-resistant ink or other permanent labeling methods on slides without frosted areas. Porous tape or adhesive labels are not adequate (often unreadable after the staining process).

□ **Do not** send slides along with formalin-containing samples or in mailers previously used to ship formalinized samples.

□ Formalin vapors alter staining characteristics of cells and may make the slides unreadable.

□ Protect slides against moisture, which can cause cell lysis.

■ Submit fluid samples in combination with glass slide smears prepared immediately after collection.

□ If sample is low in cellularity, make direct smears as well as smears from concentrating the sample in a manner similar to that used in preparing urine sediment.

□ Centrifuge sample in a conical tube, discard the supernatant, and make a smear from the resuspended pellet. Obviously, this preparation cannot be used to estimate nucleated cell count.

■ Submit fluid samples in EDTA (lavender-top) tube to prevent potential clot formation. Also submit sterile serum (red-top) tube for possible microbiologic culture and sensitivity. If prolonged transit of sample is anticipated, use microbiologic transport system, as bacterial growth has occurred in "sterile" red-top tubes over time.

PERITONEAL FLUID

■ Normal peritoneal fluid is essentially a dialysate of plasma:
  □ low volume, cellularity, and total protein
  □ Biochemical constituents are present in concentrations similar to plasma.

■ Low molecular weight substances (e.g., glucose and urea) diffuse easily across the mesothelium and equilibrate quickly between plasma, interstitial fluid, and peritoneal fluid.

■ Higher molecular weight substances (e.g., creatinine and most enzymes) are less readily diffusable and require longer for equilibration. Plasma proteins (very large molecular weight substances) are primarily limited to the vascular compartment.

- Peritoneal fluid is normally drained from the abdominal cavity by specialized lymphatic lacunae in the diaphragm that connect to the right lymphatic duct; this drainage is crucial for recirculation of protein entering the peritoneal cavity.
- Normal peritoneal fluid contains a negligible amount of fibrinogen and therefore does not clot. Blood contamination, hemorrhage, or protein exudation is accompanied by increased fibrinogen content, and the sample may subsequently clot; therefore, collect peritoneal fluid in EDTA (lavender-top) tube for cell count, total protein determination, and cytologic evaluation.

Cell Counts and Cytologic Examination

- Nucleated cell counts are performed in a manner similar to that used for blood (manual dilution with microscopic enumeration or automated cell counter).
  - □ Normal cell count is less than 5000 cells/μl
  - □ Cell counts above 10,000 cells/μl are abnormal.
  - □ Interpretation of cell counts of 5000—10,000 cells/μl is not always clear-cut.
- Normal peritoneal fluid contains very few erythrocytes and negligible erythrophagocytosis (ingestion of erythrocytes by phagocytic cells).
- Normal leukocytes found in peritoneal fluid (Fig. 38–1, see Color Plate 2).
  - □ Neutrophils: up to 70% of nucleated cell population, making fluid appear inflammatory to the inexperienced cytologist
  - □ Large mononuclear cells and macrophages: up to 50%. This group of cells includes nonreactive tissue macrophages of blood monocyte origin, activated macrophages, and mesothelial cells. The cells are often difficult to distinguish morphologically and are consequently grouped together and termed "mononuclear phagocytes."
  - □ Lymphocytes: small numbers; exhibit the same morphologic characteristics as those found in blood. These cells recirculate into the blood stream via the lymphatic lacunae in the diaphragm. Lymphoblasts are not present in normal peritoneal fluid and their presence indicates neoplasia (lymphosarcoma).
  - □ Eosinophils: the presence of more than a rare eosinophil suggests parasites; use further diagnostics to rule out parasitic infection.
- Assessment of neutrophil morphology is very important in the cytologic evaluation of most cytologic samples, including peritoneal fluid. Neutrophils entering body cavities or tissues do not return to the blood stream; therefore, aging and cell death are normal events. These cells are often hypersegmented or display pyknosis, indicating senescent changes. Leukocytophagia (ingestion of leukocytes by phagocytic cells) may be observed.
  - □ Bacterial cytotoxins may rapidly damage inflammatory cells in vivo, particularly neutrophils. This acute cell injury causes cellular disruption and nuclear degeneration.

□ Nuclear degeneration: swollen, pale-staining nuclei (karyolysis), which may fragment (karyorrhexis).

□ Karyolysis is suggestive of sepsis; examine the smear carefully for the presence of microorganisms.

□ When bacteria are present in peritoneal fluid, the prognosis is generally better with lower numbers of organisms that are highly phagocytized.

□ When all bacteria have an identical morphology it generally indicates an abdominal abscess (e.g., *Streptococcus* sp.) and not intestinal leakage.

Interpretation of Peritoneal Fluid

Enterocentesis

■ Accidental puncture of the intestine during abdominocentesis causes an inflammatory response in the peritoneal cavity but is usually without overt clinical signs or deleterious sequelae.

■ The sample generally contains gut contents and has a greenish-brown, turbid appearance, with a characteristic fermentative odor.

■ Cytologically, there may be a population of relatively normal-appearing cells with large numbers of a mixed population of extracellular bacteria (cocci and rods), or very few nucleated cells with the bacterial population. The presence of cells is dictated by whether a volume of peritoneal fluid is obtained before the enterocentesis, or whether the viscus is entered immediately so that only GI contents are sampled.

□ Protozoal organisms may be seen, depending on the area of the GI tract entered.

□ In cases where only very few nucleated cells are present, consider the clinical findings to determine whether the sample is representative of enterocentesis or GI rupture.

GI Rupture (Fig. 38–2, see Color Plate 2)

■ The site of rupture along the GI tract often influences the character of the fluid obtained via abdominocentesis.

□ Gastric and large intestinal ruptures result in widespread contamination of the peritoneal cavity. The sample is often almost acellular; very few intact inflammatory cells can survive in such a hostile environment. There is usually marked karyolytic degeneration, and large numbers of a mixed population of bacteria.

□ Small intestinal and rectal ruptures usually result in less contamination of the peritoneal cavity because of the effectiveness of the omentum in isolating the affected bowel from the rest of the abdominal cavity.

Suppurative and Septic Suppurative Inflammation

■ Suppurative inflammation is diagnosed when the nucleated cell count and total protein content are elevated. The nucleated cell population is composed of high numbers of neutrophils.

■ When bacteria can be identified intracellularly, the process is classified

as septic suppurative inflammation. The neutrophils become "degenerate," and karyolytic and karyorrhectic changes are seen.
  □ Normal neutrophil morphology does not exclude the possibility of a bacterial etiology; if only small volumes of cytotoxins are produced by the microorganisms involved, cell morphology is not greatly affected.
- Culture of the microorganisms and sensitivity testing for a variety of antimicrobial agents aids in specifically directing therapeutic efforts.

Hemorrhagic Effusions

- Hemorrhage can result from:
  □ Iatrogenic contamination at the time of collection
  □ Hemorrhagic diapedesis, usually from a compromised segment of the gastrointestinal tract
  □ Intra-abdominal hemorrhage
  □ Penetration of the spleen during the abdominocentesis procedure
- Recent hemorrhage into the peritoneal cavity or contamination of peritoneal fluid during sample collection may result in the presence of platelets microscopically. Platelets are not usually seen if hemorrhage has occurred more than several hours previously.
- Macrophages "clean up" the erythrocytes in the abdominal cavity and display erythrocytophagia. Hemoglobin from the red blood cells is broken down and the iron conserved for new heme production (Fig. 38–3, see Color Plate 2)
- Macrophages may contain iron pigment:
  □ *Hemosiderin*: refractile pigment, yellow-green to dark brown–black in color
  □ *Hematoidin crystals*: bright yellow and refractile
- The presence of erythrophagocytosis, hemosiderin pigment, or hematoidin crystals indicates previous hemorrhage. Must differentiate between pathologic process or iatrogenic causes.
- A packed cell volume (PCV) and total protein determination of the abdominal fluid are helpful in determining the amount of blood present in the fluid, as it takes relatively few erythrocytes to impart a red color to the fluid grossly.

Seminoperitoneum

- Vaginal perforation during breeding may result in a septic, nonseptic, or seminoperitoneum. With seminoperitoneum, free sperm, neutrophils, and macrophages containing phagocytosed sperm heads may be found in the peritoneal fluid sample. A mild suppurative inflammation results from exposure of the peritoneum to seminal fluid.

Uroperitoneum

- Rupture of the urinary bladder is most frequently seen in neonatal foals, although cases in adults have been described.
- Analysis of peritoneal fluid usually reveals an increased volume of clear, pale yellow fluid with low cell count and low specific gravity. A mild

suppurative inflammation may be present secondary to chemical irritation of the peritoneal surfaces.

- Calcium carbonate crystals may be identified during cytologic evaluation of the fluid sample in adults.

Neoplasia

- Most cases involving neoplasia in the horse present with chronic symptoms (weight loss, weakness, and intermittent colic); however, tumors involving the GI tract have been reported to cause acute abdominal pain.
  - □ Neoplasms involving the GI tract include lymphosarcoma, squamous cell carcinoma, fibrosarcoma, adenocarcinoma, leiomyoma, leiomyosarcoma, myxosarcoma, lipoma, mesothelioma, intestinal carcinoid, and neurofibroma.
  - □ Intra-abdominal tumors may not exfoliate cells into the peritoneal fluid; therefore, the absence of neoplastic cells does not preclude a diagnosis of neoplasia. Abdominocentesis results in a diagnosis of neoplasia in approximately 40% of positive cases.
  - □ Tumors involving serosal surfaces, particularly those that cause erosion of serosal blood vessels, may cause hemorrhage into the abdominal cavity.
  - □ Inflammation secondary to tumor necrosis or infection results in peritonitis and the associated changes in peritoneal fluid.
  - □ Reactive mesothelial cells may be mistaken for neoplastic cells because of their highly pleomorphic appearance. This can result in a difficult differentiation between a reactive/inflammatory process and neoplasia.

Incidental Findings

- Glove powder (cornstarch) can be found in cytologic specimens whenever sterile technique is used for collection (Figs. 38–4 and 38–5, see Color Plate 3). Microscopically, it appears as large, round to hexagonal particles with a central fissure or nidus. The particles usually do not take up stain and are clear or slightly blue in hue.
- Cornified squamous epithelial cells are occasionally found in samples when a sterile preparation has been performed before sampling. The cells typically are rolled up and appear as dark, deeply basophilic structures with ragged ends. These structures are commonly known as "keratin flakes."
- Microfilariae of *Setaria* spp. are occasionally observed in peritoneal fluid samples (Figs. 38–4 and 38–6, see Color Plate 3). Incidence is relatively rare since the widespread use of ivermectin anthelmintics.
- Lipemic peritoneal fluid is occasionally observed in healthy foals.

THORACIC FLUID

- Analysis is indicated with evidence of pleural effusion (auscultation, percussion, radiographic studies, or ultrasonographic evaluation).
- Normal pleural fluid is essentially a dialysate of plasma (like abdominal fluid), with low cellularity and total protein concentration.

- Volume, cellularity, and biochemical composition of pleural fluid often reflects the pathophysiologic status of the visceral and parietal pleural surfaces.
- Effusions are noted in case of:
  - ☐ Heart failure
  - ☐ Chronic hepatic disease
  - ☐ Hypoalbuminemia
  - ☐ Diaphragmatic hernia
  - ☐ Pleuropneumonia
  - ☐ Pulmonary abscesses
  - ☐ Thoracic abscesses
  - ☐ Thoracic neoplasia
  - ☐ Hemothorax
- Cell counts, total protein determinations, and cellular makeup of thoracic fluid are essentially identical to that of peritoneal fluid. Interpretation of samples is carried out in a similar manner.
- Neoplasia involving the pleura often causes a uniform red color (hemorrhage) of the peritoneal fluid. Septic pleuritis may also have a red color but is most commonly amber colored and hazy.

SYNOVIAL FLUID

- Normal synovial fluid is a dialysate of plasma modified by the secretion of hyaluronic acid, glycoproteins, and macromolecules.
- Synovial fluid functions:
  - ☐ Supplies nutrition to articular cartilage, which is avascular
  - ☐ Lubricates the joint surfaces, limiting friction and wear between opposing articular cartilage surfaces

Cell Counts and Cytologic Examination

- Samples from the more commonly sampled joints usually contain less than 500 nucleated cells per microliter.
- Neutrophils should not exceed 10% of the population of nucleated cells unless there is obvious blood contamination of the sample.
- The majority of nucleated cells present in normal synovial fluid are lymphocytes and large mononuclear cells, which include monocytes, macrophages, and synovial lining cells (synoviocytes).
- Intact clumps of synovial lining cells are occasionally aspirated.
- The size and degree of cytoplasmic vacuolization in synovial fluid macrophages is variable; some macrophages contain cytoplasmic metachromatic granules.
- Normal synovial fluid is essentially free of erythrocytes; however, almost all specimens contain some erythrocytes, commonly due to sample contamination with blood during the collection process. Erythrocytes also enter synovial fluid in a variety of disease processes involving the joint.

Interpretation of Synovial Fluid

Degenerative and Traumatic Joint Disease

- Typically less than 5000 nucleated cells/μl; usually 1000–3000 cells/μl.
- Mononuclear cells predominate. The extent of vacuolization in macrophages is of little diagnostic significance.
- Neutrophils are usually present as less than 10% of the nucleated cell population.
- It is difficult to differentiate acute traumatic injury with resultant hemorrhage from blood contamination during collection, particularly if there has been insufficient time for macrophages to phagocytize erythrocytes and/or break down hemoglobin into hemosiderin or hematoidin pigment.
  - □ The presence of platelets or platelet clumps may be helpful in suggesting blood contamination.
  - □ Phagocytized erythrocytes by macrophages suggests that the red cells are already present in the fluid at the time of collection.
- Cartilage fragments may be found in concentrated cytologic preparations with degenerative or traumatic joint disease; however, techniques describing the severity of the joint disease by examining the number and type of cartilage fragments have not gained wide acceptance.

Inflammatory Joint Disease

- Neutrophils are usually the predominant cell type.
- Two major groups of diseases that classically respond with a neutrophilic (suppurative) inflammatory response:
  - □ Septic arthritis
  - □ Immune-mediated diseases (e.g., rheumatoid arthritis and systemic lupus erythematosus).
- Septic arthritis should be the primary differential diagnosis when suppurative synovial fluid is obtained; immune-mediated arthritis is rare in horses.
- Noninfectious causes of neutrophilic inflammation include acute traumatic joint disease and chronic hemarthrosis.
- It is important to assess neutrophil morphology in synovial fluid samples:
  - □ Nuclear degeneration (karyolysis) is evident in cases of septic arthritis and can be more difficult to assess in synovial than in peritoneal or pleural fluids because of synovial fluid mucin, which may prevent neutrophils from flattening on a slide and therefore prevent a true evaluation of nuclear morphology.
- Detecting bacteria in synovial fluid is more difficult than in other fluids. Bacteria are often rare and are found either intracellularly in neutrophils or free in the fluid.
- Acute traumatic joint disease
  - □ Nucleated cell counts usually less than 5000 cells/μl
  - □ Mononuclear cells predominate.
  - □ Increased neutrophils may be present, making differentiation between sepsis and acute trauma difficult.
  - □ Nucleated cell counts greater than 30,000 cells/μl are unlikely with acute traumatic injury.

☐ Elevated cell counts secondary to trauma typically decrease within a few days to counts less than 5000 cells/μl.
- Chronic hemorrhage
  ☐ Cellular response can vary but is often characterized by neutrophilia.
  ☐ Phagocytic cells displaying erythrocytophagia or containing iron pigments such as hemosiderin or hematoidin help identify previous hemorrhage.
- Rarely, synovial fluid has nucleated cell counts greater than 5000 cells/μl, made up primarily of lymphocytes. Considerations should include *Mycoplasma* sp. or *Borrelia burgdorferi* organisms.
- A single case of eosinophilic synovitis has been described, with marked synovial hyperplasia and eosinophilic infiltration.

BRONCHOALVEOLAR LAVAGE (BAL) AND TRANSTRACHEAL ASPIRATE

- Techniques for collection of material using BAL or transtracheal aspirate are described on pages 36 & 38.
- Protein determination is not routinely performed on these samples.
  ☐ Samples are collected in saline and often contain only small amounts of protein, often in the form of mucus.
  ☐ Samples from inflamed lungs also contain plasma proteins but are diluted by saline used during sample collection.
- Cell numbers are often low in samples due to dilution, and it is therefore necessary to use methods to concentrate the cells present for microscopic evaluation.
  ☐ Adding one or two drops of serum or commercially prepared bovine serum albumin before the slides are made helps preserve cells and results in better cellular morphology.
- Slides are stained with Romanowsky stain. Additional stains may be helpful:
  ☐ Gram stain: identify and classify bacteria
  ☐ PAS stain: fungal organisms
  ☐ Perl Prussian blue or Gomori stain: iron

Microscopic Features

- Mucus appears as strands of flocculent material and stains pink to light blue with Romanowsky stains.
- Curschmann spirals of mucus: dark-staining, tight spirals of mucus:
  ☐ Do not overinterpret; these formations likely occur secondary to specific pH and protein concentrations and do not always represent inspissated mucus casts from small bronchi and bronchioles.
- Nucleated cells from the lower respiratory tract include epithelial cells and inflammatory cells:
  ☐ Epithelial cells: ciliated columnar epithelial cells (Fig. 38–7, see Color Plate 3), nonciliated epithelial cells, goblet cells
  ☐ Inflammatory cells: neutrophils, macrophages, eosinophils, lymphocytes, mast cells
- Erythrocytes are frequently present because of minor trauma to the

epithelium during collection; however, they may be present because of true hemorrhage into the respiratory tract.

- Other substances may be identified in samples:
  - □ Squamous epithelial cells from oral cavity or pharynx
  - □ Bacteria
  - □ Plant material
  - □ Pollen
  - □ Fungal elements
  - □ Starch granules from surgical gloves

Normal Cytologic Features

- The majority of nucleated cells in a transtracheal aspirate or wash without lower respiratory disease are ciliated and nonciliated columnar epithelial cells and alveolar macrophages. Small numbers of neutrophils and lymphocytes may be present. A small amount of mucus is usually present.
- BAL samples contain predominantly macrophages and relatively few columnar epithelial cells. Small numbers of lymphocytes, epithelial cells, and neutrophils are present.

Oropharyngeal Contamination

(Fig. 38–8, see Color Plate 4)

- Contamination with material from the oropharyngeal cavity occurs occasionally during sample collection. Squamous epithelial cells and a mixed population of bacteria located predominantly extracellularly and often adhering to the squamous epithelial cells are evidence of contamination.
- Evidence of oropharyngeal contamination is also found in samples obtained in cases of aspiration pneumonia.
  - □ Evidence of inflammation of the lower respiratory tract is present and should be factored into the interpretation.

Acute Inflammation

- Suppurative inflammation characterized by a majority of neutrophils is one of the most common lesions detected by examination of the lower respiratory tract. (Fig. 38–9, see Color Plate 4)
  - □ Careful examination for the presence of intracellular bacterial microorganisms, along with aerobic and anaerobic cultures of the sample, is warranted.
  - □ Alveolar macrophages and columnar epithelial cells are usually present.
  - □ With chronic inflammation, the ratio of neutrophils to alveolar macrophages decreases, and binucleate and multinucleate macrophages appear.

Chronic Obstructive Pulmonary Disease (COPD)

- Occurs because of hypersensitivity and hyperirritability of the lungs to inhaled irritants and/or allergens. Cytologic features (Fig. 38–10, see Color Plate 4):

- □ Increased amount of mucus
- □ Inflammation characterized by either predominantly neutrophils or a mixed neutrophil and macrophage exudate
- □ Hyperplastic ciliated respiratory epithelial cells and increased numbers of goblet cells may be present.
- □ Eosinophils may be present in increased numbers, but this is not consistent; the diagnosis should not be dismissed because of the absence of eosinophils.
- □ Bacterial and/or fungal component may be present, usually mild when considering the degree of inflammation present.

Eosinophilic Inflammation

- Eosinophilic inflammation suggests hypersensitivity associated with allergic bronchitis or parasite migration:
  - □ *Dictyocaulus arnfieldi* in adults
  - □ *Parascaris equorum* in foals
- Eosinophilic inflammation is usually accompanied by marked alveolar macrophage proliferation.

Smoke Inhalation

- Smoke inhalation is usually associated with a barn fire and causes severe damage to the respiratory tract.
- Upper respiratory tract is more vulnerable to the effects of heat, whereas the lower respiratory tract is affected by noxious gases and particles generated in the fire.
- The tracheal, bronchial, and bronchiolar epithelium may be destroyed or severely damaged, resulting in edema and hemorrhage into the airways.
- Alveolar macrophages may be heavily laden with erythrocytes and carbon particles.
- The mucociliary clearance mechanism of the lungs is severely damaged, and secondary bacterial and/or fungal infection occurs with resultant increased numbers of neutrophils and macrophages.

Previous Hemorrhage

- Causes:
  - □ Exercise-induced pulmonary hemorrhage (EIPH)
  - □ Severe inflammation and necrosis of small blood vessels
  - □ Trauma, including previous aspiration procedures
  - □ Neoplasia
- Cytologic findings:
  - □ Macrophages displaying erythrocytophagia or containing pigment compatible with hemosiderin or hematoidin. Special stains such as Perl Prussian blue or Gomori stains are useful in determining whether material present in macrophages contains iron.

Silicosis

- Silicosis or pneumoconiosis is best documented in affected individuals in the Monterey and Central Peninsula areas of California.
- Samples contain large numbers of macrophages; some contain cytoplasmic inclusions composed of pink crystalline material.
- Excessive mucus along with increased numbers of neutrophils and hyperplastic epithelial cells are present.

Neoplasia

- Primary lung tumors are rare in horses; it is unlikely that BAL or transtracheal wash (TTW) samples facilitate the diagnosis of primary or metastatic lung neoplasia.
- For neoplastic cells to be recovered in lower respiratory tract samples, the tumor must invade the bronchi or bronchioles in a central location in the lung so as to be sampled by the collection technique used.
- Pulmonary neoplasia has been diagnosed from BAL samples in humans; however, this does not appear to be a productive diagnostic procedure in the equine patient.

SUGGESTED REFERENCES

Meyer DJ. The management of cytology specimens. Compend Contin Educ 1987;(9)1:10–17.

Ziemer EL. Cytologic analysis of large-animal body fluids. June 1989;574–583.

Cowell RL, Tyler RD. Cytology and Hematology of the Horse. Goleta, CA, American Veterinary Publications, Inc., 1992.

Kobluk CN, Ames TR, Geor RJ, eds: The Horse; Diseases and Clinical Management. Philadelphia, WB Saunders, 1995; 265, 269, 395, 642, 708, 714, 1112, 1121–1122, 1276–1277.

3

Pharmacology and Toxicology

39. Pharmacology and Adverse Drug Reactions 565
40. Toxicology 599

39 Pharmacology and Adverse Drug Reactions

PHARMACOLOGY

Thomas J. Divers
J. Edward Kirker

This chapter provides answers to frequently asked questions regarding drugs used to treat equine emergencies.

ANTIMICROBIALS

β-Lactam Drugs (Penicillins, Cephalosporins, Carbapenems, Monobactams)

- Stability: When reconstituted, most are stable for 12–24 hours at room temperature (use sodium ampicillin and ticarcillin within 1 hour), 3–7 days when refrigerated (best), and 30 days frozen ($-20°$ C). Some precipitate may be noted at cold temperatures; if the drug goes back into solution after warming in water, it can be used.

Information for this section was drawn from personal experiences, publications, and specifically Plumb DC. Veterinary Drug Handbook. 2nd ed. Ames IA; Iowa State University Press, 1995. This Handbook is an excellent pharmacology reference for equine clinicians.

- Incompatibilities: Do not mix in the same syringe and/or solution with aminoglycosides.
- Orally administered penicillin V: Poorly absorbed in the horse and may cause diarrhea. Rarely indicated in equine practice.
- β-Lactam drugs are generally synergistic when combined with aminoglycosides in the patient.
- Activity of β-lactam drugs against anaerobic infections: Effective against many anaerobic agents (*Clostridium* spp. and *Fusobacterium*) but are generally *not* effective in treating *Bacteroides fragilis*.

Procaine Penicillin

- Heating may increase procaine reactions.
- Repeated injections in the same muscle mass increases chance of procaine reaction.
- Doses over 10,000 units/kg are poorly absorbed.

Ceftiofur

- Has been used for several years in horses IM and IV. There are a few reports of diarrhea occurring after its use. In intensive care facilities, adverse effects from ceftiofur are surprisingly rare.
- A dosage of two to five times the package insert recommendation is frequently used in critically ill patients (e.g., septic foals, pleuropneumonia) with few adverse reactions.
- Higher intramuscular doses are irritating.

Ticarcillin/Clavulanate

- An excellent drug for bacteremia in foals.
- Irritating if administered IM.

"Newer" β-Lactam Antimicrobials

CEFOPERAZONE

- Third-generation cephalosporin used to treat life-threatening bacteremia
- Dose: 30 mg/kg q8h
- Like most third-generation cephalosporins, cefoperazone has retained activity similar to first-generation cephalosporins against gram-positive organisms but has extended activity against many gram-negative organisms.
- One of the only cephalosporins routinely effective against *Pseudomonas*
- Has the potential to produce bleeding disorder similar to reports of foals treated with moxalactam
- Monitor prothrombin time (PT), partial thromboplastin time (PTT).

CARBAPENEM GROUP—IMIPENEM CILASTATIN

- Do not use with other β-lactam drugs (may antagonize activity).
- Administer in IV fluids, 15 mg/kg q4–6h.

MONOBACTAMS

- Aztreonam has activity against many gram-negative bacteria but little activity against gram-positive anaerobic bacteria.

Erythromycin

- Suspensions for oral administration:
  - □ The crushing of the enteric-coated tablets, e.g., stearate, is unlikely to be a problem if the individual is eating and/or is being treated with a H_2-antagonist or proton pump blocker. Lower gastric pHs ($<$ 4.0), as reported in anorexic horses, can inactivate erythromycin in the crushed tablets.
- Products:
  - □ Erythromycin stearate and phosphate (a poultry product) are reported to provide higher plasma concentrations of the active drug (at least in adults) than erythromycin estolate or ethylsuccinate. All have been used with clinical success in foals and none is shown to have a higher incidence of diarrhea than others.
- Mix erythromycin lactobionate for IV infusion (mostly for ileus treatment), 1 gm/450-kg adult, in a *buffered* IV fluid.
- *Use oral erythromycin cautiously in horses $>$ 5 months of age* because of increased risk of drug-induced Clostridial *colitis.*
- May alter temperature homeostasis in foals, causing hyperthermia.
- May increase serum theophylline levels to toxic concentrations when used concurrently.

4

Trimethoprim/Sulfonamides

- Differences between TMP/sulfadiazine and TMP/sulfamethoxazole:
  - □ Sulfadiazine has a more favorable pharmacokinetic profile, but little difference in clinical success between the two products.
- Enteral absorption:
  - □ Paste and commercially prepared oral suspensions are often better absorbed than suspensions of crushed tablets, with little difference in clinical success or incidence of adverse reaction (diarrhea).
- Best absorbed when administered without feed
- Toxicity:
  - □ The incidence of diarrhea after oral administration is very low. Diarrhea seems to be more common in postoperative patients that have had dramatic reductions in feed and/or have been treated with other antimicrobials before the TMP/S. If diarrhea is an adverse effect of TMP/S treatment, it usually occurs 2–6 days after treatment is started.
  - □ Safety in pregnant mares:

☐ May falsely elevate serum creatinine when administered to horses with renal dysfunction.

☐ Frequency of treatment: Generally recommended to administer q12h.

Pyrimethamine

■ Best administered without food or trimethoprim; has been used successfully in treating equine protozoal myelitis with sulfa drugs. If TMP and pyrimethamine are administered together, folic acid supplementation is not routinely indicated.

Oxytetracycline/Tetracycline/Doxycycline

■ Administration:
  ☐ Oxytetracycline administered IV can be diluted with any IV fluid except sodium bicarbonate or fluids containing calcium.
  ☐ Administer slowly IV. Nonfatal collapse and/or hemolysis rarely occur.
  ☐ *Do not administer IM or SQ.*
  ☐ Orally administered tetracycline has not been shown to be well absorbed in the horse.
  ☐ *Do not administer doxycycline IV!*
  ☐ Doxycycline, 10.0 mg/kg PO q12h.

Metronidazole

■ Anorexia directly associated with treatment is unusual in the horse but does occur.
■ Excellent distribution properties, e.g., peritoneum.
■ Safety in pregnant mares has not been demonstrated and it is frequently used without known adverse effect.
■ Neurologic signs have been reported when the recommended dose of 15–25 mg/kg q6–8h is exceeded.

Aminoglycosides

■ Incompatibilities:
  ☐ Do not mix in the same solution/syringe with β-lactam drugs.
  ☐ More effective when used in an alkaline pH
  ☐ Generally preferred to administer once daily dose (q24h).
■ Indications:
  ☐ Life-threatening gram-negative aerobic infections that cannot be treated with safer antibiotics
  ☐ Synergistic when administered with β-lactam drugs. Do not combine in the same syringe.
  ☐ Ineffective for treating anaerobic infections (add metronidazole) and most intracellular bacteria

- Contraindications:
  - □ Do not administer to dehydrated individuals, premature foals, or hypokalemic patients without fluid support.

Enrofloxacin

- Contraindications/indications:
  - □ Although cartilage damage has not been conclusively demonstrated in the horse, it is best not to use in individuals < 18 months of age.
  - □ Has been used safely in pregnant mares, but safety has not been proved.
  - □ Enrofloxacin is preferred over ciprofloxacin in the horse because of better absorption.
  - □ Fluoroquinolones are not effective against anaerobic bacteria!
  - □ Excellent distribution properties

Chloramphenicol

- Pharmacokinetics:
  - □ Chloramphenicol is poorly absorbed when administered orally to horses and has a very short half-life when administered IV. Therefore, there are only a few indications for its use in the horse. It is indicated for long-term treatment of anaerobic infections.
- Adverse effects: None reported in the horse, but there is some risk (1 in 40,000) to humans handling the drug
- **Do not use florfenicol in the horse.**

Rifampin

- Adverse effects:
  - □ It may cause urine discoloration, which is clinically important.
  - □ It may increase rate of elimination of theophylline and diazepam.

Spectinomycin HCl

- The sterile solution for injection in poultry has been successfully used in the horse, but clinical indications are limited. Dosage: 22 mg/kg IV q8h

Vancomycin

- Primary indication is life-threatening staphylococcal infection resistant to the more commonly used antistaphylococcal agents.
- The mainstay of treatment for colitis caused by *Clostridium difficile*.

Itraconazole

- Preparation for oral administration:
  - □ Empty capsules in 95% ethanol (24 capsules/4–5 ml ethanol). Let stand 3–4 minutes, then grind to paste and allow to dry.
  - □ Can be mixed with syrup and refrigerated for 35 days.

4

☐ Absorption is better than with other antifungal drugs.
☐ If nonsteroidal anti-inflammatory drugs (NSAIDs) are administered concurrently, they may increase free itraconazole.

Ketoconazole

- Absorption: *Very poor* after oral administration in the horse. Mixing with an acidic fluid (e.g., orange juice) or withholding feed improves absorption.

ANTIHISTAMINES

Diphenhydramine HCl, Doxylamine Succinate, Hydroxyzine HCl, Tripelennamine

- Administer slowly IV.
- For overdose causing hyperexcitability/seizure, DO NOT use barbiturates or diazepam; chloral hydrate is recommended.

SHORT-ACTING ANESTHETICS, TRANQUILIZERS, NARCOTICS, SEDATIVES
Diazepam

- Administration: Do not draw into plastic syringes except immediately before administration; adsorbs to plastic.
- Interactions: When used in foals receiving erythromycin, the effect may be prolonged.

Butorphanol Tartrate

- Compatibilities: can be combined in the same syringe with acepromazine or xylazine.
- Contraindications: do not use in head trauma because CSF pressure is generally increased.
- When administered before tranquilization, may produce severe head shaking. No treatment is required, and the antagonist naloxone is not indicated.
- Controlled Schedule IV.

Narcotic Agonists/Analgesics (Morphine, Meperidine, Oxymorphone)

- These produce analgesia, sedation, respiratory depression, and decreased intestinal motility.
- Administration: When administered before tranquilization, excitement may occur!

Acepromazine

- Incompatibilities: May be mixed in same syringe with xylazine but not diazepam

- Contraindications: DO NOT use in hypotensive shock and/or hypovolemia. Use barbiturates or chloral hydrate in patients with tetanus instead of acepromazine because of acepromazine's effect on the extrapyramidal system.
- Do not administer to individuals with previous history of seizure.
- Do not use within 1 month of deworming with organophosphates.
- Do not use in intact stallions unless absolutely necessary! If used in a stallion for treating laminitis, use lower dosage (10 mg/450 kg) and do not allow stallion exposure to other horses, especially mares, or excessive movement, e.g., trailering, until tranquilization is no longer apparent.
- Treatment of acepromazine-induced hypotension: Administer hypertonic saline, ephedrine, phenylephrine, or norepinephrine.
- Treatment of *paraphimosis*: See p. 405.

Xylazine

- Compatibility: May be mixed in the same syringe with acepromazine and/or butorphanol and combined with acepromazine if *both* are administered at a lower than normal dose.
- Contraindications:
  □ Do not use in patients with severe upper airway obstruction; can be used in lower airway disorders (COPD) when tranquilization is required.
  □ Xylazine has been used in pregnant mares without inducing abortions (unlike in cattle)!
  □ **Caution:** Some breeds, e.g., draft breeds, are more susceptible to sedative effects.
  □ Collapse may occur in some draft horses and in immature equines.
  □ **Caution:** Intestinal motility is inhibited, especially with repeated use.

Detomidine

- Contraindications:
  □ Heart block
  □ Critically ill patients

Guaifenesin (GG)

- Preparation/storage:
  □ Precipitation generally occurs when temperature is < 72° F (22.2° C). Prepare as a 10% solution (in sterile water or D_5W); may be stored at room temperature for 1 week. A 5% solution causes less endothelial irritation than does a 10% solution.
- Compatibilities: Can be combined with ketamine, xylazine, barbiturates

Ketamine HCl

- Compatibilities:

4

☐ Can be mixed with xylazine in the same syringe, but induction of anesthesia is best accomplished by tranquilization before administering ketamine.

☐ May precipitate when mixed with barbiturates or diazepam

☐ Can be mixed in polyionic fluids with GG and xylazine

☐ Contraindications: NOTE: **Do not use in head trauma or deep corneal wounds because CSF pressure and intraocular pressure are increased following administration.**

Barbiturates

- Compatibilities: May be mixed in polyionic IV fluid solutions
- Contraindications:
    ☐ Severe respiratory depression
    ☐ Decreases lidocaine clearance, which may result in lidocaine toxicity
    ☐ Perivascular injections results in severe inflammation (see pp. 267 and 590).
    ☐ Depresses fetal respiration
- Indications for pentobarbital/phenobarbital:
    ☐ Head trauma (may need to assist ventilation and hyperventilate to lower $PaCO_2$, which decreases cerebral vascular pressure)
    ☐ Most seizures
    ☐ Tetanus
    ☐ Has been used to stimulate bilirubin metabolism in neonatal foals

Chloral Hydrate

- Activity: Hypnotic-sedative—no analgesic properties
- Advantages:
    ☐ Inexpensive
    ☐ Minimal cardiopulmonary and GI side effects unless used at higher dosage.
- Administration
    ☐ Use after tranquilization with acepromazine; an analgesic (meperidine/morphine) is preferred.
    ☐ Administer 12% solution IV at approximately 22 mg/kg.
    ☐ Titrate to effect, 30–60 minutes after first dose.
    ☐ Duration up to 12 hours
    ☐ Can be administered orally at the same dose
    ☐ **Caution:** Do not administer perivascularly!
- Indications:
    ☐ Medical colics with severe intractable pain that cannot be controlled with NSAI drugs or tranquilizers/narcotics and when these drugs are contraindicated or are required frequently. In some cases of severe ileus and gas distention, neostigmine is administered while the individual is sedated with chloral hydrate.

Tolazine HCl

- Specific reversal agent for xylazine and detomidine.
- Recommended dose: 4.0 mg/kg administered slowly IV

DRUGS USED TO TREAT GASTROINTESTINAL EMERGENCIES

Antiulcer Treatment

Ranitidine

- Administration: Do not give orally within 2 hours of sucralfate.

Famotidine

- Administration: As for ranitidine
- Storage: Refrigerate the injectable form; it is stable at room temperature for at least 48 hours.

Cimetidine

- Administration: As for ranitidine
- Storage: Do not refrigerate.
- Drug interactions: May prolong serum half-life of drugs requiring hepatic metabolism, e.g., diazepam

Omeprazole

- Administration: As for ranitidine.
- Drug interactions: May decrease clearance of diazepam
- Generally not recommended because of difficulty administering capsules, poor bioavailability and expense.
- An improved gel formulation is available.

Sucralfate

- Administration: Administer 2 *hours apart* from *other oral medication* because it may decrease absorption of orally administered drugs.

Misoprostol

- Possible contraindications: Do not administer to pregnant mares or to individuals with chronic obstructive pulmonary disease (COPD).

Cisapride

- Dosages as high as 0.8 mg/kg PO or per rectum may be required for therapeutic effect.
- Poor bioavailability when administered per rectum
- Erythromycin and lidocaine have also been used IV to enhance intestinal motility (see pp. 189 and 567).

Metoclopramide

- Incompatibilities: Do not mix with calcium gluconate or erythromycin in same IV solution.
- Protect from prolonged exposure to light.
- CNS effects may be enhanced by some sedatives, tranquilizers, and narcotics. Diazepam has been used to help control CNS side effects.

Bethanechol

- Preparation of injectable solution from tablets (commercially available parenteral product is preferred but is expensive):
  □ Tablets are soluble in water (sterile).
  □ Can be autoclaved without loss of potency
  □ Administer through 0.2-U filter.

Dioctyl Sodium Sulfosuccinate (DSS)

- Theoretically, DSS and mineral oil should not be administered together because DSS damages epithelial cells and may increase intestinal absorption of mineral oil. These two drugs are commonly administered in combination without reported clinical problems.

Bismuth Subsalicylate

- Manure turns black after administration and is of no clinical concern.
- Sufficient salicylate may be absorbed so that metabolism of salicylic acid may affect platelet function; therefore, additional aspirin therapy to alter platelet function may not be required.

Neostigmine

- Contraindications:
  □ *Do not* use in individuals with intestinal displacement.
  □ *Do not* use in individuals with severe COPD.
- Indications:
  □ Foals or adults with ileus and severe large intestinal tympany after an obstruction (e.g., radiographs) has been ruled out
  □ Adults with gravel obstruction of the rectum
  □ Atropine toxicity
- Neostigmine should always be used cautiously; analgesics may be required.

STEROIDAL/NONSTEROIDAL ANTI-INFLAMMATORY DRUGS

Aspirin

- Contraindications: Do not administer to patients with bleeding disorders.
- Indication: Administer 60–90 gr/450-kg adult every 2 or 3 days PO or rectally to inhibit platelet function.

- Platelet function is inhibited in normal individuals; in vitro aggregation is not inhibited after in vitro endotoxin stimulation.

Flunixin Meglumine

- Administration: Irritating when administered perivascularly. Occasionally associated with clostridial myositis after IM injection
- Indications/possible contraindications:
  □ Preferred NSAID (0.25–0.3 mg/kg) to treat cardiopulmonary effects of endotoxemia
  □ Should not be used in foals with gastric ulceration or dehydration
  □ Has minimal effect on platelet function
  □ Use with caution in foals with diarrhea or dehydration, duodenal ulceration may result!

Phenylbutazone

- Administration: Irritating when administered perivascularly; do not administer IM.
- Use lower dosage in ponies.
- Indications/possible contraindications:
  □ Preferred NSAID by many clinicians to treat musculoskeletal disorders
  □ Avoid using when treating ulcerative colitis, gastric ulceration, acute renal failure, and in dehydrated patients.
  □ Minimal effect on platelet function
  □ May help to normalize intestinal motility in endotoxemia.

Ketoprofen

- Reported to have lower incidence of adverse effects, e.g., GI ulceration, than phenylbutazone
- Use: Reported to inhibit prostanoids and leukotrienes, but superiority in treating endotoxemia has not been demonstrated.
- Significance of L-arginine component unproven.

Meclofenamic Acid

- Use: Compared with other NSAID, infrequently used in practice
- May affect platelet function
- Adverse effects are rarely reported.

Dipyrone

- Indications: Generally believed to be the safest NSAID and is predominantly used in the treatment of hyperthermia and mild colic. Has not been associated with gastric ulcers in foals; currently not available.

Additional Cautions on the Use of All NSAIDs

- All NSAIDs are highly protein-bound and can displace other drugs from protein-binding sites, which

□ Increases free drug levels of the displaced drugs
□ Enhances/speeds the displaced drugs' therapeutic effect/toxicity
□ Speeds elimination of displaced drugs
- Use with caution in individuals with COPD, because inhibition of prostaglandin E may worsen airway function.

DRUGS USED IN TREATING EMERGENCY RESPIRATORY DISORDERS

Bronchodilators

Atropine

- Administration:
  □ Caution: Use only at low dosage for bronchodilation effect, 7–10 mg/450-kg adult IV, IM, or SQ q12–24h for only 1 day.
- Incompatibility: Do not mix with sodium bicarbonate.
- Contraindications:
  □ Severe tachycardia
  □ Ileus
  □ When combined with epinephrine, may increase risk of arrhythmia

Albuterol

- Contraindications:
  □ Do not use in hypokalemic patients.
  □ May delay labor in term pregnant mares or uterine involution during the postpartum period

Aminophylline

- Drug interaction: Should be used with **caution** in foals treated with erythromycin because hepatic metabolism of theophylline may be delayed, causing toxicity (CNS signs). Rifampin may increase rate of elimination.
- Administration: If administered IV, aminophylline can be mixed in most IV fluid solutions. NOTE: Therapeutic index to toxic range is very narrow in the horse.

Glycopyrrolate

- Administration: Has a pH of 2–3; do not mix in solution with alkaline drugs/fluids.

Doxapram HCl

- Compatibility: Do not mix with alkaline solutions (e.g., sodium bicarbonate or aminophylline).
- Use: Controversial, main indication is for primary apnea, and most apneas are believed secondary to asphyxia or drug overdose. Regardless, it is reported to be used successfully in many apneic foals. It can be used

for apnea when mechanical ventilation is impractical but should *not* be used if mechanical ventilation is available or if oxygen is not available because as the respiratory rate and depth of breathing increases, the oxygen demand increases.
- Can be administered by injection in umbilical vessels, jugular vein, and so on, or placed on tongue.

Inhalation Drug Therapy

- Beclomethasone is the preferred corticosteroid inhalant: 3750 μg/450-kg adult q12h, combined with ipratropium bromide, 75 μg/ml, 4 ml/100 kg BW (see p. 434 for additional information on inhalation therapy).

CORTICOSTEROIDS

- Administered IV, corticosteroids are best administered as a bolus rather than mixed in IV solutions.
- May cause hepatic lipidosis and elevations in serum gamma-glutamyl transferase (GGT) when used for prolonged periods
- May cause late-term abortions in mares only when administered in very high doses (e.g., dexamethasone, 0.2 mg/kg for 3 consecutive days)
- If used to treat CNS inflammation or septic shock (empirical), a rapid-acting water soluble agent (e.g., dexamethasone sodium phosphate or prednisolone sodium acetate) should be used.

Dexamethasone

- Store only at room temperature.
- Administration: IV or IM in emergency situations because oral bioavailability is erratic.
- Indications: Commonly used corticosteroid in practice for treating
  □ Acute, noncardiogenic edema
  □ Nonseptic respiratory disease
  □ Severe COPD
  □ Interstitial pneumonia
  □ Cerebrospinal trauma and/or inflammation—efficacy not demonstrated!
  □ Shock—efficacy not demonstrated!

  NOTE: It is occasionally reported to cause laminitis; therefore, use with caution in individuals with laminitis. It is frequently used for cortisol suppression test (dexamethasone suppression test) without adverse effects, to test for pituitary adenoma.

Prednisone/Prednisolone

- Metabolism: Prednisone is converted to the active drug prednisolone by the liver.
- NOTE: Do not use prednisone in individuals with severe hepatic dysfunction.

4

Triamcinolone

- Adverse effects: For unknown reasons, triamcinolone is reported to have a higher incidence of laminitis after its use than other corticosteroids.

INTRAVENOUS FLUIDS

Calcium Salts

- Compatibility: Calcium gluconate and calcium chloride are compatible with most fluids and drugs, *except* tetracyclines, intravenous lipids, and sodium bicarbonate.
- Adverse effects: Calcium gluconate is considered to be less irritating and safer than calcium chloride.
- Contraindications: There is some evidence that calcium is contraindicated in resuscitation therapy because it may enhance cellular death.
- **SQ, IM, or perivascular administration causes severe local injection site reactions.**

Dimethyl Sulfoxide (DMSO)

- Storage: Airtight container away from light
- Incompatibility: If mixed with water, heat is produced, which may cause local irritation/blistering when applied to wet skin and bandaged tightly or covered with plastic.
- *Do not administer* IV with water or D_5W because hemolysis can be severe.
- *Always* dilute to concentrations of less than 10% for parenteral administration.
- Hemolysis and hemoglobinuria may occur in some adults even with proper dilution—usually of no concern.
- NOTE: **Use only medical grade DMSO.**

Magnesium

- Administer *slowly* IV as a 10% solution (100 gm $MgSO_4$/liter water).
- Can be mixed with calcium borogluconate for treating hypomagnesemia.

Hyperimmune Serum

- Administer slowly IV.
- Adverse effects, probably resulting from endotoxin in the product, are reported.

Equine Plasma

- Administration: Administered at a moderately fast rate, 20–40 ml/kg/h, if monitored closely for signs of adverse reaction (trembling, rapid respiration). *Adverse reactions are rare.*

- Pretreatment with antihistamines may prevent adverse reactions and maintains albumin in the intravascular space for a longer period of time, but this is generally not performed.
- Indications:
  □ Ideal fluid for most emergency/life-threatening conditions
  □ Shock
  □ Hypoalbuminemia/edema
  □ Synergistic with polyionic crystalloids
  □ Heparin, 100 mg/kg BW as total initial dose, can be mixed in plasma before administration to activate antithrombin III.

Phosphorus

- Available in most bovine milk fever preparations

Hypertonic Saline

- Frequently used for severe hypovolemia/hypotension
- Has beneficial effects of rapid and dramatic intravascular expansion with only small administration volume, 4–8 ml/kg
- Added advantage of
  □ Decrease in pulmonary arterial pressure, which inhibits pulmonary edema formation
  □ Rapid diuresis
- Do not use in chronically dehydrated patients, since intracellular water is severely depleted in these patients.
- Additional polyionic crystalloids recommended simultaneously or within 1.5 hours after hypertonic saline to prevent "rebound" intravascular volume depletion.
- Do not use, or use only as last resort, in individuals with uncontrolled bleeding.

Sodium Bicarbonate

- Can be administered as a hypertonic (e.g., 5%, 8.4%) solution to individuals with severe metabolic acidosis (pH < 7.1) and intravascular volume depletion
- For severe metabolic acidosis without intravascular volume depletion, best administered as an isotonic solution, 1.25% (100 gm sodium bicarbonate in 8 liters of sterile water).
- Do not use
  □ When hypokalemia is present
  □ In respiratory acidosis
  □ In head trauma
- Controversial for use in resuscitation

Dextrose

- Frequently added to crystalloids for IV fluid treatment of foals (solution generally 5%–10% dextrose)

- Do *not* use as sole source of fluid replacement in dehydrated individuals.
- Avoid excessive administration and prolonged or severe hyperglycemia.
- Not recommended to use in resuscitation unless hypoglycemia is present.

CARDIAC DRUGS

β₁-Agonist

Dobutamine

- Stability: Use diluted solutions within 24 hours.
- Compatibility: With most IV fluid solutions except sodium bicarbonate, and is compatible with most other β- and α-agonists in the same solution. Do not mix with other drugs, including calcium chloride/gluconate, heparin, furosemide, and digoxin.
- Indications: To improve cardiac output when fluid therapy is unsuccessful or cannot be used. Synergistic when administered with nitroprusside or other venodilators to improve peripheral circulation.
- Solution preparation:
  □ 1 vial (250 mg) in 1000 ml = 250 μg/ml
  □ Minidrip set = 60 drops/1 ml
  □ Normal drip set = 10 drops/1 ml
- *Caution* when calculating the dosage rate (generally 2–10 μg/kg/min) because of the potency of dobutamine. Monitor for tachycardia/arrhythmia and discontinue if necessary.

β₁- and β₂-Agonist

Isoproterenol

- Compatible with most fluids but not with sodium bicarbonate and aminophylline
- Indications: Because of many adverse effects on the heart and blood pressure, rarely indicated except for the purpose of increasing ventricular rate

β₁- and α-Agonist

Dopamine

- Solution stability: Use diluted solutions within 24 hours.
- Compatible with most other β- and α-agonists and with mannitol
- *Incompatibilities:* Furosemide and potassium penicillin. More likely than dobutamine to be compatible with other drugs
- Preparation of solution:
  □ Add 5 ml vial (80 mg/ml) to 1 liter of 0.9% NaCl, D₅W, etc. = 400 μg/ml.
  □ Minidrop set = 60 drops/ml
  □ Normal drop set = 10 drops/ml
- Pharmacology/indications:
  □ At lower dosage, 1–5 μg/kg/min dopamine may act primarily at renal dopaminergic receptors (use in renal failure with normal cardiac output).

- At medium dose, 5–10 μg/kg/min dopamine stimulates β_1-adrenergic receptors (use in renal failure without normal cardiac output or noncardiogenic shock with normal or high normal CVP).
- At higher doses, > 10 μg/kg/min stimulates α effects and causes increased vascular tone (increased blood pressure with possible decrease in renal, splenic, and coronary blood flow). Use in severe hypotension unresponsive to fluid therapy.
- Use with caution. If heart rate increases 50% above normal, arrhythmias develop and/or hypertension occurs. Discontinue administration.

β_1-, β_2-, and α-Agonist

Epinephrine

- Incompatible with sodium bicarbonate, hypertonic saline, and aminophylline. NOTE: Does not need to be diluted in adults when administered via the jugular vein.
- Indications:
  - Anaphylaxis—drug of choice
  - Cardiac resuscitation—drug of choice
- Routes of administration:
  - IV—immediate effect
  - Intratracheal—effect within 5 minutes; larger dosage (2–10×) may be required
  - Intramuscular—effect within 5–10 minutes
  - Subcutaneous—10 minutes
  - Intracardiac (injection above left lateral thoracic vein on left chest)—*rarely indicated*. Effect—immediate
- Contraindications:
  - Shock due to causes other than anaphylaxis (may increase oxygen demand and undesirable peripheral perfusion associated with β- and α-responses.
  - Do not inject undiluted into a small vessel.

α_1-Adrenergics

Phenylephrine

- Compatible with all common IV preparations, including sodium bicarbonate
- Indications:
  - Splenic contraction (3 μg/kg/min) to correct left colon displacement
  - Increase blood pressure during general anesthesia when dopamine or dobutamine may not be desirable due to their arrhythmogenic properties and *after* IV fluids have been unsuccessful.
  - Topically as a hemostatic agent

Phenylpropanolamine HCl

- Indications: Used commonly in the horse to increase urethral sphincter tone (0.5–2.0 mg/kg q12h)
- Adverse effects: Restlessness, sweating, tachycardia

Phenoxybenzamine

- An alpha-antagonist
- May be used to relax urethral tone in herpes myelitis

VASODILATOR DRUGS

Nitroprusside

- Storage: *Protect from light!* Solutions for injection are stable for 24 hours *if* protected from light (cover the infusion bag; the tubing can be left exposed to light).
- Solution preparation for IV administration: D_5W without added medications
- Indications:
  □ Rarely indicated in practice
  □ Shock after restoration of cardiac output and systemic arterial pressure returned to normal or elevated, with continued evidence of hypoperfusion, e.g., abnormal hematocrit.
  □ Acute heart failure to decrease preload and afterload
- Contraindications:
  □ Systemic hypotension! Note: Administer only with specific indication and careful monitoring of blood pressure and heart rate.

Isoxsuprine

- Administered orally does **not** increase digital blood flow.

Hydralazine

- Compatible with most isotonic IV fluid solutions and dobutamine
- Indications:
  □ In heart failure, to decrease afterload and improve cardiac output. Primary effect is to decrease arteriolar smooth muscle contractions and arteriolar resistance to blood flow (see p. 138).
- Monitor heart rate carefully.

Nitroglycerin

- Use topically over digital arteries for treatment of laminitis.
- Apply 2% cream, approximately 15 mg q12h and cover.
- **Caution:** Wear gloves for application.

Enalapril (Angiotensin-Converting Enzyme Inhibitor)

- Compatibility: Most IV isotonic fluids, and stable in solution for 24 hours
- Indications: Same as for hydralazine above

Acepromazine (see p. 570)

Phenoxybenzamine (see p. 582)

ANTIARRHYTHMIC DRUGS

Lidocaine

- Compatible with most IV solutions
- Incompatible with dopamine, epinephrine, isoproterenol, norepinephrine, ampicillin, and cefazolin
- Indications:
  - Antiarrhythmic (see p. 123)
  - Enhances intestinal motility (see p. 189)
- Adverse effects (see p. 126)
- CAUTION: When administered IV, make certain lidocaine product does *not* contain epinephrine.

Quinidine

- Drug interactions:
  - Increases digoxin levels
  - Sodium bicarbonate decreases excretion
- Indications (see p. 124)
- Adverse effects (see pp. 112 and 126)
  - Potentiated with hypokalemia

Propranolol (β-Blocker)

- Administration: Do not combine with sodium bicarbonate.
- Indications (see p. 124)
- Adverse effects (see p. 126)
  - Do not use in horses with COPD.

Phenytoin

- Administration: If solution for IV use is needed, it can be prepared, filtered, and administered with sodium bicarbonate.
- Indications:
  - Digitalis-induced ventricular arrhythmias
  - Anticonvulsive therapy—generally administered orally
  - Myopathy—generally administered orally

Magnesium Sulfate

- Calcium channel blocker
- Use to treat ventricular tachycardia
- 4 mg/kg bolus q2min up to 50 mg/kg total dose.

Bretylium Tosylate

- Use for ventricular arrhythmias unresponsive to lidocaine
- May cause severe hypotension!

Positive Inotropic Drugs for Treating Heart Failure

Digoxin (for Injection)

- Compatible with most IV solutions of near-normal pH (dilute in at least 4× volume). Incompatible with dobutamine
- Orally administered digoxin is best used as follow-up therapy after IV digoxin or in a nonemergency situation
- Indications: Heart failure (*except ionophore toxicity*) and supraventricular tachycardias. (See p. 119.)
- Contraindications: Do not use with ionophore toxicity.
- Adverse effects (see p. 126)
- Drug interactions:
  □ Diazepam, tetracycline, quinidine, and erythromycin may increase the serum levels of digoxin.
  □ Hypokalemia (e.g., furosemide [Lasix] administration) may increase toxicity.

Digitoxin

- Indications, adverse effects, and drug interactions same as for digoxin.
- Digitoxin may be used instead of digoxin with renal insufficiency because digitoxin is metabolized by the liver.

DIURETICS

Furosemide

- Storage: A precipitate occurs with refrigeration but the drug resolubolizes after warming without loss of potency.
- May turn brown when exposed to air but is usable if not past expiration date.
- Compatible with all IV fluids. Incompatible with dobutamine, epinephrine, and aminoglycosides.
- Indications:
  □ Congestive heart failure
  □ Pulmonary edema
  □ Edema—especially noninflammatory
  □ Oliguric renal failure when used with dopamine/dobutamine and/or mannitol
  □ Inflammatory/septic shock—controversial because it decreases cardiac output
  □ COPD
- Contraindications:
  □ Hypokalemia
  □ Dehydration
  □ May enhance digitalis, aminophylline, and aminoglycoside toxicity

Acetazolamide

- Compatible with all IV fluid solutions
- Oral administration is most common.
- Indication: Hyperkalemia
- May increase gastric pH

Trichlormethiazide/Dexamethasone

- Indication: Use orally for nonseptic inflammatory edema, e.g., vasculitis

Mannitol

- Precipitation occurs if cooled and/or mixed with high chloride-containing fluids.
- Indications:
  □ Cerebral edema
  □ Renal failure—controversial
  □ To decrease ocular pressure
- Contraindications:
  □ Progressive cerebral hemorrhage
  □ Anuric renal failure

DRUGS SPECIFICALLY FOR MUSCLE DISORDERS

Methocarbamol

- Administration: Drug should be precipitate-free for intravenous injection. Do not administer SQ or perivascular.
- Sedation and ataxia may occur.

Dantrolene Sodium

- Storage: Use reconstituted product for injection within 6 hours and protect from light.
- Do not mix with saline or dextrose.

NEUROMUSCULAR BLOCKING AGENTS

Succinylcholine

- Administration: Incompatible with sodium bicarbonate
  □ Do NOT use in Quarter Horses with genetic defect for hyperkalemia.
  □ If used for C-section, mechanical ventilation may be required for the foal.
  □ Do NOT use in debilitated, exhausted, or excited horse or in individuals recently treated with organophosphates.
- Doses higher than 0.088 mg/kg cause respiratory depression.
- Does not provide analgesia!
- Indications:
  □ For muscle relaxation during surgery with mechanical ventilation and when atracurium is not available

□ For muscle relaxation to remove entrapped horse when general anesthesia is not indicated and/or unavailable
□ Do not use if severe hemorrhage is occurring.
□ In combination with euthanasia solution to prevent agonal movements (gasping)

Atracurium

- Neuromuscular blocking drug, preferred in the horse because of minimal cardiovascular side effects.
- Onset of action is slower than that of succinylcholine.
- Indications:
  □ Muscle relaxation during surgery with mechanical ventilation
  □ Muscle relaxation in foals on ventilator
- Can be reversed with neostigmine, 0.06 mg/kg IV, after atropine, 0.02 mg/kg.

MISCELLANEOUS DRUGS

Aminocaproic Acid

- Administration: Dilute in IV fluids
- Frequently used for uncontrolled bleeding when surgery is not an option

Cyproheptadine

- Safety—reproductive safety has not been demonstrated but it has been used frequently in pregnant mares without reported adverse effects.
- Frequently used for treatment of pituitary adenoma
- Used to treat photophobic head shaking

Heparin Sodium

- Administration: Do not mix in solutions containing aminoglycosides.
- Can be mixed with fresh frozen plasma (100–125 U/kg BW) before administration of plasma to activate antithrombin III activity as part of shock therapy
- Compatible with TPN solutions
- Contraindications: Do not administer IM.
- NOTE: Blood gas values may be erroneous if heparin is > 10% of the sample.

Insulin (Regular)

- Administration: Adheres to bottles, bags, and tubing unless "rinsed" first with other fluids
- Compatible with TPN, dextrose, KCl, and other IV fluids (*except sodium bicarbonate*), but bag should be mixed intermittently.
- Indications:
  □ Hyperlipemia—controversial

□ Septic/inflammatory shock (used with glucose, KCl, and Mg)—controversial
- Contraindications are hypoglycemia and hypokalemia.

Naloxone

- Administration: Do not mix in alkaline pH fluids.

Vasopressin

- Administration: Dilute in saline or D_5W and administer slowly, in aqueous suspension only.

Oxytocin

- Administration: Doses > 20 IU/450-kg mare may cause "colicky" signs.

Prostaglandin Analgesics

Fluprostenol Sodium, Dinoprost Tromethamine

- Contraindications: Do not use in individuals with COPD.
- CAUTION: Abortifacient! (both human and horse)

CONSIDERATIONS FOR DRUG THERAPY IN THE NEONATAL FOAL

- Renal excretion of most drugs is approximately equal to that of adults by 1 week of age.
- Premature foals and foals less than 1 week of age may require increased treatment intervals if drug is excreted predominantly by kidneys—particularly drugs with potential toxicity, e.g., aminoglycosides.
- Hepatic metabolism is slower in the foal than in the adult; time of delayed metabolism varies owing to drug-induced enhanced activity. Sulfonamides, phenobarbital, trimethoprim, NSAIDs, diazepam, and theophylline may require prolonged dosing intervals, and, in the case of inhalant anesthesia, lower concentrations.
- The albumin concentration in young foals is approximately that of adults: protein binding is not very different between age groups. If hypoalbuminemia, as from enteritis, is present, highly protein-bound drugs such as diazepam, sulfas, and NSAIDs may have enhanced effect; may be partially offset by more rapid elimination.
- Extracellular fluid volume in neonatal foals is nearly double that of adults, resulting in decreased blood concentrations and prolonged excretion of many drugs. In treating life-threatening infections, it may be advisable to administer a larger loading dose (approximately 30%–50% larger than adult dose), with prolonged treatment intervals to compensate for delayed metabolism or elimination.
- Oral absorption of many drugs may be different in foals than in weanlings, yearlings, or adults.

4

ADVERSE DRUG REACTIONS

Thomas J. Divers

IMPORTANT DRUG REFERENCE INFORMATION

FDA/DVM Drugs, Devices, Feeds:
Department of Epidemiology and Surveillance
(301) 594 1722
Drug Interaction
1-888-FDAVETS (toll free)
Director of Center for Veterinary Medicine
(301) 594 1740

United States Department of Agriculture:
Veterinary Biologics and Diagnostics Hotline:
(800) 752 6255; weekdays, 7:30 A.M.–4:00 P.M. CT
(message service after hours)

National Animal Poison Control Center Hotline:
(800) 548 2423

Veterinary Practitioners' Reporting Program:
(800) 487 7776

FDA Internet Home Page:
www.cvm.fda.gov

INTRACAROTID INJECTIONS

Many of the immediate adverse reactions to parenterally administered xylazine, detomidine, phenylbutazone, and trimethoprim/sulfadiazine (no longer available) are probably the result of inadvertent intracarotid injections.

Water-Soluble Intracarotid Drugs

These include acepromazine, detomidine, some barbiturates, and xylazine.

Clinical Signs

- Immediate *hyperexcitability* and possibly *collapse*.
- Seizure or coma may follow.

Treatment

- Usually can be successfully managed by sedation with pentobarbital or phenobarbital, 5–12 mg/kg IV (or to effect) q12h or as needed.
- Alternatively, administer chloral hydrate IV to effect as a relatively safe sedative.

- Administer anti-inflammatory, edema-reducing drugs (e.g., DMSO), 1 gm/kg, or dexamethasone, 0.5 mg/kg.
- Some individuals may remain recumbent for several hours or days before rising.
- Treat wounds and corneal trauma that may occur as a result of the seizure.
- Cortical blindness may occur in some cases.
- Additionally, include antiedema therapy:
  □ DMSO, 1 mg/kg IV diluted in polyionic crystalloid fluid
  □ Dexamethasone, 0.2 mg/kg IV
  □ Mannitol (20%), 0.25–2.0 gm/kg slowly IV

Oil-Based Intracarotid Drugs

These include propylene glycol, trimethoprim-sulfadiazine, diazepam, procaine penicillin, and phenylbutazone.

Clinical Signs

- Seizure, collapse, and rapid death
- Contralateral cortical blindness is a frequent finding in surviving individuals.
- Cerebral hemorrhage is often present.

Treatment

- If the patient does not immediately die, administer treatment as for water-soluble drugs.

FLUNIXIN MEGLUMINE

Intracarotid injection does not produce as severe signs as some of the drugs listed earlier, may produce neurologic signs such as ataxia and hysteria, hyperventilation, and muscle weakness. However, these signs are transient, according to the package inserts, and require no antidote.

NOTE: When a 20-gauge needle is used to penetrate the carotid artery, blood may not spurt from needle hub.

THE FOLLOWING DOES NOT IMPLY THAT ALL REACTIONS TO THE DRUGS MENTIONED ARE THE RESULT OF INADVERTENT INTRACAROTID INJECTIONS. For example, procaine penicillin may cause procaine reactions when the drug is inadvertently administered in a small vessel. This is more common in patients receiving long-term injections in the same muscle mass. Similarly, acute tachypnea may follow xylazine or detomidine injections. This reaction is usually not fatal, but in a rare case may cause fatal pulmonary edema. When injectable trimethoprim-sulfadiazine was available, fatal reactions were reported when detomidine was given IV following the trimethoprim-sulfadiazine. Please see the drug list that follows this section.

ACUTE ANAPHYLAXIS, POSSIBLE WITH ANY DRUG

Most common with vaccines, occasionally penicillin, IV *selenium*, IV phytonadione (vitamin K), and other vitamins and minerals administered IV. In most cases, this is not a result of prior sensitization and antigen/antibody reaction but is instead an immediate "triggering" of the complement/kinin system caused by some part of the drug.

Mild Forms

- Mild forms of anaphylaxis cause urticaria and/or minor increases in respiratory rate. May be simply treated with antihistamines:
  □ Doxylamine succinate, 0.5 mg/kg, OR
  □ Pyrilamine maleate, 1.0 mg/kg *slowly* IV or IM/SQ, OR
  □ Tripelennamine, 1.1 mg/kg with close monitoring
- NOTE: Administer all antihistamines slowly IV as excitement and hypotension are occasional adverse effects. Alternatively, epinephrine can be administered IM, 5–8 ml/450-kg adult.

Severe Forms

(see p. 446)

- Epinephrine, 3–7 ml (1:1000 undiluted) slowly IV to 450-kg adult. May be administered IM in less severe cases at same dosage or 2 times this dosage IM for severe anaphylaxis (intratracheal route, 5 × IV dosage, may be used when IV access is not possible or limited)
- Provide patent airway if needed by intubation. This is imperative when laryngeal edema becomes severe. It is also of some benefit in treating pulmonary edema when the upper airway is edematous and compromised. Remember, stridor may not appear until 80% of the upper airway is obstructed.
- Furosemide, 1 mg/kg IV
- Use plasma as an oncotic volume expander if pulmonary edema is believed to be progressive. If other fluids are required for hypotension, administer hypertonic saline, 4 ml/kg.
- Corticosteroids. Although of no demonstrated benefit, dexamethasone, 0.2–0.5 mg/kg, is frequently administered to prevent delayed edema formation.
- Intranasal oxygen

SPECIAL CONSIDERATIONS

Perivascular Injections

- Perivascular injections with irritating drugs are common.
- The most irritating drugs are those with high or low pH.

- Clinical signs include pain, swelling, cellulitis, and vessel necrosis. Vessel necrosis may occur several days after the perivascular injection and can be fatal.
- Recommendations:
  - □ Stop the infusion.
  - □ Infiltrate the area with 10 ml saline mixed with 1 ml procaine penicillin.
  - □ Apply heat to the area.
  - □ If a large volume of irritating drug is administered, ventral drainage and flushing may be indicated.

Drug Overdose

What to do if an *overdose* of a drug has occurred:

- Keep records and provide proper communication.
- Review clinical/physiologic effects from overdose.
- Provide specific therapy if indicated.
- General treatment for most overdoses includes
  - □ IV fluids
  - □ Activated charcoal PO (0.5 kg/450-kg adult). NOTE: Even when the overdose has been administered parenterally, the oral charcoal may act as a "sink" and "pull" some of the drug into the GI tract for excretion.
  - □ If overdose was administered orally, give $MgSO_4$, 0.5 kg/450-kg adult PO, in addition to fluids and charcoal.

Broken Jugular Catheters

Although alarming, breaking off a jugular catheter in an adult is often not a life-threatening occurrence. The catheter usually passes through the right side of the heart and lodges in the pulmonary circulation, where it is walled off and causes no clinical problems. Via ultrasound, confirm passage of the catheter into the lungs. In foals, the catheter is often too large to pass out of the right side of the heart and must be removed. For a foal or the rare adult in which the catheter is lodged in the heart, consult vascular surgeons regarding techniques for retrieval of the catheters. Location of the broken end is important because some lodge at the thoracic inlet and can be removed surgically.

Acute Drug Reactions

These are alphabetically tabulated for drugs from acepromazine to xylazine and are listed in Table 39–1.

SUGGESTED REFERENCES

Kauffman VG, Soma L, Divers TJ, Perkons SZ. Extrapyramidal side effects caused by fluphenazine decanoate in a horse. J Am Vet Med Assoc 1989;195(8):1128–1130.
References continued on page 598

TABLE 39–1. **Specific Acute Drug Reactions and Recommended Treatments**

Drug	Clinical Signs/Overdose Information	Treatment
Acepromazine	Weakness, sweating, pale membranes, death, lower PCV (chronic), penile paralysis	4 ml/kg hypertonic saline IV for hypotension; for paraphimosis, see p. 405
Albuterol	Tremors, tachycardia, CNS excitement, some of which may be caused by hypokalemia	Usually requires no treatment, but serum K+ should be checked and if hypokalemia present, supplemental K+ provided
Altrenogest, oral	Colic, sweating rarely reported. Avoid human skin exposure	Symptomatic
Aminoglycoside antibiotics	A single dose of even 10× normal dose is unlikely to cause clinical problems. Treatment of a dehydrated patient with aminoglycosides is most common predisposing factor for aminoglycoside toxicity. Weakness due to neuromuscular blockade may rarely occur, unless other neuromuscular blocking drugs are administered or a neuromuscular disease, e.g., *botulism*, is present	IV fluid therapy (see p. 463); monitoring serum creatinine levels and urine production is advisable for prevention. If neuromuscular blockage occurs, it may be reversed if necessary with neostigmine, 0.01 mg/kg SQ, and/or slowly administered calcium IV mixed in polyionic fluids
Amitraz	Accidental exposure (see p. 601)	See p. 602
Amphotericin B	Rarely recommended in the horse, but may cause renal failure unless sodium diuresis administered during treatment	See p. 464
Anthelmintics	Colic, diarrhea	Supportive; in most cases do not treat with atropine unless an organophosphate is used *and other clinical signs of organophosphate toxicity are present* (miosis, salivation)!
Atropine	Colic, abdominal distention	Analgesics plus neostigmine, 0.01–0.02 mg/kg SQ q2h and/or cecal trocharization
Barbiturates	Respiratory depression, hypothermia; irritating when administered perivascularly	Assisted respiration

Table continued on opposite page

TABLE 39–1. **Specific Acute Drug Reactions and Recommended Treatments** Continued

Drug	Clinical Signs/Overdose Information	Treatment
Bethanechol	Rarely produces adverse effects, other than salivation	None
Butorphanol	Head tremors, excitement, ataxia, death (rare). Most often occurs when used without tranquilizers	Xylazine
Detomidine	Do not administer with IV trimethoprim-sulfa; sweating, cardiovascular and respiratory depression, collapse	Yohimbine, 0.07–0.1 mg/kg or tolazoline, 2.2 mg/kg IV
Diazepam	Ataxia	None
Dichlorvos	Colic and/or signs of organophosphate toxicity (salivation, miosis, diarrhea); rarely neuromuscular weakness	NSAID for colic. Atropine only if certain organophosphate toxicity has occurred
Digoxin	See p. 141	See p. 141
Dimethyl sulfoxide (DMSO)	Hemolysis—do not use in concentrations greater than 10% dextrose	No treatment required unless severe. Transfusion
Dinoprost tromethamine (prostaglandin $F_{2\alpha}$)	Colic, sweating	Usually none required
Dobutamine	Heart rate increases greater than 30%–50%. Arrhythmias	Usually none required except decrease rate of administration or stop infusion
Dopamine	Tachycardia, very irritating if perivascular	Usually none required except decrease rate of administration
Doxapram HCl	Seizures	Pentobarbital to effect, intranasal oxygen
Doxycycline	Collapse, death, supraventricular tachycardia, hypertension when administered IV	DO NOT USE IV
Embutramide, mebezonium and tetracaine	CNS signs, hyperactivity	Sedation rarely needed
Epinephrine	Collapse	Usually none—monitor cardiac rhythm and blood pressure. A β-blocker proponent should be used only if hypertension demonstrated

Table continued on following page

TABLE 39–1. **Specific Acute Drug Reactions and Recommended Treatments** *Continued*

Drug	Clinical Signs/Overdose Information	Treatment
Flunixin meglumine	Injection site swelling most common. Collapse if administered intracarotid	If swelling occurs, monitor closely for sepsis (see pp. 267 and 268)
Fluprostenol sodium	Sweating, colic	Treatment generally not required
Fluphenazine Decanoate (prolixin decanoate)—a phenothiazine derivative that blocks dopamine receptors	Bizarre behavior, restlessness (refractory to treatment with xylazine), recumbency, seizure	Phenobarbital, 12 mg/kg, administered in 1 liter over 20 minutes rather than by bolus; antihistamines (e.g., diphenhydramine). Supportive therapy, hypnotic therapy. Chloral hydrate to effect IV may be used in place of barbiturates
Glycopyrrolate	Tenesmus, small colon impaction, possible cardiovascular effects	Analgesics, oral and IV fluids for impaction
Guaifenesin	Toxic at high dosage (3× normal), causes hypotension	IV fluids
Halothane	Respiratory/cardiac depression, arrhythmia	See p. 125; stop anesthesia; CPR if arrest occurs
Heparin	Anemia	Discontinue treatment; PCV should return to pretreatment values within 2–4 days
Hyaluronate sodium	Swollen joints, lameness. See *Polysulfated Glycosaminoglycan* in this table	NSAIDs, joint lavage, hydrotherapy, antibiotics (especially if swelling does not occur for several hours)
Iron	In newborn foals, produces acute hepatic failure and death when administered PO before colostrum. May cause acute collapse followed by hepatic or renal disease in some individuals when administered IV	Fluids
Isoflurane	Respiratory/cardiac depression	See p. 125; CPR if arrest occurs, O₂ therapy, stop anesthesia
Isoxsuprine	When administered IV, may cause hyperexcitability and hypotension	Diazepam and IV fluids

Table continued on opposite page

TABLE 39–1. **Specific Acute Drug Reactions and Recommended Treatments** *Continued*

Drug	Clinical Signs/Overdose Information	Treatment
Ivermectin (oral)	Rare severe systemic reaction, ventral abdominal swelling caused by death of *Onchocerca* microfilaria not unusual. Injection of ivermectin (SQ or IM) can result in severe local swelling	For *Onchocerca* reaction—symptomatic usually. If severe, steroids
Ketamine (see p. 649)	Respiratory depression	Mechanical/physical ventilation
Ketoprofen	Injection site reactions; collapse and death if intracarotid administration	None
Lidocaine (see p. 583). *Do not use lidocaine with epinephrine IV*	CNS signs/hypotension	Diazepam, hypertonic saline for hypotension
Lincomycin	*Contraindicated* in the horse—severe colitis	IV fluids; metronidazole, 25 mg/kg PO q12h
Magnesium toxicity	Rare, may produce weakness and respiratory distress when administered to oliguric individuals	Slow IV fluids with calcium borogluconate
Meperidine HCl	Overdose may produce respiratory depression and hypotension. Excitement may occur when used without tranquilization!	Naloxone, 0.01 mg/kg IV, repeated if necessary, and IV fluids
Methocarbamol	Sedation and ataxia	Supportive
Metoclopramide HCl	Bizarre behavior, head tremors, ataxia	Diphenhydramine and *phenobarbital, do not use tranquilizers.* Chloral hydrate can be administered to effect as a sedative
Monensin (oral)	Increased heart rate, diarrhea, recumbency, death	Supportive (see p. 148)
Morphine sulfate, oxymorphone, and pentazocine	After IV administration, hyperexcitability, ataxia may occur when pretreatment with tranquilizers has not been administered. Large doses may depress respiration	Naloxone, 0.01 mg/kg IV, repeated if necessary. Efficacy of naloxone in treating drugs (pentazocine, butorphanol) with both opiate agonist and antagonist properties is unknown; therefore, use it cautiously

Table continued on following page

TABLE 39–1. **Specific Acute Drug Reactions and Recommended Treatments** *Continued*

Drug	Clinical Signs/Overdose Information	Treatment
Neostigmine	Colic	Analgesics and fluids
Nitroglycerin ointment	If used for laminitis in a hypotensive patient, hypotension could worsen	Fluids IV, remove ointment. *Avoid human contact*
Organophosphate anthelminthics, e.g., trichlorofon	Rarely causes signs, loose feces, diarrhea, increased salivation, sweating, colic, ataxia, death	Supportive treatment, fluids and analgesics. If classic signs (salivation, miosis) of organophosphate poisoning are present and overdosing is known to have occurred, administer atropine, 0.22 mg/kg. *Do not use atropine unless certain of organophosphate toxicity*
Oxytetracycline	Rapid IV infusion may cause collapse and hemolysis	Treatment usually not required
	Large doses (3 gm) administered to foals only to treated contracted/deformed tendons and rarely results in renal failure. Do not use >15 mg/kg/daily for prolonged periods.	IV fluid diuresis (see p. 464)
Oxytocin	Colic	Treatment usually not required
Penicillin	Procaine penicillin reactions are more common in patients receiving long-term injections in the same muscle mass. **Heating procaine penicillin increases procaine toxicity.** Rarely, immune-mediated anaphylaxis or hemolytic anemia. IV penicillin salts may cause salivation, "smacking" lips, head movement. (No treatment required)	Prevent injury to the individual by removing dangerous objects from the area. Humans should leave the stall to prevent bodily harm unless the patient is persistently circling, in which case an experienced person may walk *carefully* with the horse. Diazepam has no effect after excitability has occurred. For anaphylaxis, see p. 590. For hemolytic anemia, see p. 284
Phenoxybenzamine	May cause hypotension when administered IV (little or no indication for IV use in horse)	Hypertonic saline IV, if Na fluid loading not indicated, administer phenylephrine. *Epinephrine contraindicated with any α-adrenergic-blocking agent adverse reaction.*

Table continued on opposite page

TABLE 39–1. **Specific Acute Drug Reactions and Recommended Treatments** *Continued*

Drug	Clinical Signs/Overdose Information	Treatment
Phenylpropanolamine	Relatively safe in the horse; gross overdosing may cause CNS signs and cardiovascular collapse.	IV fluids and oral charcoal and $MgSO_4$ if treatment within last hour
Phenytoin	Ataxia, depression, weakness, recumbency	Treatment usually not required but may administer IV fluids
Piperazine	Gross overdosing has occurred in the horse and caused paralysis, salivation, and CNS signs. As with any anthelmintic effective against *Parascarid equorum*, it may cause colic if large numbers of the worms are killed	IV fluids and oral charcoal and $MgSO_4$ for overdose
Plasma/whole blood	Tremors, pyrexia, agitation, tachypnea, tachycardia, piloerection	If hemolysis does not occur, slow plasma/blood infusion and administer antihistamine; if severe
Polysulfated glycosaminoglycan	When administered intra-articularly, may cause subacute (within hours) swelling and pain. This is usually a nonseptic inflammatory response; sepsis is always a concern and should be ruled out via arthrocentesis and cytology if pain/lameness does not occur for 12–24 hours or more	Phenylbutazone systemically and cold hydrotherapy. Joint lavage if swelling is severe and/or sepsis suspected. If sepsis is suspected, therapy should be directed against the most common organism, *Staphylococcus aureus*
Procainamide	Rarely used in the horse, but when used may cause hypotension	IV hypertonic saline
Promazine	See Acepromazine	Fluids or pressor drugs for hypotension
Propantheline bromide	GI ileus, colic	Dipyrone or low dose flunixin meglumine, 0.3 mg/kg IV; cecal trocarization if needed; neostigmine, 0.01–0.02 mg/kg SQ; and IV fluids
Propranolol	Rarely used in the horse, but may cause severe bradycardia and collapse	Atropine, 0.07 mg/kg IV, fluids
Pergolide	Overdose may cause CNS signs similar to those seen with metoclopramide	Sedation (barbiturates) and fluid therapy

Table continued on following page

4

TABLE 39–1. **Specific Acute Drug Reactions and Recommended Treatments** *Continued*

Drug	Clinical Signs/Overdose Information	Treatment
Quinidine	Tachycardia, sweating, collapse, hypotension, ataxia (usually mild), mild nasal stridor	Digoxin, 1 mg IV per 450-kg adult. Fluids, HCO_3 IV to increase excretion, and KCl
Selenium	Collapse occurs occasionally with IV injections, death, colic, ataxia	Supportive; do not administer IV
Sodium bicarbonate	Gross overdosage either IV or PO may cause alkalosis and synchronous diaphragmatic flutter	0.9% NaCl with KCl and calcium borogluconate
Succinylcholine chloride	Respiratory paralysis	Mechanical ventilation
Terbutaline	Excitement, tachycardia, sweating, tremors	IV fluids containing potassium
Trimethoprim/sulfa	Oral, rarely diarrhea; IV, rarely collapse. Fatal if administered intracarotid	Diarrhea (see p. 235)
Vasopressin	If administered IV, may cause CNS signs	Treatment usually not required
Warfarin	See p. 629.	Treat with charcoal and $MgSO_4$ PO; Vitamin K
Xylazine	Hyperventilation, death from pulmonary edema on rare occasion (when pre-existing respiratory disease present)	Do not use with upper respiratory obstruction. Treat with yohimbine, 0.075 mg/kg IV, or preferably tolazoline, 2.2 mg/kg IV. Use diazepam rather than xylazine when possible in foals < 1 week of age
	Intracarotid administration (see p. 588)	
	Some horses (breeds: e.g., draft breeds, warm bloods; age: foals) may become recumbent with recommended dose	Treatment usually not required, but if severely hypotensive, administer IV fluids

Note: For any adverse drug reaction, *read the package insert.*
PCV, packed cell volume.

Riond JL, Riviere JE, Duckett WM, Atkins CE. Cardiovascular effects and fatalities associated with intravenous administration of doxycycline to horses and ponies. Equine Vet J 1992;24(1):41–45.

Gabel AA, Koestner A. The effects of intracarotid artery injection of drugs in domestic animals. J Am Vet Med Assoc 1993;142(12):1397–1403.

40 Toxicology

Thomas J. Divers, Larry J. Thompson, and
Mary C. Smith

A poisoning or toxicosis should be suspected if

- Many horses are sick with no known exposure to infectious disease;
- The affected individual(s) has been exposed recently to a new environment;
- There has been a recent change in the feed;
- There are unusual weather conditions;
- The individual has limited feeds or pasture;
- An uncommon clinical condition exists;
- An unexplained death(s) has occurred.

If toxicosis is suspected, a complete history is imperative in addition to a complete physical examination, laboratory testing, and a detective-like inspection of the premises. If unexplained deaths occur, a complete postmortem examination should be performed on all suspect cases, including thorough gross inspection of the entire body and all intestinal contents.

Collect specimens from all major organs and tissues, fix them in formalin, and submit for histopathologic examination. Ancillary tests may include serologic testing, microbiologic culturing of suspect tissue or lesions, or virus isolation.

For toxicologic testing, the most important specimens to collect are liver, kidney, body fat, spleen (200 gm of each), whole EDTA blood (10 ml), stomach and intestinal contents (500 gm of each), urine (50 ml), half of the brain, feed samples (1–2 kg) and water (1 liter), and any suspect plant or toxic substances in the environment.

Clearly label samples and package individually in sealable plastic bags or clean plastic containers. Tissues can be frozen, and whole blood should be *refrigerated.* Double-bag samples and package them in an insulated container to avoid breakage or leakage and deliver to the laboratory by overnight or second-day delivery service.

A letter of transmittal should accompany the specimens to the laboratory with specific identification of the affected individuals and a list of all samples submitted. Include pertinent facts concerning background, history, clinical signs, and gross postmortem findings, with an explanation of any treatments given. NOTE: *No toxicologic screen can test for all poisons,* and a complete and accurate history helps the toxicologist test for the most likely toxicants.

Clinicians should strive to be as complete as possible in their examination, to document their findings, and to keep an open mind.

Additional help on the diagnosis and management of suspected poisoning cases can be obtained by calling the National Animal Poison Control Center hotlines:

- ■ **1 (800) 548 2423**. The fee is $30 per case unless product is covered by a sponsoring company; credit cards and the 800 access only; follow-up calls are included.
- ■ **1 (900) 680 0000**. The fee is $20 for the first 5 minutes, $2.95 for each additional minute ($20 minimum); if product is covered by a sponsoring company, call is transferred to the 800 line and no fee charged.

Utilize regional laboratories for diagnostic testing when possible because the regional laboratory is more likely to have information on common toxicants in the area. A list of these laboratories follows:

California Veterinary Diagnostic Laboratory System
School of Veterinary Medicine—UC Davis
West Health Science Drive
Davis, CA 95616; (916) 752 8700

Veterinary Diagnostic and Investigational Laboratory
University of Georgia
P.O. Box 1389
Tifton, GA 31793

Laboratories of Veterinary Diagnostic Medicine
College of Veterinary Medicine—UIUC
2001 S. Lincoln Avenue
Urbana, IL 61801

Animal Disease Diagnostic Laboratory
School of Veterinary Medicine—Purdue University
West Lafayette, IN 47907

Veterinary Diagnostic Laboratory
College of Veterinary Medicine—ISU
Ames, IA 50010

Veterinary Diagnostic and Research Center
Murray State University
P.O. Box 2000 North Drive
Hopkinsville, KY 42240

Animal Health Diagnostic Laboratory
Michigan State University
P.O. Box 30076
Lansing, MI 48909–7576; (517) 355 0281

Veterinary Diagnostic Medicine
University of Minnesota
1943 Carter Avenue
St. Paul, MN 55101

Veterinary Medical Diagnostic Laboratory
University of Missouri

P.O. Box 6023
Columbia, MO 65205

Veterinary Diagnostic Laboratory
College of Veterinary Medicine—Cornell University
Upper Tower Road
Ithaca, NY 14853; (607) 253 3900

Animal Disease Diagnostic Laboratory
College of Veterinary Medicine
Oklahoma State University
Stillwater, OK 74078; (405) 744 6623

Veterinary Medical Diagnostic Laboratory
Texas A&M University
P.O. Box 3200
Amarillo, TX 79106

Texas Veterinary Medical Diagnostic Laboratory
College Station, TX; (409) 845 3414

Poisonous Plants Research Laboratory
Utah State University
1150 East 1400 North
Logan, UT 84341

Animal Disease Diagnostic Laboratory
Washington State University
P.O. Box 2037, College Station
Pullman, WA 99165

PADLS-NBC Toxicology
382 West Street Road
Kennett Square, PA 19348
Phone: (610) 444 5800 ext 2217
FAX: (610) 444 4617

Phone numbers of other laboratories that are occasionally used by the Veterinary Diagnostic Laboratory—Cornell University:

Barrow Agee	(901) 332 1590
Woodson Tennet	(901) 521 4500
Hazelton	(608) 241 4471
A&L Laboratories	(901) 527 2781
Southwest Laboratories	(800) 592 0503

COMMON TOXINS PREDOMINANTLY AFFECTING THE GASTROINTESTINAL TRACT

Amitraz

A formamidine insecticide, available in the United States as an acaricide dip/spray for cattle and hogs and used in treating canine demodectic mange. Horses are very sensitive to this drug; *it should not be used on horses.*

Clinical Signs

- Impaction colic, depression, incoordination
- All occur within 24 hours of exposure.

Treatment

- If dermal exposure, soap and water bath
- If oral exposure, activated charcoal 1–5 gm/kg PO
- IV fluids
- Flunixin meglumine, 1 mg/kg q24h

Atropine Toxicosis

Most commonly occurs when atropine has been administered (often incorrectly) for suspected organophosphate poisoning. Plants such as jimsonweed *(Datura stramonium)*, nightshades *(Solanum nigra, S. dulcamara, S. eleagnifolium)*, and belladonna *(Atropa belladonna)* contain related tropane alkaloids. Foliage of potatoes and tomatoes contains tropane and steroidal glycoalkaloids and can also be toxic.

Clinical Signs

- Bloat, colic, dry membranes, and dilated pupils
- Steroidal glycoalkaloids cause gastroenteritis.

Treatment

- Flunixin meglumine, 1.0 mg/kg, and neostigmine, 0.01 mg/kg SQ
- Activated charcoal following plant ingestion, 1–5 gm/kg PO.

Black Locust *(Robinia pseudoacacia)*

Toxic principle, robin, is a toxalbumin that inhibits protein synthesis. Ingestion of young sprouts, bark, or pruned or fresh leaves can cause illness.

Clinical Signs

- Anorexia, diarrhea (may be bloody), colic, depression, weakness, irregular pulse
- Rarely fatal, laminitis can be a severe sequela.

Treatment

- Activated charcoal, 1–5 gm/kg PO, IV fluids, and nutritional support

Blister Beetle (Cantharidin)

Toxicosis is due to ingestion of the blister beetle *(Epicauta* spp., see p. 223), which can be found in alfalfa that has been simultaneously cut and crimped.

Blister beetles are usually found in the Plains states and the Midwest, occasionally in other parts of the country.

Clinical Signs

- Mucous membrane irritation, including oral, GI tract, and urinary tract
- Colic, hypocalcemia with synchronous diaphragmatic flutter, frequent urination, shock, and death
- Cardiac damage is possible.
- Neurologic signs only in a few cases
- Acute death

Diagnosis

- Compatible clinical signs, postmortem lesions (erythema and occasionally erosions of GI mucosa)
- Identification of blister beetles in hay or GI contents
- Submit GI contents and urine for analysis for cantharidin. Several laboratories commonly performing this test:

Texas Veterinary Medical Diagnostic Laboratory (409) 845 3414
Michigan State University Diagnostic Laboratory (517) 355 0281
University of California at Davis Diagnostic Laboratory (916) 752 8700
Animal Disease Diagnostic Laboratory, Oklahoma State University (405) 744 6623

Treatment

- Remove suspect feed, administer 1 gallon of mineral oil PO/450-kg adult and fluid therapy.
- Monitor serum calcium.
- Supportive care!
- Mucosal ulcerations may develop.
- There is no known antidote.

Prognosis

- Guarded
- Poor with neurologic signs

Buttercups (*Ranunculus* spp.)

Plentiful in many pastures, fortunately horses almost never eat the plant in a pasture setting, and drying renders the plant nontoxic. Toxic principle is ranunculin, which releases protoanemonin when damaged.

Clinical Signs

- Irritated oral mucous membranes, colic, anorexia, diarrhea, muscle tremors that may proceed to excitement and convulsions

■ Contact with crushed plant may cause skin irritation.

Treatment

■ Activated charcoal 1–5 gm/kg PO; symptomatic and supportive care

Castor Bean *(Ricinus communis)*

Seeds and foliage are poisonous.

Clinical Signs

■ Colic, profuse and watery diarrhea, fever, incoordination, depression, sweating, terminal convulsions, death
■ Signs may be delayed 12 hours or more after ingestion.

Diagnosis

■ Identification of seeds in GI contents, evidence of consumption, and compatible clinical signs

Treatment

■ Sedation if needed (xylazine, 0.4 mg/kg), fluids (hypertonic saline), followed by polyionic isotonic fluids
■ Flunixin meglumine, 1.0 mg/kg
■ Activated charcoal, 1–5 gm/kg PO

Horse Chestnut *(Aesculus hippocastanum)*
(Fig. 40–1)
Buckeye *(A. glabra)*

The toxic principle is esculin, a saponin glycoside present in the leaves and nuts.

Clinical Signs

■ Ingestion may cause colic, inflamed mucous membranes, hyperesthesia, and ataxia, followed by muscle tremors, paresis, dyspnea, convulsions, and death.

Treatment

■ Activated charcoal 1–5 gm/kg PO, analgesics (parenterally), supportive fluids (IV), and symptomatic treatment

Oak *(Quercus* spp.)

Toxic principles are gallotannins. Rarely causes poisoning in horses as opposed to cattle, although poorly fed individuals may eat leaves, acorns, or oak buds.

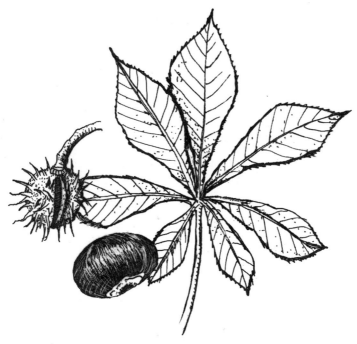

FIGURE 40–1. Horse Chestnut.

Clinical Signs

- Anorexia, colic, sometimes bloody diarrhea, depression followed by frequent urination and constipation
- May develop dependent edema

Treatment

- Fluids, nutritional and other supportive care
- Evaluate for possible kidney damage.

Organophosphate (OP) and Carbamate Insecticides

Poisoning with these usually causes clinical signs of nervous and GI dysfunction. The most likely source of the poisoning is an inappropriate or accidental oral or topical administration of an insecticide or anthelmintic containing OPs (see p. 596) or carbamates. Clinical signs for both insecticides are similar.

Clinical Signs

- Colic, hypersalivation, sweating, diarrhea, muscle tremors, miosis, weakness, dyspnea, and/or convulsions

- Organophosphates and carbamates cause an increase in the peristaltic activity of the intestines, as well as a bradycardia.

Diagnosis

- History of exposure and compatible clinical signs
- Exposure confirmed by measurement of whole blood cholinesterase activity or plasma pseudocholinesterase activity. If significant OP or carbamate exposure has occurred, the patient's cholinesterase or pseudocholinesterase activity is much lower (<25%) than the normal value for the referring laboratory. If submitting to a human laboratory, also submit a control (nonexposed) equine sample. A postmortem sample of brain or eyeball shows decreased cholinesterase activity in OP or carbamate exposure.
- If submittal to the laboratory is delayed, all samples of carbamate insecticides can exhibit a "regeneration" of active cholinesterase, resulting in a normal value.
- Submit GI contents and liver for insecticide screen.

Treatment

- Atropine, 0.01–0.05 mg/kg IV and 0.05 mg/kg SQ as needed (up to four times daily) to control clinical signs of OP and carbamate poisoning
- There should be an obvious improvement in the muscarinic effects (salivation, miosis and sweating) soon after the treatment begins.
- 2-PAM (pralidoxime hydrochloride) is specific for OPs and does not help in carbamate poisoning. Administer 20 mg/kg IV every 4–6 hours, if needed.
- Pass a stomach tube to remove any gastric reflux.
- Administer activated charcoal 1–5 gm/kg PO, along with supportive care such as replacement fluids.

> - Accurate diagnosis of organophosphate or carbamate poisoning in the horse is imperative because of the possible adverse effects from atropine administration. High-dose atropine used in OP or carbamate poisoning therapy should never be administered without clear historical, clinical, and preferably laboratory evidence that OP or carbamate poisoning is responsible for the clinical signs!

- Transient abdominal pain following oral administration of organophosphate anthelmintics is not uncommon; however, it is unusual that atropine treatment is required.

Red Clover *(Trifolium pratense)*

Under certain environmental conditions a fungus, *Rhizoctonia leguminicola*, can grow on the clover and produce a mycotoxin, slaframine, which increases saliva production and causes *slobbering*. The fungus is seen as black/brown spots on the clover. More commonly affects individuals grazing pastures containing some red clover or, less commonly, when red clover is in the hay. The same fungus may produce clinical signs in horses when grown on other legumes, e.g., white clover *(Trifolium repens)*, alfalfa *(Medicago sativa)*.

Clinical Signs

- Excess salivation; duration can be several hours for mild cases or can be continuous.
- In severe cases, diarrhea and anorexia occur.

Treatment

- Remove affected individual from the pasture
- Provide water and salt

Tobacco (*Nicotiana* spp.)

Toxic principles are nicotine and other alkaloids. Tobacco plants (commercial, wild, and ornamental) are extremely unpalatable; therefore, poisoning is unusual. It may occur if horses are housed where tobacco is stored or where wild tobacco plants grow and there is little else to eat. Nicotine first stimulates, then blocks, nervous activity.

Clinical Signs

- Initial excitement, colic, diarrhea, incoordination, muscle tremors, excess salivation followed by muscle weakness, recumbency, stupor
- Death from respiratory paralysis

Treatment

- Activated charcoal 1–5 gm/kg PO
- Fluids and symptomatic treatment

Miscellaneous Toxic Plants

Those predominantly affecting the GI tract include

- *Delphinium* spp. (larkspur)
- Rotten potatoes
- *Berteroa incana* (see p. 264), producing fever, limb edema, diarrhea, mainly in northeastern, north central United States and Canada

Other Gastrointestinal Poisonings

Salt Poisoning

May cause diarrhea, colic, and neurologic signs when salt-deprived horses are fed salt and do not have adequate water available.

DIAGNOSIS

- Elevated serum or cerebrospinal fluid (CSF) sodium

TREATMENT

- Fluid therapy, 2.5% dextrose/0.45% saline, polyionic crystalloid; DMSO, 1 gm/kg IV
- Do not use 5% dextrose!

Arsenic and Mercury

Can produce sudden death with severe GI erosions

CLINICAL SIGNS

- Salivation
- Diarrhea
- Depression

DIAGNOSIS

- History plus GI contents, liver, and kidney for arsenic or mercury concentrations
- Clinical signs plus hepatic and kidney arsenic concentrations—>10 ppm are compatible with arsenic intoxication

TREATMENT

- Dimercaprol, 3–5 mg/kg IM q8h on day 1 and 1 mg/kg IM q6h on days 2 and 3.

TOXINS PREDOMINANTLY AFFECTING THE NERVOUS SYSTEM

Ammonia Intoxication

This should be strongly considered in individuals with signs of acute encephalopathy, severe acidosis, normal liver enzymes, and hyperglycemia. Supportive treatment may result in complete recovery. Colic and diarrhea may also be present.

Australian Dandelion (Hypochoesis radicata)

This causes outbreaks of stringhalt and roaring in horses in Australia. Similar outbreaks of unknown etiology are reported in the western and southeastern United States. Stringhalt may also occur acutely associated with injury to the rear leg(s) or from hypocalcemia.

Treatment

- For severely affected individuals, phenytoin, 7.5 mg/kg PO q12h, may eliminate clinical signs.
- Acupuncture

Avocado *(Persea americana)*

Found mainly in Florida and California. Toxic principle is unknown; however, all parts of the tree are believed to be toxic. Poisoning most commonly occurs when affected individuals have access to pruned branches, which remain toxic when dried.

Clinical Signs

- Noninfectious mastitis, depression, mild tremors, and colic
- Death is unusual.

Treatment

- Symptomatic and supportive care.
- The mastitis subsides within 1 week; however, no additional milk is produced during the lactation.

Botulism (see p. 348)

Caused by *Clostridium botulinum*, this is mainly a clinical problem in foals 2–8 weeks of age but can affect adults. In Kentucky, Pennsylvania, Maryland, New Jersey, and Virginia, it is usually caused by *C. botulinum* toxin type B. There are 8 toxin types with variable regional distribution. Types A and C may also occur sporadically. In adults, it is most often a result of ingestion of preformed toxin in vegetative matter. In foals, it is a toxicoinfectious process due to ingestion of the *C. botulinum* type B spores. Wound botulism does occur in the horse but is uncommon.

Clinical Signs

- Dysphagia, trembling; mydriasis (type C); weak tail, tongue, and eyelid tone; recumbency

Diagnosis

- Although it is difficult to isolate the toxin, submit samples of serum, gastric/intestinal contents, feces, and suspect feed. A laboratory for testing is at the University of Pennsylvania, New Bolton Center; (610) 444 5800 ext 2321 or 2383.
- In foals, culture of *Clostridium* type B from the feces is strongly supportive of the diagnosis in the presence of dysphagia and weakness.

Treatment

- Antiserum (see p. 349)

Bracken Fern *(Pteridium aquilinum)*
(Fig. 40–2)

Although frequently listed in textbooks, this poisoning is uncommon in the horse because a large quantity of the unpalatable plant must be consumed. Toxic principle is a thiaminase that causes a thiamine deficiency.

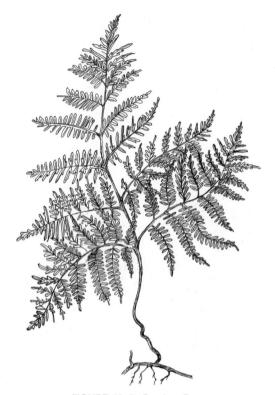

FIGURE 40–2. Bracken Fern.

Clinical Signs

- Unthriftiness, lethargy, ataxia, blindness, recumbency, and convulsions
- Polioencephalomalacia can be found on postmortem examination.

Treatment

- Thiamine hydrochloride, 5 mg/kg slowly IV or IM q6h for 5 days.
- Response to early treatment is dramatic.

Fumonisin B_1/B_2

Fumonisins are mycotoxins produced by the *Fusarium* species of fungus, mainly found on corn, and can be in high concentration in corn screenings. Fumonisin causes equine leukoencephalomalacia (moldy corn poisoning).

Clinical Signs

- Occur after the affected individuals eat the feed for several days
- Anorexia, ataxia, blindness, head pressing, occasionally icterus, and death

Diagnosis (see p. 359)

- Can be toxic if over 5 ppm fumonisin is in the feed for several days to several weeks.
- Malacia of the white matter in the cerebral cortex and in some cases hepatosis with elevation of serum hepatic enzymes.
- The contaminated corn usually appears normal on inspection. Many diagnostic laboratories test for fumonisin.

Treatment

- Supportive. Affected individuals rarely completely recover.

Horsetail (*Equisetum hyemale* and *E. arvense*)

Rarely reported as a toxicosis in horses and can occur if little else is available to eat. Toxic principle is a thiaminase, similar to bracken fern.

Clinical Signs

- Unthriftiness, lethargy, ataxia, blindness, recumbency, and convulsions
- Polioencephalomalacia can be found on postmortem examination.

Treatment

- Thiamine hydrochloride (see Bracken Fern)

Insulin

Hypoglycemic shock has been reported in horses inappropriately treated with insulin. High-pressure liquid chromatography (HPLC) is used to identify the source of insulin in the serum, performed by drug-testing centers.

Treatment

- Continuous 5%–10% dextrose administration, polyionic crystalloids with 40 mEq/L KCl, and dexamethasone, 0.2 mg/kg IV initially followed by a decreasing dosage for 2–3 additional days

Prognosis

- Poor

Lead

Lead poisoning is rare but may occur from ingestion of lead paint, old batteries, or lead weights.

Acute Signs

- Weakness, ataxia, depression, and convulsions
- Laryngeal paresis, especially with exercise or excitement, may be present with chronic lead poisoning.

Diagnosis

- Whole blood lead greater than 0.6 ppm (or above 0.3 ppm with compatible clinical signs)
- Liver or kidney, 5–10 ppm (wet weight*) or greater

Treatment

- Calcium-EDTA, 75 mg/kg/day slowly IV, divided q12h. Treat for 2 or 3 days and then stop for 2 or 3 days, and repeat if needed.
- Thiamine, 5 mg/kg IV or IM
- Magnesium or sodium sulfate, 1 gm/kg PO, helps remove lead from GI tract.
- Maintain adequate hydration of affected individual during treatment period.

Locoweed (Certain *Astragalus* spp. and *Oxytropis* spp.)
(Fig. 40–3)

Grows in central and western rangelands of North America. A large amount of the plant must be ingested (30% of BW over 6–7 weeks). Toxic principle is swainsonine, which causes an accumulation of oligosaccharides in neural tissue.

Clinical Signs

- Depression, ataxia, dysphagia, hyperexcitability, apparent blindness, stringhalt-like gaits, paraplegia, and death
- Affected individuals may become dependent and seek the plant.

Treatment

- None demonstrated to be effective; reserpine, 3.0 mg/450 kg IM or 1.25 mg/450 kg PO for 6 days, has been reported to eliminate the clinical signs.
- Recovery may occur in mild cases.

Marijuana, Hemp *(Cannabis sativa)*

Occasionally fed to horses and may cause excitement, incoordination, sweating, salivation, and subsequent weakness and depression.

Treatment

- Activated charcoal, 1–5 gm/kg PO, if ingestion within previous 2 hours
- Symptomatic and supportive care.

---

*To convert liver and kidney wet weight concentration to dry weight, multiply ppm ×4.

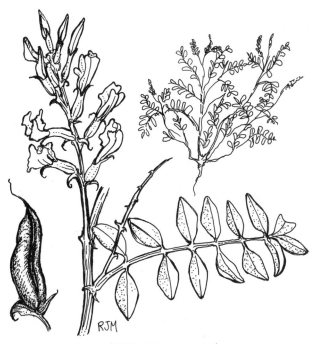

FIGURE 40–3. Locoweed.

4

Ryegrass *(Lolium perenne)*

A common pasture grass of southeastern United States and western coast that can be parasitized by an endophytic fungus. Tremors and ataxia are seen in horses, caused by ingestion of endophytic fungus in the grass. Occasionally seen during certain years that are apparently conducive to the fungal growth. May be seen with other grasses rarely, e.g., Bermuda and Dallis grasses.

Clinical Signs

- Tremors, weakness, incoordination
- Death is usually accidental, e.g., falling into water and drowning.

Treatment

- Remove from pasture and recovery occurs.

Selenium Toxicosis

Acute form from inappropriate selenium injections (see p. 598) or feeding toxic amounts. Errors in feed formulation can occur but rarely cause problems.

Toxicity reported in horses administered 3.3 mg/kg PO (smaller amounts may be toxic).

Clinical Signs

- Acute form can exhibit excess salivation, tremors, ataxia, apparent blindness, respiratory distress, diarrhea, inability to stand, and death.
- Chronic form may exhibit hair or hoof abnormalities, coronary band separation, and joint stiffness.
- If poisoning is suspected, measure selenium levels in the blood and/or liver samples.

Treatment

- Symptomatic and supportive care
- Acetylcysteine beginning at 140 mg/kg IV, then 70 mg/kg IV q6h, is suggested for acute poisonings.

Sudan Grass (*Sorghum vulgare* var. *sudanense*)

In addition to the potential for acute cyanide poisoning, the grazing of Sudan grass for several weeks may cause equine cystitis/ataxia syndrome. It has occurred in the central and southern Great Plains of North America on pastures almost exclusively composed of sorghum species. Problems do not occur from eating dry hay.

Clinical Signs

- Ataxia of the rear limbs, a hopping gait, dribbling of urine (the bladder is enlarged)
- Acute poisoning (cyanide) frequently causes death.

Diagnosis

- Clinical signs, exposure, cyanide levels in gastric contents

Treatment

- Remove from pasture and treat any bladder infection with antibiotics.
- Full recovery is unusual.
- Use sodium thiosulfate 30–40 mg/kg IV q12h to treat acute poisoning.

White Snakeroot (*Eupatorium rugosum*)
(Fig. 40–4)

Toxic principle is unknown (older texts list tremetol) and is cumulative and can be passed in the milk. Grows in shady areas and is a problem in late summer or fall; remains toxic after frost or when dried.

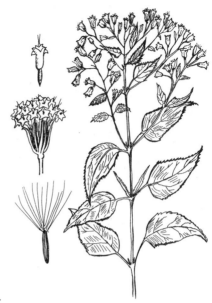

FIGURE 40–4. White Snakeroot.

Clinical Signs

- Weakness, depression, trembling, sweating, salivation, and recumbency.
- Dependent edema and cardiac damage are possible.

Treatment

- Symptomatic and supportive care
- Remove from source.
- May have long-term cardiac compromise

Yellow Star Thistle *(Centaurea solstitialis)*
(Fig. 40–5)

Grows predominantly in the western United States. **Russian knapweed** *(Centaurea repens)* causes identical signs.

Clinical Signs

- Begin suddenly after chronic ingestion of the plant(s)
- Affected individuals can prehend food with their incisors but cannot move the food back into the mouth. Difficulty in drinking water and may immerse head deep into the water to swallow. The lips may be retracted from hypertonic facial muscles, and the tongue may protrude.
- Depression, ataxia, circling, and starvation.
- May have secondary aspiration pneumonia.

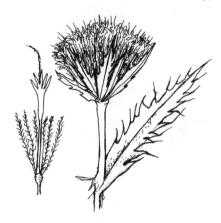

FIGURE 40–5. Yellow Star Thistle.

- Nigropallidal encephalomalacia is found at autopsy.
- Oxidative stress may play a role in the toxicity.

Treatment

- No specific treatment; Vitamin E should be administered. Affected individuals do not recover and if not severely affected may learn to accommodate.

TOXINS PREDOMINANTLY AFFECTING THE LIVER

Aflatoxicosis

Metabolites B_1, B_2, G_1, G_2, and M_1, M_2 from *Aspergillus flavus*, which grows on corn, peanuts, and so on, with warm, wet conditions. Has been reported to cause acute hepatic failure (neurologic signs and icterus) in horses; it is apparently rare.

Diagnosis

- Evidence of exposure (have feed tested for mycotoxins), clinical signs, laboratory findings of liver disease and failure.
- Most laboratories can test for aflatoxin metabolites in urine (submit 1 liter) or liver.

Treatment

- Remove from suspect feed.
- General treatment for hepatic failure (see p. 283)
- L-Methionine, 25 mg/kg PO
- Vitamin E, 6000–10,000 units q24h PO, in adult

Alsike Clover *(Trifolium hybridum)*

A pasture legume found mostly in Canada and northeastern United States. A cluster of cases may occur in individuals grazing alsike clover grown on clay soils during certain years, probably due to wet weather conditions. Alsike must be predominant feed for several days to several weeks. Toxic principle is believed to be a steroidal saponin.

Clinical Signs
- Photosensitivity, icterus

Treatment
- General treatment for liver failure
- Remove alsike from diet.

Prognosis
- Good if identified early in the syndrome before significant liver damage has occurred.

Iron Toxicosis

May occur in individuals associated with acute administration of a large dose (overuse of a hematinic; oral or injectable) or from chronic accumulation (hemochromatosis). Foals receiving even small-dose iron supplements before nursing may develop fatal hepatopathy.

Clinical Signs
- In acute exposures, colic signs predominate.
- Clinical signs of liver failure generally do not occur unless more than 60%–75% of hepatic function is lost.

Diagnosis
- Signs of liver failure, laboratory findings of liver disease (increased serum gamma-glutamyl transaminopeptidase), and failure (increased serum conjugated bilirubin).
- Liver iron concentration > 300 ppm (most horses with iron toxicosis have values threefold or more above the upper normal range). Liver iron can be abnormally high without liver disease (hemosiderosis) e.g., vitamin E deficiency
- Serum iron is frequently normal with chronic hemochromatosis and may be increased with acute toxicosis.
- Elevations in serum iron is *not* specific for iron toxicosis and is frequently found in a variety of liver disorders.

Treatment
- Supportive for hepatic failure
- Following oral exposure, magnesium hydroxide (milk of magnesia) to precipitate iron in the GI tract

4

- Vitamin C, 0.5 gm/kg PO, and desferroxamine, 10 mg/kg IM or slowly IV twice, 2 hours apart
- If urine is reddish gold in color, additional treatment may be needed to hasten excretion in acute cases.

Kleingrass and Fall Panicum (*Panicum* spp.)

Kleingrass poisoning is primarily a problem in Texas and the southwestern United States, whereas fall panicum occasionally is a problem in the mid-Atlantic states. Toxic principle is a steroidal saponin.

Clinical Signs

- Depression, icterus, photosensitivity, and neurologic signs of hepatoencephalopathy

Treatment

- General treatment for hepatic failure (see p. 283)

Prognosis

- Guarded if signs of hepatic failure are present

Pyrrolizidine Alkaloids (PA)

Contained in the following plants: *Senecio* spp. (ragwort, groundsel), *Crotalaria* spp. (rattlebox), *Amsinckia* spp. (fiddleneck) (Fig. 40–6), *Echium vulgare* (viper's bugloss), *Heliotropium europaeum* (heliotrope), *Cynoglossum officinale* (hound's tongue), and others. Toxicity from PA-containing plants is a clinical problem mostly in the western United States, although some areas of eastern Canada and the United States have reported cases. Toxicity occurs from chronic ingestion of the plants, mostly in spring-cut alfalfa hay. PAs produce a chronic hepatic disease, and the onset is often acute several weeks after ingestion.

Clinical Signs

- Head pressing, circling, blindness, ataxia, icterus, photosensitivity, and weight loss

Diagnosis

- Inspection of the hay
- Liver biopsy with characteristic findings of megalocytosis, necrosis, and fibrosis
- Suspect feed can be analyzed for alkaloids (Poisonous Plant Research Laboratory, Logan, UT 84341).
- See p. 280 for additional information on diagnosis including the use of GGT in detecting subclinical cases.

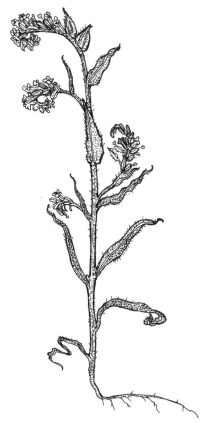

FIGURE 40–6. Fiddleneck.

4

Treatment

- Supportive for hepatic failure (see p. 283); most affected individuals have signs of liver failure and die within days to several months later.

Sensitive Fern *(Onoclea sensibilis)*

Found throughout eastern North America in open woods and meadows. Poisoning is rare as quantities must be ingested over long periods.

Clinical Signs

- Incoordination, anorexia, hyperesthesia
- Affected individuals develop liver disease (fatty degeneration) and cerebral edema with neuronal degeneration.
- **Blue-Green Algae** (see p. 631)

TOXINS PREDOMINANTLY AFFECTING THE SKIN

Lower Limb Dermatitis

An acutely developing dermatitis of one or more lower limbs on a horse is common under certain conditions, usually due to excessive moisture (from wash racks or wet pasture). It appears more noticeably on white legs. The limb is swollen, has many scabs, and is painful. **Rule out** *Dermatophilus*!

Treatment

- Systemic corticosteroids, e.g., prednisone, 0.5–1.0 mg/kg PO q24h
- Clean the leg and apply chlorhexidine cream.

Snow-On-The-Mountain *(Euphorbia marginata)*
(Fig. 40–7)

This and other *Euphorbia* spp. are in the spurge family. Spurges contain an irritant milky sap that causes *contact irritation* of the skin, mouth, and GI tract.

Treatment

- Wash skin with water; apply topical steroid or antihistamine emollients.
- Demulcents or mineral oil PO

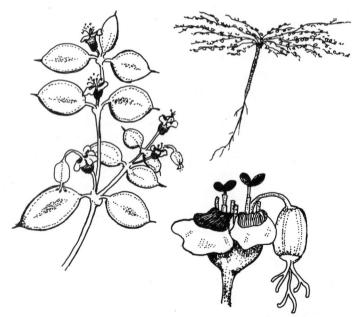

FIGURE 40–7. Snow-On-The-Mountain. The prostrate growth form is top right.

- ■ If severe clinical signs: steroids, antihistamines, and analgesics

Stinging Nettle (*Urtica dioica* and others)

Plants have stinging hairs containing formic acid, histamine, serotonin, and other constituents that cause local irritation. Affected individuals have been reported to exhibit ataxia, distress, and muscle weakness for several hours following a large contact with nettle, the mechanism is unknown.

Treatment

- ■ Steroids, antihistamines, analgesics, local cleansing of affected area, and topical emollients as needed

St. John's Wort *(Hypericum perforatum)*

Found throughout the United States along roadsides and in abandoned fields and open woods. Toxic principle is hypericin, a pigment that directly reacts with light to cause primary photosensitization, often within 24 hours after ingestion. Buckwheat *(Fagopyrum esculentum)* also causes primary photosensitivity but exposure is unusual. Both plants remain toxic when dried.

Clinical Signs

- ■ Dermatitis, pruritus, ulceration, all of which are more severe in nonpigmented areas of skin and those areas of the body with more exposure to sunlight
- ■ May also find lacrimation, conjunctival erythema, corneal ulceration, and anorexia due to irritation around the mouth.

Treatment

- ■ Remove the affected individuals from plant exposure and sunlight.
- ■ Topical treatment of the dermatitis (e.g., silver sulfadiazine cream), antihistamines, or systemic corticosteroids if pruritus is severe.
- ■ Ophthalmic antibiotics as needed
- ■ Oral antibiotics (e.g., TMP/S) in cases with severe dermatitis.

PHOTOSENSITIZATION (SECONDARY)

In *primary photosensitization* (e.g., St. John's Wort), there is no biochemical evidence of liver disease. Rule-outs for secondary or hepatogenous photosensitivity include hepatic failure (use biochemical tests, gamma-glutamyl transaminopeptidase, bilirubin) and other plants such as alsike clover, and panicum, and pyrrolizidine alkaloid plants. *Secondary photosensitization* involves the failure of the liver to excrete a normal metabolite of chlorophyll and the subsequent accumulation of phylloerythrin, a pigment that causes photosensitization. Prognosis for individuals with secondary photosensitization is worse than for primary photosensitization because of the severe liver disease.

TOXINS PREDOMINANTLY AFFECTING THE MUSCULOSKELETAL SYSTEM

Black Walnut *(Juglans nigra)*

The toxic principle of black walnut shavings is unknown.

Clinical Signs

- Laminitis often occurs within 12–24 hours of bedding on fresh black walnut shavings. As little as 5% black walnut shavings in the bedding may cause clinical disease.
- There may be marked edema of all four limbs and mild pyrexia.
- Laminitis with edema of all four limbs affecting more than one individual on the farm should arouse suspicion of black walnut shaving toxicity.

Diagnosis

- Rule out other causes of laminitis.
- Black walnut can be identified in shavings by diagnostic laboratories or wood technologists.

Treatment

- Remove from the shavings.
- Wash legs with mild soap and hydrotherapy.
- Treat for laminitis, e.g., analgesics such as phenylbutazone, 4.0 mg/kg; flunixin meglumine, 1.0 mg/kg; or ketoprofen, 2.2 mg/kg (see p. 323).
- Apply frog pads or place in sand bedding.
- Support wraps
- Pentoxifylline, 8.4 mg/kg q12h, and aspirin, 60–90 grains PO every other day for a 450-kg adult

Prognosis

- Generally better than for other causes of laminitis

Day-Blooming Jessamine *(Cestrum diurnum)*

Toxic principle is cholecalciferol glycoside, causing hypervitaminosis D. Found in southeastern United States, Texas, California, and Hawaii.

Clinical Signs

- Lameness, loss of weight, stiffness, and reluctance to move
- Acute poisoning does not occur, but chronic ingestion may cause calcification of tendons, ligaments, arteries, and kidneys.
- Serum calcium is elevated.

Treatment

- Remove from source.
- Symptomatic and supportive care
- Evaluate kidney function.

Fescue Foot in Foals

Arterial constriction of a limb(s) is a rare occurrence in otherwise healthy foals grazing on fescue pasture. Most reported cases occurred during one summer, suggesting unusual environmental conditions are needed. Ergotism produced from the growth of *Claviceps purpurea* on grains has a similar presentation.

Treatment

- None demonstrated
- Nitroglycerin cream can be applied over affected arteries.

Hoary Alyssum *(Berteroa incana)*
(Fig. 40–8)

A plant in the mustard family found throughout the midwest and northeastern United States. Often grows in older alfalfa fields where significant winterkill occurs; remains toxic and palatable in dried hay.

FIGURE 40–8. Hoary Alyssum.

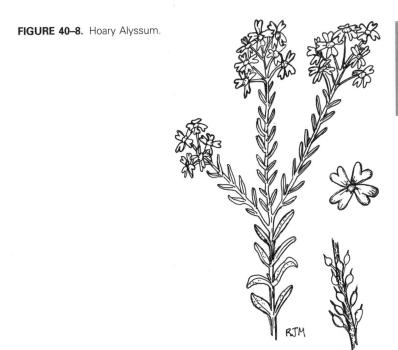

4

RJM

Clinical Signs

- Acute onset of limb edema, along with lethargy, fever, and sometimes diarrhea
- Joint stiffness, laminitis, and hematuria may develop.
- Death is unusual.
- Clinical signs develop 18–36 hours after ingestion.

Treatment

- Symptomatic and supportive care
- When plant is removed from diet, remission of signs generally occurs within 2–4 days.

TOXINS PREDOMINANTLY AFFECTING THE CARDIOVASCULAR SYSTEM

Foxglove *(Digitalis purpurea)* (Fig. 40–9), **Milkweed** (*Asclepias* spp.), **Yellow Oleander** *(Thevetia peruviana)*, **Dogbanes** (*Apocynum* spp.), *Lily-Of-The-Valley (Convallaria majalis)* (Fig. 40–10)

These are all potentially toxic plants that contain cardiac glycosides. Poisoning of horses by these plants is uncommon but may occur if they are mixed in hay and the affected individuals have little else to eat.

Clinical Signs and Treatment

- As for Oleander below.

Ionophore Antibiotic Poisoning

Ionophore antibiotics are used in cattle and poultry feeds to improve feed efficiency and as coccidiostats. They are capable of carrying ions across biologic membranes. Common ionophores include monensin (Rumensin, Coban), lasalocid (Bovatec, Avatec), narasin, and salinomycin. Horses are extremely susceptible to ionophore antibiotics; the minimal lethal dose of monensin may be as low as 1 mg/kg BW.

Clinical Signs

- Vary depending upon the amount ingested and ionophore involved: Anorexia, colic, diarrhea, depression, sweating, labored breathing, prostration, and death
- Hyperventilation, jugular pulsation, tachycardia, and bright red membranes are found with cardiac failure (especially monensin).
- Acute death has also been reported, presumably from cardiac failure (especially monensin).
- Recumbency occurs in some cases without signs of heart failure (especially lasalocid). The cause for the recumbency has not been demonstrated.

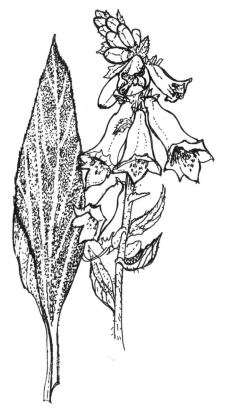

FIGURE 40–9. Foxglove.

4

- Stranguria (straining) and excess urination (polyuria) are reported in some individuals.

Diagnosis

- Send the suspect feed or intestinal (stomach and colon) contents to a laboratory. Most diagnostic laboratories can test for ionophores. Texas A&M, California at Davis, Michigan State University, and Cornell Diagnostic Laboratories are sites that test for ionophores.
- Serum concentration of muscle enzymes generally is increased.

Treatment

- Remove the suspect feed.
- Administer activated charcoal.
- Nasogastric intubation with mineral oil PO q2 hours after activated charcoal.

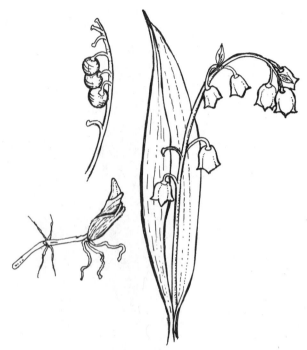

FIGURE 40–10. Lily-Of-The-Valley.

- IV polyionic fluids
- Vitamin E and selenium injection (IM)
- Other supportive care
- Do not administer digoxin!

Japanese Yew *(Taxus cuspidata)*

A common ornamental shrub throughout the United States, the toxic principle is taxine, which interferes with nerve conduction in the heart. Also contains cardioactive glycosides. Horses are most commonly exposed to yew plants when they are allowed to graze around show barns, offices, homes, or when clippings from the bushes are thrown into the pasture. Japanese yew is extremely toxic—1.0 kg may kill a 450-kg adult. The English yew *(T. baccata)* is also toxic.

Clinical Signs

- Ataxia, muscle trembling, and collapse are seen. The heart rate is abnormally low.
- Acute death, within 1–5 hours of ingestion, may occur. If the individual survives, mild colic and diarrhea develop.

Diagnosis
- Compatible history and clinical signs
- Identification of needle fragments in the stomach contents

Treatment

If ingestion is suspected and no clinical signs are exhibited, administer activated charcoal and place in a quiet area.

Administering any treatment *after clinical signs* are exhibited may lead to excitement-induced death.

Oleander *(Nerium oleander)*

Introduced into the United States and grows mostly in the southern states from California to Florida. Can be a potted house plant in northern climates. Affected individuals become exposed from browsing on plants around buildings or eating dried leaves in the hay. All parts of the plant are toxic, and as little as 1 ounce of leaves can be lethal to a 450-kg adult. Toxic principle is a cardiac glycoside, which remains when plant is dried.

Clinical Signs
- Colic, muscle tremors, hemorrhagic diarrhea, recumbency, arrhythmias, weak pulse, and signs of cardiac failure.
- Onset of clinical signs may be delayed several hours after ingestion.
- Signs may persist for 1–2 days after last ingestion.

Diagnosis
- Evidence of consumption, compatible clinical signs
- Identification of leaf fragments in the stomach or GI contents. Some laboratories (California Veterinary Diagnostic Laboratory) test for cardiac glycosides in the stomach contents.
- Histologic evidence of cardiac necrosis

Treatment
- Activated charcoal PO
- Magnesium sulfate PO
- Supportive care and confine in a quiet area.
- Evaluate cardiac irregularities and treat with appropriate antiarrhythmic drugs; if arrhythmia is severe, see p. 102.

TOXINS PREDOMINANTLY CAUSING HEMOLYSIS OR BLEEDING

Moldy Yellow Sweet Clover *(Melilotus officinalis)*
Moldy White Sweet Clover *(M. alba)*

Grown as forage crops, especially in northwestern United States and western Canada. Only when moldy are these plants toxic; the mold converts normal plant constituents to dicoumarol, an anticoagulant. Occurrence is rare in horses because they are less likely than cattle to be chronically fed or ingest the moldy sweet clover hay.

Clinical Signs

- Bleeding abnormalities, as seen in warfarin poisoning

Diagnosis

- History and clinical signs
- Prolonged prothrombin time or other abnormalities in coagulation profile
- Liver function is otherwise normal.

Treatment

- Remove from suspect hay.
- Treat as for warfarin below.

Red Maple *(Acer rubrum)*
(Fig. 40–11)

A common tree throughout eastern North America, also known as the swamp maple. This is the most common cause of hemolytic anemia in adults in eastern United States. The poisoning most commonly follows a storm that causes limbs to fall into the pasture or when cut trees are left lying in the pasture. Wilted leaves are the most toxic, and toxicity slowly decreases on drying. The toxic

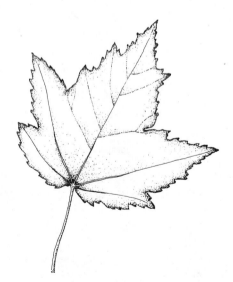

FIGURE 40–11. Red Maple.

principle is unknown, but it causes oxidative damage to the red blood cells. (Also see p. 284.)

Clinical Signs

- Depression, red urine, jaundice, ataxia, and sometimes acute death
- Hemolysis and methemoglobinemia occur, although one may predominate. If hemolysis is the primary clinical finding of the disease, the course of the disease is 2–10 days; if methemoglobinemia predominates, then acute death may occur.

Diagnosis

- History and clinical signs
- Clinical pathology reveals Coombs-negative hemolytic anemia, with Heinz bodies and variable degree of methemoglobinemia (8%–50%).

Treatment

- Blood transfusions if packed cell volume (PCV) is less than 11% over 2 or more days or if it is less than 18% in 1 day (see p. 294)
- Large doses of vitamin C (1 gm/kg PO) may be of some benefit but efficacy not demonstrated.
- Methylene blue, 8.8 mg/kg slowly IV, for individuals with methemoglobin over 20%, but results may not be dramatic because of relatively low methemoglobin reductase activity in the horse.
- IV polyionic fluids are important to prevent hypovolemia, dilute RBC fragments that may trigger disseminated intravascular coagulation (DIC), and prevent tubular necrosis. Although the PCV decreases with fluids, the number of RBCs remains the same, and may improve function.

Warfarin Poisoning

This occurs from overzealous administration of warfarin in treating navicular disease and from ingestion of anticoagulant rodenticides (e.g., warfarin, indanediones, brodifacoum). Newer anticoagulant rodenticides are 40–200 times as potent as warfarin.

Clinical Signs

- Excessive bleeding from wounds, failure of blood to coagulate. Often pale mucous membranes from intraabdominal bleeding. May have hematoma formation or exhibit dyspnea from intrapleural bleeding.
- Clinical signs are delayed for 1–5 days following ingestion.

Diagnosis

- History and clinical signs
- Prolonged prothrombin time or other abnormalities in coagulation profile (submit citrate sample with control)
- Liver function is otherwise normal.

Treatment

- Administer vitamin K_1, 0.5–1 mg/kg SQ every 4–6 hours for the first 24 hours. *Do not administer vitamin K_1 IV.*
- Follow with oral vitamin K_1, 5 mg/kg/day with food for an additional 7 days. Newer anticoagulants (indanediones, brodifacoum) are recommended for a minimum of 21 days.
- Administer fresh-frozen plasma in affected individuals with clinical hemorrhage.
- Avoid steroid use or other drugs that are highly protein bound, as they may exacerbate the anticoagulant effects.
- *Do not use vitamin K_3 in horses.*

Wild Onions (*Allium* spp.)
Domestic Onions *(A. cepa)*

Wild onions are found in moist areas of most states, and the feeding of cull onions is associated with clinical problems. Onions cause a Heinz body hemolytic anemia in horses ingesting large quantities of the plant or bulbs. The toxic principle is *n*-propyl disulfide, which causes hemoglobin denaturation.

Clinical Signs

- Vary from a mild anemia to acute hemolytic anemia
- Other signs as with red maple poisoning
- Affected individuals often have a sulfur or onion odor to breath.

Treatment

- Remove onions from diet.
- Symptomatic and supportive
- Generally not life threatening; anemia is unusual.

TOXINS PREDOMINANTLY AFFECTING THE URINARY SYSTEM
Aminoglycosides

Toxicity especially common when used in dehydrated or hypotensive patients. See p. 462.

Mercury

Inorganic mercury may be ingested in toxic amounts when horses lick mercury poultices or blisters (mercuric iodide, mercuric oxide) applied to the legs. If ingested, severe tubular nephrosis and gastrointestinal ulceration occur (see p. 608).

Clinical Signs

- Anorexia, weight loss, colic, stomatitis, and diarrhea
- Progressive signs of renal failure, laboratory findings of azotemia

Treatment
- IV fluids (see p. 464)
- Acute cases are treated with oral sodium thiosulfate, 30–500 mg/kg slowly IV, and dimercaprol (BAL), 2.5 mg/kg IM q6h for 2 days, and continue q12h for an additional 8 days.
- Supportive care with GI protectants: sucralfate, 4 gm PO q6h

Vitamin K₃ (Menadione)

Signs of depression and renal failure may occur in affected individuals 3–4 days after receiving vitamin K_3 parenterally (no longer commercially available).

Treatment
- IV fluids (see p. 464)

SUDDEN AND UNEXPECTED DEATH IN HORSES WITHOUT CLINICAL SIGNS

This is one of the most frustrating emergency calls for clinicians. Rather than treating a medical emergency, it is now the clinician's role to decide why death occurred. This becomes especially urgent when there is a chance of foul play, the affected individual is insured, and/or there is a possibility of other individuals being affected. A complete history is imperative, including

- Use of the horse
- Any management changes, including personnel, at the stable
- Changes
  - Feed
  - Pasture
  - Treatments
  - Ownership
  - Insurance
  - Weather

Perform a complete postmortem examination initially, looking for obvious causes of death: hemorrhage, gastric rupture, or cardiac abnormalities as discussed in the following sections. If the cause of death is not obvious, obtain samples of all appropriate tissues for histopathologic evaluation as well as toxicologic testing, as listed at the beginning of this chapter. If there is the suspicion of foul play, take photographs or video footage of the affected individual and surroundings. Label all samples, and document all reports regarding the case.

The most common causes of sudden death in horses (defined as death which occurs acutely without prior illness or illness of only a few minutes) are presented.

TOXIC CAUSES OF SUDDEN DEATH (VIA INGESTION)

Blue-Green Algae (*Microcystis* spp. and Others)

Rarely reported in horses but may cause sudden death, especially in the Plains states in summer months when horses drink from ponds in full bloom with algae. Algae are often concentrated at the side of the pond by the wind. Affected individuals may have sudden onset of gastroenteritis and hemorrhagic diarrhea, with acute liver failure and seizures preceding death.

Diagnosis

- Preserve algae water with 10% formalin (9 parts water to 1 part 10% formalin) for testing for the pathogenic algae.
- Freeze samples of stomach/intestinal contents.

Treatment

- For other exposed individuals: activated charcoal
- Symptomatic and supportive care

Cyanide Poisoning

Has been reported as a cause of acute death in horses ingesting wild cherry (*Prunus* spp.) leaves, saplings, or bark

Diagnosis

- Cyanide in stomach contents or blood. Freeze stomach contents immediately in airtight container.

Treatment

- For known exposed individuals on the farm: 16 mg/kg sodium nitrate (1%), followed by sodium thiosulfate, 30–40 mg/kg slowly IV

Monensin Poisoning

See p. 624.

Oleander Poisoning

See p. 627.

Red Maple

See p. 628. Sudden illness and rapid death may result from acute methemoglobinemia and for some unexplained reason; seen more commonly late in the leaf season. Death may precede jaundice, but urine is dark black.

Taxus

See p. 626.

Diagnosis

- Plants found in stomach

Cardiac Defects and Exercise-Induced Death

A variety of cardiac abnormalities have been blamed for sudden and unexpected death in horses either during or immediately after exercise:

- **Aortic valve thickening**
- **Ruptured chordae tendineae**—more commonly results in acute respiratory distress and signs of heart failure
- **Occlusion of the coronary artery**
- **Lacerated coronary artery** in foals, associated with fractured ribs
- **Cardiac arrhythmias** and/or **myocarditis**, as in humans, results in some unexplained and unexpected deaths associated with exercise.
- **White muscle disease** in young foals <8 months of age should be considered in areas with severe selenium deficiency (e.g., Canada, Northeast, Ohio, and others). Measure liver and/or heart blood selenium concentrations.
- **Air emboli**—unlikely to cause problems in the horse unless large volumes are rapidly injected
- **Electrolyte abnormalities** (hypocalcemia, hypercalcemia, hypokalemia, hyperkalemia) and cardiac arrhythmia are a common cause of acute death and generally occur in individuals with severe predisposing illness.

Hemorrhage as a Cause of Sudden and Unexpected Death

- **Ruptured uterine artery** in mares, more common in older brood mares in late pregnancy or at the time of foaling
- **Lacerated iliac artery**, may or may not be associated with a fractured pelvis
- **Ruptured kidney**, history of trauma and/or rib fracture in many cases
- **Ruptured aorta**, most common in middle-aged or older breeding stallions, frequently occurring immediately after breeding
- **Ruptured spleen or liver**, in most cases associated with trauma
- **Rupture of the internal carotid or maxillary artery** in association with guttural pouch mycosis (massive external hemorrhage is seen)
- **Pulmonary hemorrhage** in the racehorse rarely results in sudden death.
- **Acute hemolytic anemia** rarely causes sudden death in horses without prior clinical signs. Sudden death rarely occurs in foals with neonatal isoerythrolysis.

Neurologic Causes of Sudden Death

- **Trauma**
    - □ Rearing and falling backward, fracturing the junction between the

basisphenoid and basioccipital bones resulting in cerebral trauma, hemorrhage, and acute death. Evidence of blood in the external ear canal or from the nostrils supports this premise.

□ Fractured cervical vertebrae
□ Other traumatic events causing severe head injury (i.e., kicks)

- **Botulism** causes sudden death if a large amount of preformed toxin (e.g., as from silage) is ingested.
- **Accidental feeding of 4-aminopyridine** (a bird-repellent agent) produces severe neurologic signs and/or sudden death in horses fed 2–3 mg/kg. Diagnosis is by testing (chromatography) of the feed and history of exposure.
- **Heat stroke, hypothermia, and hypoglycemia** causes coma and sudden death.
- **Organophosphate poisoning** causes acute paralysis and death if horses are exposed to sufficient quantities of the toxin (seed corn) (see p. 605).

Intestinal Causes of Sudden and Unexpected Death

Intestinal diseases rarely cause acute death without evidence of illness (colic, diarrhea, toxemia) preceding the death. In some cases these signs may be brief:

- **Gastric rupture**, most commonly from tympany and from impaction in a few peracute cases or in foals with perforating ulcer.
- **Colitis** rarely causes death from endotoxemia with only a brief clinical illness (e.g., <1 hour).
- **Ruptured cecum**—in most cases there is some evidence of mild discomfort for hours or days preceding the death and in a few cases following foaling
- **Rupture of the colon** rarely occurs without mechanical displacement.
- **Blister beetle poisoning** (see pp. 223 and 602)
- **Volvulus of the small intestine**—acute abdominal signs and/or evidence of colic usually precede death.

Septicemia/Bacteremia/Endotoxemia as a Cause of Sudden Death

This is more common in young foals, in which death occasionally occurs within 1 hour of clinical signs. In 8–42-day-old foals, Tyzzer's disease is a primary differential. In a 2–4-day-old foal, *Actinobacillus* is a primary differential.

Respiratory Causes of Sudden and Unexpected Death

- **Pneumothorax**—most are associated with trauma, although some are idiopathic.
- **Pulmonary hemorrhage**—most common in racehorse during or immediately following a race. In most cases blood is seen at the nares or on the ground.
- **Airway obstruction**—acute laryngeal obstruction caused by edema, food bolus, paralysis, or spasms (postoperatively after removing an endotra-

cheal tube) may result in sudden death. Rarely horses with hyperkalemic periodic paralysis die from laryngeal obstruction.

- **Acute pulmonary edema**—most common causes are:
  - □ *acute heart failure* (e.g., monensin, ruptured chordae tendineae, acute myocarditis associated with a viral infection)
  - □ *anaphylaxis*
  - □ *endotoxemia*
  - □ *laryngeal obstruction.*

In most cases clinical signs are noticeable before death.

- **Smoke inhalation** (see p. 447)

Other Causes of Sudden and Unexpected Death

- **Lightning strike or electrocution**. History of a storm, evidence of exposed electrical wires support the diagnosis. A *select few* affected individuals may have linear burn marks on the body.
- **Gunshot wounds**. Look for penetrating wounds entering and/or exiting the body. The bullet is found in the body in some cases.
- **Black fly swarms** occasionally kill horses.
- **Drowning**

Adverse Drug Reactions

See p. 588.

Causes of Malicious or Criminal Death

- **Electrocution**. Examine the skin closely for injury from placement of needles or clamps used to electrocute the individual. The head, especially lips; back; and tail or perineal area are the most common sites used for malicious electrocution.
- **Insulin injections**. Collect serum from the heart blood clot and determine insulin concentration and type by high-performance liquid chromatography (see p. 611).
- **Potassium injections**. Examine the jugular veins closely for evidence of needle insertion.
- If **deliberate feeding of a poison** is suspected, collect the gastric contents, remaining feed and water, kidney, urine, liver, and fat and test as the minimum the following: monensin, arsenic, strychnine, chlorinated hydrocarbons, and organophosphates.

SUGGESTED REFERENCES

Toxicities
Galey FD. Disorders caused by toxicants. *In* Smith BP (ed): Large Animal Internal Medicine. 2nd ed. St. Louis, CV Mosby, 1996, pp 1874–1919.
Galey FD. Toxicology. *In* Robinson NE (ed): Current Therapy in Equine Medicine III. Philadelphia, WB Saunders, 1992, pp 337–377.

4

*Galey FD, Holstege DM, Plumlee KH, et al. Diagnosis of oleander poisoning in livestock. J Vet Diagn Invest 1996; 8:358–364.

Given BD, Mostrom MS, Tully R, et al. Severe hypoglycemia attributable to surreptitious administration of insulin in a mare. J Am Vet Med Assoc 1988; 193(2):224–226.

*Goer RJ, Becker RL, Kanara EW, et al. Toxicosis in horses after ingesting hoary alyssum. J Am Vet Med Assoc 1992; 201:63–67.

*Guglick MA, MacAllister CG, Panciera R. Equine cantharidiasis. Comp Cont Educ Pract Vet 1996; 18:77–83.

*Hall JO, Buck WB, Cote J. Natural Poisons in Horses. 2nd ed. Urbana, IL, National Animal Poison Control Center, University of Illinois, 1995.

*Knight AP. Plant poisoning of horses. *In* Lewis L (ed): Equine Clinical Nutrition: Feeding and Care. Media, PA, Williams & Wilkins, 1995, pp 447–502.

Roberts MC, Seawright AA. Experimental studies of drug-induced impaction colic in the horse. Equine Vet J 1983; 15:222–228.

Acute and Unexpected Death

Brown CM, Taylor J, Flint R, Shaker MR. Sudden and unexplained death in adult horses. Comp Cont Educ Pract Vet 1987; 9(1):78–85.

Platt H. Sudden and unexplained deaths in horses. A review of 69 cases. Br Vet J 1982; 138:417–429.

---

*Pictures of plants included in article.

Management of Special Problems

41. Disaster Medicine   **638**
42. Anesthesia for Field Emergencies and Euthanasia   **646**
43. Nutritional Guidelines for the Injured Horse   **658**

5

41 Disaster Medicine

Richard A. Mansmann

INDIVIDUAL SITUATIONS

Frequently, clinicians equate emergencies with "disasters," or at a minimum, some complex emergencies are referred to as "disasters"! The difference between an emergency and a disaster is the number of people involved:

- In an emergency, the clinician and staff work with the owner to help the patient.
- In a disaster, additional people are needed to help the patient.

This is true for individual disasters involving small numbers of individuals or disasters with large numbers of individuals.

Individual Disasters
- Trailer accident (1–2 horses)
- Fall, or isolation in an inaccessible area
- Competition accident

Group Disasters
- Van accident (2–16 horses)
- Barn fire
- Natural disasters
- Hazardous spills

Veterinarians are creative and independent; this creativity allows clinicians to help horses in difficult situations by being able to process the many "helpful" suggestions. However, their independence frequently results in humane destruction of patients that could have been helped by a well-organized team.

Preparation

Preplanning for disasters is difficult and requires detailed protocols at several **levels.** *The basis of disaster medicine is sharpening standard emergency skills rehearsed in routine clinical emergencies.* Written emergency protocols are mandatory, with "emergency kits" prepared.

The emergency kit contents is everything required for a *specific emergency*; it is portable, clearly marked, and readily accessible. These kits can serve several functions in the routine practice:

- *Crash kit* for chemical restraint, resuscitation, or euthanasia, with dosages of each drug listed. This kit is most valuable at the side of anesthetized patient and in adverse drug reactions (see Chapter 39).
- *Catheter kit* contains all the materials for placing an intravenous (IV) catheter and fluid administration, with several boxes of fluids readily available. The catheter kit saves valuable time in an emergency situation and makes routine catheter placement in nonemergency situations easy (see p. 12).

- *Respiratory kit* contains tracheotomy equipment and instruments and includes tubing for oxygen delivery, a humidifier, and a small oxygen tank (see p. 40).
- *Splint kit* contains precut polyvinyl chloride (PVC) pieces, tape, bandage material, hack saw, and cast material, all of which can be tailored to the specific type of limb problem (see p. 298).

These emergency kits can be a part of the ambulatory clinician's vehicle and/or stored as part of the hospital's inventory.

Disaster Equipment

Very little specialized or researched disaster equipment is commercially available. Cotton ear plugs and a blindfold are simple pieces of equipment that can be "designed" on site. Larger equipment needs for a particular community should be proposed and purchased by the community and used under the direction of veterinarians in the community.

Two slings used extensively are:

- The Anderson sling (CDA Products, P.O. Box 53, Potter Valley, CA 95461. Phone: (707) 431 1300; fax: (707) 443 2530), used in helicopter rescues and in hospitals
- The plastic mesh sling

Ropes are important in disasters:

- Strong lead rope(s) with a nonbreakable halter and snaps
- Chain shank long enough to place over the nose or used as a lip chain—invaluable in leading a patient from a terrifying situation
- Tail rope tied into the tail to aid in moving an individual (Fig. 41–1)
- A length of cotton rope for restraining a patient while moving it from a trailer accident or a narrow space. A video detailing trailer rescue is commercially available (see References).
- Two rope(s) for pulling a recumbent individual or another vehicle

A surcingle placed around the chest just behind the withers and elbows, with preplaced rings to attach ropes to, is useful. This equipment is used in situations when the individual needs to be slid on a surface not accessible to a vehicle, such as mud, a hill, ice. NOTE: *A patient should only be slid, never lifted, with a surcingle.*

A mat made from durable material such as conveyor belting, approximately $9' \times 5'6''$, is used for moving recumbent individuals. The head end has a bar attachment for towing, with several holes on its edge to secure a patient. It can be folded and stored easily. Portable screens for isolating an emergency at a competition or public event are useful. They can be made from canvas and hung on PVC tubing.

Additional equipment:

- Cutting saws, axes, shovels
- 1-Ton (minimum) winch
- Water for drinking or cooling carried in 5-gallon jugs
- A hand sprayer for cold water application
- Blankets

5

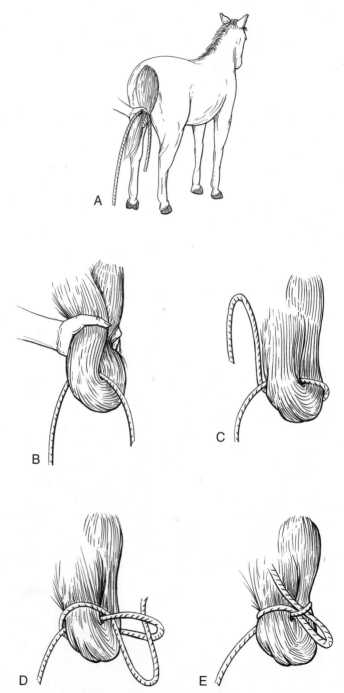

FIGURE 41–1 *See legend on opposite page*

Vehicle equipment:

- 4-Wheel drive with towing accessory
- Wrecker with appropriate boom
- Mobile command center, for large-scale events or disasters
- "Ambulances," such as a converted horse trailer adapted for IV fluids, specially designed trailers, or sophisticated commercial trucks

Personnel

- Disaster preplanning is positive and nonthreatening and brings together many different people working as a team.
- Area veterinarians can exchange ideas on how to respond to various problems.
- Volunteer groups, similar to volunteer fire companies, colic or foal teams in academic institutions, can be organized.
- Any volunteer group is a means to involve various talents, including county, emergency professionals.
- Practice drills for various emergency situations train an emergency team and maintain interest in disaster skills current.

Chronologic Walk-Through an Individual Disaster

Steps Where Decisions Need to be Made	Specific Considerations at Each Step
Assessment during initial contact	Access to patient—need an escort? Additional equipment needs

Develop a mental protocol on way to the scene	Restraint
	   Calming techniques:
	     Physical: Cotton in ears, blindfold, twitch, massaging, and the like.
	     Chemical: Drugs and dosages
	 Physical examination of the patient
	   What to do under special circumstances?
	 "Onlooker" recruitment or dispersement
	   Jobs needed
	   Traffic control, rope pulling, etc.

Immediate arrival on the scene	Contact chief emergency person
	   Who is in charge?
	 Assess overall situation
	   Is the patient the center of attention?

5

FIGURE 41–1. *A–E,* The technique for making a tail tie to secure a rope to horse's tail.

Assess situation of the patient(s)

> Or secondary problem in large disaster?
> Dead or alive
> Attitude:
>> Quiet
>> Struggling: coordinated or incoordinated?
>> Does individual have concept of self-preservation?
> Obvious medical problems
>> Wounds, shock, etc.
> Assess less obvious problems
>> TPR, neurologic and musculoskeletal systems

Finalize plans

> Specific equipment and personnel needed
>> Ropes, jaws of life, particularly for patient's feet caught in cattle guards
> Specific restraint
>> None, sedation, anesthesia, or euthanasia—*when in doubt, be conservative!*

Rescue

> *Don't stop in middle of rescue unless something is seriously wrong!*

Post rescue

> Examination/Assessment
> Treatment
>> The disaster is now an emergency!

Debriefing/Review of emergency procedures

> Share written information
>> "Thank you" to all personnel
> Review the entire protocol
>> Mentally and/or written procedure
> Schedule follow-up examinations

PRACTICE/COMMUNITY INVOLVEMENT

Dealing with the effects of large-scale natural or man-made disasters involves more personnel than an individual emergency.

- Emergency system procedures in place are a help.
- Preplanning and knowledge learned from personal experiences and previous disasters can save human and animal lives.
- Avoid counter productive thinking: *"These things happen in other places, not here!"*
- The primary goal is for veterinarians to be facilitators and help owners help themselves and their animals.

A clinician involved in disaster planning needs to understand four specific points:

- The present level of interest and organizational skills of the equine community.

- The office of emergency planning, community response, and its relationship to other emergency response groups (e.g., fire, police, emergency medical technicians and hospitals)
- What veterinary skills are available at the local, state, and national level that can help in a disaster
- Learn what national, state, and local emergency preparedness and response system(s) are in place.

To accomplish disaster preparedness and response successfully, all four areas need to be carefully assessed and the most common types of disasters that could occur in the community prioritized. Use the disaster curve (Fig. 41–2), to prioritize the time needed for specific disasters.

Involvement of the Horse Community

Veterinarians are ideal leaders in a community's animal disaster planning. Individuals interested in disaster preparedness and response organize their practices or are involved in routine emergencies at all levels of disaster preparedness.

- Groups require 6–12 owners with basic skills to form an organization of other local owners.
- Models for organizations are available
- Shared experiences with emergency personnel owning horses can help the beginning organization.

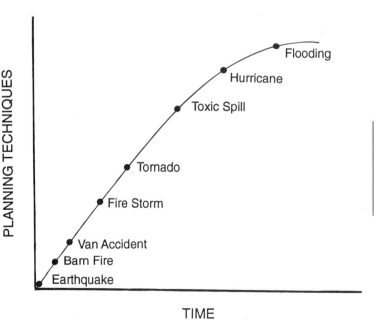

FIGURE 41–2. The disaster curve for intelligent planning.

- Disaster response can be a unifying experience for different horse groups.

Involvement of the Local Office of Emergency Services

To be successful, a strong interaction and trust must be developed between local volunteer groups of animal owners and the office of emergency planning for the community.

- This is the most critical component for any animal group doing community emergency work.
- The veterinary/animal issue of incorporating animals in disaster planning can be organized into local planning by representatives attending emergency service meetings.
- Owners and veterinarians must learn the protocols for emergency preparedness and responses.
- Organizations such as humane societies or American Red Cross are excellent resources for training and help.
- Large facilities such as race tracks, fairgrounds, and show facilities can develop shared needs in an emergency.
- Insurance for volunteers used in a disaster might be available through county emergency services.

Available Emergency Services

- The American Veterinary Medical Association (AVMA) is heavily involved in veterinary disaster preparedness and response and has published an excellent guide.
- In cooperation with the United States Department of Public Health, the AVMA is helping organize VMATs (Veterinary Medical Assistance Teams) that can be used in a national disaster.
- The VMAT system is an excellent model to integrate several county organizations and therefore act as a regional group.
- The American Academy of Veterinary Disaster Medicine has cross-over with the human disaster preparedness groups and significant organizational skills. For additional information, contact:

Lyle Vogel, DVM, Secretary/Treasurer, AAVDM
1931 N. Meacham Road, Suite 100
Schaumburg, IL 60173

- Several state veterinary medical associations are involved in their state's emergency planning. Contact your association for specifics.
- The American Humane Association and the Humane Society of the United States are designated as the animal arm of the American Red Cross.
- FEMA (Federal Emergency Management Agency) has an educational campus:

Emergency Management Institute
16825 South Seton Avenue
Emmitsburg, MD 21727

A catalog of activities and several self-study and on-campus courses are available from this agency (see References).

A complete definition of funding and roles of all animal-related organizations in various disasters is presently undetermined. It is the responsibility of every veterinarian, horse owner, and community to work within the framework of existing emergency planning to help reduce losses in disasters and identify the necessary funding and role played by everyone involved in emergency management.

SUGGESTED REFERENCES

**Auf der Heide E. Disaster Response: Principles of Preparation and Coordination. Baltimore, CV Mosby, 1989.

***Bertone JJ (ed): Emergency treatment in the adult horse. Vet Clin North Am Equine Pract Dec. 1994; 10(3).

**Catalog of Activities of the Emergency Management Institute, 16825 South Seton Avenue, Emmitsburg, MD 21727.

**Dey S. Equine Trailer Rescue. Horse Park of New Jersey, P.O. Box 548, Allentown, NJ 08501. FILM.

***Duffy JC (ed). Health and Medical Aspects of Disaster Preparedness. New York, Plenum Publishing Corp., 1990.

*Filkins ME (ed). Veterinary Medicine for Back Country Horsemen. Kern Sierra Unit of the Backcountry Horsemen of California, P.O. Box 11095, Bakersfield, CA 93389, 1994.

*Goodman J, Abronson S. Emergency—Red Alert! What Do I Do with My Horse in Fire, Flood, and/or Earthquake? E.T.I. Corral 63, 543 Cold Canyon Road, Monte Nido, CA 91302–2206, 1993.

*Hamilton JM, Scheve NK. Hawkins Guide—Equine Emergencies on the Road. Bluegreen Publishing Co., P.O. Box 1255, Southern Pines, NC 28327, 1994.

**Lundin CS (ed). AVMA Emergency Preparedness and Response Guide. American Veterinary Medical Association, 1931 N. Meacham Road, Schaumburg, IL 60173–4360, 1994.

**Mansmann RA, McCurdy B, O'Connor K, Collins T, et al. Disaster planning model for an equine assistance and evacuation team. J Equine Vet Sci 1992; 12(5):268–271.

**Natural Hazards Observer (monthly newsletter). Natural Hazards Research and Application Information Center, Institute of Behavioral Science #6, University of Colorado at Boulder, Campus Box 482, Boulder, CO 80309–0482.

***Prehospital and Disaster Medicine. (Human disaster medical journal.) Jems Communications, P.O. Box 2789, Carlsbad, CA 92018.

**Proceedings of the First International Conference on Equine Rescue. J Equine Vet Sci 1993; 13(5).

**Proceedings of the Second International Conference on Equine Rescue. J Equine Vet Sci 1995; 15(4).

*Sakach E (ed). Disaster Relief: Designing a Disaster Plan for Your Community. The Humane Society of the United States, 700 Professional Drive, Gaithersburg, MD 20879, 1996.

---

*Basic for client distribution
**Organizers
***Medical personnel

5

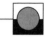

42 Anesthesia for Field Emergencies and Euthanasia

A. ANESTHESIA FOR FIELD EMERGENCIES

Ann Townsend Sturmer and Robin D. Gleed

Emergencies requiring field anesthesia occur often and require the practitioner to be familiar with current techniques. The focus of this section is on methods to provide short-term (<40 minutes) general anesthesia when analgesia, unconsciousness, and complete immobility are needed and inhalant anesthesia is not practical. Emergencies requiring only sedation and tranquilization are not discussed.

The goal of emergency anesthesia is usually one or more of the following:

- To enable acute, definitive treatment to be given on site (e.g., suture laceration, control of bleeding)
- To permit life-threatening conditions to be stabilized before and during transportation to a surgical facility (e.g., long bone fractures)
- To prevent further injury to the patient and/or persons while the patient is evaluated and plans made for treatment

Normal risks associated with general anesthesia are amplified when anesthesia is administered in an emergency away from the hospital. Increased risk may be due to

- The compromised condition of the patient
- Unsatisfactory environment for administering anesthesia
- Minimal time for planning

Increased risk can be reduced by preparing standard emergency anesthetic protocols that are understood by everyone involved, with preassembly of all needed materials for easy transportation. "Up front" investment in time and resources results in quality emergency care.

BASIC EMERGENCY ANESTHESIA KIT

Suggested Equipment

- Halter for restraining head during induction, made from webbing with 1″ cotton rope braided to it (Equa-Sport, Monument, CO)

- Two 30′ × 1″ cotton ropes:
  - Tail rope
  - General
- Protective hood (Top Floor and Pad, Maryville, TN)
- Body sling (CDA Products, Potter Valley, CA)
- Endotracheal tubes with intact cuffs (Cook Veterinary Products, Bloomington, IN)
- Syringe, 60 ml (to inflate and deflate cuff)
- Tracheotomy tubes, 8–26-mm inner diameter (ID) with functional cuffs (Bivona Veterinary Products, Gary, IN)
- Oxygen, medical grade, size E tanks with transport dolly
- Oxygen regulator (two-stage, downstream pressure set at 60 psi for use with the demand valve)
- Quick release adaptor for oxygen regulator
- Oxygen demand valve (Model-LSP, 160 L/min capacity, Chesapeake Breathing Services, Ephrata, PA)
- Oxygen hose, 20–40 ft
- Adaptor (to connect demand valve to the endotracheal tubes larger than 22-mm ID)*
- Portable ECG (battery-operated, telemetry preferred)
- Cable hoist puller/come along (Mini Mule, Deuer, Dayton, OH)
- Hobbles
- Space blankets
- General surgical pack
- 2″ Brass pipe for mouth gag (wrapped with porous white tape)
- Cordless clippers
- Injection pole (Simmons heavy duty syringe pole, Zulu Arms Co., Omaha, NE, distributed by Furhman Diversified Inc., LaPorte, TX)
- Tackle box (containing needles, syringes, injection caps, over-the-needle catheters (22–10-gauge), 4×4 gauze, heparinized saline and drugs (Tables 42–1 and 42–2). Prelabeling of essential syringes minimizes confusion during emergency anesthesia (Time Med Label Systems, Burr Ridge, IL)
- Oscillometric sphygmomanometer (Dynamap, Critikon, Tampa, FL)
- Roller pump for fluids (Watson-Marlow, distributed by Baxter Healthcare, Deerfield, IL)
- Extension cord, 100 ft

ANALGESIC, ANESTHETIC, AND RESTRAINT DRUGS
(See Table 42–1)

- Atracurium (Tracrium), 0.10–0.20 mg/kg IV, blocks neuromuscular transmission and causes apnea. **Equipment for controlling ventilation must be readily available when this drug is used.** It is a nondepolarizing neuromuscular blocking agent without anesthetic or analgesic properties, used to enhance muscle relaxation. The palpebral reflex is diminished or

---

*This adaptor needs to be machined to match the tapered connections on the demand valve and endotracheal tubes. Delrin, a plastic, is suitable because it can be turned easily, is biologically inert, and can be sterilized by steam or ethylene oxide.

TABLE 42–1. **Analgesic, Anesthetic and Restraint Drugs for the Tackle Box**

	No. Vials or Bags	Volume and Concentration
Atracurium	3 vials	5 ml (10 mg/ml)
Butorphanol	1 vial	50 ml (10 mg/ml)
Detomidine	1 vial	20 ml (10 mg/ml)
Diazepam	3 vials	10 ml (5 mg/ml)
Edrophonium	6 vials	10 ml (10 mg/ml)
Guaifenesin	2 bags	1000 ml (50 mg/ml) (5% soln)
Ketamine	5 vials	10 ml (100 mg/ml)
Thiopental sodium	2 vials	5 gm
Xylazine	1 vial	50 ml (100 mg/ml)
Euthanasia solution	1 vial	250 ml

absent, making depth of anesthesia difficult to assess. Consider judicious use in individuals in which severe CNS depression is part of the presenting problem and, hence, large doses of centrally active drugs are contraindicated. Duration of action of the initial dose (0.20 mg/kg) is approximately 20 min. Subsequent doses are 0.05–0.10 mg/kg. Dehydration, hypothermia, and some antibiotics (e.g., aminoglycosides, gentamicin) prolong its effects. Reverse the effects of atracurium with edrophonium.

■ Butorphanol (Torbugesic), 0.01–0.04 mg/kg IV, is an opioid that produces unreliable analgesia when used alone. It has opioid agonist and antagonist properties. It may produce excitement or dysphoria in some individuals. It potentiates α_2-agonist drugs and may be used in conjunction with

TABLE 42–2. **Resuscitation Drugs for the Tackle Box**

	No. Vials or Bags	Volume and Concentration
Atropine	1 vial	100 ml (0.5 mg/ml)
Dextran 70 in 0.9% saline	10 bags	500 ml
Dobutamine	1 vial	20 ml (12.5 mg/ml)
Doxapram	1 vial	20 ml (20 mg/ml)
Epinephrine	2 vials	30 ml (1 mg/ml)
Flunixin meglumine	1 vial	50 ml (50 mg/ml)
Hetastarch	10 bags	500 ml
7% Hypertonic saline	6 vials	1000 ml
Lactated Ringer's solution (or other crystalloid electrolyte solutions)	6 bags	5000 ml
Lidocaine	1 vial	100 ml (20 mg/ml)
Prednisolone sodium succinate	3 vials	10 ml (500 mg/vial)
Tolazoline HCl	1 vial	100 ml (100 mg/ml)

xylazine to produce analgesia and chemical restraint (butorphanol, 0.01–0.02 mg/kg plus xylazine, <0.6 mg/kg IV).

- Detomidine (Domosedan), 0.005–0.02 mg/kg IV, 0.02–0.04 mg/kg IM, is an α_2-agonist that produces reliable sedation and analgesia. It has a long duration of action (up to 2 hours). Because of its profound cardiovascular depressant effects, use carefully in patients with cardiovascular compromise. **Draft breeds** are more susceptible to its effects than other horses and rarely require more than 0.01 mg/kg IV to produce sedation. Conversely, mules may require greater doses, 0.03 mg/kg IV, and donkeys usually sedate with 0.02 mg/kg IV. Donkeys may assume sternal recumbency.

- Diazepam (Valium), 0.1–0.2 mg/kg IV, is a sedative frequently administered to promote muscle relaxation with drugs such as ketamine. It may produce excitement in adults when used on its own. In foals up to 4 weeks old, it has sedative effects and may be used as a preanesthetic. Its primary use is to treat seizures.

- Edrophonium (Enlon), 0.5 mg/kg IV, is used to reverse nondepolarizing neuromuscular blockers competitively, e.g., atracurium. Preferred to neostigmine for this purpose because it produces less bradycardia and, therefore, does not require atropine administration. Administer slowly (over >2 min) to avoid excitement and bradycardia.

- Guaifenesin, 40–80 mg/kg to effect IV, is a centrally acting muscle relaxant used in conjunction with the anesthetic drugs ketamine and thiopental to induce and/or maintain anesthesia. No analgesic or anesthetic properties. **Overdose causes apnea.** NOTE: Mules and donkeys may be more sensitive to it than horses. It is usually administered as a 5% or 10% solution. Precipitates during storage, therefore make solutions fresh. Peak effect is reached 10 min after administration.

- Ketamine (Ketaset/Ketaject), 2.2 mg/kg IV, is a dissociative anesthetic that may be preferred to a barbiturate because of its relatively benign effects on the cardiovascular system. It increases heart rate and overrides the bradycardia caused by xylazine and detomidine tranquilization. **It causes increased cerebral and ocular pressure and may be contraindicated when cerebral and intraocular pressures are a primary concern.** May cause excitement and even seizure-like activity if administered without pre-existing CNS depression, hence precede by a sedative (e.g., xylazine or diazepam).

- Thiopental sodium (Pentothal), 4–10 mg/kg IV alone, or 3–4 mg/kg IV, with 5% guaifenisen. An ultrashort-acting barbiturate used for rapid anesthesia induction after bolus administration. Transient apnea often occurs. **Use with caution in emergency situations because it depresses ventilation, cardiac output, and systemic blood pressure.** It may also be used at 3–4 mg/kg, either mixed with guaifenisen or as a bolus after pretreatment with guaifenesin.

- Xylazine (Rompun), 0.2–1.1 mg/kg IV, is an α_2-agonist that produces reliable sedation and analgesia. It also causes bradycardia and reduces cardiac output, therefore use with caution in patients with cardiovascular compromise. To some extent the adverse effects of xylazine on the cardiovascular system are ameliorated by ketamine. **Draft breeds are**

more sensitive to xylazine than other horses. Mules may require higher doses than either donkeys or horses.

- Romifidine, 40–100 μg/kg IV, is an α₂-agonist used in Europe. It has similar preanesthetic and tranquilizing effects to other α₂-agonists. It can be combined with diazepam and ketamine for short-duration intravenous anesthesia. The sedation and analgesia achieved with romifidine are not as great as with detomidine.

- Euthanasia solution (e.g., Beuthanasia, >0.2 ml/kg IV). **Used for humane destruction only!** Because this solution often produces transient motor activity and gasping, it is occasionally advised to anesthetize the horse before administering it (e.g., with xylazine and ketamine).

RESUSCITATION DRUGS AND SUPPORT DRUGS
(See Table 42–2)

- Atropine, 0.01–0.02 mg/kg IV, is used to treat sinus bradycardia. It may produce ileus at higher doses.

- Dextran 70 (Gentran 70) in 0.9% saline, 5–10 ml/kg/h, is a colloidal solution used as a blood volume expander. Indicated in hypovolemia and when total plasma protein is decreased. **CAUTION**: During the first minutes of infusion, observe for signs of an adverse reaction (tachycardia, tachypnea, etc.) due to antigenic properties.

- Dobutamine (Dobutrex), 0.001–0.008 mg/kg/min IV, is a β₁-agonist that increases mean cardiac output and arterial blood pressure. It has a short half-life and is best used as an infusion (mix 50 mg in 500 ml of 0.9% saline equals 0.01% solution or 0.1 mg/ml). Overdose produces tachycardia, tachydysrhythmias, and hypertension. In hypovolemic individuals, do not use dobutamine as a substitute for blood volume replacement. It produces severe sinus tachycardia when used with atropine.

- Doxapram (Dopram), 0.2 mg/kg IV, is a respiratory stimulant that is contraindicated if severe hypoxia has already occurred. In an emergency situation, resuscitation by positive-pressure ventilation with 100% oxygen is the preferred treatment for apnea.

- Epinephrine (adrenaline), 0.02 mg/kg intracardiac or into a jugular vein and repeat as necessary, is the drug of choice in cardiopulmonary resuscitation. It is a mixed α- and β-sympathomimetic, producing peripheral vasoconstriction and cardiac stimulation. By jugular vein, inject in conjunction with fluid therapy to ensure that the drug is flushed centrally.

- Flunixin meglumine (Banamine), 0.25–1.0 mg/kg IV, is a nonsteroidal anti-inflammatory agent used to treat endotoxic shock.

- Hetastarch (Hespan), 10–20 ml/kg/h, is a colloid solution with a higher molecular weight and less antigenic properties than dextran. Presently, it is three times the cost of dextran.

- 7% Hypertonic saline, 4 ml/kg/5 min (**3 liters maximum dose to a 450-kg adult**), is used principally as a blood volume expander to treat shock. It causes hypernatremia. It is contraindicated in cardiogenic shock. Its mechanism of action is to shift intracellular and interstitial water into the intravascular space. Therefore, it is viewed as an emergency treatment only; administer in conjunction with conventional replacement fluids.

- Lactated Ringer's solution (and other "balanced" electrolyte solutions),

10–40 ml/kg/h, is an isotonic crystalloid solution used to correct hypovolemia, dehydration, shock, and acidosis. It may be used with colloidal and/or hypertonic saline solutions.

- Lidocaine, 0.5 mg/kg IV, is used to treat ventricular tachydysrhythmias. These are relatively uncommon in horses, but prompt treatment is crucial when present.
- Prednisolone sodium succinate (Solu-Delta Cortef), 2–5 mg/kg, is used to stabilize cell membranes during shock and after resuscitation.
- Yohimbine (Yobine), 0.1 mg/kg IV, or Tolazoline HCl (Tolazine), 4 mg/kg slowly IV, is used to reverse the effects of α_2-agonists, xylazine, and detomidine. Yohimbine can cause excitement; minimize this by administering half the calculated dose slowly. Administer the second half of the dose only if necessary. Use when early termination of an α_2-agonist is desirable or to treat inadvertent α_2-agonist overdosage. Repeat doses may be needed.

GENERAL ANESTHETIC CONSIDERATIONS

Depth of Anesthesia

Distressed individuals in emergency situations are likely to have different sensitivity to anesthetics compared with nondistressed individuals. Therefore, depth of anesthesia should be monitored closely by trained personnel.

Pain and distress cause an increase in sympathetic tone and circulating catecholamine levels. These, in turn, may cause a hyperdynamic cardiovascular state characterized by increased cardiac output (CO). Drug requirements may markedly increase under these circumstances, but use caution to prevent an overdose when catecholamine levels decline. In hypovolemic individuals the reduced volume for distribution of injected drugs may cause increased susceptibility. Exhaustion can also complicate an emergency situation, because it is often associated with muscle damage, dehydration, electrolyte imbalance, and decreased circulating catecholamines.

Monitoring

A portable ECG monitor detects dysrhythmias and monitors their response to treatment. A telemetry unit (Hewlett Packard, Andover, MA 01810 [Recorder and Monitor/Holter]) is particularly useful.

Systemic arterial hypotension indicates cardiovascular collapse due to a primary problem or anesthetic overdose. Modern portable oscillometric sphygmomanometers help the anesthetist by warning of hypotension.

An accurate anesthetic record is the best defense against charges of negligence. The best way to ensure safe anesthesia and an accurate record is to designate someone to be solely responsible for anesthesia and supportive care.

Respiratory Support

Orotracheal intubation is the best method to ensure airway patency and is mandatory if ventilation is controlled. A demand valve attached to a two-stage regulator valve and type E oxygen cylinder is suitable for controlling ventilation with oxygen. Demand valves allow spontaneous ventilation to be supplemented with oxygen. Larger horses may require adjusting the regulator to 60 psi in order to maintain sufficiently high inspiratory flows. E cylinders contain approximately 660 gaseous liters, therefore 3–4 cylinders may be needed to ventilate a 450-kg adult for 30 minutes. A 30-ft length of hose allows isolation of the compressed gas cylinder from the patient. A dolly also helps secure the cylinder.

Cardiovascular Support

A 14-gauge (or larger) 5.5-inch over-the-needle catheter should be secured (with superglue and/or suture [2-0 Ethilon]) in a peripheral vein; the jugular vein is preferred. In hypovolemic patients, give balanced electrolyte solutions at a rate of 10–20 ml/kg IV. Use hypertonic saline, 7%, at a rate of 4–6 ml/kg/10 min in severe hypovolemia. A 450-kg adult should receive no more than 3 liters of 7% hypertonic saline. Dextran 70 in 0.9% saline can also be used to treat hypovolemia. Infuse dobutamine in conjunction with fluid therapy when necessary.

Positioning and Padding

Pad pressure points (shoulder, hips) and large muscle groups during anesthesia. Protect the eyes, especially when moving the patient.

Ileus

Individuals requiring emergency anesthesia may have a full GI tract. The reduction in GI motility caused by anesthetic drugs may predispose these patients to ileus and colic. A full GI tract may complicate ventilation and result in hypoxemia during anesthesia. Many anesthetic and tranquilizing drugs decrease gut motility, therefore consider the potential for postanesthetic colic. Minimize positional changes while the patient is recumbent to decrease the chances of torsion.

Hyperkalemic Periodic Paralysis

HYPP is a genetic disorder of Quarter Horses. Stress is a primary factor in the disease. In the emergency setting and under anesthesia it is important to recognize and treat HYPP immediately (see p. 353).

Hypothermia

Usually a problem associated only with foals. However, monitor body temperature in all emergency situations when shock and environmental temperature extremes are possible.

Euthanasia

Humane or economic considerations may require destruction of the patient. Anesthesia (see Protocol 1, p. 657) makes euthanasia easier to accomplish and more humane.

SPECIFIC CASES

In most cases requiring emergency anesthesia, consider sedation or tranquilization and local anesthesia initially. Reserve general anesthesia for patients requiring complete immobilization. Minimizing down time decreases the incidence of complications.

Severe Lacerations

- Often difficult to determine the volume of blood lost after a laceration. Presume tachycardia (heart rate > 50 bpm) to be secondary to hypovolemia until proved otherwise, and treat by blood volume replacement with crystalloid or colloidal solutions.
- When possible, control severe bleeding before anesthesia.
- Cardiodepressant effects of α_2-agonists and barbiturates are dangerous in hypovolemic patients. Diazepam, 0.1 mg/kg IV, and ketamine, 2 mg/kg IV (see Protocol 4, p. 656) are preferred for induction because they cause minimal depression of the cardiovascular system.

Fractures

- Often necessary to stabilize fractures before transport to a surgical facility
- Same considerations as for Severe Lacerations apply.
- Ameliorate anxiety associated with pain with butorphanol.
- When hypovolemia is not evident, use α_2-agonists for analgesia.

Seizures

- Treat a seizuring patient with 0.1–0.2 mg/kg of diazepam IV.
- If anesthesia is needed for immediate transport and diagnostic tests, a thiopental bolus or thiopental with 5% guaifenisen (Protocol 2, see p. 656) is the protocol of choice.
- Avoid ketamine because it produces seizure-like activity of the CNS and increases intracranial pressure.

Dystocia

- General anesthesia can produce enough vaginal and uterine relaxation to facilitate manipulation of malpresented foals.
- Elevating the caudal end of the anesthetized mare allows abdominal viscera to move cranially and improves the ease of fetal manipulation. Do not maintain this Trendelenburg (head down) position for long periods because it is associated with reduced ventilation and cardiac output. Controlling ventilation with a demand valve minimizes ventilatory compromise.
- Protocol 1 (see p. 654) is satisfactory for these situations, followed by maintenance with "triple drip."
- General anesthesia for field cesarean section rarely results in a live foal and places the mare at increased risk; extensive manipulation per vaginum increases the chances of complications during cesarean section.

5

Colic

- Individuals with colic are frequently unresponsive to analgesics and are unmanageable to the point at which they injure themselves and are dangerous to transport. Injectable anesthesia may be needed before definitive therapy or transportation to a surgical facility.
- IV fluids and other supportive treatment is usually needed in these situations.
- Diazepam with ketamine combination is a suitable induction technique.
- Abdominal distention may require controlled ventilation.
- Correct nephrosplenic entrapment in the field by "rolling" from right to left lateral recumbency under general anesthesia. Protocol 1 (see below) is usually used for this purpose. Appropriate medical therapy is important in conjunction with "rolling" providing phenylephrine and exercise do not correct the problem.

Extrications/Entrapments

- Horses may need to be anesthetized for safe removal from dangerous situations.
- Often impossible to assess accurately the physiologic status
- Sometimes difficult or unsafe to get close to the patient. A pole syringe may permit IM drugs.
- Skills and equipment needed for safe removal of horses are important in disasters like hurricanes, floods, and trailer accidents. See p. 638.

Cardiopulmonary Resuscitation

- Emergency field anesthesia can result in respiratory and cardiac arrest from hypovolemia, upper airway obstruction, pneumothorax, hypokalemia, and so on.
- Careful continuous monitoring and early intervention are the keys to success in cardiopulmonary resuscitation. Figure 42–1 is a guide for patient evaluation.
- Table 42–3 is a guide for CPR.

SELECTED PROTOCOLS FOR EMERGENCY ANESTHESIA

PROCEDURE Protocol 1

Premedication: Xylazine, 0.3–0.6 mg/kg IV, and butorphanol, 0.01–0.02 mg/kg IV. Wait 3–5 minutes for peak effect.

Induction: Ketamine, 2.2 mg/kg IV, with diazepam, 0.05–0.10 mg/kg IV

Maintenance: "Triple drip," 1 liter 5% guaifenesin, 1–2 gm of ketamine, and 250–500 mg of xylazine in solution. Titrate carefully to approximately 1–2 ml/kg/h to produce the desired level of anesthesia. (With a standard 10 drops/ml administration set, this equates to 1–2 drops per second for a 450-kg adult.)

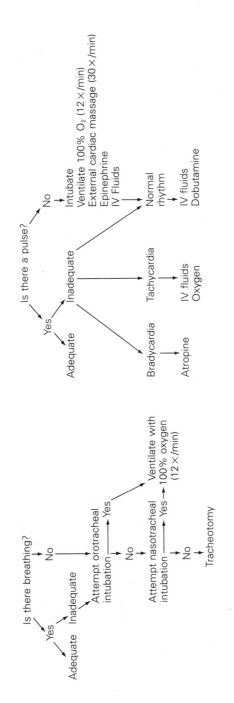

TABLE 42–3. **Cardiopulmonary Resuscitation**

Verify Arrest, Discontinue Anesthetics, Note Time of Arrest

A. Airway—Pass orotracheal or nasotracheal tube

B. Breathing—Start positive-pressure ventilation with 100% oxygen

C. Circulation—Establish external cardiac massage 30/min by knee drops on chest

Epinephrine—0.02 mg/kg IV, intratracheal, or IC

Administer fluids (LRS, PSS) at shock dosage so heart has something to pump (40 ml/kg)

IC, intracardiac; LRS, lactated Ringer's solution; PSS, physiologic saline solution.

PROCEDURE Protocol 2 (**CAUTION:** This protocol is not recommended in cases of hypovolemia and shock.)

Premedication: Xylazine, 0.2–0.4 mg/kg IV; wait 3–5 minutes for peak sedation.
Induction: 5% guaifenesin in 1 liter 5% dextrose or sterile water; administer until patient becomes ataxic (after approximately 0.6–1.0 ml/kg IV), then administer a bolus of thiopental, 3–4 mg/kg IV.
Maintenance: 2 gm thiopental in 1 liter of 5% guaifenesin titrated to approximately 1–1.8 ml/kg/h

PROCEDURE Protocol 3 (For foals ≤ 4 weeks of age)

Premedication: Diazepam, 0.1 mg/kg IV, wait for peak sedation to take effect. The foal may lie down.
Induction: Ketamine, 2.2 mg/kg IV
Maintenance: Modified "triple drip," 1 liter 5% guaifenesin with 125–250 mg of xylazine and 1 gm of ketamine. Titrate to approximately 0.5–1.0 ml/kg/h.

PROCEDURE Protocol 4 (**CAUTION:** In healthy individuals, induction may cause excitement. This protocol is indicated *only* in cases of severe hypovolemic, endotoxic shock or CNS depression.)

Premedication: None
Induction: Diazepam, 0.1–0.2 mg/kg IV, followed immediately by ketamine, 2.2 mg/kg IV.
Maintenance: See Protocol 1. Treat shock with large-volume fluid therapy.

B. EUTHANASIA

Thomas J. Divers

Properly performed euthanasia is important to ensure humane destruction of terminally ill or suffering individuals and is particularly important when viewed by the client. Before administering any euthanasia solution:

- Properly identify the patient being euthanized and **recheck**.
- Consider the venue, distracting noise, surface, surrounding objects, condition of the jugular veins, placement of the needle or catheter, location of burial, condition of the halter, and shank and holder.

PERFORMING EUTHANASIA WHEN EXPENSE IS A PRIMARY CONCERN

Insert a 12-gauge, 2-inch, nondisposable needle or 14-gauge, 5.25-inch IV catheter in the jugular vein. Prepare two 60-ml syringes of euthanasia solution, with one syringe containing 40 mg of succinylcholine. After aspiration to ensure that the needle is properly positioned in the vein, *rapidly* inject the syringe with the succinylcholine and 50 ml of the euthanasia solution into the jugular vein. Immediately attach the second syringe (60 ml) to the needle and administer rapidly. The individual usually falls within 30 seconds after injection of the two doses.

PERFORMING EUTHANASIA WHEN EXPENSE IS NOT A PRIMARY CONCERN

To ensure a tranquil state during the administration of the euthanasia solution, heavily sedate the patient with detomidine, 0.01–0.02 mg/kg IV, or xylazine, 0.5–1.0 mg/kg IV. Once sedation is established, administer the solutions, as in preceding paragraph, through a 12-gauge needle or a 14-gauge, 5.25-inch catheter properly placed in the jugular vein.

NERVOUS OR NEEDLE-SHY PATIENT

Heavily sedate the individual with detomidine, 10 mg IV or 40 mg IM (via injection pole if necessary); place a 14-gauge, 3.5- or 5.25-inch catheter in the jugular vein, and administer euthanasia/succinylcholine solution rapidly.

EUTHANASIA UNDER ANESTHESIA

This can be performed by administering euthanasia solution.

EUTHANASIA OF PATIENTS WITH THROMBOSED JUGULAR VEINS

Place a 14- or 16-gauge, 3.5-inch catheter in the lateral thoracic vein. Tranquilize the individual and administer the euthanasia/succinylcholine solution. If the lateral thoracic vein cannot be catheterized, use detomidine, 20 mg IV, injected into the cephalic vein, or 40 mg IM. Once sedated, intracardiac administration of euthanasia solution or concentrated KCl (500 mEq) and succinylcholine can be administered with an 18-gauge, 3.5–6.0-inch needle and 30–60 ml syringe. The immediate need for euthanasia can cause a crisis when no euthanasia solution is available. An alternative is sedation with detomidine and administration of KCl (lite salt) mixed with 40–80 mg of succinylcholine.

5

43 Nutritional Guidelines for the Injured Horse

Jonathan M. Naylor

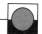

The only true nutritional emergency is *hypoglycemia*, which is discussed in Chapter 35.

NUTRITION FOR SICK HORSES

The clinician usually chooses the diet for an individual as part of the therapeutic regimen; this important decision is made early in the patient care cycle. Different feeding regimens are presented in this chapter.

Some practitioners feed only complete feeds or alfalfa hay cubes as the standard hospital diet. These are convenient but usually lead to stall chewing (boredom, no long-stem fiber) and may increase the incidence of colic.

In general, most patients can be fed a diet of a high-quality grass hay or a grass-alfalfa hay mixture, given either free choice or at a minimum of 1.5% of body weight. A salt block and free-choice water should also be available. Some individuals are not accustomed to automatic waterers, so monitor closely for the first 24 hours to be sure the affected individual is drinking.

Hay is usually supplemented with approximately 1 kg of whole oats twice a day. Feeding oats helps maintain acclimation to grain, thus making it easier to return to a high-grain diet when recovered. Whole oats are palatable and relatively unlikely to cause digestive problems because the thick, fibrous capsule is intact. If the patient is thin, the usual remedy is to feed more grain and avoid poor quality hay. The general rule for changing grain is to increase it by no more than 0.5 kg/day.

Specific disease problems require modified approaches, which are outlined in Table 43–1.

NUTRITION FOR PHYSIOLOGIC STRESS

Normal physiologic changes increase nutrient requirements. The two most important situations are *heavy lactation* and *growth*. Growing or lactating individuals usually require high-quality hay, grain, and a mineral supplement (Table 43–2).

NUTRITION OF NURSING FOALS

Nursing foals require special attention. If the mare is present, the foal can be encouraged to nurse the mare, or the mare can be milked out and the foal fed by hand. A general guideline: *The foal should receive 10%–12% of body weight*

TABLE 43–1. **Dietary Guidelines for Specific Disease Conditions**

Disease	Nutritional Objectives	Dietary Recommendations
Cervical vertebral malformation (Wobbler)	To maintain steady growth without excessively rapid periods of growth	Balanced diet including adequate copper so that nutritional objectives are met
Choke (esophageal obstruction)	Soft diet to avoid further obstruction at site of spasm or stricture	Following removal, feed soft, short-particle-size feeds—e.g., soak complete feed pellets to make a soft mash or give fresh, tender grass. Continue until esophageal ulceration and inflammation repaired
Colic (following surgical or medical treatment)	Return to normal diet	If no GI reflux, start feed with small quantities of high-quality hay or grass to promote intestinal contractions. Gradually increase amounts
COPD (heaves)	Avoid fungi associated with hay and bedding Some pastures in the southeastern US are also associated with COPD	Keep outside if possible; if not, keep in well-ventilated, clean stall at end of barn. Feed alfalfa cubes from feeder on ground. Complete pelleted feeds can be fed but the fiber length is shorter. Use shredded paper or wood shavings for bedding
Diarrhea: Without weight loss	Increase water and electrolyte absorption	Good quality hay—fiber may bind water, loose salt, both free-choice water and electrolyte solutions
With weight loss	Reduce maldigestion	Small amounts of grain frequently—monitor for signs of aggravation of diarrhea. Loose salt, water, and electrolytes
Enterolithiasis	Decrease large intestine pH, calcium, magnesium, phosphorus	Grass hay, grain (up to 50% of diet) Vinegar appears to reduce enterolith formation
Extensive large colon resection	Increase carbohydrates, protein, minerals	Alfalfa hay, grain, B vitamin supplements, phosphate (5–10 gm/day)
Extensive small intestinal resection	Increase soluble fiber, decrease bulk	Slurry of pelleted feed or alfalfa pellets. After 7–10 days, gradually change to alfalfa hay or pellets and feed small amounts of grain. B vitamin supplement

Table continued on following page

TABLE 43–1. **Dietary Guidelines for Specific Disease Conditions** *Continued*

Disease	Nutritional Objectives	Dietary Recommendations
Geriatric (>20 years)	Increase protein, phosphorus. Decrease fiber. Goal is for a calcium:phosphorus ratio of 1:1 to 3:1	High-quality grass hay and grain. Pelleted feeds (12%–14% CP). May supplement with linseed or soybean meal (200–400 gm), B vitamins, ascorbic acid (10 gm), phosphate (5 gm). Can feed mashes or slurries if teeth problems
Hepatic encephalopathy	Reduce protein, increase branched-chain amino acids, simple sugars, B vitamins	Grass hay (8% CP). Corn grain, milo. Avoid lush spring grass, feed small amounts of carbohydrates frequently
Hyperakalemic periodic paralysis (HYPP)	Decrease serum potassium	Avoid lush green feeds, lush hay made from young grass, molasses. Feed late-cut grass hays, sugar beet pulp, grain. Supplement with sodium bicarbonate, 15–30 gm/day (500-kg adult). Proprietary HYPP feed available from Montana Pride, Dillon, MT
Rectal or vaginal surgery	Low-bulk, laxative diet	Green grass, finely ground pelleted feed (alfalfa or complete feed)
Renal disease with azotemia	Increase water, salt; reduce protein, if BUN:Cr ratio > 15, calcium	Loose salt. Grass hay (8% CP). Feed grain (oats, corn) as necessary to maintain condition or reduce hypercalcemia
Right dorsal colitis	Low bulk, anti-inflammatory prostanoids	Pelleted feeds, miprostonol, sucralfate, 1–2 oz of dietary linseed oil

CP, Crude protein.
Reprinted with permission. Copyright 1998 Jonathan M. Naylor.

as mare's milk. Healthy, hand-fed foals drink no more than 12% of body weight as milk, and it has been suggested that this is the most the foals' stomachs can accommodate on a hand-feeding regimen. However, foals nursing mares ingest smaller amounts at much more frequent intervals and can drink more. In the first few days of life, feed foals every 2 hours; the frequency can be slowly decreased over a 10-day period.

If the foal is tube-fed, it is important to check for reflux through the tube before each feeding. Reflux suggests ileus and is a reason for discontinuing or decreasing the amounts of milk fed.

Human indwelling 12 F. enteral feeding tubes (Flexiflo enteral feeding tube, Ross Laboratories, Columbus, OH) are successfully used to feed foals placing a tube with the tip in the distal esophagus. Tape a plastic collar to the

TABLE 43–2. **Nutritional Guidelines for Pregnant, Lactating, or Growing Horses**

Condition	Hay (% of Body Weight)	Grain (% of Body Weight)
Mares, late gestation	1.0 to 1.5	0.5 to 1.0
Early lactation	1.0 to 2.0	1.0 to 2.0
Late lactation	1.0 to 2.0	0.5 to 1.5
Foals, nursing, 3–6 month	0	1.0 to 2.0
Weanling, 6–12 month	0.5 to 1.0	1.5 to 3.0
Weanling, 12–18 month	1.0 to 1.5	1.5 to 3.0
Long yearling, 18–24 month	1.0 to 1.5	1.0 to 1.5
2-Year-olds	1.0 to 1.5	1.0 to 1.5

In general, try to feed a good-quality hay and restrict grain to the lower end of the recommended ranges. Alfalfa or grass-alfalfa mix hays are preferred because they are good sources of the calcium and protein required to support growth and lactation. Feed a mineral block containing appropriate amounts of trace minerals (especially copper), and calcium and phosphorus if needed. Mineral blocks should contain salt to promote and control intake. Only feed one type of block—horses can eat plain salt blocks and ignore the trace mineral–fortified block.
Reprinted with permission. Copyright 1998 Jonathan M. Naylor.

halter to reduce the risk of dislodgement in active foals. In sick foals it is important to check for ileus and potential reflux of food. Connect the tube to a fluid delivery set (e.g., Flexitainer-500, Ross Laboratories, Columbus, OH), and the liquid meal is slowly delivered over a period of an hour.

If a lactating mare is not available, the foal can be fed commercial foal milk replacers, which use only milk proteins (casein, whey) as the protein source. These are likely to be closer in composition to mare's milk and have been used more extensively on foals than human enteral preparations. Often, the amounts recommended on the package have to be divided into several smaller meals for sick foals. Some foals are raised on goat's milk, but 2% fat cow's milk is actually closer in composition to mare's milk.

After a foal is healthy, it can go to a nurse mare or be trained to drink from a bucket. In the latter case, milk can be made up several times a day and left out for the foal to drink. It is a good idea to weigh the amount of powder added to water, because there is a lot of variation in the amount of powder scooped into a cup, and overconcentrated solutions can result.

Mare's milk is about 12% dry matter, and foals are successfully hand-fed on 14% milk replacer. The slight increase in concentration over mare's milk helps compensate for the reduced volume intake of hand-fed foals.

With good management and early provision of high-quality hay and creep feed (a mixture of grain and protein supplement), foals can be weaned at 7 weeks of age. Socialization is very important, so provide access to a role model (e.g., an old quiet pony) as early as possible.

Fostering onto a mare is usually accomplished using the principles of restraint and time. Rubbing the dead foal's placenta or skin onto the foal to be fostered and putting Vicks vaporizing ointment on the mare's nostrils helps.

Tranquilize and hobble or twitch the mare as necessary (see p. 431). The foal can then be helped to nurse. Some mares readily accept a foster foal; others require a week or more of continuous observation and restraint.

FEEDING BY TUBE

Some individuals are unable or unwilling to eat normal diets and require tube feeding with liquid diets or slurries. Three basic types of diet can be fed:

Pelleted Feed. Some clinicians soak pelleted feeds made from finely ground ingredients and feed the liquid gruel through a large-bore stomach tube. Typically, about 500 gm of pellets, 50 ml of vegetable oil, and 3 liters of water are mixed together. A blender aids in grinding and mixing the diet. Initially, a 500-kg adult might receive about four to eight 3-liter meals a day. Over the course of a week, the volume fed can be increased to 6–8 liters a meal and the number of feedings gradually reduced to four per day. A wide-bore tube and large funnel or high-capacity hand pump—such as a marine bilge pump—helps move the gruel flow through the tube. This approach is inexpensive, but it can be difficult to get sufficient gruel down the tube to meet requirements.

Defined Diet. Another approach is to make a defined diet from a mixture of electrolytes, glucose, and casein. It is important to add some alfalfa meal because addition of a fiber source appears to reduce the incidence of diet-induced diarrhea. The ingredients for this approach are inexpensive, but weighing out the components is time consuming (Table 43–3).

Commercial Human Diet. A third approach is to buy a commercial enteral diet designed for human use. These commercial diets are expensive, and

TABLE 43–3. **Alfalfa, Casein, Dextrose Slurry**

Individual Feeding (Four Feeds per Day)

Alfalfa meal	500 gm
Casein*	225 gm
Dextrose*	225 gm
Electrolyte mixture (see below)	58 gm
Water	5.25 L

Electrolyte Mixture (One Day's Supply)

Sodium chloride (NaCl)	10 gm
Sodium bicarbonate (NaHCO$_3$)	15 gm
Potassium chloride (KCl)	75 gm
Potassium phosphate (dibasic anhydrous) (K$_2$HPO$_4$)	60 gm
Calcium chloride (CaCl$_2$2H$_2$O)	45 gm
Magnesium oxide (MgO)	25 gm
Total, gm	230 gm

*Initially feed only 100-gm amounts of dextrose and casein in the slurry; slowly increase the amounts to the levels in the table over 5–7 days.

Casein or dehydrated cottage cheese = 82% crude protein with less than 2% lactose.

Adapted from data in Naylor JM, Freeman DE, Kronfeld DS: Alimentation of hypophagic horses. Compend Cont Educ Pract Vet 1984;6(2):S93–S100.

Reprinted with permission. Copyright 1998 Jonathan M. Naylor.

individuals fed solely on these diets often develop diarrhea. Mature individuals have been satisfactorily maintained on Osmolite HN (Ross Laboratories, Columbus, OH), administered at a total daily caloric intake of 155 kcal × (body weight in kg)$^{0.75}$ or approximately 16 Mcal for a 500-kg adult. The solution comes at an energy density of 1 Mcal/L, so the total volume fed is about 16 liters for a 500-kg adult, and this is divided among three feeds. Additional water is usually added to each feed to provide a total daily water intake of 45 ml/kg. Deliver each meal over a period of an hour using a drip system *or* adding a fiber source such as ground alfalfa meal (1 kg per feeding) is likely to reduce the risk of digestive upsets. Introduce the diet at 25% of caloric needs on day 1, 50% of caloric needs on day 2, 75% on day 3, and 100% of maintenance requirements thereafter. Another equine enteral diet is Nutri Prime (Ken Vet, Ashland, OH).

Comments on Tube Feeding

Whichever approach is used, it is important to introduce the diet gradually and to monitor hydration, electrolyte balance, and GI function carefully.

Tube feeding can be highly successful when lack of food intake is due to a temporary functional or painful problem in the mouth or pharynx. Individuals with these conditions can be maintained satisfactorily for several weeks on a liquid diet.

When anorexia is secondary to systemic disease, anticipate some degree of weight loss. Forced feeding becomes more important with chronic inappetence (more than 3 days) and poor body condition.

FASTING

Deliberate underfeeding is often practiced in veterinary medicine to empty or rest the gut—e.g., before surgery or following major abdominal surgery. Since prolonged fasting predisposes individuals to gastric ulcers and diarrhea, which can be severe in some cases, it may be better to allow patients with digestive tract problems access to small amounts of food when possible rather than to err on the side of complete food restriction.

5

Appendices

APPENDIX I: *Equine Emergency Drugs:*
               Approximate Dosages *666*

APPENDIX II: *Reference Values* *678*

APPENDIX III: *Anthelmintics* *695*

APPENDIX IV: *Vaccination Schedule* *700*

APPENDIX V: *Product Manufacturers* *704*

APPENDIX VI: *Registry Information for the Breeds of Horses* .. *711*

6

Equine Emergency Drugs: Approximate Dosages

Drug	Dose	Route	Precautions/Comments
Acepromazine	0.02–0.05 mg/kg q8h	IV/IM	Lowers seizure threshold and produces hypotension
Acetazolamide	2–4 mg/kg q6h	PO	Used for hyperkalemia
Acetylcholine	6 mg/kg	IC	Use for ventricular fibrillation
Acetylcysteine	140 mg/kg	IV	
N-Acetyl-L-cysteine (powdered)	Add 8 gm powder and 1.5 tbsp of sodium bicarbonate (baking soda) to 200 ml water; infuse 4–6 oz (120–180 ml)	Per rectum	Used for refractory meconium impactions
Albuterol*	0.02 mg/kg q12h	PO	Do not use in hypokalemic patients
Altrenogest	0.044–0.088 mg/kg q24h	PO	For pregnant mares experiencing toxemia
Amikacin	6.6 mg/kg q8h or 15–25 mg/kg q24h	IV/IM	Preferred over gentamicin in foals
Aminocaproic acid	10–20 mg/kg	IV diluted in 1–3 L 0.9% saline and administered slowly	Used for uncontrollable bleeding when surgery is not an option

*Bioavailability unknown in the horse.

Drug	Dose	Route	Comments
Aminophylline	0.5 mg/kg q12h; can be substituted for theophylline; 1 mg aminophylline = 0.8 mg theophylline	IV diluted or PO	May improve glomerular filtration rate; rarely recommended as a bronchodilator
Antacids (Maalox; Di-Gel)	30–100 ml q3–4h	PO	Buffers acid for a brief period
Aspirin	5–20 mg/kg	PO/per rectum	May not inhibit platelets stimulated by endotoxins
Atracurium	0.1–0.2 mg/kg	IV	Paralytic agent
Atropine	0.005–0.01 mg/kg for sinus bradycardia; 0.04–0.06 mg/kg (repeat in 5 min if indicated)—preanesthetic; 0.014–0.02 mg/kg for bronchodilatation; 0.02–0.05 mg/kg	IV	Tachycardia, arrhythmia, ileus, mydriasis. Administer once only and observe closely for signs of abdominal pain. Use high dose only with confirmed organophosphate toxicity
Beclomethasone	8 µg/kg	Nebulization	
Benztropine mesylate	8 mg/450 kg	IV	
Bethanechol	0.03 mg/kg q8h	SQ	
	0.16–0.2 mg/kg q8h	PO	
Beuthanasia solution	> 0.2 mg/kg	IV	Euthanasia ONLY
Bismuth subsalicylate	0.5–2 ml/kg q4–6h	PO	
Bovine hemoglobin	30 ml/kg	IV slowly	Used in life threatening anemia when an equine donor transfusion is impossible

Table continued on following page

6

Equine Emergency Drugs: Approximate Dosages *Continued*

Drug	Dose	Route	Precautions/Comments
Bretylium	5.0–10.0 mg/kg (every 10 min)	IV	Do not exceed 30.0–35.0 mg/kg total dose
Butorphanol tartrate	0.01–0.1 mg/kg	IV/IM	Ataxia/head tremors when used without prior tranquilization
Ca-EDTA	75 mg/kg/day divided q12h	IV slowly	
Caffeine	10 mg/kg loading dose, then 2.5–3 mg/kg q24h maintenance dose; therapeutic range = 5–20 mg/L	PO	Toxic level ≥ 40 mg/L
Calcium borogluconate (23%)	0.2–0.4 mg/kg	IV slowly	
Calcium gluconate	4 mg/kg; 0.1–0.2 mEq/kg	IV slowly	Monitor cardiac rate and rhythm
Calcium chloride	5–7 mg/kg		
Carbon disulfide (CDs)			
Carprofen	1.4 mg/kg q24h	PO	
Cefoperazone	30 mg/kg q8h	PO	
Cefotaxime	50 mg/kg q6–8h	IV	
Ceftazidime	20–30 mg/kg q12h	IV or IM	
Ceftiofur	1–5 mg/kg q6h or 2–5 mg/kg q12h	IV or IM	Varies with severity of disease
Charcoal	0.5 gm/kg	PO	
Chloral hydrate	22 mg/kg	IV, 12% solution	Administered perivascularly
Cimetidine	30–60 mg/kg titrated	IV slowly or PO	Phlebitis
	6.6 mg/kg q6–8h, or 16–20 mg/kg q8h	IV	
Cisapride	0.1 mg/kg q4–8h	PO	Poor bioavailability per rectum
Clavulanic acid/ticarcillin	50 mg/kg q6h	IV	
Clenbuterol	0.8–1.6 µg/kg q12h	IV, PO, nebulization	Not approved for use in the United States

Drug	Dosage	Route	Comments
Cromolyn	0.2–0.5 mg/kg	Nebulization	
Cyproheptadine	0.25–0.5 mg/kg q12h	PO	
Desferrioxamine	10 mg/kg	IM or slowly IV	
Detomidine hydrochloride	5–40 µg/kg	IV/IM	Higher dosage for IM only; breed variation in dosage
Dexamethasone	0.02–0.05 mg/kg q24h	IV/IM/PO	Anti-inflammatory—lower
	0.05–0.25 mg/kg	IV/IM	Anti-inflammatory—higher
	0.5 mg/kg q6–24h	IV	Antiedema
Dexamethasone/ trichlormethiazide	5 mg/200 mg boluses q24h	PO	
Dextran 70	5–10 ml/kg/h	IV	
Dextrose	5% or 10% solution at 4–8 mg/kg/ min; 0.5 ml/kg	IV	
Diazepam	0.05–0.44 mg/kg	IV	Respiratory depression may occur
Dichlorvos (DDVP)	0.1–0.2 mg/kg, foal	IV	
	20 mg/kg	PO	
Diclazuril	2.5 g/450 kg	PO	
Digoxin	0.0022–0.0075 mg/kg q12h;	IV	Depression, anorexia, colic may be seen
	0.011–0.0175 mg/kg q12h	PO	
Dimercaprol	2.5–5.0 mg/kg	IM	
10% dimethyl sulfoxide (DMSO)	10%–20% solution at 0.5–1.0 gm/kg slowly over 1 hour	IV in crystalloid solution	Antiedema
DMSO	10%–20% solution at 100 mg/kg q8h	IV in electrolyte solution	Postoperative treatment/anti-inflammatory
Dinoprost tromethamine	0.011–0.022 mg/kg	IM	Early and midgestation; abortifacient
Dioctyl sodium sulfosuccinate (DSS)	10–20 mg/kg; up to 2 doses, 48 hours apart	PO	May cause mild abdominal pain and diarrhea

Table continued on following page

6

669

Equine Emergency Drugs: Approximate Dosages *Continued*

Drug	Dose	Route	Precautions/Comments
Diphenhydramine hydrochloride	0.5–2.0 mg/kg	IV/IM	
Dipyrone	10–22 mg/kg	IV/IM	
Dobutamine	1.0–20.0 µg/kg/min	IV	
Dopamine	1.0–20.0 µg/kg/min	IV	
Doperidone	1.1 mg/kg q12h	PO	For agalactia
Doxapram	0.2 mg/kg	IV	
Doxycycline	3 mg/kg q12h	PO	
Doxylamine succinate	0.5 mg/kg q6–12h	Slowly IV, IM, or SQ	
Edrophonium	0.5–1.0 mg/kg	IV	Antagonist for atracurium
Enalapril	0.25–0.5 mg/kg q12h or q24h	PO	
Enrofloxacin	2.5–3.3 mg/kg q12h/5–7.5 mg/kg q24h	PO	Safety not demonstrated in foals
Epinephrine	0.01–0.02 mg/kg (approx. 4.5–9 ml/450 kg); anaphylaxis	IV/IM	
	0.1–0.5 mg/kg anaphylaxis	IT-intratracheal	
	0.03–0.05 mg/kg—asystole	IV	
	0.03–0.5 mg/kg—asystole	IT	
Equine plasma	1 or more liters	IV	
Erythromycin	1–2.5 mg/kg q6h as 1 hour infusion	IV	To improve intestinal motility; observe for colic/diarrhea/intussusception
Erythromycin stearate/phosphate or estolate	25–30 mg/kg q8–12h	PO	
Famotidine	1.0–2.0 mg/kg q24h	IV	
	2.8 mg/kg q24h	PO	
Febantel (FBT)	6 mg/kg	PO	
Fenbendazole (FBZ)	5–10 mg/kg	PO	

Drug	Dosage	Route	Comments
Fluconazole	4 mg/lb q24h loading dose; 2 mg/lb q24h maintenance dose	PO	
Flumazenil	0.01–0.02 mg/kg	IV slowly	
Flunixin meglumine	0.25 mg/kg q8h	IV	
	0.25–1.1 mg/kg	IV/IM	
Fluprostenol sodium	2.2 µg/kg	IM	Induce parturition
Furosemide	1.0–2.0 mg/kg for acute edema; 0.25–1.0 mg/kg q12–24h (maintenance)	SQ/IM/IV/PO	
	Administer small amounts (0.25–0.5 mg/kg q30–60 min) during dopamine infusion or begin continuous infusion (0.25–2.0 mg/kg/h)	IV	Protect solution from light
Gentamicin	2.2 mg/kg q8h	IV/IM	Nephrotoxic; use cautiously and only in well-hydrated foals
	6.6 mg/kg q24h	IV	
Glycopyrrolate	0.005–0.01 mg/kg	IV	Tachycardia, arrhythmia, ileus, mydriasis
	0.005 mg/kg q8–12h	IV, IM, SQ	
Guaifenesin	40–80 mg/kg	IV as 5% solution	
Haloperidol decanoate	0.01 mg/kg	IM	May cause sedation for 5–7 days
Heparin	40–100 IU/kg q6h	IV/SQ, and/or mixed in equine plasma	Monitor for RBC agglutination and decreasing hematocrit
Hetastarch	10–20 ml/kg/h	IV	
Hydralazine	0.5–1.5 mg/kg q12h	PO	
Hydrochlorothiazide	250 mg q6h	IM/IV	
Hydroxyzine hydrochloride	1.0–1.5 mg/kg q8–12h	IV or IM slowly	
Hyperimmune plasma	2–4 L/450 kg	IV	
Imidocarb	2.2–4.0 mg/kg	IM	
Imipenem	15 mg/kg q6–8h	IV in fluids	
Imipramine	1 mg/kg q12h	PO	

Table continued on following page

6

Equine Emergency Drugs: Approximate Dosages *Continued*

Drug	Dose	Route	Precautions/Comments
Insulin, Protamine Zinc	0.4 IU/kg q24h	SQ	
Insulin, Regular	0.1 IU/kg	IV	
Insulin, Ultralente	0.4 IU/kg q24h	IV or IM	Dose and duration of treatment variable
Ipratropium bromide	0.5–3 µg/kg	Nebulization	
Isoproterenol	0.05–0.2 µg/kg/min	IV	
Isoxsuprine	1–2 mg/kg q 12h	PO	
Itraconazole	2.6 mg/kg q12h	PO	
Ivermectin	200 µg/kg	PO	
Kaolin	4–8 ml/kg q12h	PO	
Ketamine	1.0–2.0 mg/kg, adult	IV	
	1.0 mg/kg, foal		
Ketoprofen	1.1–2.2 mg/kg	IV	
Lidocaine	20–50 µg/kg/min; 0.25 mg/kg (bolus); 0.5 mg/kg (very slowly)	IV	For ventricular arrhythmias, excitement, seizures
	1.3 mg/kg, followed by 0.05 mg/kg/min	IV slowly	Ataxia may occur if administered too fast
	1.5 mg/kg (repeat in 5 min; then 8–10 min later with 0.5 mg/kg)	IV	} To improve intestinal motility
Loperamide	4–16 mg/foal q6h; then increase by 2-mg increments every 2–3 doses	PO	Do not exceed 3.0 mg/kg total dose Enhances toxin absorption in cases of acute, infectious enteritis
Magnesium sulfate	1.0–2.5 gm/450 kg/min; 14.0–28.0 mg/kg diluted to 10 ml in 5% dextrose in water;	IV	Do not exceed 25 gm IV total dose; for ventricular tachycardia
		IV	
	6 mg/kg	IV	
Magnesium sulfate (Epsom salts)	0.2–1 gm/kg diluted in warm water q24h	PO	Do not use longer than 3 days to avoid enteritis and magnesium intoxication

Drug	Dosage	Route	Comments
Mannitol	20% solution at 0.25–2.0 g/kg over 15–40 min	IV	May exacerbate cerebral hemorrhage
Mebendazole (MBZ)	8.8 mg/kg	PO	
Meperidine hydrochloride	1.1–2.2 mg/kg	IV/IM	IV administration may cause severe hypotension
Metamucil	400 gm/500 kg q6–12h	PO	
L-Methionine	25 mg/kg	PO	
Methylene blue	5–8.8 mg/kg	IV slowly	
Metoclopramide	0.25–0.5 mg/kg q4–8h as a 1-hour infusion; 0.6 mg/kg q4–6h	IV	
Metronidazole	15–25 mg/kg q6h	PO or per rectum / PO or suppository	Suppository bioavailability is 50% of orally administered drug
Milk of magnesia	6–8 L/500 kg	PO	
Milrinone	10 µg/kg/min; 0.5–1.0 mg/kg q12h	IV / PO	
Mineral oil	6–8 L/450 kg; 120–160 oz	PO / PO (via nasogastric tube)	
Misoprotol	1–4 µg/kg q12h	PO	
Morphine sulfate	0.3–0.66 mg/kg	IV	Use only with xylazine (0.66–1.1 mg/kg IV) to avoid CNS excitement
Moxidectin	400–500 µg/kg	PO	
Mucomyst	Add 40 ml of 20% solution to 160 ml water to make 4% solution	Per rectum	Rarely used for meconium impaction
Naloxone	0.01–0.02 mg/kg	IV	
Neomycin	8 mg/kg q8h	PO	Prolonged (3–4 doses) may cause diarrhea

Table continued on following page

6

Equine Emergency Drugs: Approximate Dosages *Continued*

Drug	Dose	Route	Precautions/Comments
Neostigmine	0.005–0.01 mg/kg	SQ/IM	
Nitric oxide	20–80 ppm	Inhalation	
Nitroglycerin cream	15 mg over each digital artery (1″ strip) q24h	Topical	Do not exceed 60 mg/day
Norepinephrine	0.05–1.0 µg/kg/min	IV	Do not exceed 2.0 µg/kg/min
Omeprazole	0.5 mg/kg q24h/1–4 mg/kg q24h	IV/PO	May require 2–3 days to effectively raise pH
Oxfendazole (OFZ)	10 mg/kg	PO	
Oxibendazole (OBZ)	10–15 mg/kg	PO	
Oxytocin	2.5–20 units/450 kg	IV/IM/SQ	Higher doses produce pain
Paromomycin	100 mg/kg q24h × 5 days	PO	Efficacy unproven in foals; for *Cryptosporidia*
Pectin	4–8 ml/kg q12h	PO	
Penicillin/Na⁺ or K⁺	15,000–44,000 IU/kg q6h, or q12h	IV	
Penicillin/Procaine		IM	
Pentazocine	0.3–0.6 mg/kg q12h	PO/IV	
Pentobarbital	3–10 mg/kg	IV	To effect for sedation or seizure control
Pentoxifylline	8.4 mg/kg q8–12h	PO	
Pergolide	0.0017–0.01 mg/kg q24h	PO	
Perphenazine	0.3–0.5 mg/kg q8h	PO	
Phenobarbital	2–10 mg/kg q8–12h	IV/PO	Respiratory depression, hypotension; monitor serum levels (15–40 µg/ml)
Phenoxybenzamine	0.4 mg/kg q6h	PO	
Phenylbutazone	2.2–4.4 mg/kg q12h	PO/IV	
Phenylephrine hydrochloride	0.1–0.2 µg/kg/min	IV	
	10 mg diluted to 10 ml for nasal spray	Intranasal	

Drug	Dose	Route	Comments
Phenylpropanolamine	0.5–2.0 mg/kg q12h	PO	
Phenytoin	5.0–10.0 mg/kg (first 12 hours), then 1.0–5.0 mg/kg q12h;	IV	Sedation, drowsiness, lip and facial twitching, gait deficits, seizures, rhabdomyolysis
	1.82 mg/kg q8h, may increase to 2.27 mg/kg after 2–3 days, and to 2.73 mg/kg after 2–3 more days;	IM	
	7.5 mg/kg q12h	PO	
Piperazine (PPZ)	1 oz/100 lb	PO	Erratic absorption may cause weakness
Polymyxin	600 U/kg	PO	For endotoxemia
Potassium chloride	1 mEq/kg	IV slowly	Use for ventricular fibrillation
	0.5 mEq/kg/h	IC	
	0.1 gm/kg	IV	
Pralidoxime (2-PAM)	20 mg/kg q4–6h	PO	
Prednisolone	0.4–1.6 mg/kg q24h	IV	Anti-inflammatory
Prednisolone Na succinate	2–5 mg/kg	PO	
Prednisone	0.5–2.0 mg/kg q24h	IV	Anti-inflammatory
Procainamide	1.0 mg/kg/min;	PO	Do not exceed 20 mg/kg IV total dose; GI, neurologic signs—similar to quinidine
	25–35 mg/kg q8h	IV	
Progesterone (in oil)	0.8 mg/kg q24h	IM	For pregnant mares in late gestation experiencing endotoxemia
Propafenone	0.5–1.0 mg/kg in 5% dextrose (slowly to effect over 5–8 min);	IV	GI, neurologic signs—similar to quinidine; bronchospasm may occur
	2 mg/kg q8h	PO	

Table continued on following page

6

Equine Emergency Drugs: Approximate Dosages *Continued*

Drug	Dose	Route	Precautions/Comments
Propofol	4 mg/kg	IV after tranquilization	
Propranolol	0.03 mg/kg;	IV	Lethargy, worsening of COPD
	0.38–0.78 mg/kg q8h	PO	
Prostaglandin E₁ (PGE₁)	4 µg/kg q8–12h	PO	
Psyllium hydrophilic mucilloid (Metamucil)	400 gm/450 kg q6–12h	PO	
Pyrantel (PRT)	3 mg/lb	PO	
Pyrimethamine	0.25–2 mg/kg q24h	PO	
Quinidine gluconate	0.5–2.2 mg/kg (bolus q10min to effect)	IV	Do not exceed 12 mg/kg IV total dose; depression, paraphimosis, urticaria, wheals, nasal mucosal swelling, laminitis, neurologic, GI
Quinidine sulfate	22 mg/kg q2h until converted, toxic, or plasma [quinidine] > 4.0 µg/ml; continue q6h until converted or toxic	NG tube	Do not exceed 6 doses q2h; depression, paraphimosis, urticaria, wheals, nasal mucosal swelling, laminitis, neurologic, GI
Ranitidine	6.6 mg/kg q8h, or	PO	
	1.5 mg/kg q8h	IV	
Rifampin	5 mg/kg q12h	PO	
5 or 7% normal saline	4 ml/kg	IV	
Selenium	0.05 mg/kg	**IM only**	
Sodium bicarbonate	1 mEq/kg;	IV	For hyperkalemia
	0.5–1.0 mEq/kg (over 1–2 min; repeat in 5–10 min if indicated)	IV	
Sodium nitrate 1%	16 mg/kg	IV	
Sodium thiosulfate	30–500 mg/kg	IV slowly	

Drug	Dose	Route	Comments
Sucralfate	20–40 mg/kg q6h	PO	
Tetracycline	6.6 mg/kg q12h	IV slowly	
Theophylline	Loading dose of 5–6 mg/kg administered slowly q12h; therapeutic levels = 6–12 mg/L	IV	Seizures, colic, hyperesthesia, tachycardia; toxic level > 20 mg/L
Thiabendazole (TBZ)	50–100 mg/kg	PO	
Thiamine	1–10 mg/kg	IV, IM	
Thiopental Na	3–10 mg/kg	IV	
Timentin (ticarcillin clavulanate)	50 mg/kg q6h	IV	
Timolol maleate	0.5% ophthalmic q8h	Topical	
Tolazine	4.0 mg/kg	IV slowly	α_2 antagonist
Tolazoline	Foal dose: 1–2 mg/kg over 10 min, then infuse at 0.2 mg/kg/h; for each 1 mg/kg pulse dose administered	IV	
Torbugesic tartrate	0.01 mg/kg	IV	
Trichlormethiazide/ dexamethasone	2 boluses	PO	Administer as suspension
Trimethoprim/sulfa	20–30 mg/kg q12h	PO	Do not use with ileus
Vancomycin	4.3–7.5 mg/kg q8h	IV Slowly	
Verapamil	0.025–0.05 mg/kg q30min	IV	Do not exceed 0.2 mg/kg IV total dose
Vitamin C	0.5–1.0 gm/kg q24h	PO	
Vitamin E	20,000 IU q24h	PO	
Vitamin K$_1$	0.5–1 mg/kg	SQ	
Xylazine hydrochloride	0.2–1.1 mg/kg q8–12h	IV slowly or IM	Do not administer IV
Yohimbine	0.1 mg/kg	IV slowly	

6

Reference Values

REFERENCE VALUES FOR NORMAL BLOOD CHEMISTRY

Test	Normal Values
Acetylcholinesterase	450–790 IU/L
Adrenocorticotrophic hormone (ACTH)	8–35 pg/ml—horse
	8–20 pg/ml—ponies
Alanine aminotransferase*	3–23 IU/L (14 ± 11)
Alkaline phosphatase*	86–285 IU/L
Albumin	2.9–3.8 gm/dl
	29–38 gm/L
Ammonia (on ice)	7.63–63.4 μmol/L (35.8 ± 17.0)
	13–108 μg/dl (61 ± 29)
Amylase	75–150 IU/L
Anion gap	6–15 mEq/L
Arginase	0–14 IU/L (11 ± 18)
Aspartate aminotransferase*	138–409 IU/L (296 ± 70)†
Bicarbonate	20–28 mmol/L
Bile acids (total)	5–15 μmol/L
	Up to 20 μmol/L in anorexia
Bilirubin (conjugated)*	0–6.48 mmol/L (1.71)
	0–0.4 mg/dl (0.1)
Bilirubin (unconjugated)*	3.42–34.2 mmol/L (17.1)
	0.2–2.0 mg/dl (1.0)‡
Bilirubin (total)*	7.1–34.2 mmol/L (17.2)
	0–2.0 mg/dl (1.0)
Butyrylcholinesterase	2000–3100 IU/L
Calcium*	2.80–3.40 mmol/L (3.10 ± 0.14)
	11.2–13.6 mg/dl (12.4 ± 0.58)
Carbon dioxide, pCO_2 (venous and arterial)	38–46 mmHg (42.4 ± 2.0)
Carbon dioxide (total)*	24–32 mmol/L (28)
Chloride*	99–109 mmol/L (104 ± 2.6)
Cholesterol (ester)	(81.1) mg/dl
Cholesterol (free)	(0.41) mmol/L
	15.7 mg/dl
Cholesterol (total)*	1.94–3.89 mmol/L (2.88 ± 0.47)
	75–150 mg/dl (111 ± 18)
Cortisol	36–81 nmol/L
	1.30–2.93 μg/dl
Creatine phosphokinase	119–287 IU/L
Creatinine*	106–168 μmol/L
	1.2–1.9 mg/dl
Fibrinogen*	2.94–11.8 μmol/L (7.65 ± 2.35)
	1.0–4.0 gm/L (2.6 ± 0.8)
	100–400 mg/dl (260 ± 80)
Glucose*	4.16–6.39 mmol/L (5.30 ± 0.47)
	75–115 mg/dl (95.6 ± 8.5)

REFERENCE VALUES FOR NORMAL BLOOD
CHEMISTRY *Continued*

Test	Normal Values
Glutamate dehydrogenase	0–11.8 IU/L (5.6 ± 4.2)
Gamma-glutamyl transaminopeptidase	0–44 IU/L
Globulin, alpha-1*	7–13 gm/L
Globulin, alpha-2*	7–13 gm/L
Globulin, beta*	4–12 gm/L
Globulin, gamma*	9–15 gm/L
Hemoglobin*	110–190 gm/L (144 ± 17)
Icterus index	5–20 IU
Insulin§	10–30 μIU/mL
Iodine	394–946 nmol/L
	5–12 μg/dl
Iodine, protein bound	1.5–3.5 μg/dl
Iron	13.1–25.1 μmol/L (19.9 ± 1.97)
	73–140 μg/dl (111 ± 11)
Iron binding capacity, total*	(59.1 ± 5.73) μmol/L
	330 ± 32 μg/dl
Iron binding capacity, unbound*	35.8–46.9 μmol (39.0 ± 3.78)
	200–262 μg/dl (218 ± 21)
Isocitrate dehydrogenase	4.8–18.0 IU/L (10.0 ± 3.3)
Ketones, acetoacetate	(0.029 ± 0.003) mmol/L
Ketones, β-hydroxybutyric acid	(0.06 ± 0.006) mmol/L
	(0.67 ± 0.006) mg/dl
Lactate	1.11–1.78 mmol/L
	10–16 mg/dl
Lactate dehydrogenase	162–412 IU/L (252 ± 63)
LDH-1	6.3–18.5% (11.5 ± 4.0)
LDH-2	8.4–20.5% (14.8 ± 3.2)
LDH-3	41.0–65.9% (50.2 ± 7.2)
LDH-4	9.5–20.9% (16.2 ± 3.8)
LDH-5	1.7–16.5% (7.3 ± 4)
Lead	0.24–1.21 μmol/L
	5–25 μg/dl
Magnesium*	0.90–1.15 mmol/L (1.03 ± 0.13)
	2.2–2.8 mg/dl (2.5 ± 0.31)
Ornithine carbomyl transferase	(3.3 ± 4.2) IU/L
Osmolality	270–300 mOsm/kg
pH (venous and arterial)	7.32–7.44 (7.38 ± 0.03)
Phosphorus	3.1–5.6 mg/dl
Potassium	2.4–4.7 mmol/L (3.51 ± 0.57)
Protein (total)*	52–79.0 gm/L (63.5 ± 5.9)
Albumin*	26.0–37.0 gm/L (30.9 ± 2.8)
Globulins (total)*	26.2–40.4 gm/L (33.3 ± 7.1)
Alpha₁*	0.6–7.0 gm/L (1.9 ± 2.6)
Alpha₂*	3.1–13.1 gm/L (6.5 ± 1.3)
Beta₁*	4.0–15.8 gm/L (9.2 ± 3)
Beta₂*	2.9–8.9 gm/L (5.7 ± 1.1)
Gamma*	5.5–19.0 gm/L (10.0 ± 1.4)
Albumin/globulin ratio*	0.62–1.46 (0.96 ± 0.17)

§Fasting range

Table continued on following page

6

REFERENCE VALUES FOR NORMAL BLOOD
CHEMISTRY *Continued*

Test	Normal Values
Selenium	15–25 mg/dl
Sodium*	132–146 mmol/L (139 ± 3.5)
Sorbitol dehydrogenase*	0–8 IU/L (3.3 ± 1.3)
Thyroxine (T_4)	11.6–36.0 nmol/L (24.5)
	0.9–2.8 µg/dl (1.9)
Triiodothyronine (T_3)	0.3–0.9 ng/mL
Urate	53.5–65.4 mmol/L
	0.9–1.1 mg/dl
Urea	3.57–8.57 mmol/L
Urea nitrogen*	10–24 mg/dl
Vitamin A	20–175 µg/dl (100)
β-carotene	150–397 µg/dl
Vitamin E (α-tocopherol)	>1.5 µg/mL

Some values affected by hemolysis.
*Indicates that values for these parameters are given for foals at various ages in subsequent tables.
†Reported upper limit considered abnormal.
‡May be higher in some normal horses.
Numbers in parentheses = mean ± standard deviation.
Data from Smith BP. Large Animal Internal Medicine. 2nd ed. St. Louis, Mosby–Year Book, 1996.

REFERENCE VALUES FOR NORMAL URINE CHEMISTRY

	Adult	Foal
Allantoin	5–15 mg/kg/d	
Hydrogen ion, pH (venous and arterial)	7.0–9.0	5.5–8.0
Total nitrogen	100–160 mg/kg/d	
Specific gravity	1.020–1.050	1.001–1.027
Uric acid	1–2 mg/kg/d	
Urine volume	3–18 ml/kg/d	
Creatinine	156–232.5 mg/dl	26.5 ± 13.7 mg/dl
Osmolality	727–1456 mOsm/kg	101.7 ± 24 mOsm/kg
Alkaline phosphatase	10.2 ± 4 IU/L	2.3 ± 1.8 IU/L
Gamma-glutamyl transaminopeptidase	3.3–40.7 IU/L	2.4 ± 2 IU/L
Protein	Neg. to 30	Neg. to 30
Glucose	Neg.	Neg.
Crystals/Ca Carbonate	None	None
Casts	Neg.	Neg.
Hemoprotein	Neg. to +2	Neg. to +2
Bacteria	Neg.	Neg.
Epithelial cells	Squamous or caudate	Squamous or caudate
RBCs	Neg.	Neg.
WBCs	3 per high power field	3 per high power field
Mucus	Neg. to abundant	Neg. to abundant

Data from Smith BP. Large Animal Internal Medicine. 2nd ed. St. Louis, Mosby–Year Book, 1996.

REFERENCE VALUES FOR PLEURAL FLUID

Measurement	Observed Range	Comments
RBC count	22,000–540,000/μl	≤370,000/μl
	22–540 × 10⁹/L	(≤370 × 10⁹/L) in 94% of horses
Total nucleated cell count	800–12,100/μl	≤8000/μl
	0.8–12.1 × 10⁹/L	(≤8.0 × 10⁹/L) in 94% of horses
Differential cell count		
Neutrophils	450–10,290/μl	450–7120/μl
	0.5–10.3 × 10⁹/L	(0.5–7.1 × 10⁹/L) in 94% of horses
	32–91%	
Lymphocytes	0–680/μl	0–10% in 94% of horses
	0–0.7 × 10⁹/L	
	0–22%	
Large mononu- clear cells	50–2620/μl	
	0.1–2.6 × 10⁹/L	
	5–66%	
Eosinophils	0–170/μl	No eosinophils observed in 89% of horses;
	0–0.2 × 10⁹/L	0–1% in 94% of horses
	0–9%	
Specific gravity	1.008–1.031	
Total protein	0.2–4.7 gm/dl	≤2.5 gm/dl (25 gm/L) in 83% of horses;
	2–47 gm/L	≤3.4 gm/dl (≤34 gm/L) in 94% of horses

From Cowell RL, Tyler RD. Cytology and Hematology of the Horse. Galeta, CA, American Veterinary Publications, Inc., 1992.

6

BIOCHEMISTRY REFERENCE VALUES FOR PERITONEAL FLUID (PF)

	Blood	PF
Albumin, gm/dl	1.7–3.9	0.3–1.0
Albumin, gm/L	17–39	3–10
Globulin, gm/dl	3.9–4.6	0.7–1.4
Globulin, gm/L	39–46	7–14
Total protein, gm/dl	4.7–8.9	0.1–2.8
Total protein, gm/L	47–89	1–28
Amylase, IU/L (37° C)	14–35	0–14
AP, IU/L	28–543	0–161
AST, IU/L	133–459	25–213
Total bilirubin, mg/dl	0–5.3	0–1.2
Total bilirubin, μmol/L	0–90	0–20
Creatinine, mg/dl	1.5–1.8	1.8–2.7
Creatinine, μmol/L	130–160	160–240
GGT, IU/L (37° C)	9–29	0–6
Glucose, mg/dl	45–167	74–203
Glucose, mmol/L	2.5–9.3	4.1–11.3
Inorganic phosphorus, mg/dl	0.6–6.8	1.2–7.4
Inorganic phosphorus, mmol/L	0.2–2.2	0.4–2.4
Lactate, mg/dl	6.3–15.3	3.6–10.8
Lactate, mmol/L	0.7–1.7	0.4–1.2
LDH, IU/L	151–590	0–355
Lipase, IU/L (37° C)	23–87	0–36
Urea (BUN), mg/dl	8.1–24.9	10.9–23.2
Urea (BUN), mmol/L	2.9–8.9	3.9–8.3

AP, alkaline phosphatase; AST, aspartate transaminase; GGT, gamma-glutamyl transaminopeptidase; LDH, lactate dehydrogenase; BUN, blood urea nitrogen.

From Cowell RL, Tyler RD. Cytology and Hematology of the Horse. Galeta, CA, American Veterinary Publications, Inc., 1992.

NORMAL HEMATOLOGIC VALUES

Hg*	11.0–19.0 gm/dl
PCV*	32–53%
RBC*	$6.7–12.9 \times 10^6/\mu l$
MCV*	37.0–58.5 fl
MCH*	12.3–19.7 pg
MCHC*	31.0–38.6 gm/dl
Thrombocytes	$1.0–3.5 \times 10^5/\mu l$
WBC*	5400–14300/μl
Neutrophils, mature*	2260–8580/μl
Neutrophils, band	0–100/μl
Lymphocytes*	1500–7700/μl
Neutrophil/lymphocyte ratio	0.8–2.8
Monocytes*	0–1000/μl
Eosinophils*	0–1000/μl
Basophils*	0–290/μl
Platelet count	$100–600 \times 10^3/L$
Plasma proteins*	5.8–8.7 gm/dl
Fibrinogen	200–400 mg/dl
RBC diameter	5.0–6.0 m

*Indicates that values for these parameters are given for foals at various ages in subsequent tables.
HG, hemoglobin; PCV, packed cell volume; MCV, mean corpuscular volume; MCH, mean corpuscular hemoglobin; MCHC, mean corpuscular hemoglobin concentration.
From Blood DC, Radostits OM. Veterinary Medicine, 7th ed. Philadelphia, Bailliere Tindall, 1989.

CAUSE OF ALTERED LEUKOCYTE COUNTS

Neutrophilia

Physiologic	Fear, excitement, brief but strenuous exercise
Corticosteroid-associated	Drugs, severe stress
Inflammation	Various causes
Infection	Bacterial, viral, fungal
Granulocytic leukemia	Very rare

Neutropenia

Defective neutrophil production in bone marrow	Drugs, irradiation, bacterial bone marrow necrosis, myelophthisis, myelofibrosis, osteopetrosis, disseminated granulomatous inflammation, neoplasia
Excessive tissue demand for neutrophils (margination)	Septicemia/endotoxemia (salmonellosis, foal septicemia), severe bacterial infection, blister beetle toxicosis, cecal perforation, colic, chronic enteritis, monocytic ehrlichiosis (Potomac horse fever), phenylbutazone toxicity, immune-mediated neutropenia

Lymphocytosis

Physiologic	Especially high-strung light breeds
Chronic infection	Bacterial, viral
Postvaccination	
Lymphosarcoma/lymphocytic leukemia	Unusual to rare

Lymphopenia

Corticosteroid-associated	Drugs, severe stress
Acute infection	Bacterial, viral
Combined immunodeficiency	Especially Arabian horses

Monocytosis

Suppuration, tissue necrosis	
Hemolysis, hemorrhage	
Potomac horse fever	
Pyogranulomatous inflammation	
Nonhematopoietic neoplasia	
Monocytic/myelomonocytic leukemia	Very rare

From Cowell RL, Tyler RD. Cytology and Hematology of the Horse. Galeta, CA, American Veterinary Publications, Inc., 1992.

REFERENCE VALUES FOR CELLULAR COMPOSITION OF BONE MARROW

Cell Type	Range (%)	Mean (%)
Myeloblasts	0.0–5.0	1.0
Promyelocytes	0.5–3.5	1.7
Neutrophilic myelocytes	1.0–7.5	3.2
Eosinophilic myelocytes	0.0–0.3	0.05
Neutrophilic metamyelocytes	1.5–15.0	5.6
Eosinophilic metamyelocytes	0.0–0.3	0.1
Basophilic metamyelocytes	0.0–0.3	0.08
Band neutrophils	6.0–26.5	15.7
Neutrophils	3.0–16.5	8.4
Eosinophils	0.0–5.0	1.8
Basophils	0.0–1.0	0.3
Total myeloid cells	26.5–45.0	35.7
Rubriblasts	0.0–2.0	0.7
Prorubricytes	1.0–9.5	3.6
Rubricytes	14.5–44.0	28.2
Metarubricytes	14.0–36.0	23.2
Total erythroid cells	47.0–69.0	58.0
Monocytes	0.0–1.0	0.2
Lymphocytes	1.5–8.5	3.8
Plasma cells	0.0–0.2	0.6
Megakaryocytes	0.0–1.0	0.3
Mitotic figures	0.0–3.5	8.0
Myeloid-erythroid ratio	0.48–0.91:1	0.71:1

From Jain NC. Schalm's Veterinary Hematology. 4th ed. Philadelphia, Lea & Febiger, 1986.

6

SERUM ELECTROLYTE CONCENTRATIONS IN FOALS (MEAN ± 2 S.D.)

Age	Na⁺ (mEq/L)	K⁺ (mEq/L)	Cl⁻ (mEq/L)	CO_2 (mEq/L)	HPO_4^- (mg/dl)	Ca^{2+} (mg/dl)	Mg^{2+} (mg/dl)	Anion Gap (mEq/L)
Hours								
<12	148 ± 15	4.4 ± 1.0	105 ± 12	25 ± 5	4.7 ± 1.6	12.8 ± 2.0	1.5 ± 0.8	21 ± 12
Days								
1	141 ± 18	4.6 ± 1.0	102 ± 12	27 ± 6	5.6 ± 1.8	11.7 ± 2.0	2.4 ± 1.8	16 ± 8
3	142 ± 19	4.8 ± 1.4	101 ± 11	28 ± 12	6.4 ± 2.6	12.1 ± 4.4	2.1 ± 0.9	23 ± 4
5							2.2 ± 2.0	
7	142 ± 12	4.8 ± 1.0	102 ± 8	28 ± 4	7.4 ± 2.0	12.5 ± 1.2	2.0 ± 0.6	17 ± 8
14	143 ± 8	4.6 ± 0.8	103 ± 6	26 ± 7	7.8 ± 1.8	12.4 ± 1.2	2.1 ± 1.1	18 ± 6
21	144 ± 8	4.6 ± 1.0	104 ± 11	27 ± 6	7.6 ± 0.8	12.3 ± 1.0	2.3 ± 3.0	18 ± 8
28	145 ± 9	4.6 ± 0.8	103 ± 6	27 ± 5	7.1 ± 2.2	12.2 ± 1.2	2.0 ± 1.0	19 ± 6
Months								
2	148 ± 12	4.8 ± 1.0	105 ± 12	27 ± 5	7.4 ± 1.4	12.3 ± 0.6	2.0 ± 0.8	21 ± 10
3	148 ± 8	4.6 ± 1.2	106 ± 4	27 ± 3	7.3 ± 1.0	12.2 ± 1.0	2.2 ± 0.6	20 ± 8
4	147 ± 12	4.8 ± 1.0	105 ± 11	27 ± 4	6.7 ± 1.8	12.3 ± 1.6	2.4 ± 0.7	21 ± 8
5	145 ± 12	4.5 ± 1.4	107 ± 7	27 ± 5	6.3 ± 1.6	11.8 ± 1.4	2.4 ± 0.6	16 ± 10
6	143 ± 10	4.2 ± 1.4	105 ± 7	26 ± 4	6.2 ± 1.4	11.8 ± 1.6	2.4 ± 0.7	17 ± 8
9	143 ± 5	3.7 ± 1.0	102 ± 6	28 ± 4	6.0 ± 1.4	12.0 ± 1.2	2.3 ± 0.4	16 ± 8
12	146 ± 12	3.8 ± 1.6	104 ± 5	29 ± 2	6.0 ± 0.8	12.7 ± 1.4		17 ± 12
Adults	139 ± 8	4.2 ± 1.0	101 ± 6	26 ± 4	4.5 ± 1.4	12.0 ± 1.2	2.2 ± 0.6	18 ± 8

From Koterba AM, Drummond WH, Koseh PC. Equine Clinical Neonatology. Philadelphia, Lea & Febiger, 1990.

SERUM IRON AND RELATED PARAMETERS

Age	Iron (μg/dl)	UIBC (μg/dl)	TIBC (μg/dl)	Iron Saturation (%)	Ferritin (ng/ml)
Hours					
<1	345–592	4–156	386–663	73–99	34–161
<12	262–488	10–133	339–535	69–98	
Days					
1	78–348	28–416	208–620	22–90	79–263
3	29–191	47–494	175–552	6–66	52–200
5	21–258	129–460	250–581	7–59	54–170
Weeks					
1	30–273	35–503	222–619	10–72	57–173
2	22–215	168–643	337–706	4–52	21–136
3	46–241	228–669	408–745	7–46	27–117
Months					
1	49–288	250–668	437–777	9–50	33–140
2	43–340	201–529	397–716	19–57	32–144
3	61–306	163–478	410–596	12–63	33–223
4	44–236	215–441	356–573	10–49	53–278
5	52–229	185–444	322–591	13–50	30–304
6	85–264	159–467	341–635	16–58	81–331
9	82–277	139–392	320–570	20–62	103–362
12	96–249	159–402	321–584	22–55	103–278
Adults	74–209	177–379	305–542	21–48	58–365

UIBC, unbound iron-binding capacity; TIBC, total iron-binding capacity.
From Koterba AM, Drummond WH, Koseh PC. Equine Clinical Neonatology. Philadelphia, Lea & Febiger, 1990.

6

NORMAL HEMATOLOGIC VALUES IN FOALS

Age	Total Plasma Protein (gm/dl)	Fibrinogen (mg/dl)	Haptoglobin (mg/dl)	Icterus Index (units)	Platelets ($\times 10^3/\mu l$)
Hours					
<1	4.4–5.9	100–500		20–100	
<12	5.1–7.6	100–350	8–120	15–50	105–446
Days					
1	5.2–8.0	100–400	0–136	10–75	129–409
3	5.3–7.9	150–500	8–162	10–50	105–353
5	5.4–7.6	100–500		15–50	
Weeks					
1	5.2–7.5	150–450	0–143	5–25	111–387
2	5.2–7.2	150–600	0–202	5–25	133–457
3	5.2–6.8	150–600	11–184	5–20	134–442
Months					
1	5.1–7.1	200–700	0–214	5–20	136–468
2	5.2–6.8	150–650	15–214	5–25	152–456
3	5.5–7.1	100–800	23–187	5–25	200–376
4	5.9–7.5	250–800	53–182	5–20	140–388
5	6.1–7.3	300–800	32–198	5–20	132–376
6	5.9–7.1	200–550	0–125	5–20	128–368
9	5.6–6.8	200–550	16–127	5–20	105–337
12	5.4–7.0	200–550	0–179	5–20	120–316
Adults	6.2–8.0	100–600	19–177	5–20	100–350

From Koterba AM, Drummond WH, Koseh PC. Equine Clinical Neonatology. Philadelphia, Lea & Febiger, 1990.

RENAL FUNCTION

	2–4-Day-Old Foal	Adult
GFR (ml/kg/min)	2.3–2.8	1.5–2.2
ERPF (ml/kg/min)	15.2–18.2	12.1
FF (GFR/ERPF)	0.15	0.14–0.16

GFR, glomerular filtration rate; ERPF, effective renal plasma flow; FF, filtration fraction.
From Koterba AM, Drummond WH, Koseh PC. Equine Clinical Neonatology. Philadelphia, Lea & Febiger, 1990.

SERUM ENZYME ACTIVITIES (Range, IU/L)

Age	ALP	GGT	SDH	AST*	ALT	CK*
Hours						
<12	152–2835	13–39	0.2–4.8	97–315	0–47	65–380
Days						
1	861–2671	18–43	0.6–4.6	146–340	0–49	40–909
3	283–1462	9.0–40	0.6–3.7	80–580	0–52	21–97
5	156–1294	8.0–89	0.8–5.3			29–208
7	137–1169	14–164	0.8–8.2	237–620	4.0–50	52–143
14	182–859	16–169	0.6–4.3	240–540	1.0–9	46–208
21	146–752	16–132	1.0–8.4	226–540	0–45	44–210
28	210–866	17–99	1.2–5.9	252–440	5.0–47	81–585
Months						
2	201–741	8.0–38	1.1–4.6	282–484	7.0–57	50–170
3	206–458	0–27	1.1–3.9	282–480	8.0–65	57–204
4	124–222	0–27	1.5–4.4	280–520	8.0–65	60–266
5	105–239	0–30	1.3–4.8	225–420	0–65	60–125
6	155–226	0–26	0.3–3.3	300–620	7.0–20	97–396
9	158–232	0–26	0.3–3.3	246–728	4.0–27	97–396
Adults	64–214	5.0–28	0.5–3.0	149–267	4.0–10	69–272

ALP, alkaline phosphatase; GGT, gamma-glutamyl transaminopeptidase; SDH, sorbitol dehydrogenase; AST, aspartate aminotransferase; ALT, alanine transaminase; CK, creatine kinase.

From Koterba AM, Drummond WH, Koseh PC. Equine Clinical Neonatology. Philadelphia, Lea & Febiger, 1990.

*Upper range may be considered abnormal.

LEUKOCYTE COUNTS (× 10³/UL)

Age	Total Leukocytes	Neutrophils	Lymphocytes	Monocytes	Eosinophils	Basophils
Hours						
<12	6.9–14.4	5.55–12.38	0.46–0.43	0.04–0.43	0–0	0–0.02
Days						
1	4.9–11.7	3.36–9.57	0.67–2.12	0.07–0.39	0–0.02	0–0.03
3	5.1–10.1	3.21–8.58	0.73–2.17	0.08–0.58	0–0.22	0–0.12
Weeks						
1	6.3–13.6	4.35–10.55	1.43–2.28	0.03–0.54	0–0.09	0–0.18
2	5.2–11.9	3.99–9.08	1.32–3.12	0.07–0.58	0–0.10	0–0.10
3	5.4–12.4	3.16–8.94	1.47–3.26	0.06–0.69	0–0.16	0–0.09
Months						
1	5.3–12.2	2.76–9.27	1.73–4.85	0.05–0.63	0–0.12	0–0.08
2	5.4–13.5	2.70–9.46	2.37–4.72	0.05–0.61	0–0.28	0–0.10
3	6.7–16.8	3.92–10.35	2.88–7.15	0.12–0.76	0–0.55	0–0.07
4	6.2–14.2	3.01–7.48	2.80–7.32	0.08–0.66	0–0.99	0–0.07
5	6.4–14.6	1.70–8.40	2.37–7.88	0.09–0.51	0–0.58	0–0.06
6	7.8–11.6	2.89–5.56	3.20–6.01	0.04–0.45	0–0.55	0–0.06
9	6.3–11.1	2.60–5.38	2.98–6.59	0.05–0.42	0–0.70	0–0.07
12	6.5–11.8	2.66–5.90	2.01–6.53	0.04–0.44	0–0.78	0–0.09
Adults	5.4–14.3	2.26–8.58	1.50–7.70	0–1.00	0–1.00	0–0.40

From Koterba AM, Drummond WH, Koseh PC. Equine Clinical Neonatology. Philadelphia, Lea & Febiger, 1990.

SERUM PROTEIN VALUES (gm/dl)

Age	Total Protein*	Albumin	Total Globulin	Albumin:Globulin
Hours				
<12	4.0–7.9	2.7–3.9	1.1–4.8	0.7–2.8
Days				
1	4.3–8.1	2.5–3.6	1.5–4.6	0.6–1.9
3	4.4–7.6	2.8–3.7	1.6–4.5	0.7–2.1
5				
7	4.4–6.8	2.7–3.4	2.7–3.4	0.7–1.8
14	4.8–6.7	2.6–3.3	2.6–3.3	0.7–1.7
21	4.7–6.5	2.6–3.2	2.6–3.2	0.8–1.8
28	5.0–6.7	2.7–3.4	2.7–3.4	0.8–1.5
Months				
2	5.2–6.5	2.7–3.5	1.9–3.8	0.7–1.6
3	5.5–7.0	2.8–3.5	2.6–4.1	0.7–1.7
4	5.7–7.3	2.8–3.7	2.7–3.9	0.7–1.3
5	6.0–6.9	2.9–3.4	2.7–4.0	0.8–1.2
6	6.0–6.9	3.0–3.5	2.8–3.7	0.8–1.4
9	5.6–6.7	3.0–3.6	2.2–3.1	1.0–1.6
12	5.8–6.6	3.1–3.8	2.2–3.5	1.0–1.6
Adults	5.5–7.9	2.8–4.8	1.9–3.8	0.7–1.9

From Koterba AM, Drummond WH, Koseh PC. Equine Clinical Neonatology. Philadelphia, Lea & Febiger, 1990.
*Some values within these reported ranges may be considered abnormal.

ERYTHROCYTE PARAMETERS

Age	PCV	Hg (gm/dl)	RBC (× 10⁶/μl)	MCV (ff)	MCHC (gm/dl)
Hours					
<1*	40–52	13.4–19.9	9.3–12.9	37–45	33–39
<12†	37–49	12.6–17.4	9.0–12.0	36–45	32–40
Days					
1	32–46	12.0–16.6	8.2–11.0	36–46	32–40
3	30–46	11.5–16.7	7.8–11.4	35–44	34–40
5	30–44	11.0–16.6	7.2–11.6	35–45	34–40
Weeks					
1	28–43	10.7–15.8	7.4–10.6	35–44	35–40
2	28–41	10.1–15.3	7.2–10.8	35–41	34–40
3	29–40	10.5–14.8	7.8–10.6	34–41	34–40
Months					
1	29–41	10.9–15.3	7.9–11.1	33–40	34–40
2	31–44	11.6–16.0	9.1–13.2	32–38	33–40
3	32–42	11.7–15.3	9.2–12.0	31–38	34–40
4	32–43	11.6–17.2	8.9–12.7	31–37	34–40
5	29–41	10.5–15.2	8.8–11.4	32–38	34–41
6	29–41	10.8–15.4	7.9–11.6	32–39	33–40
9	31–44	10.9–15.9	8.0–11.2	36–43	32–40
12	31–42	11.0–15.4	7.7–10.9	35–44	34–40
Years					
>4	31–47	11.0–18.0	5.9–9.9	41–51	33–41

*Before nursing.
†After nursing.
PCV, packed cell volume; Hg, hemoglobin; RBC, red blood cells; MCV, mean corpuscular volume; MCHC, mean corpuscular hemoglobin concentration; ff, free fraction.
From Koterba AM, Drummond WH, Koseh PC. Equine Clinical Neonatology. Philadelphia, Lea & Febiger, 1990.

SERUM CHEMISTRY CONCENTRATIONS: SMALL ORGANIC MOLECULES (Range, mg/dl)

Age	Glucose	BUN	Creatinine	TBR	CJBR	UNCJBR	Cholesterol	Triglycerides
Hours								
<12	108–190	12.0–27	1.7–4.2	0.9–2.8	0.3–0.6	0.8–2.5	111–432	24–88
Days								
1	121–233	9.0–40	1.2–4.3	1.3–4.5	0.3–0.7	1.0–3.8	110–562	30–193
3	101–226	2.0–29	0.4–2.1	0.5–1.2	0.2–0.8	0.2–3.3	142–350	63–342
5				1.2–3.6	0.1–0.7	0.8–2.8	127–361	52–340
7	121–192	4.0–20	1.0–1.7	0.8–3.0	0.3–0.7	0.5–2.3	139–445	30–239
14	137–205	6.0–13	0.9–1.8	0.7–2.2	0.3–0.6	0.5–1.6	164–287	39–200
21	130–240	6.0–14	0.6–2.0	0.5–1.6	0.2–0.5	0.2–1.1	74–276	34–124
28	130–216	6.0–21	1.1–1.8	0.5–1.7	0.1–0.6	0.4–1.2	83–233	45–155
Months								
2	119–204	6.0–11	1.1–1.2	0.5–2.0	0.2–0.5	0.3–1.5	98–242	10–148
3	88–179	7.0–20	0.7–2.2	0.4–2.0	0.1–0.7	0.4–1.4	110–226	28–151
4	113–196	9.0–25	1.3–2.1	0.3–1.0	0.1–0.6	0.2–0.4	91–207	14–148
5	95–210	11.0–33	1.2–2.1	0.3–1.8	0.1–0.7	0.1–1.1	51–137	14–57
6	110–210	15–30	1.2–2.1	0.3–1.3	0.1–0.7	0.1–0.6	83–173	35–76
9	104–207	16–26	1.1–2.2	0.3–1.1	0.1–0.7	0.2–0.6	11–187	38–86
12	105–165	15–24	1.3–2.1	0.4–1.4	0.1–1.0	0.2–0.6		
Adults	57–96	12.0–24	0.9–2.0	0.5–1.8	0.2–0.7	0.3–1.0	58–109	6.0–44

From Koterba AM, Drummond WH, Koseh PC. Equine Clinical Neonatology. Philadelphia, Lea & Febiger, 1990.
BUN, blood urea nitrogen; TBR, total bilirubin; CJBR, conjugated bilirubin; UNCJBR, unconjugated bilirubin.

APPENDIX III

Anthelmintics

Class	Generic Name	Trade Name	Source	Route of Administration	Dosage
Avermectins					
	Ivermectin	Eqvalan	Merck	liquid, paste	200 µg/kg
		Zinecrin	Farnam	paste	
		Rotectin	TRC Anim. Health	paste	
	Moxidectin	Quest	Fort Dodge Animal Health	paste	0.4 mg/kg
Benzimidazoles					
	Fenbendazole (FBZ)	Panacur	Hoechst	liquid, feed, paste	5–10 mg/kg
		Safeguard	Hoechst	paste	
	Mebendazole (MBZ)	Telmin	Mallinckrodt	tube, feed, paste	1 gm/125kg
	MBZ + TCF	Telmin B	Mallinckrodt	liquid, feed, paste	
	Oxfendazole (OFZ)	Benzelmin	Syntex/Roche	liquid, feed, paste	10 mg/kg
	OFZ + TCF	Benzelmin Plus	Syntex/Roche	liquid, paste	
	Oxibendazole (OBZ)	Anthelcide EQ	Pfizer Animal Health	liquid, feed, paste	10–15 mg/kg
	Thiabendazole (TBZ)	Equipar	Coopers	liquid, paste	
		Equizole	Merck	liquid	
	TBZ + PIP	Equizole A	Merck	liquid	

Table continued on following page

6

695

Anthelmintics *Continued*

Class	Generic Name	Trade Name	Source	Route of Administration	Dosage
Phenylguanidines					
	Febantel (FBT)	Rintal	Bayer	liquid, feed, paste	6 mg/kg
		Cutter horse dewormer	Cutter	paste	
	FBT + TCF	Combotel	Bayer	paste	
Organophosphates					
	Dichlorvos (DDVP)*	Equiguard	Squibb	feed	20 mg/kg
	Trichlorfon (TCF)*	Combotel	Bayer	liquid, paste	
Piperazines					
	Piperazine (PPZ)	Several	Several	liquid	1 oz/45 kg
	PPZ + PTZ + TCF*	Dyrex, T. F.	Ft. Dodge	tube formula	
Pyrimidines					
	Pyrantel (PRT)	Strongid T	Pfizer	liquid	6.6 mg/kg
		Strongidpaste	Pfizer	paste	
		Strongid C	Pfizer	feed	
Other					
	Phenothiazine (PTZ)*	several	several	feed	
	Carbon disulfide (CDS)*	several	several	tube	
	Imidocarb*	Imizad	Coopers	injection	

*No longer available in the United States.
From Smith BP: Large Animal Internal Medicine. 2nd ed. St. Louis, Mosby–Year Book, 1996.

ANTHELMINTIC ACTIVITY ACCORDING TO CLASS OF DRUG

	Large Strongyles	Small Strongyles	Ascarids	Pinworms	Gasterophilus Sp. (Bots)
Avermectins*	X	X	X	X	X
Benzimidazoles	X	X	X	X	
Phenylguanidines	X	X	X	X	
Organophosphates					
Dichlorvos			X	X	X
Trichlorfon			X	X	X
Piperazines		X	X	X	
Pyrimidines	X	X	X	X	
Phenothiazines	X	X		X	
Carbon Disulfide			X		X

*Also rids threadworms, cutaneous onchocerciasis, and summer sores.
From Smith BP: Large Animal Internal Medicine. 2nd ed. St. Louis, Mosby–Year Book, 1996.

SAMPLE ANTHELMINTIC PROGRAMS FOR FOALS 8 WEEKS OR OLDER

Month	Program A	Program B
March/April	Anthelcide EQ	Eqvizole A
May/June	Eqvalan	Eqvalan
July/August	Rintal	Panacur
September/October	Strongid T, paste	Strongid T, paste
November/December	Eqvalan, Benzelmin Plus, or Telmin B	Eqvalan, Benzelmin Plus, or Telmin B

From Koterba AM, Drummond WH, Koseh PC. Equine Clinical Neonatology. Philadelphia, Lea & Febiger, 1990.

SAMPLE ANTHELMINTIC PROGRAM FOR OLDER HORSES

Month	Program A	Program B	Program C
February	Equizole, Panacur, Telmin, or Rintal (alone or with piperazine or trichlorfon)	None	None
April	Eqvalan	Eqvalan	Eqvalan
June	Equiguard	Equizole A or Anth. EQ	None
August	Anthelcide EQ	Strongid T, paste (double dose)	None
October	Strongid T, paste (double dose)	None	None
December	Eqvalan, Equiguard, Telmin B, or Quest	Eqvalan, Equiguard, Dyrex T.F., Telmin B, Combotel, or Quest	Eqvalan, Dyrex T.F., Telmin B, Combotel, or Quest

Do not treat mares within 1 month of foaling.
From Smith BP. Large Animal Internal Medicine. 2nd ed. St. Louis, Mosby–Year Book, 1996.

APPENDIX IV

Vaccination Schedule

SUGGESTED VACCINATION SCHEDULE FOR HORSES*

Disease/ Etiologic Agent	Foals/ Weanlings	Yearlings	Performance Horses	Pleasure Horses	Brood Mares	Comments
Anthrax/ *Bacillus Anthracis*	2 doses, 2–3 weeks apart	Annual	Annual	Annual	Annual	Vaccinate 4 weeks before potential exposure. Placing a horse in a dark stall for 10 days may be beneficial. Local reactions may occur. Do not administer antibiotics within 1 week of vaccination **Not used in United States**
Botulism/ *Clostridium botulinum* Type B toxin	3-dose series at 30-day intervals. Age at first injection dependent on local factors	Annual	Annual	Annual	Annual; 4 weeks prepartum	Only in endemic areas or if travel to endemic area is planned

Encephalomyelitis/ EEE, WEE	First dose: 3–4 months. Second dose: 4–5 months	Annual; spring	Annual; spring	Annual; spring	Annual; 4–6 weeks prepartum	In endemic areas, booster every 6 months
Encephalo-myelitis/VEE	First dose: 3–4 months. Second dose: 4–5 months	Annual; spring	Annual; spring	Annual; spring	Annual; 4–6 weeks prepartum	Only needed when threat of an outbreak exists. This antigen is only available as a combination vaccine with EEE and WEE
Equine influenza/ equine influenza A-equine-1 and A-equine-2	First dose: 3–6 months. Second dose: 4–7 months. Third dose: 5–8 months. Repeat at 3-month intervals	Every 3 months	Every 3 months	Annual, with added boosters prior to likely exposure	At least biannual; with 1 booster 4–6 weeks prepartum	A series of at least 3 doses is recommended for primary immunization of foals Vaccination response might not be seen in foals < 7 months

Table continued on following page

6

701

SUGGESTED VACCINATION SCHEDULE FOR HORSES* Continued

Disease/ Etiologic Agent	Foals/ Weanlings	Yearlings	Performance Horses	Pleasure Horses	Brood Mares	Comments
Equine viral arteritis/equine arteritis virus					Annual; vaccinate mares that plan to be bred to a positive stallion at least 3 weeks before breeding. Pregnant mares should not be vaccinated the last 2 months of gestation	Vaccination of stallions at least 3 weeks before breeding season is occasionally performed. Prior authorization by state veterinarian is required. Permit may be necessary. Regulations vary with state. Vaccinated horses may be ineligible for export due to seroconversion
Potomac horse fever/*Ehrlichia risticii*	First dose: 3–4 months. Second dose: 4–5 months	Biannual	Biannual	Biannual	Biannual; with 1 dose 4–6 weeks prepartum	Booster during May to June in endemic areas
Rabies/rabies virus	First dose: 3–6 months. Second dose: 6–7 months	Annual	Annual	Annual	Annual; before breeding	Rabies vaccination recommended in endemic areas

Disease/Agent	Primary Series				Broodmare	Comments
Rhinopneumonitis/ equine Herpesvirus Type 1	First dose: 2–3 months. Second dose: 3–4 months. Third dose: 4–5 months. Repeat at 3-months intervals	Every 3 months	Every 3 months	Optional: biannual if elected	Fifth, seventh, ninth month of gestation (inactivated EHV-1 vaccine) Vaccinate mares before breeding and 4–6 weeks prepartum	If primary series is started before 3 months of age, a 3-dose primary series is preferred
Strangles/ *Streptococcus equi*	First dose: 8–12 weeks. Second dose: 11–15 weeks. Third dose: 14–18 weeks (depending on product use). Fourth dose: weaning (6–8 months)	Biannual	Optional; biannual if risk is high	Optional; biannual if risk is high	Biannual, with 1 dose 4–6 weeks prepartum	Vaccines containing M-protein extract may be less reactive than whole-cell vaccines. Can be used when endemic conditions exist or risk is high
Tetanus/ *Clostridium tetani*	First dose: Before 3–4 months. Second dose: 4–5 months	Annual	Annual	Annual	Annual; 4–6 weeks prepartum	Booster at time of penetrating injury or surgery if last dose not administered within the last 6 months

As with administration of all medications, read the label and product insert before administration of all vaccines. Stallion schedules should be consistent with the vaccination program of the adult population on the farm and modified according to risk.

EEE, Eastern Equine Encephalomyelitis; WEE, Western Equine Encephalomyelitis; VEE, Venezuelan Equine Encephalomyelitis.

Modified from Smith BP: Large Animal Internal Medicine. 2nd ed. St. Louis, Mosby–Year Book, 1996.

*Varies between regions and farms.

6

Product Manufacturers

Abbott Hospitals, Inc.
North Chicago, IL 60064
Abbocath-T radiopaque FEP Teflon IV catheter (14-gauge, 2-inch-long)

Abbott Laboratories
North Chicago, IL 60064
Extension Set (7- or 30-inch)

Air Vet (Bivona) Inc.
5425 Raines Road, Suite 3
Memphis, TN 38115
(800) 343 6237
Silicone cuffed endotracheal tubes (sizes 7, 9, 10, 12 mm, 55-cm-long)

A.J. Buck and Son, Inc.
See under Buck.

Arrow International, Inc.
P.O. Box 12888
3000 Bernville Road
Reading, PA 19612
(610) 378 0131
Central venous catheter (16-gauge, 8-inch)

Ayerst Laboratories, Inc.
New York, NY 10017
Fluor-I-Strip (fluorescein sodium ophthalmic strip)

Baker Cummins Pharmaceuticals, Inc.
Miami, FL 32178
(800) 374 4774
Baker's biopsy punch

C.R. Bard, Inc.
Covington, GA 30209
(800) 526 4455
Bard Monopty biopsy instrument

Baxter Healthcare Corporation
Deerfield, IL 60015
Jamshidi disposable bone marrow biopsy/aspiration needle

Baxter Healthcare Corporation
Pharmaseal Division
Valencia, CA 91355–8900
Tru-Cut biopsy needle
Pharmaseal K75 3-way stopcock

Becton-Dickinson
Franklin Lakes, NJ 07417
Spinal needles

Becton-Dickinson Microbiology Systems
Cockeysville, MD 21030
Culturette collection and transport system
Port-a-Cul

Becton-Dickinson Vacutainer Systems
Rutherford, NJ 07070
Vacutainer needles
Vacutainer cuffs
Vacutainer blood tubes

Bivona, Inc.
Gary, IN
(800) 348 6064
Cuffed silicone nasotracheal tube, 7–10-mm diameter, 55-cm-long

Boehringer Mannheim
9115 Hague Road
Indianapolis, IN 46250
(800) 858 8072
Dextrometer (ACCU-CHEK III—Chemstrip bG)

Breathing Services, Inc.
P.O. Box 817
931 East Main Street
Ephrata, PA 17522
(800) 732 0028
Flowmeter/humidifier
Hudson Model 5040 demand valve
Adult human Ambu bag, PMR-2 manual resuscitator (self-inflating bag with accumulator)

A.J. Buck and Son, Inc.
11407 Cronhill Drive
Owings Mills, MD 21117
(800) 638 8672
FAX: (410) 581 1809
Jacobs chuck

The Butler Company
5000 Bradenton Avenue
P.O. Box 7153
Dublin, OH 43017–0753
Ideal udder infusion cannula

CDA Products
P.O. Box 53
Potter Valley, CA 95461
(707) 431 1300
FAX: (707) 443 2530
Anderson sling

6

Cook Veterinary Products
   127 South Main Street
   P.O. Box 266
   Spencer, IN 47460
   (800) 826 2380
   Cuffed endotracheal tubes
   Cuffed foal nasotracheal tubes
   Thal-Quick chest drainage catheter set (24–36 F., 41-cm-long)
   Heimlich chest drainage valve
   Stallion Foley catheter (28 F. Foley)
   Uterine flushing tube (33 F., 80-cm-long)

Cook Veterinary Products
   P.O. Box 489
   Bloomingham, IN 47402
   (800) 826 2380
   Silicone cuffed endotracheal tubes (sizes 7, 9, 10, 12 mm, 55-cm-long)

Critikon, Inc.
   5820 West Cypress, Suite B
   Tampa, FL 33634
   (813) 887 2000
   Noninvasive blood pressure monitor

Datascope Corporation
   580 Winters Avenue
   Paramus, NJ 07632
   (800) 288 2121
   Noninvasive blood pressure monitor
   Electrocardiogram

Davol Inc.
   100 Sockanosset Crossroad
   Cranston, RI 02920
   (401) 463 7000
   Intranasal O_2 tubing (16 F. Levin, 127-cm tubing)

Deseret Medical Inc.
   Becton-Dickinson and Co.
   Sandy, UT 84070
   Intracath intravenous catheter placement unit

Hartford Veterinary Supply
   9100 Persimmon Tree Road
   Potomac, MD 20854
   Double-guarded uterine swab

High Horse, Inc.
   Reno, NV 72851–1217
   Velcro foam leg wraps
   Velcro foam helmet

Howmedica Inc.
359 Veterans Blvd
Rutherford, NJ 07070
Surgical Simplex P (polymethylmethacrylate)

IMED Corporation
9775 Businesspark Avenue
San Diego, CA 92131–1192
(800) 854 2033
IV pumps (Gemini PC-1)

Immvac
6080 Bass Lane
Columbia, MO 65201
(573) 443 5363
Endoserum

International Win, LTD
340 North Mill Road, Suite 6
Kennett Square, PA 19348
(800) 359 4946
Large animal extension set (large-bore, 7-inch)
Stat large animal IV set (large-bore, 10-feet-long)

J.A. Webster, Inc.
See under Webster.

Johnson and Johnson Medical, Inc.
Arlington, TX 76004–3130
Elasticon
K-Y lubricating jelly

Jorgensen Laboratories, Inc.
1450 North Van Buren Avenue
Loveland, CO 80538
(970) 669 2500
Jackson uterine biopsy forceps
Tracheotomy tube (18- or 28-mm internal diameter)
Metal bitch urinary catheter

Karl Storz Veterinary Endoscopy-America, Inc.
177 Cremona Drive
Goleta, CA 93117
(800) 955 7832
Flexible Fiberoptic Endoscopes: 11-mm outer diameter, 100-cm-long; 12-mm
    outer diameter, 160-cm-long; 8-mm outer diameter, 150-cm-long

Laerdal Medical Corporation
1 Labriola Court
Armonk, NY 10504
(800) 431 1055
Laerdal Silicone resuscitator (adult size, 1600 ml; with O_2 reservoir bag,
    2600 ml)
Compact suction unit

6

Lake Immunogenics
  348 Berg Road
  Ontario, NY 14519
  (800) 648 9990
  HiGamm Equi: [IgG] = 2500 mg/dl
  Plasma products

Mila International, Inc.
  510 West Sixth Street
  Covington, KY 41011
  (606) 261 6631
  Milacath polyurethane catheter-over-needle
  Guidewire catheters (14- or 16-gauge, 8-inch). Single and double lumen
    styles available

Mill-Rose Labs, Inc.
  7310 Corporate Boulevard
  Mentor, OH 44060
  (216) 255 7995
  Darien microbiological aspiration catheter

Monoject
  Sherwood Medical
  St. Louis, MO 63103
  Dose syringe with catheter tip

Olympus America Inc.
  2 Corporate Center Drive
  Melville, NY 11747
  (516) 844 5000
  Flexible Videoendoscopes:
  GIF 130 Gastroscope (9.8-mm outer diameter, 200- or 300-cm-long)
  SIF 100 (11.2-mm outer diameter, 300-cm-long)
  CF 100 TL (12.9-mm outer diameter, 200- or 300-cm-long)

Pall Biomedical Products Corporation
  Glen Cove, NY 11542
  (800) 645 6578
  HME filter (heat-moisture exchange filter)

Physiocontrol Corporation
  P.O. Box 97006
  Redmond, WA 98073–9706
  Defibrillator with ECG (Life Pak-10)

Puritan Bennett Corporation
  9410 Indian Creek PKY#300
  Shawnee Mission, KS 66225–5905
  (913) 661 0444
  Bubble-jet humidifier

Roche Diagnostic Systems
  Nutley, NJ 07110–1199
  Septi-Check, BB blood culture bottle

Rusch Inc.
53 West 23rd Street
New York, NY 10010
(212) 675 5556
Silicone cuffed endotracheal tubes (sizes 7, 9, 10, 12-mm, 55-cm-long)

Rusch, Inc.
Duluth, GA 30136
(800) 553 5214/50
Nasal catheter "Levin tubes" 235200-160

Safe and Warm, Inc.
Boulder City, NV 89005
(800) 421 3237
Intratherm (warm IV fluid pouch)
Safe and Warm reusable instant heat, $7'' \times 9''$

Schein Pharmaceutical
Florham Park, NJ 07932
Progesterone Injection USP

Sherwood Medical
1915 Olive Street
St. Louis, MO 63103
(800) 428 4400
Monoject 60-ml syringe with catheter tip
Polypropylene catheter
Feline indwelling catheter (20-gauge)

StatPal II—PPG Industries
Biomedical Systems Division
11077 Torrey Pines Road
La Jolla, CA 92037
(800) 369 3457
Blood gas analyzer

Stortz Instrument Co.
St. Louis, MO 63122
Dow-Corning Silastic tubing

Synthes (USA)
P.O. Box 1766
1690 Russell Road
Paoli, PA 19301–0800
(800) 523 0322
Steinmann pin (sizes 2.5, 3.2, 4.5, 6.34-mm)

Thomas Register of American Manufacturers
5 Penn Plaza
New York, NY 10001
(212) 290 7277 or (800) 222 7900, Ext 200
Information on every manufacturer in the United States

The Upjohn Co.
Kalamazoo, MI 49001

Veterinary Dynamics, Inc.
P.O. Box 2406
Chino, CA 91708–2406
(800) 654 9743
Polymune Plus: [IgG] = 2500 mg/dl

VWR Scientific
200 Center Square Road
Bridgeport, NJ 08014
(609) 467 3333
O_2 line (clear vinyl tubing 3/8″ ID, 1/2″ OD, 1/16″ thick)

J.A. Webster, Inc.
86 Leominster Road
Sterling, MA 01564–2198
(800) 222 7911
400-ml nylon dose syringe

Registry Information for the Breeds of Horses

AMERICAN ALBINO

International American Albino Association
Route 1, Box 20
Naper, NE 68755
(402) 832 5560

American White. must have pink skin and true white coloring, no slight pigmentation of hair allowed. May have a few small scattered spots only on the skin and not the hair. These spots are usually found around eye and chest and genital areas. All eye colors accepted. Will reproduce 50% white when bred to colored stock.

American Cream. must also have pink skin but its coat color may vary from a pale ivory to a deep rich creme. Mane and tail may vary from true white through varying shades of creme to a rich cinnamon-buff. Eyes are usually pale, but all eye colors are accepted. Will reproduce its color 100% when bred to a Creme. When bred to colored stock, it will dilute its color, i.e., Chestnut × Creme = Palomino; Bay × Creme = Buckskin or Dun.

AMERICAN PAINT HORSE

American Paint Horse Association
P.O. Box 961023
Fort Worth, TX 76161–0023
(817) 439 3400
FAX: (817) 439 3484

American Paint Horse has a unique combination of white and any one of the colors of the equine rainbow: black, bay, brown, chestnut, dun, grulla, sorrel, palomino, gray, or roan.

ANDALUSIAN

International Andalusian Horse Association
1201 S. Main, #D-7
Boerne, TX 78006
(512) 249 4027

Of Spanish descent: usually white, gray, or bay. Stands about 15.2 hands.

6

APPALOOSA

Appaloosa Horse Club
5070 Hwy. 8 West
P.O. Box 8403
Moscow, ID 83843
(208) 882 5578

Noted for its spotted coat, which may be an all-over spotted pattern, consisting of dark spots on a white background (leopard); light spots on a dark background (snowflake); and spots on the quarters and loins only (spotted blanket). Any color combination permissible. Skin of the nose, lips, and genitalia is mottled, and there is white sclera around the eye. Hooves are often vertically striped. Sparse mane and tail. Usually about 15.2 hands.

ARABIAN

Arabian Horse Trust
12000 Zuni Street
Westminster, CO 80234
(303) 450 4710

Typical characteristics: dished profile, prominent eyes, large nostrils, and small teacup muzzle. Graceful arched neck arising out of a long sloping shoulder and broad chest. Short, strong back. Usually gray, chestnut bay, or roan and occasionally solid black. Most between 14.2 and 15.2 hands and 800–1000 pounds.

BELGIAN

Belgian Draft Horse Corporation of America
P.O. Box 335
Wabash, IN 46992–0335
(219) 563 3205

Native of the country of Belgium. A heavy, powerful, drafty breed. Usually stands between 16 and 17 hands. Short back, deep girth, and short legs. Often a pronounced thick, crested neck and feathered fetlocks.

BUCKSKIN

American Buckskin Registry Association
P.O. Box 1125
Anderson, CA 96007
International Buckskin Horse Association
P.O. Box 268
Shelby, IN 46377
(219) 552 1013

A color designation: horses with tan or light brown coats.

CHINCOTEAGUE PONY

The National Chincoteague Pony Association
Gale Park Frederick
2595 Jensen Road
Bellingham, WA 98226
(206) 671 8338

Small, hardy, and compact. These wild ponies live on the islands of Chincoteague and Assateague off the coast of Virginia and Maryland.

CLEVELAND BAY

The Cleveland Bay Horse Society of North America
P.O. Box 211
South Windham, CT 06266

"The English Warmblood." The oldest established breed of English horse. Has been bred free of outcrosses since 1884, resulting in a very "pure" breed, with remarkable uniformity of size, conformation, soundness, stamina, disposition, and color. Large, convex head and longish neck, good shoulders, deep girth, and strong, though fairly long back. Strong quarters and short legs. Usually bay-colored and between 16 and 16.2 hands. Noted for their intelligence, temperament, strength, stamina, and longevity.

CLYDESDALE

Clydesdale Breeders of the USA
17378 Kelley Road
Pecatonica, IL 61063
(815) 247 8780

A breed of heavy draft horse originating in Scotland. Large, open forehead (broad between the eyes), a flat, neither Roman-nosed nor dished profile, a wide muzzle, well-arched long neck, oblique shoulder, and high withers. Short back, sharp hocks, and broad, flat knees. Most range in size from 16.2 to 18 hands and weight between 1600 and 1800 pounds. Most common color is bay but black, brown, chestnut, and roan are also seen. Preferred markings include four white socks to the knees and hocks and a well-defined blaze or bald face.

CONNEMARA PONY

American Connemara Pony Society
P.O. Box 513
Goshen, CT 06756–0513
(540) 722 2277

Native of Ireland. Usually 13–14.2 hands; sturdy, general purpose riding pony.

6

DARTMOOR PONY

The American Dartmoor Pony Association
1005 Pearlwood Road
Albany, OH 45710

Sensible and surefooted, with a reputation as a naturally good jumper. Native to Britain. Short, compact body. Black, brown, and bay with only a small amount of white markings are the acceptable colors, and the height limit is 12.2 hands.

DUTCH WARMBLOOD

In the Americas:

Koninklijk Warmbloed (USA)
P.O. Box 956
Winchester, OR 97495–0956
(503) 672 8145
FAX: (503) 672 1721

Outside the Americas:

KWPN
Postbus 382
3700 AJ Ziest
The Netherlands 03404–32004
FAX: 03404-31455

EXMOOR PONY

American Exmoor Pony Registry
American Minor Breeds Conservancy
Box 477
Pittsboro, NC 27312–0477
(919) 542 5704

An exceptionally tough, strong pony noted for its endurance. Highly intelligent and independent. The height limit is 12.2 hands for mares and 12.3 hands for stallions. Colors may be bay, brown, and a mousy dun, with no white markings permitted. They have unique "toad" eyes—heavy top lids, which give a hooded look.

FRIESIAN

The Friesian Horse Association of North America
4127 Kentridge Dr., SE
Grand Rapids, MI 49508–3705
(616) 455 7913

One of Europe's oldest breeds. Relatively small in stature, standing around 15 hands. It is compact and muscular, with a fine head, strong body, short legs, with some feathers at the fetlock. The color is exclusively black with no white markings.

HACKNEY

American Hackney Horse Society
4059 Iron Works Pike
Lexington, KY 40511–8462
(606) 255 8694

Originated in Great Britain, a descendant of both Arabian and Thoroughbred lines. Usually used as a driving horse, it boasts an extravagant, elevated trot. Spirited disposition, neat head, well-arched neck and high-set tail. The usual colors are bay, brown, black, and chestnut, and the average height is about 15 hands.

HANOVERIAN

Purebred Hanoverian Association of American Breeders and Owners, Inc.
P.O. Box 429
Rocky Hill, NJ 08553
(409) 466 9543

The foremost German warmblood. Big and strong, usually between 16 and 17 hands. Primarily in demand as a dressage horse and in show jumping. All colors are permissible, the most common being brown, chestnut, bay, and black.

HOLSTEINER

The American Holsteiner Horse Association
222 East Main Street, Suite 1
Georgetown, KY 40324
(502) 863 4239

Another German warmblood. Strong, steady, and reliable, ideally suited as a sport horse in dressage, jumping, driving, and eventing. Medium frame and usually between 16 and 17 hands, powerful hind end, strong back and loin.

ICELANDIC

United States Icelandic Horse Federation
38 Park Street
Montclair, NJ 07042
(201) 783 3429

Small and stocky, deep through the girth, and with a rather large head set on a short, thick neck. One of the toughest pony breeds, noted for their intelligence, independence, and homing instinct. They have an abundance of mane and tail hair and feather on the fetlocks. Usually gray or dun and between 12 and 13 hands.

6

LIPIZZAN

United States Lipizzan Registry
13351 Chula Road
Amelia, VA 23002

Sturdy, intelligent, and docile. Born dark, black-brown, brown, or mousy gray, they turn white somewhere between the ages of 6 and 10 years. A smallish horse, averaging 14.3 to 15.3 hands. Heavy shoulders and short, strong legs with well defined tendons and joints. Tail carried high, and long and thick, like the mane.

MINIATURE

American Miniature Horse Association, Inc.
2908 SE Loop 820
Fort Worth, TX 76140
(817) 293 0041

American Miniature Horse Registry
6748 N. Frostwood Pkwy.
Peoria, IL 61615–2402
(309) 263 4132

A small, sound, well-balanced horse; must measure not more than 34″ at the base of the last hair on the mane for Division A, and not more than 38″ for Division B.

MORAB

International Morab Breeders Association (IMBA)
S. 101 W. 34828 Hwy. 99
Eagle, WI 53119–1857
(414) 594 3667
FAX: (414) 594 5136

Combines the best genetic traits of its parents' breeds, the Arabian and Morgan horse.

MORGAN

American Morgan Horse Association
P.O. Box 960
Shelburne, VT 05482–0960
(802) 985 4944

Stands up to 15.2 hands and makes an ideal all-around pleasure horse. Frequently shown both under saddle and in harness. Strong shoulders, and short, strong back legs. Usual colors are bay, chestnut, brown, and black.

PAINT

American Paint Horse Association
P.O. Box 96102
Fort Worth, TX 76161–0023
(817) 439 3400

To register, must prove parentage from one of three approved registries: AQHA, TB, or APHA, as well as meet a minimum color requirement.

PALOMINO

Palomino Horse Breeders of America
15253 E. Skelly Drive
Tulsa, OK 74116–2637

A color registry. Horses stand between 14 and 17 hands and exhibit a coat color with variations, from light to dark of a United States 14-karat gold coin. The skin is usually gray, black, brown, or motley, without underlying pink skin or spots except on the face and legs. The eyes are usually black, hazel, or brown. The mane and tail must be white, with not more than 15% dark, sorrel, or chestnut hairs. There are three basic divisions of Palomino horses. The stock type are western horses predominantly represented by Quarter Horses. The Golden American Saddlebred is typically represented by Saddlebreds, and the pleasure type exemplified by Morgan, Arabian, and Tennessee Walking Horses.

PASO FINO

The Paso Fino Horse Association
P.O. Box 600 F
Bowling Green, FL 33834
(813) 375 4331

What distinguishes this breed is what is felt to be a genetically inherent gait. It is a lateral four-beat gait in which the horse's feet fall in a natural lateral pattern instead of the more common diagonal pattern. The gait is evenly spaced, with each foot contacting the ground independently. They range in size from 13.2 to 15.2 hands, with any color permissible.

PERCHERON

Percheron Horse Association of America
P.O. Box 141
Fredericktown, OH 43019
(614) 694 3602

A more high-strung horse than the other draft-type horses. It is a well proportioned, gray or black heavy horse, standing between 15.2 and 17 hands.

PINTO

National Pinto Horse Registry
P.O. Box 486

6

Oxford, NY 13830–0486
(607) 334 4964

Pinto Horse Association of America, Inc.
1900 Samuels Avenue
Fort Worth, TX 76102–1141
(817) 336 7842

This is a color registry, and Pintos may be of any breed.

PONY OF THE AMERICAS

Pony of the Americas Club, Inc.
5240 Elmwood Ave.
Indianapolis, IN 46203–5990
(317) 788 0107

A relatively recent breed, founded by crossing a Shetland stallion and an Appaloosa mare. A small, useful child's pony with plenty of substance. The height must be between 11.2 and 13 hands, and any of six Appaloosa colors are permissible.

QUARAB

The United Quarab Registry
P.O. Box 12754
Ogden, UT 84412–2754

QUARTER HORSE

American Quarter Horse Association
P.O. Box 200
Amarillo, TX 79168
(806) 376 4811

Used as an all-purpose riding and harness horse and raced over short distances. A compact horse with a kind disposition, massive, powerful quarters, strong shoulders, and a short muscular back. The average height is about 15.2 hands, and any solid color is permissible. An exceptionally good mount for working cattle.

SADDLEBRED

The American Saddlebred Horse
4093 Iron Works Pike
Lexington, KY 40511
(606) 259 2742

Primarily bred for the show ring, where they can compete in three types of classes: in light harness, as a three-gaited saddler, or as a five-gaited saddler. Small head set on a long muscular neck with strong shoulders, back, and quarters and an artificially high tail carriage. Predominant colors are bay, brown, black, and chestnut, and the average height is 15 to 16 hands.

SELLE FRANCAIS

North American Selle Francais Horse Association, Inc
P.O. Box 646
Winchester, VA 22601-0646
(703) 662 2870

A good-quality type of hunter horse, whose registry dates back only to 1965. It stands between 15.2 and 16.3 hands and is a strong horse of good conformation and temperament, well suited to competitive sports such as show-jumping, eventing, and dressage. Any color is permissible, but chestnut is predominant.

SHETLAND PONY

American Shetland Pony Club
6748 N. Frostwood Pkwy.
Peoria, IL 61615–2402
(309) 691 9661

SHIRE

The American Shire Horse Association
2354 315 Court
Andel, IA 50003
(515) 993 3113

One of the largest horses in the world. It stands up to 18 hands and may be bay, brown, black, or gray. An immensely strong, big barrelled horse, although a gentle, good-natured agricultural and draft worker.

SPANISH BARB

Spanish Barb Breeders Association
188 Springridge Rd
Terry, MS 39170
(601) 372 8801

STANDARDBRED

US Trotting Association
750 Michigan Ave.
Columbus, OH 53215
(614) 224 2291
(614) 228 1385

Among the world's finest harness racehorses. May be raced as trotters or as pacers. A medium-sized horse standing between 15.2 and 16 hands, and the predominant colors are bay, brown, black, and chestnut.

6

TARPAN

American Tarpan Studbook Association
  1658 Coleman Ave.
  Macon, GA 31201-6602
  (912) 741 2062

TENNESSEE WALKING HORSE

Tennessee Walking Horse Breeders' & Exhibitors' Association
  P.O. Box 286
  Lewisburg, TN 37091
  (615) 359 1574

Claimed to be the most comfortable ride in the world. A characteristic feature of the breed is its peculiar four-beated gait that is half walk and half run. A notably good-tempered horse, with particularly powerful shoulders and strong limbs. It stands around 15 to 15.2 hands and is usually black, bay, and chestnut.

THOROUGHBRED

The Jockey Club
  821 Corporate Drive
  Lexington, KY 40503–2794
  (606) 224 2700

Bred extensively for flat racing but its athleticism allows it to be successful in all equestrian sports. Any color is permissible, and the height can vary from as little as 14.2 to well over 17 hands.

TRAKEHNER

American Trakehner Association
  1520 West Church Street
  Newark, OH 43055
  (614) 344 1111

A large horse standing between 16 and 17 hands. Characterized by great substance and bone, yet refined. An excellent performance horse, particularly in dressage and show jumping.

WELSH PONY AND COB

Welsh Pony and Cob Society of America
  P.O. Box 2977
  Winchester, VA 22604
  (703) 667 6195

A courageous and intelligent riding pony. The height limit is 13.2 hands, and any color is permissible except piebald or skewbald.

Index

Note: Page numbers in *italics* refer to illustrations; page numbers followed by t refer to tables.

Abaxial sesamoid nerve block, of distal limb, 66, *66*
"ABCD," of cardiopulmonary resuscitation, 125
Abdomen, examination of, in newborn foal, 476–478
Abdominal muscles, rupture of, 428–429
Abdominal pain, 156. See also *Colic.*
  analgesics for, 158t
    response to, 160
  associated with colitis, treatment of, 220–223
  signs of, 157
Abdominal quadrants, auscultation of, for intestinal borborygmi, 158–159
Abdominocentesis, 55–59
  complications of, 57, 59
  equipment for, 55–56
  in assessment of gastrointestinal emergencies, 161
  in newborn foal, 478
  peritoneal fluid following, 57, 58t
  procedure for, 56
Abortion, 211
  induced, for hydrops of fetal membranes, 420
Abrasion(s), corneal, 390–393
  penile, 409
Abscess, as complication of abdominocentesis, 57
  as complication of cecal trocharization, 60
  as complication of intramuscular drug administration, 9
  as complication of paranasal trephination, 49
  cerebral, 361–363
Accidental intra-arterial injection, as complication of intravenous drug administration, 9
ACE (angiotensin-converting enzyme) inhibitors, 582
  for congestive heart failure, 138

Acepromazine, 570–571
  dosage of, 666
  for duodenitis/jejunitis, 189
  for laminitis, 326
  for tetanus, 355
  overdose of, treatment for, 592t
Acetazolamide, 585
  dosage of, 666
  for hyperkalemic periodic paralysis, 354
Acetylcholine, dosage of, 666
  for ventricular fibrillation, 128t
Acetylcysteine, dosage of, 666
  for corneal ulcers, 394
N-Acetyl-L-cysteine, dosage of, 666
Acetylpromazine, for laminitis, 326
  for orthopedic emergencies, 298t
Acute renal failure, 462–465
  causes of, 462–463
  nephropathy in, 463–464
  treatment of, 464–465
α-Adrenergic drugs, 581–582
Aflatoxicosis, 616
Agalactia, 430–431
  treatment of, in foal, 430–431
    in mare, 431
α-Agonists, 580–581
β-Agonists, 580–581
Airway, clearance of, during birth resuscitation, 532
  endoscopic examination of, 31–32
  establishing, in foals, 510, *511–512,* 512
  intubation of, complications of, 36
    via mouth, 35–36
    via nose, 34–35
  obstruction of, 435–443
  patency of, in cardiopulmonary resuscitation, 126, 128t
Albumin, normal values of, 697
Albuterol, dosage of, 666
  for bronchointerstitial pneumonia, 455
  for respiratory disorders, 576
  for smoke inhalation, 448
  for viral respiratory distress syndrome, 451

Albuterol *(Continued)*
    overdose of, treatment for, 592t
Alfalfa, in diet, 662t
Algae poisoning, 631–632
Alkaloid poisoning, pyrrolizidine, 280,
    438, 618–619, *619*
Alpha-adrenergic drugs, 581–582
Alpha-agonists, 580–581
Alsike clover poisoning, causing liver
    failure, 283, 617
Altrenogest, dosage of, 666
    overdose of, treatment for, 592t
Ambu bag, ventilation using, in foals, 43,
    513
American albino horse, registry
    information for, 711
American paint horse, registry information
    for, 711, 717
Amikacin, dosage of, 666
    for bacterial pneumonia, 454
    for esophageal perforation, 169
    for infections, in newborns and foals,
        334t
    for lacerations, 315t
    for necrotizing enterocolitis, 228
    for peritonitis, 217
    for salmonellosis, 230
    for septicemia, 489
Aminocaproic acid, 586
    dosage of, 666
Aminoglycosides, 568–569
    overdose of, treatment for, 592t
    toxicity of, 630
Aminophylline, dosage of, 667
    for renal failure, 465
    for respiratory disorders, 576
Amitraz, overdose of, treatment for, 592t
    toxicity of, 601–602
Ammonia intoxication, 608
Amphotericin B overdose, treatment for,
    592t
Ampicillin, for lacerations, 315t
Analgesic drugs, for abdominal pain, 158t,
    163
    response to, 160
    in field emergencies, 647–650, 648t
Anaphylaxis, 435–436
    causing edema, 266–267
    drug-induced, 590
    pulmonary edema secondary to, 446–
        447
Andalusian horse, registry information for,
    711
Anemia, and wound healing, 243
    classification of, *286*
    diagnosis of, 284–285

Anemia *(Continued)*
    hemolytic, 284–291
        immune-mediated, 287–288
        other causes of, 289–291
        toxin-induced, 285, 287
    infectious, 265, 290–291
Anesthesia, for eyelid laceration repair,
    385
    in field emergencies, 646–656
        analgesic, anesthetic, and restraint
            drugs for, 647–650, 648t
        cardiovascular support with, 652
        depth of anesthesia and, 651
        equipment for, 646–647
        euthanasia and, 652
        for cardiopulmonary resuscitation,
            654, *655*, 656t
        for colic, 654
        for dystocia, 653
        for extrications and entrapments, 654
        for fractures, 653
        for seizures, 653
        for severe lacerations, 653
        hyperkalemic periodic paralysis and,
            652
        ileus and, 652
        monitoring of, 651
        positioning and paddling for, 652
        respiratory support with, 651–652
        resuscitation and support drugs for,
            648t, 650–651
        selected protocols for, 654, 656
    local. See *Local anesthesia.*
    topical, for ocular emergencies, 380
Anesthesia bag, ventilation with, for foals,
    513
Anesthesia kit, emergency, 646–647
Anesthetic drugs, in field emergencies,
    647–650, 648t
    short-acting, 570–572
Aneurysm, sinus of Valsalva, ruptured,
    154–155
Angiotensin-converting enzyme (ACE)
    inhibitors, 582
    for congestive heart failure, 138
Anhydrosis, 544
Anoplocephala perfoliata infestation, 185
Antacids, dosage of, 667
Antebrachial nerve block, of proximal
    forelimb, 68, *68*
Anthelmintics, 686–687
    activity of, according to class of drug,
        688
    for foals 8 weeks and older, 689
    for older horses, 690
    overdose of, treatment for, 592t

Anthelmintics *(Continued)*
  respiratory distress after, in foals, 455–456
Anthrax, vaccination schedule for, 700
Antiarrhythmic therapy, 583–584. See also
      specific agent, e.g., *Dexamethasone.*
  adverse effects of, 125t
  indications for and dosages of, 124t
Antibiotics, 565–570. See also specific
      antibiotic, e.g., *Penicillin.*
  diarrhea induced by, 218
    in weanlings and yearlings, 235–236
    treatment of, 222
  for acute abdominal pain, 164
  for bacterial pneumonia, 454
  for cellulitis, 268
  for cholangiohepatitis, 277
  for corneal abrasions, 393
  for corneal ulcers, 393, 394
  for esophageal perforation, 169
  for infections, in newborns and foals, 334t
  for lacerations, 315t
  for lymphangitis, 269
  for paraphimosis, 406
  for penile hematoma, 407
  for pericarditis, 148
  for purpura hemorrhagica, 263
  for retained placenta, 426
  for *Rhodococcus equi* pneumonia, 452–453
  for salmonellosis, 230
  for septic shock and SIRS, 541
  for septicemia, 489–490
  for smoke inhalation, 448
  for traumatic pneumothorax, 444
  for Tyzzer's disease, 281
  prophylactic, for choke, 167
Antiendotoxin therapy, for acute
      abdominal pain, 163
Antihistamines, 570
  for anaphylactic reactions, 266
  for bites, 271
  for stings, 271, 442
Anti-inflammatory drugs, 574–576
  nonsteroidal. See *Nonsteroidal anti-
      inflammatory drugs (NSAIDs).*
Antimicrobials. See *Antibiotics.*
Antipyretics, for anhydrosis, 544
Antiseptics, for skin preparation, 246
  for wound lavage, 246–247
Antiserum, botulism, 349
  for duodenitis/jejunitis, 189
  for peritonitis, 216
Antitoxin, tetanus, 355
Aorta, rupture of, 293

Aortic regurgitation, clinical signs of, 135t
  echocardiogram of, *139*
Aortic root, rupture of, 152–155
  clinical signs of, 152
  diagnosis of, 152, *153–155,* 154
  prognosis in, 154–155
  treatment of, 154
Aortic-iliac thrombosis, trembling with, 358
Apgar score, modified, for foal, 532t
Apnea, in newborn foal, 476
  development of, 531
Appaloosa horse, registry information for, 712
Arabian horse, registry information for, 712
Arrhythmia(s), 102–125
  bradyarrhythmias as, 102–107. See also
      specific type, e.g., *Sinus bradycar-
      dia.*
  drug treatment of, 124t
  electrolyte disturbances causing, 129–134. See also specific disorder,
      e.g., *Hyperkalemia.*
  quinidine-induced, 113, 115, *116*
    treatment of, 113t
  tachyarrhythmias as, 107–125. See also
      specific type, e.g., *Ventricular
      tachycardia.*
Arsenic poisoning, 608
Arterial pulse, during resuscitation, of
      foals, 515–516
Arteritis, viral, vaccination schedule for, 702
Artery(ies). See also named artery, e.g.,
      Iliac artery.
  puncture of, blood collection via, 4, *5,
      6*
Arthritis, septic, in newborn foal, 481
Arthrocentesis, 77–78
Arytenoid chondritis, 436
Ascarid impaction, of small intestine, 186–187
Asphyxia, in neonate, 530
  peripartum, 491–496
    CNS disturbances in, treatment of, 492–493
    diagnosis of, 491–492
    persistent fetal circulation pulmonary
        vasoconstriction in, treatment of, 494–495
    prognosis of, 496
    renal failure in, treatment of, 493–494
    respiratory compromise in, treatment
        of, 495–496

Asphyxia *(Continued)*
    treatment of, 492–496
Aspiration, bone marrow, 28
  meconium, in foals, 459–460
  transtracheal, 36–37, *38*
    complications of, 37–38
    material collected by, microscopic features of, 560–563
Aspiration pneumonia, 458–460
Aspirin, 574–575
  dosage of, 667
  for heart disease, 119t
  for jugular vein thrombosis, 442
  for laminitis, 326
  for nonstrangulation infarction, 190
  for septic shock and SIRS, 541
  for uveitis, 402
Assisted ventilation, 41–43
  complications of, 43
  using ambu bag, in foals, 43
  with demand valve, 42–43
  with nasogastric tube and demand valve, 43
Asystole, cardiopulmonary resuscitation of patient with, 127, 128t
Ataxia, 337–348
  in cervical stenotic myelopathy, 339–340
  in equine herpes virus–1 myeloencephalitis, 340–342
  in equine protozoal myelitis, 338–339
  in rabies, 344–346
  in spinal cord trauma, 366–368
  in verminous encephalitis, 346–347
  in vestibular disease, 343–344
  physical examination for, 337–338
  plant-induced, 347–348
  quinidine-induced, 118
Atlanto-occipital space, cerebrospinal fluid collection from, 87, 89, *89*
Atracurium, 586
  dosage of, 667
  used in field emergencies, 647–648, 648t
Atresia, intestinal, 203–204
Atresia coli, 203–204
Atrial fibrillation, 107–119
  congestive heart failure and, *118,* 118–119
    treatment of, 119, 119t
  electrocardiogram of, 107, *108*
  treatment of, 108–110
    adverse effect(s) and toxicity of, 110, 111t, 112
      congestive heart failure as, 117
      electrocardiographic monitoring for, 112–113, *114*

Atrial fibrillation *(Continued)*
      gastrointestinal signs of, 118
      hypotension as, 116
      laminitis as, 118
      neurologic signs of, 118
      paraphimosis as, 117
      sudden death as, 115–116
      supraventricular tachycardia as, 112–113, *114–115*
      upper respiratory tract obstruction as, 117
      urticaria as, 117
      ventricular arrhythmias as, 113, 115, *116*
      wheals as, 117
  patient preparation for, 108, *109*
Atrioventricular (AV) block, second-degree, 94, 105, *105–106*
  third-degree, 102–105
    electrocardiogram of, 102–103, *102–103*
    treatment of, 103–105, *104*
Atropine, adverse effects of, 125t
  dosage of, 124t, 667
  for cardiopulmonary resuscitation, 518t, 521–522
  for heaves, 449
  for respiratory disorders, 576
  for sinus bradycardia, 106
  for smoke inhalation, 448
  for third-degree AV block, 103
  in birth resuscitation, 534
  indications for, 124t
  overdose of, treatment for, 592t
  to relieve choke, 167
  toxicity of, 602
  used in field emergencies, 648t, 650
Auriculopalpebral nerve block, 379
  needle placement for, 83, *84*
Auscultation, abdominal, for intestinal borborygmi, 158–159
  in newborn foal, 476
  of heart, 94–95, 95t, *96,* 97t, 97–98
    in left-sided congestive failure, 136
    in right-sided congestive failure, 139–140
Australian dandelion poisoning, 608
Autotransfusion, 295. See also *Blood transfusion(s).*
Avocado poisoning, 609
Avulsion, of brachial plexus, 375
Azotemia, dietary guidelines for, 660t

Babesia caballi infection, 289–290

Babesia equi infection, 289–290
Babesia infection (piroplasmosis), 289–290
Bacteremia, causing sudden and unexpected death, 634
Bacterial pneumonia, in foals, 453–454
Bacterial samples, collection of, equipment for, 17
  procedure in, 18–19
Bag-valve device, self-inflating, ventilation using, in foals, 43, 513
BAL (bronchoalveolar lavage), 38–39
  material collected by, microscopic features of, 560–563
Bandage(s), as wound support, 258
  in wound healing, 248–250
  Robert Jones. See *Robert Jones bandage.*
Barbiturates, 572
  overdose of, treatment for, 592t
Basioccipital fracture, 366
Basisphenoid fracture, 366
Basophil count, 696
Bean poisoning, castor, 604
Beclomethasone, dosage of, 667
  for respiratory disorders, 577
Bee stings, 271–272, 442
Beetle, blister, *223*
  toxicity of, 223–225, 602–603
Behavior, bizarre, drug-induced, 372
  nursing, in newborn foal, 481–482
Belgian horse, registry information for, 712
Benzimidazole, 686
Benztropine mesylate, dosage of, 667
Beta-lactam drugs, 565–567
Bethanechol, dosage of, 667
  for equine herpes virus–1 myeloencephalitis, 341
  for ulcers, 574
  for urinary incontinence, 472
  overdose of, treatment for, 593t
Bile duct(s), distention of, 277, *278*
  obstruction of, 281–282
Biopsy, 21–30
  of bone marrow, 27–28
  of cyst, 22–23
  of endometrium, 29–30
  of kidney, 24–25
  of liver, 25–26, 283
  of lung, 26–27
  of lymph node, 23–24
  of mass, 22–23
  of muscle, 28–29
  of nodule, 22–23

Biopsy *(Continued)*
  of skin, 21–22
Birth resuscitation, 528–537
  airway clearance in, 532
  assessment in, 531–532, 532t
  cardiovascular support in, 533
  drug therapy in, 534
  fluid therapy in, 534–535
  in neonatal hypercapnia, 536
  in neonatal hypoxia, 535–536
  in persistent pulmonary hypertension, 535
  overview of, *529*
  respiratory support in, 533
    during dystocia, 536–537
  steps in, 531–537
  tactile stimulation in, 532
  thermal management in, 533–534
Bismuth subsalicylate, dosage of, 667
  for enteritis, 503
  for ulcers, 574
Bite(s), fly, 272
  snake, 271–272, 442–443
  spider, 271–272
Black locust poisoning, 602
Black walnut poisoning, 622
Bladder, prolapsed, 471
  ruptured, 469–471
    in foals, 469–470
Bleeding. See *Hemorrhage.*
Blepharitis, acute, 382–383
Blind biopsy, of kidney, 25
Blind-end atresia, of intestines, 203
Blister beetle, *223*
  toxicity of, 223–225, 602–603
Blood chemistry, reference values for, 678–680
Blood collection, 2–6
  by arterial puncture, 4, *5*, 6
  by venipuncture, 2–4, *5*
Blood gases, evaluation of, in gastrointestinal emergencies, 160
Blood loss, and wound healing, 243
Blood samples, bacterial, collection and transport of, 19
  from newborn foal, 482
  viral, collection and transport of, 20
Blood supply, and wound healing, 250
Blood transfusion(s), administration of blood in, 295
  blood volume needed in, calculation of, 296
  choice of donor for, 295
  collection of blood in, 295
  comments on, 294–296
  for anemia, 285, 287, 288–289

Blood transfusion(s) *(Continued)*
  side effects of, 295
Blood tubes, for diagnostic procedures, 3t
Blood urea nitrogen (BUN), serum
    concentration of, 699
Blood vessels. See also specific artery and
    vein.
  laceration of, 317–318
Blue green algae poisoning, 631–632
Blunt trauma, to eye, without laceration or
    rupture, 381, Color Plate 1
  to head, 380–381
Board splint, for flexor tendon lacerations,
    application of, *314,* 314–315
  materials for, 314
Body cavity, hemorrhage into, 291–294
Bone(s). See also named bone, e.g.,
    Sesamoid bone.
  long, fracture of. See *Forelimb, fracture
    of; Hindlimb, fracture of.*
Bone marrow, biopsy of, 27–28
  cellular composition of, reference val-
    ues for, 685
Bony trauma, to head, 381–382, Color
    Plate 1
Borborygmi, intestinal, auscultation for,
    158–159
Botulism, 348–350, 609
  in adults, 349
  in foals, 348–349
  vaccination schedule for, 700
Botulism antiserum, 349
Bovine hemoglobin, dosage of, 667
Brace, Leg-Savr, 302
Brachial plexus, avulsion of, 375
Bracken fern poisoning, 609–610, *610*
Bradyarrhythmia(s), 102–107
  second-degree AV block as, 105, *105–
    106*
  sick sinus syndrome as, 107
  sinoatrial arrest as, 106–107
  sinoatrial block as, 105–106
  sinus bradycardia as, 105–106
  third-degree AV block as, *102–104,*
    102–105
Brain stem trauma, as complication of
    cerebrospinal fluid collection, 91
Breathing, initiation of, in
    cardiopulmonary resuscitation, 126
Breeding injury(ies), in stallion,
    paraphimosis as, 405–408
  penile abrasions and lacerations as,
    409
  ruptured corpus spongiosum penis as,
    408–409
  testicular trauma as, 410

Breeds of horses, registry information for,
    711–720
Bretylium tosylate, 584
  adverse effects of, 125t
  dosage of, 124t, 668
  for cardiopulmonary resuscitation, 518t,
    523–524
  for quinidine-induced arrhythmias, 113t
  for ventricular fibrillation, 128t, 129
  for ventricular tachycardia, 126
  indications for, 124t
Bronchial foreign bodies, 441
Bronchoalveolar lavage (BAL), 38–39
  material collected by, microscopic fea-
    tures of, 560–563
Bronchodilators, 576–577
Bronchointerstitial pneumonia, in foals,
    454–455
Buckeye poisoning, 604
Buckskin horse, registry information for,
    712
BUN (blood urea nitrogen), serum
    concentration of, 699
Burn(s), 258–262
  classification of, 259–260
  complications of, 261–262
  full-thickness, 259–260
  life-threatening shock associated with,
    260–261
  management of, 260–261
  partial thickness, 259
  superficial, 259
  to eyelid, 261–262
Butorphanol, 570
  dosage of, 668
  for abdominal pain, 158t
  for antibiotic-induced diarrhea, 235
  for hematoma, 270
  for meconium impaction, 499
  for necrotizing enterocolitis, 228
  for orthopedic emergencies, 298t
  overdose of, treatment for, 593t
  used in field emergencies, 648t, 648–
    649
Buttercup toxicity, 603–604

Ca-EDTA, dosage of, 668
Caffeine, as respiratory support for
    septicemia, 488
  dosage of, 668
  for neonatal hypercapnia, 536
  for respiratory compromise, in peripar-
    tum asphyxia, 495
Calcium borogluconate, dosage of, 668

Calcium borogluconate *(Continued)*
for hyperkalemic periodic paralysis, 131
for tetanic hypocalcemia, 351–353
Calcium chloride, dosage of, 668
for cardiopulmonary resuscitation, 518t,
522–523
postresuscitation administration of, 129
Calcium gluconate, dosage of, 668
for hyperkalemia, 130
for hyperkalemic periodic paralysis, 354
for hypocalcemia, 133
postresuscitation administration of, 129
Calcium salts, intravenous administration
of, 578
Cannulation, of nasolacrimal duct, 82
Cantharidin intoxication, 223–225
Carbamate insecticides, toxicity of,
605–606
Carbon disulfide, dosage of, 668
Cardiac. See also *Heart* entries.
Cardiac arrest, establish circulation in,
126–127
Cardiac compression(s), technique of, in
foals, 514–515, *515*
Cardiac drugs, 580–582
Cardiac massage, in cardiopulmonary
resuscitation, 127
Cardiac output, measuring effectiveness
of, during resuscitation, of foals, 515
Cardiac pacemaker, implantation of, for
third-degree AV block, 103–105, *104*
Cardiac rhythm, in congestive heart
failure, 136
in newborn foal, 475
Cardiopulmonary failure, in foals, reasons
for, 506
recognition of, 506–509
Cardiopulmonary resuscitation (CPR),
126–129
administration of drugs in, 127, 128t,
129
administration of fluids in, 129
airway in, patency of, 125
anesthesia for, in field emergencies,
654, *655,* 656t
breathe for patient in, 125–126
cardiac arrest and, establishing circulation in, 126–127
cardiac massage in, 127
of foals, 503–537
arterial pulse during, 515–516
cardiac compression during, 514–515,
515
cardiac output during, effectiveness
of, 515
chest compression during, complications of, 516

Cardiopulmonary resuscitation (CPR)
(Continued)
clinical approach to, 507, *508–509,*
510–514
defibrillation during, 525
drug therapy during, 517, 518t, 519–
524
end-tidal CO_2 during, 516
equipment required for, 504t, 505t
establishing airway in, 510, *511–512,*
512
establishing circulation in, 514–517
facts in, 503–506
fluid therapy in, 519
humane aspects of, 505–506
postresuscitation treatment in, 525–
528
pupil size and, 516
vascular access during, 516–517
ventilation during, 513–514
ventilatory aids for, 513
of patient with asystole, 127, *128,* 128t
of patient with ventricular fibrillation,
127, *128,* 128t
postresuscitation treatment in, 129
Cardiovascular support, during birth
resuscitation, 533
in field emergencies, 652
Cardiovascular system, 94–155. See also
specific part, e.g., *Heart.*
disorder(s) of, aortic root rupture as,
152–155
arrhythmias as, 102–125. See also
specific arrhythmia, e.g., *Atrial
fibrillation.*
congestive heart failure as, 134–142.
See also *Congestive heart failure.*
electrolyte disturbances as, 129–134.
See also specific disorder, e.g.,
Hyperkalemia.
ionophore toxicity as, 148–151
pericarditis/pericardial effusion as,
142–148
electrocardiographic examination of, 98,
99t, *100–101*
of newborn foal, 475
physical examination of, 94–98
resuscitation of, 125–129. See also *Cardiopulmonary resuscitation (CPR).*
toxins affecting, 624–627
Carotid artery, puncture of, 4, 6
Carpal joint, anesthesia of, 70, *71*
incomplete ossification of, *335,* 336

Carprofen, dosage of, 668
  for antibiotic-induced diarrhea, 236
Casein, in diet, 662t
Cast(s). See also *Splint-cast.*
  as wound support, 258
  for pediatric orthopedic emergencies,
    328–329
  "slipper," for hoof wall lacerations,
    319, *319*
Castor bean poisoning, 604
Castration, complications following,
    410–411
Catheter(s), intravenous placement of,
    12–15
  equipment for, 13
  procedure in, 13–14
  jugular, broken, 591
  subpalpebral placement of, 83–85
    complications of, 84–85
    equipment for, 83
    procedure in, 83–84, *84–85*
  use and maintenance of, 14–15
Catheterization, of newborn foal, 482
  of urinary tract, 61–63
    complications of, 63
    in females, 62
    in males, 61–62
Caudal root, disorders of, 377
Cecocolic intussusception, 196
Cecum, impaction of, 191–192
  perforation of, 192–193
  trocharization of, 59–60
Cefoperazone, 566
  dosage of, 668
Cefotaxime, dosage of, 668
  for septicemia, 489
Ceftazidime, dosage of, 668
Ceftiofur, 566
  dosage of, 668
  for acute colitis, 221
  for aspiration pneumonia, 459
  for bacterial pneumonia, 454
  for botulism, 349
  for bronchointerstitial pneumonia, 455
  for cholangiohepatitis, 277
  for equine herpes virus–1 myeloencepha-
    litis, 342
  for infections, in newborns and foals,
    334t
  for lacerations, 315t
  for limb edema, 264
  for meconium aspiration, 460
  for paraphimosis, 406
  for penile hematoma, 407
  for pleuropneumonia, 457
  for salmonellosis, 230

Ceftiofur *(Continued)*
  for septicemia, 489
  for smoke inhalation, 448
  for testicular trauma, 410
  for vaginal hemorrhage, 423
  for viral respiratory distress syndrome,
    451
  postdystocia, 415
Celiotomy, exploratory, candidates for,
    164
  indications for, 162t
  for uterine torsion, 212–213
Cellulitis, 267–268
  as complication of intravenous cathe-
    ters, 15
Centesis, needle placement for, 321, *321*
Central nervous system, disorders of,
  correlation of cerebrospinal fluid
    parameters and, 90t
    in peripartum asphyxia, treatment of,
      492–493
  toxins affecting, 608–616
Cerebral abscess, 361–363
Cerebral trauma, 363–366
Cerebrospinal fluid, 86–91
  analysis of, 89, 90t, 91
  collection of, complications of, 91
    equipment for, 86–87
    indications for, 86
    procedure for, from atlanto-occipital
      space, 87, 89, *89*
      from lumbosacral space, 87, *88*
Cervical esophagotomy, for choke,
    167–168
Cervical stenotic myelopathy, 339–340
Cervical vertebral malformation, dietary
  guidelines for, 659t
Charcoal, activated, for acute colitis, 221
  for ionophore toxicity, 151
  dosage of, 668
Chest compression, during resuscitation,
  complications of, 516
Chest tube(s), placement of, 51–52
Chincoteague pony, registry information
  for, 713
Chloral hydrate, 572
  dosage of, 668
  for abdominal pain, 158t
Chloramphenicol, 569
Chlorhexidine diacetate solution, for
  wound lavage, 247
Choke, diagnosis of, 166
  dietary guidelines for, 659t
  esophageal, 437
  medical treatment of, 166–167
  prognosis and complications of, 168

Choke *(Continued)*
  surgical treatment of, 167–168
Cholangiohepatitis, 277–278
Cholelithiasis, 277–278
Cholesterol, serum concentration of, 699
Chondritis, arytenoid, 436
Chronic obstructive pulmonary disease
      (COPD), 449–451, 561–562
  dietary guidelines for, 659t
Cimetidine, dosage of, 668
  for gastric ulcers, in foals, 173
  for ulcers, 573
Circulation, establishing, in cardiac arrest,
      126–127
      of foals, 514–517
  fetal, 528–530
Cisapride, dosage of, 668
  for duodenitis/jejunitis, 189
  for gastrointestinal dysmotility, in peri-
      partum asphyxia, 494
  for ileus, 500
  for ulcers, 573
Clavulanic acid. See *Ticarcillin/clavulanic
      acid.*
Clenbuterol, dosage of, 668
  for bronchointerstitial pneumonia, 455
  for *Rhodococcus equi* pneumonia, 453
  for smoke inhalation, 448
  for viral respiratory distress syndrome,
      451
Cleveland Bay horse, registry information
      for, 713
Clostridial myositis, 268–269
Clostridium, diarrhea caused by, 219, 220
  treatment of, 222, 228
Clostridium botulinum, 349. See also
      Botulism.
Clostridium perfringens, in duodenitis,
      187, *188*
Clostridium piliformis infection, 281
Clostridium tetani, 354. See also *Tetanus.*
Clover poisoning, moldy sweet, 166,
      627–628
  red, 606–607
Clydesdale horse, registry information for,
      713
Coffin joint, anesthesia of, 70, *70*
Coggins test, for anemia, 285, 291
Colic, 156–236. See also *Abdominal pain.*
  anesthesia for, in field emergencies, 654
  auscultation for intestinal borborygmi
      in, 158–159
  causes of, in newborn foal, 476–477
  classification of, 156–157
  clinicopathologic evaluation of, 160–
      161

Colic *(Continued)*
  diagnosis of, physical examination in,
      157–160
    previous and recent history in, 157
    rectal examination in, 159
  diarrheal diseases causing, in adults,
      217–225
    in foals, 225–234
    in weanlings and yearlings, 234–236
  dietary guidelines for, 659t
  in late-term pregnant mare, 211–215
  in newborn foal, 498–503
    enteritis causing, 501–503
    ileus causing, 499–501
    intussusception causing, 501
    meconium impaction causing, 498–
      499
  large intestinal disorders causing, 191–
      204. See also specific disorder,
      e.g., *Impaction.*
  management of, 162–164
    analgesics in, 158t, 163
      response to, 160
    antibiotics in, 164
    antiendotoxin therapy in, 163
    fluid therapy and cardiovascular sup-
      port in, 163
    laxatives in, 163
    medical vs. surgical, 161–162, 162t
    nutritional support in, 164
  nasogastric intubation for, 159
  pathophysiology of, 156–164
  peritonitis causing, 215–217
  postfoaling, 415
  quinidine-induced, 118
  small colon and rectal disorders caus-
      ing, 201–211
  small intestine disorders causing, 175–
      191. See also specific disorder,
      e.g., *Intussusception.*
Colitis, acute, 217–218
    diagnostic tests for, 219–220
    prognosis of, 223
    treatment of, 220–223
  dietary guidelines for, 660t
Colitis X, 219
Collapse, sudden, 363–372
      basisphenoid/basioccipital fractures
        causing, 366
      cranial trauma causing, 363–366
      drug-induced hyperexcitability caus-
        ing, 370–372
      seizures causing, 368–370
      spinal cord trauma causing, 366–368
Colloids, for septic shock and SIRS, 540
Colon, large, displacements of, 196–198,
      198–200, 201

Colon *(Continued)*
    impaction of, 193–194
    volvulus in, 201, *202, 203*
  resection of, dietary guidelines for, 659t
  small, disorder(s) of, 204–208
    enterolithiasis as, 205–206
    foreign body obstruction as, 204–205
    impaction as, 204–205
    meconium impaction as, 206–207, *207*
    mesocolic rupture as, 207–208
Commercial diet, enteral, 662–663
Compartmentalization syndrome, 356
Complete AV block. See *Atrioventricular (AV) block, third-degree.*
Complete blood count, in gastrointestinal emergencies, 160
Congestive heart failure, 117, 134–142
  left-sided, auscultation in, 136
    clinical signs of, 135t, 135–136
    echocardiogram in, 136–137, *137–140*
    treatment of, 119t, 136–138
  right-sided, 138–142
    auscultation in, 139–140
    clinical signs of, 139
    treatment of, 119t, 140–142
Conjunctival flap(s), for corneal ulcers, 395
Connemara pony, registry information for, 713
Contamination, of wounds, 252
Contraction, in wound healing, 242
Contracture, limb, in newborn foal, 481
COPD (chronic obstructive pulmonary disease), 449–451, 561–562
  dietary guidelines for, 659t
Cord atresia, of intestines, 203
Corneal abrasion(s), 390–393
Corneal edema, 398–399, Color Plate 2
Corneal foreign body(ies), 397–398
Corneal lacerations, 388–390
Corneal ulcer(s), 390–395
  as complication of burns, 261–262
  as complication of subpalpebral catheter placement, 85
  clinical signs of, 390–391
  complicated, debridement of, 394–395, Color Plate 1
    surgical intervention for, 395
    treatment of, 394
  diagnostic steps in, 391–393, Color Plate 1
  simple, treatment of, 393–394
Corneoscleral transposition, for corneal ulcers, 395

Coronary band, lacerations to, 318
Corpus spongiosum penis, ruptured, 408–409
Corticosteroids, 577–578. See also specific corticosteroid, e.g., *Prednisone.*
  and wound healing, 244
  for bites and stings, 271
  for dermatitis, 272
  for heaves, 449
  for hypercalcemia, 134
  for limb edema, 264
  for pericarditis, 148
  for purpura hemorrhagica, 263
  for third-degree AV block, 103
  for urticaria, 267
  for uveitis, 402
Corynebacterium pseudotuberculosis, 270
Coxofemoral joint, anesthesia of, 75, *75*
Coxofemoral luxation, 311
CPR. See *Cardiopulmonary resuscitation (CPR).*
Cranial fracture, 307–308
Cranial gluteal nerve, disorders of, 377
Cranial trauma, 363–366
  clinical examination for, 364
  neurologic examination for, 364
  poor prognostic indications in, 365–366
  treatment of, 365
Creatinine, serum concentration of, 699
Criminal death, causes of, 635
Cromolyn, dosage of, 669
Cryptosporidium parvum–associated diarrhea, in nursing foals, 232–233
Crystalloids, for septic shock and SIRS, 539–540
  for septicemia, 486–487
Cuboidal bones, incomplete ossification of, *335,* 336, 497, 498
Cutaneous/transdermal administration, of medications, 11
Cyanide poisoning, 632
Cyathostomiasis, 218–219
  treatment of, 222
Cycloplegics, for corneal ulcers, 393, 394
Cyproheptadine, 586
  dosage of, 669
  for hyperlipidemia, 279
Cyst, biopsy of, 22–23
Cytologic specimen(s), 550–552
  glass slides for, preparation of, 550
  interpretation of, 551–552
  microscopic evaluation of, 551
  obtaining, 550
  staining of, 550–551
  submission of, 552–553

Dandelion poisoning, 608
Dantrolene sodium, 585
Dartmoor pony, registry information for, 714
Day-blooming jessamine poisoning, 622–623
Death, exercise-induced, cardiac defects and, 633
  malicious or criminal, causes of, 635
  sudden and unexpected, hemorrhage causing, 633
    in horses, 631
    intestinal causes of, 634
    neurologic causes of, 633–634
    quinidine-induced, 115–116
    respiratory causes of, 634–635
    toxic causes of, 631–635
Debility, paraphimosis secondary to, 408
Debridement, of corneal ulcers, 394–395, Color Plate 1
  of wounds, 247–248
Debridement phase, of wound healing, 241
Defibrillation, in cardiopulmonary resuscitation, 525
Deformity, angular limb, as pediatric orthopedic emergency, 334, *335*, 336, 497, 498
Degloving injuries, 317
  antibiotics for, 315t
Dehydration, and wound healing, 250
  assessment of, 160
Demand valve, and nasogastric tube, ventilation with, 43
  ventilation with, 42–43
Dermatitis, acute, 272
  lower limb, 620
Dermis, 238–239, *240*
Desferrioxamine, dosage of, 669
Detomidine, 571
  dosage of, 669
  for abdominal pain, 158t
  for orthopedic emergencies, 298t
  overdose of, treatment for, 593t
  used in field emergencies, 648t, 649
Dexamethasone, 577
  dosage of, 124t, 669
  for anaphylactic reactions, 267
  for aspiration pneumonia, 458
  for bee stings, 442
  for bites and stings, 271
  for blister beetle poisoning, 225
  for bronchointerstitial pneumonia, 455
  for cerebral abscess, 362
  for cervical stenotic myelopathy, 340
  for cranial trauma, 365

Dexamethasone *(Continued)*
  for equine herpes virus–1 myeloencephalitis, 342
  for heart disease, 119t
  for heaves, 449
  for hyperexcitability, 371
  for laryngeal edema, 436
  for laryngeal spasm, 437
  for meconium aspiration, 459
  for mycotoxic encephalopathy, 359
  for neonatal isoerythrolysis, 289
  for pericarditis, 148
  for plant-induced ataxia, 348
  for pulmonary edema, secondary to anaphylaxis, 447
  for purpura hemorrhagica, 263
  for ruptured corpus spongiosum penis, 409
  for septic shock and SIRS, 541
  for sinoatrial arrest, 107
  for spinal cord syndrome, 368
  for third-degree AV block, 103
  for tibial paralysis, 376–377
  for verminous encephalitis, 347
  for vestibular disease, 344
  for viral encephalitis, 361
  indications for, 124t
Dextran 70, dosage of, 669
  used in field emergencies, 648t, 650
Dextrose, dosage of, 669
  for hyperkalemia, 130
  intravenous administration of, 579–580
Dextrose slurry, in diet, 662t
Diaphragmatic herniation, *183*, 183–184, 294
Diarrhea. See also *Colitis.*
  acute, 217–223
  antibiotic-induced, 218
    in weanlings and yearlings, 235–236
    treatment of, 222
  causes of, 218–219
  dietary guidelines for, 659t
  fetal, 233–234
  in newborn foals, 233–234, 501–503
  in nursing foals, 225–234
    Cryptosporidium parvum–associated, 232–233
    Escherichia coli–associated, 233
    necrotizing enterocolitis causing, 225–229
    rotavirus causing, 231–232
    salmonellosis causing, 229–231
  in weanlings and yearlings, 234–236
    antibiotic-induced, 235–236
    Rhodococcus equi–associated, 234–235

Diarrhea *(Continued)*
  quinidine-induced, 118
Diazepam, 570
  dosage of, 669
  for CNS disturbances, in peripartum
    asphyxia, 492
  for cranial trauma, 365
  for seizures, 370
  for ventricular tachycardia, 123
  for viral encephalitis, 361
  overdose of, treatment for, 593t
  used in field emergencies, 648t, 649
Dichlorvos, dosage of, 669
  overdose of, treatment for, 593t
Diclazuril, dosage of, 669
Diet, commercial enteral, 662–663
  defined, 662, 662t
Dietary guidelines, for specific disease
    conditions, 659t–660t
Digital flexor tendon, superficial, luxation
    of, 330
Digoxin, 584
  adverse effects of, 125t
  dosage of, 669
  for atrial fibrillation, 110
    with congestive heart failure, 119
  for congestive heart failure, 137, 138,
    140–141
  for heart disease, 119t
  for pulmonary edema, 446
  for quinidine-induced arrhythmias, 113t
  for quinidine-induced congestive heart
    failure, 117
  for supraventricular tachycardia, 112
  overdose of, treatment for, 593t
  toxicity of, 110, *112*, 141
Dimercaprol, dosage of, 669
Dimethyl sulfoxide (DMSO), dosage of,
    669
  for aspiration pneumonia, 459
  for bronchointerstitial pneumonia, 455
  for cerebral abscess, 362
  for CNS disturbances, in peripartum
    asphyxia, 493
  for cranial trauma, 365
  for duodenitis/jejunitis, 189
  for equine herpes virus–1 myeloencepha-
    litis, 340
  for equine protozoal myelitis, 339
  for hyperexcitability, 371
  for jugular vein thrombosis, 442
  for laryngeal spasm, 437
  for mycotoxic encephalopathy, 359
  for plant-induced ataxia, 348
  for seizures, 370
  for spinal cord syndrome, 368

Dimethyl sulfoxide (DMSO) *(Continued)*
  for tibial paralysis, 376–377
  for vestibular disease, 344
  for viral encephalitis, 361
  overdose of, treatment for, 593t
Dinoprost, dosage of, 669
  overdose of, treatment for, 593t
Dioctyl sodium sulfosuccinate, dosage of,
    669
  for acute abdominal pain, 163
  for ulcers, 574
Dipyrone, 575
  dosage of, 670
  for abdominal pain, 158t
  for antibiotic-induced diarrhea, 235
  for limb edema, 264
  for meconium impaction, 499
  for necrotizing enterocolitis, 228
Disaster medicine, 638–645
  available emergency services in, 644–
    645
  individual situations in, 638–642
    chronologic walk-through of, 641–
      642
    equipment for, 639, *640,* 641
    personnel involved with, 641
    preparation for, 638–639
  involvement of horse community in,
    643–644
  involvement of local office of emer-
    gency services in, 644
  involvement of practice/community in,
    642–645
Displacement(s), of large colon, 196–201
    left dorsal, 197
      treatment of, 197–198, *198–200,*
      201
    right dorsal, 196–197
      treatment of, 197
Diuretics, 584–585
DMSO. See *Dimethyl sulfoxide (DMSO).*
Dobutamine, 580
  dosage of, 670
  for congestive heart failure, 137
  for heart disease, 119t
  for necrotizing enterocolitis, 228
  for renal failure, 465
    in peripartum asphyxia, 493
  for sepsis-induced hypotension, 487
  for septic shock and SIRS, 540
  overdose of, treatment for, 593t
  postresuscitation administration of, 129
  potency of, 527t
  used in field emergencies, 648t, 650
Domestic onion poisoning, 630
Domperidone, dosage of, 670

Donor, choice of, in blood transfusions, 295
Dopamine, 580–581
  dosage of, 670
  for necrotizing enterocolitis, 228
  for renal failure, 465
    in peripartum asphyxia, 493
  for sepsis-induced hypotension, 487
  overdose of, treatment for, 593t
  potency of, 527t
Dorsal metatarsal nerve block, of proximal hindlimb, 68, 69
Doxapram, dosage of, 670
  for respiratory disorders, 576–577
  in birth resuscitation, 534
  overdose of, treatment for, 593t
  used in field emergencies, 648t, 650
Doxycycline, 568
  overdose of, treatment for, 593t
Doxylamine succinate, dosage of, 670
  for anaphylactic reactions, 266
  for bee stings, 442
  for bites and stings, 271
  for grain overload, 171
Drain(s), in wound closure, 256
Dressing(s), and wound healing, 248–250
Drug(s). See Medication(s); specific drug or drug group.
Drug overdose, 591
  recommended treatment for, 592t–598t
Drug reaction(s), adverse, 588–598
  recommended treatment for, 592t–598t
  reference information for, 588
Drug-induced hyperexcitability, 370–372
Drug-induced hypotension, 371–372
Duodenitis, 187–189, 188
Duodenum, perforation of, 175
Dutch warmblood horse, registry information for, 714
Dysmaturity. See Prematurity/dysmaturity.
Dysphagia, causes of, 372–374
Dystocia, 411–415
  anesthesia for, in field emergencies, 653
  causes of, corrective measures for, 412–414
  respiratory support during, 536–537
  treatment of, 412

Ear tick, 357
Echocardiography, of acute aortic regurgitation, 139
  of monensin toxicosis, 149, 150
  of pericarditis/pericardial effusion, 142–144, 143–145

Echocardiography (Continued)
  of ruptured aortic root, 152, 153–155
  of ruptured chordae tendineae of mitral valve, 138, 140
  of ventricular cardiomyopathy, 137
  of ventricular tachycardia, 120, 123
Edema, 262–272
  acute, in one horse in group, 264–266
  acute onset of, in four limbs, 264
  anaphylactic reactions causing, 266–267
  bites and stings causing, 271–272
  cellulitis causing, 267–268
  cerebral, 363–366
  corneal, 398–399, Color Plate 2
  ehrlichiosis causing, 265
  hematoma causing, 270
  idiopathic, 266
  in wound healing, 250
  laryngeal, 435–436
  Lyme disease causing, 265–266
  lymphangitis causing, 269–270
  malignant, 268–269
  nutritional myopathy causing, 270–271
  onchocerciasis causing, 266
  pulmonary, 445–447
    treatment of, 136
  purpura hemorrhagica causing, 262–264
  ventral, pre- or postfoaling, 266
Edrophonium, dosage of, 670
  used in field emergencies, 648t, 649
Effusion, hemorrhagic, peritoneal fluid in, 556
  pericardial, 142–148
    echocardiogram for, 142–144, 143–145
    etiology of, 147t
    treatment of, 144, 146, 148
Ehrlichiosis, 265, 290–291, 348
Elbow joint, anesthesia of, 72, 72
Electrocardiography, 98, 99t, 100–101
  of asystole, 128
  of atrial fibrillation, 108, 109
    after treatment with quinidine sulfate and digoxin, 112
    and quinidine toxicity, 112–113, 114
    with congestive heart failure, 118
  of monensin toxicosis, 149, 150
  of patient with hyperkalemia, 130, 130
  of patient with hypokalemia, 131, 132
  of patient with hypomagnesemia, 132, 132
  of ruptured aortic root, 152, 153
  of second-degree (AV) block, 105, 105–106
  of third-degree (AV) block, 102–103, 102–103

Electrocardiography *(Continued)*
with pacemaker, *104*
of ventricular fibrillation, *128*
of ventricular tachycardia, 120, *121–122*
Electrode(s), placement of, for 12-lead
electrocardiogram, 99t
sites of, *100–101*
Electrolyte(s), assessment of, in
gastrointestinal emergencies, 160–161
disorders of. See also specific disorder,
e.g., *Hyperkalemia.*
causing arrhythmias, 129–134
in diet, 662t
Embolization, as complication of
intravenous catheters, 15
Embolus, fibrocartilaginous, 348
Embutramide, overdose of, treatment for,
593t
Emergency(ies), field, anesthesia for,
646–656. See also *Anesthesia, in field
emergencies.*
Emergency anesthesia kit, 646–647
Emergency grain overload, 171
Emergency services, availability of, in
disaster medicine, 644–645
local office involvement of, in disaster
medicine, 644
Empyema, guttural pouch, 437
Enalapril, 582
dosage of, 670
for congestive heart failure, 138
for heart disease, 119t
for ruptured aortic root, 154
Encephalitis, verminous, 346–347
viral, 360–361
Encephalomyelitis, vaccination schedule
for, 701
Encephalopathy, hepatic, 358
dietary guidelines for, 660t
management of, 283–284
hypoxic-ischemic, in newborn foal, 480
mycotoxic, 358–360
Endometrial biopsy, 29–30
Endoscopy, of airway, 31–32
of gastrointestinal tract, 32–33
of urinary tract, 33
Endotoxemia, causing sudden and
unexpected death, 634
shock due to, 538–542
vaccination schedule for, 701
Endotracheal tube, placement of, in foals,
510, 512, *512*
Enemas, for meconium impaction, 499
Enrofloxacin, 569
dosage of, 670
for cholangiohepatitis, 277

Enteritis, bacterial causes of, 501–502
colic due to, in newborn foal, 501–503
parasitic causes of, 502
treatment of, 503
viral causes of, 502
Enterocentesis, as complication of
abdominocentesis, 57, 59
peritoneal fluid in, 555
Enterocolitis, necrotizing. See *Necrotizing
enterocolitis.*
Enterolithiasis, dietary guidelines for, 659t
in small colon, 205–206
Entrapments, anesthesia for, in field
emergencies, 654
Eosinophil count, 696
Eosinophilic keratitis, 395–397, Color
Plate 2
Epidermis, 238, *239*
Epidural administration, of medications,
11–12
Epiglottitis, 441
Epinephrine, 581
dosage of, 670
for anaphylactic reactions, 266–267
for asystole, 127, 128t
for bee stings, 442
for bites and stings, 271
for cardiopulmonary resuscitation, 517,
518t, 519
for laryngeal edema, 435–436
for pulmonary edema, secondary to anaphylaxis, 446
for sepsis-induced hypotension, 487
overdose of, treatment for, 593t
potency of, 527t
used in field emergencies, 648t, 650
Epinephrine challenge, in anhydrosis, 544
Epiphysis, disproportionate growth of, in
angular limb deformity, 336
Epiploic foramen herniation, 178–179
Epistaxis, 460–462
as complication of nasogastric intubation, 55
as complication of paranasal trephination, 49
due to thrombocytopenia, 461
Epithelialization, in wound healing, 241
Epsom salt. See *Magnesium sulfate.*
Equine infectious anemia, 290–291
Equine plasma, dosage of, 670
intravenous administration of, 578–579
Erythrocyte parameters, 698
Erythromycin, dosage of, 670
for gastrointestinal dysmotility, in peripartum asphyxia, 494
for ileus, 500

Erythromycin *(Continued)*
  for *Rhodococcus equi* pneumonia, 452
  for *Rhodococcus equi*–associated diarrhea, 234
Escherichia coli–associated diarrhea, in nursing foals, 233
Esophageal obstruction, 437
  diagnosis of, 166
  dietary guidelines for, 659t
  medical treatment of, 166–167
  prognosis and complications of, 168
  surgical treatment of, 167–168
Esophageal perforation, causes of, 168
  complications and prognosis of, 169
  treatment of, 169
Esophagotomy, cervical, for choke, 167–168
Ethmoid hematoma, 461
Euthanasia, 656–657
  in field emergencies, anesthesia for, 652
  of patients with thrombosed jugular veins, 657
Evisceration, postcastration, 411
Exercise-induced death, cardiac defects and, 633
Exercise-induced pulmonary hemorrhage, 461
Exhaustive disease syndrome, 544–546
  diagnosis of, 545
  prognosis of, 546
  treatment of, 545–546
Exmoor pony, registry information for, 714
Exophthalmos, acute, 386–387
Extensor tendon(s), lacerations to, management of, *316,* 316–317
Extrications, anesthesia for, in field emergencies, 654
Eye(s), blunt trauma to, without laceration or rupture, 381, Color Plate 1
Eyelid(s), 382–386
  burns to, 261–262
  injury to, facial nerve damage resulting in, 383–384
  lacerations to, 384–386
    acute injury in, 385–386
    anesthesia and wound preparation for, 385
    subacute or chronic injury in, 386
  swollen, as complication of subpalpebral catheter placement, 84

Facial artery, puncture of, 6
Facial nerve, damage to, resulting in eyelid injury, 383–384

Facial nerve *(Continued)*
  disorders of, 377–378
Facial vein, transverse, venipuncture via, 3
Fall panicum, causing liver failure, 282–283, 618
Famotidine, dosage of, 670
  for gastric ulcers, in foals, 173
  for ulcers, 573
Fasting, 663
Febantel, dosage of, 670
Fecal samples, collection and transport of, 19
Feces, "milk," 476
Feed, pelleted, 662
Feeding by tube, 662t, 662–663
  comments on, 663
Femoral nerve, disorders of, 375
Fenbendazole, dosage of, 670
  for verminous encephalitis, 347
Fern, sensitive, toxicity of, 619
Fern poisoning, bracken, 609–610, *610*
Fescue poisoning, 430, 623
Fetal circulation, 528–530
Fetal diarrhea, 233–234
Fetal membranes, hydrops of. See *Hydrops of fetal membranes.*
Fetal/neonatal transition, 528
  unsuccessful, 530–531
Fetlock joint, anesthesia of, 70, *70*
Fetotomy, equipment for, 412–413
  notes on, 414–415
Fibrillation, atrial. See *Atrial fibrillation.*
  ventricular, cardiopulmonary resuscitation of patient with, 127, 128t, 129
Fibrinogen, normal, in foals, 693
Fibrocartilaginous embolus, 348
Fibroplasia, in wound healing, 242
Field emergencies, anesthesia for, 646–656. See also *Anesthesia, in field emergencies.*
Flank celiotomy, for uterine torsion, 212–213
Flatulence, quinidine-induced, 118
Flexor tendon(s), lacerations to, management of, 313–315, *314,* 315t
  laxity of, in newborn foal, 481
  superficial digital, luxation of, in foals, 330
Fluconazole, dosage of, 670
Fluid therapy, for acute abdominal pain, 163
  for acute colitis, 221
  for acute renal failure, 464
  for blister beetle poisoning, 225
  for cardiopulmonary resuscitation, 519
  for exhaustive disease syndrome, 545

Fluid therapy *(Continued)*
  for grain overload, 171–172
  for salmonellosis, 230
  for septicemia, 486–487
  for shock, 539–540
  in birth resuscitation, 534–535
  intravenous, 578–580
  in cardiopulmonary resuscitation, 129
Flumazenil, dosage of, 670
Flunixin meglumine, 575
  dosage of, 671
  for abdominal pain, 158t
  for acute colitis, 220–221
  for antibiotic-induced diarrhea, 236
  for bites and stings, 271
  for blister beetle poisoning, 225
  for cerebral abscess, 362
  for corneal ulcers, 394
  for duodenitis/jejunitis, 189
  for grain overload, 171, 172
  for laminitis, 326
  for meconium impaction, 499
  for nonstrangulation infarction, 190
  for paraphimosis, 405
  for penile hematoma, 407
  for peritonitis, 216
  for pulmonary edema, 446
  for ruptured corpus spongiosum penis, 409
  for seizures, 370
  for septic metritis, 427
  for septic shock and SIRS, 541
  for snake bites, 443
  for testicular trauma, 410
  for uveitis, 402
  for vaginal hemorrhage, 423
  for viral encephalitis, 361
  overdose of, treatment for, 594t
  used in field emergencies, 648t, 650
Fluorescein staining, 81
Fluphenazine, overdose of, treatment for, 594t
Fluprostenol sodium, dosage of, 671
  overdose of, treatment for, 594t
Fly bites, 272
Foal(s), agalactia in, treatment of, 430–431
  ambu bag ventilation in, 43
  bacterial pneumonia in, 453–454
  botulism in, 348–349
    prognosis for, 350
  bronchointerstitial pneumonia in, 454–455
  cardiopulmonary failure in, reasons for, 506
    recognition of, 506–509

Foal(s) *(Continued)*
  cardiopulmonary resuscitation of, 503–537. See also *Cardiopulmonary resuscitation (CPR), of foals.*
  fescue foot in, 623
  gastric ulcers in, 173–175. See also *Gastric ulcer(s).*
  hematologic values in, 693
  hyperkalemic periodic paralysis in, 353–354
  laryngeal paralysis in, 438–439
  maternal rejection of, 431
  meconium aspiration in, 459–460
  newborn. See *Newborn foal.*
  nursing, behavior of, 481–482
    diarrhea in, 225–234, 501, 503. See also *Diarrhea, in nursing foals.*
  nutrition for, 488–489, 497, 658, 660–662
  respiratory distress in, after anthelminthic therapy, 455–456
  resuscitation of, at birth, 528–537. See also *Birth resuscitation.*
  Rhodococcus equi pneumonia in, 452–453
  ruptured bladder in, 469–470
  serum electrolyte concentrations in, 691
  strangles with retropharyngeal lymph node involvement in, 438
Foaling, urinary incontinence associated with, 472
Foreign body(ies), bronchial, 441
  corneal, 397–398
  in small colon, 204–205
  tracheal, 441
Forelimb, fracture of, immobilization following, 299–303, *300, 303*
  levels in, 299
  prognosis of, 304–305, 306t
  transportation of patient following, 303–304
  proximal, intrasynovial anesthesia of, 70, *71*
  perineural anesthesia of, sequential sites for, 67–68, *67–68*
Fracture(s), 298–310
  anesthesia for, in field emergencies, 653
  basioccipital, 366
  basisphenoid, 366
  cranial, 307–308
  forelimb and hindlimb, immobilization following, 299–303, *300–301, 303–304*
  level of, 299
  prognosis of, 304–305, 306t
  transportation of patient following, 303–304

Fracture(s) *(Continued)*
  jaw, 373
  mandibular, 305, 307
  nasofacial, 309–310
  orbital, 308–309
  pediatric, 330–333, *331–332*
  periorbital, 308–309
  premaxillary, 305, 307
  rib, 293
    during chest compression, 515
  Salter-Harris classification of, *332*
  styloid bone, 373
  temporomandibular, 307
  transportation of patient following, 303–
    304
Friesian horse, registry information for,
    714–715
Frontal nerve block, 379–380
Frontal sinus, trephination of, 46. See also
    Paranasal sinus trephination.
Frostbite, 546–547
Fumonisin poisoning, 610–611
Fungal meningitis, 363
Fungal samples, collection of, equipment
    in, 18
  procedure for, 18
Fungal ulcer(s), as ocular emergencies,
    395
Furosemide, 584
  dosage of, 671
  for anaphylactic reactions, 267
  for blister beetle poisoning, 225
  for congestive heart failure, 138
  for cranial trauma, 365
  for heart disease, 119t
  for hypercalcemia, 134
  for lymphangitis, 269
  for paraphimosis, 406
  for penile hematoma, 407
  for pulmonary edema, 136, 446
    secondary to anaphylaxis, 447
  for purpura hemorrhagica, 263
  for quinidine-induced congestive heart
    failure, 117
  for renal failure, 465
    in peripartum asphyxia, 493

Gastric dilation, acute, 169–170
Gastric impaction, 170–171
Gastric perforation, 175
Gastric ulcer(s), in adults, 172–173
  in foals, 173–175
    prevention of, 174–175
    prophylaxis for, 228

Gastric ulcer(s) *(Continued)*
    treatment of, 173–174
Gastrocnemius tendon, ruptured, as
    pediatric orthopedic emergency,
    329–330
Gastrointestinal tract. See also specific
    part, e.g., *Stomach.*
  emergency(ies) of, 156–236
    colic as, 156–164
      in late-term pregnant mare, 211–
        215
    colonic and rectal disorders as, 204–
      211
    diarrhea as, in adults, 217–225
      in foals, 225–234
      in weanlings and yearlings, 234–
        236
    drugs for, 573–574
    esophageal disorders as, 166–169
    large intestine disorders as, 191–204
    peritonitis as, 215–217
    ptyalism as, 164–166
    small intestine disorders as, 175–191
    stomach disorders as, 169–175
  endoscopic examination of, 32–33
  rupture of, peritoneal fluid in, 555
  toxins affecting, 601–608
Gastroscopy, in newborn foal, 478
Gentamicin, dosage of, 671
  for aspiration pneumonia, 459
  for cellulitis, 268
  for esophageal perforation, 169
  for infections, in newborns and foals,
    334t
  for lacerations, 315t
  for nonstrangulation infarction, 190
  for paraphimosis, 406
  for penile hematoma, 407
  for pericarditis, 148
  for peritonitis, 217
  for pleuropneumonia, 457
  for septicemia, 489
  for Tyzzer's disease, 281
  postdystocia, 415
Geriatric years, dietary guidelines for,
    660t
Glans penis, lesions of, 408
Glass slides, for cytologic specimens,
    preparation of, 550
Glaucoma, 403–404
  treatment of, 403
Globe, emergencies involving, 386–390
  fibrous coat of, lacerations of, 388–390
    full-thickness, 388–389
    partial thickness, 390
Globulin, normal values of, 697

Glucose, serum concentration of, 699
Glycopyrrolate, dosage of, 124t, 671
  for heaves, 450
  for respiratory disorders, 576
  for sinus bradycardia, 106
  for third-degree AV block, 103
  indications for, 124t
  overdose of, treatment for, 594t
Glycosaminoglycan, overdose of,
    treatment for, 597t
Grain overload, emergency, 171
  symptomatic, 171–172
Granulation tissue, exuberant, in wound
    closure, 257–258
  in wound healing, 242
Granulocytic ehrlichiosis, 265
Grove poisoning, 348
Growing horses, dietary guidelines for,
    661t
Guaifenesin, 571
  dosage of, 671
  overdose of, treatment for, 594t
  used in field emergencies, 648t, 649
Guttural pouch empyema, 437
Guttural pouch mycosis, 460–461
Guttural pouch tympany, 441

H$_2$-blockers, for gastric ulcers, 173–174
Hackney horse, registry information for,
    715
Haloperidol, dosage of, 671
  for tetanus, 355
Halothane, overdose of, treatment for,
    594t
Hanoverian horse, registry information for,
    715
Haptoglobin, normal, in foals, 693
Head trauma, 380–382
  blunt, 380–381
  bony, 381–382, Color Plate 1
  in newborn foal, 480
Heart. See also *Cardiac; Cardio-* entries.
  auscultation of, 94–95, 95t, *96,* 97t,
    97–98
  diseases of, drug therapy for, 119t
Heart failure, congestive. See *Congestive
    heart failure.*
  pulmonary edema secondary to, 446
Heart murmurs, characterization of, 97t
  duration of, 95, 97
  grading of, 95
  in congestive heart failure, 136
    and atrial fibrillation, *118,* 118–119
    drug treatment of, 119

Heart murmurs *(Continued)*
  drug treatment of, 119t
  left-sided, 135–138
    auscultation and, 136
    clinical signs of, 135t, 135–136
    echocardiogram of, 136, *137–139*
    treatment of, 136–138
  quinidine-induced, 117
  right-sided, 138–142
    auscultation and, 139–140
    clinical signs of, 139
    treatment of, 140–142
  in newborn foal, 475
  intensity of, 94–95
    point of maximal, 97
  quality of, 97
  radiation of, 97–98
  shape of, 97
  timing of, 95
Heart rate, in newborn foal, 475
  normal, 94
Heart sounds, 95t
Heat stroke, 543–544
Heaves, 449–451
  dietary guidelines for, 659t
Heinz body, in red maple poisoning, 285
Heinz body anemia, 285, 287
Hematologic values, in foals, 693
  normal, 683
Hematoma, 270
  and wound healing, 248
  as complication of venipuncture, 4
  ethmoid, 461
  penile, 406–407
Hematuria, 467–468
Hemoglobin, bovine, dosage of, 667
Hemolysis, toxins causing, 627–630
Hemolytic anemia, 284–291. See also
    Anemia.
  immune-mediated, 287–288
Hemorrhage, as complication of bone
    marrow biopsy, 28
  as complication of liver biopsy, 26
  as complication of renal biopsy, 25
  causing sudden and unexpected death,
    633
  external, 294
  into body cavity, 291–294
  nasal. See *Epistaxis.*
  postcastration, 410–411
  previous, 562
  pulmonary, exercise-induced, 461
  toxins causing, 627–630
  uterine, 424, 425
  vaginal, during late pregnancy, 423
    following natural service delivery,
      423

Hemorrhage *(Continued)*
    postpartum, 422
        treatment of, 423–424
    with trauma, 292
Hemorrhagic effusions, peritoneal fluid in, 556
Hemothorax, as complication of thoracocentesis, 52
Heparin, 586
    dosage of, 671
    overdose of, treatment for, 594t
Hepatic. See also *Liver* entries.
Hepatic encephalopathy, 358
    dietary guidelines for, 660t
    management of, 283–284
Hepatitis, serum, 276–277
Hepatoencephalopathy, 276
Herniation, diaphragmatic, *183,* 183–184, 294
    inguinal, 182–183
    of epiploic foramen, 178–179
    of gastrosplenic ligament, 180
    of mesentery, 180–181
    of small intestine, 178–184
    omental, as complication of abdomi-nocentesis, 59
    ventral, 428
Herpes virus–1 myeloencephalitis, 340–342
    equine, 340–342
Hetastarch, dosage of, 671
    used in field emergencies, 648t, 650
Hindlimb, fracture of, immobilization following, 299–303, *301, 304*
    levels in, 299
    prognosis of, 304–305, 306t
    transportation of patient following, 303–304
    luxation of, 310
    proximal, intrasynovial anesthesia of, 73, *73*
    perineural anesthesia of, sequential sites for, 68, *69*
Hip, luxation of, 311
Hoary alyssum poisoning, limb edema due to, 264, *623,* 623–624
Holsteiner horse, registry information for, 715
Hoof wall, lacerations to, 318–319, *319*
Horner syndrome, 367
Horsetail poisoning, 611
Hyaluronate sodium, overdose of, treatment for, 594t
Hydralazine, 582
    dosage of, 671
    for congestive heart failure, 138

Hydralazine *(Continued)*
    for heart disease, 119t
    for ruptured aortic root, 154
Hydrallantois, 419
Hydramnion, 419
Hydrochlorothiazide, dosage of, 671
Hydrogen peroxide, for wound lavage, 247
Hydrops of fetal membranes, 419–422
    diagnosis of, 420
    induction of parturition for, 421–422
        complications of, 422
    treatment of, 420–421
Hydrotherapy, for lymphangitis, 269
Hydroxyzine hydrochloride, dosage of, 671
    for bites and stings, 271
    for urticaria, 267
Hyperammonemia, 282
Hyperbilirubinemia, 276–277
Hypercalcemia, causing arrhythmias, 133–134
Hypercapnia, neonatal, birth resuscitation in, 536
Hyperexcitability, drug-induced, 370–372
Hyperimmune plasma, dosage of, 671
    intravenous administration of, 578
Hyperkalemia, causing arrhythmias, 129–131, *130*
    treatment of, 130–131
Hyperkalemic periodic paralysis, 131, 353–354, 439–440
    dietary guidelines for, 660t
    in field emergencies, anesthesia and, 652
Hyperlipemia, 278–280
Hypertonic saline, intravenous administration of, 579
Hyphema, acute, 399
Hypocalcemia, 436
    causing arrhythmias, 132–133
    in newborn foal, 480
    tetanic, 351–353
Hypoglycemia, nutritional support for, 488
Hypokalemia, causing arrhythmias, 131–132, *132*
Hypomagnesemia, causing arrhythmias, 132, *132*
Hyponatremia, in newborn foal, 480
Hypotension, drug-induced, 371–372
    quinidine-induced, 116
    sepsis-induced, treatment of, 487
Hypothermia, in field emergencies, anesthesia for, 652
    in foals, 497
Hypovolemia, as complication of thoracocentesis, 52

Hypoxia, neonatal, birth resuscitation in, 535–536
Hypoxic ischemic encephalopathy, 480, 491, 493

Icelandic horse, registry information for, 715
Icterus (jaundice), 273, *274,* 275
  diagnostic tests for, 275
Icterus index, in foals, 693
Ileum, impaction of, 185–186
Ileus, colic due to, in newborn foal, 499–501
  in field emergencies, anesthesia and, 652
  treatment of, 500–501
Iliac artery, rupture of, 424–428
Imidocarb, dosage of, 671
Imipenem, 567
  dosage of, 671
  for septicemia, 490
Imipramine, dosage of, 671
Immobilization, following forelimb and hindlimb fractures, at levels 1 to 3, 299–303, *300–301, 303–304*
Impaction, ascarid, 186–187
  cecal, 191–192
  ileal, 185–186
  large colon, 193–194
  meconium, of small colon, 206–207, *207*
  small colon, 204–205
Inanition, paraphimosis secondary to, 408
Incarceration, of intestine, 156
Incontinence, urinary, associated with foaling, 472
Infarction, nonstrangulating, of small intestine, 189–191
Infection(s), 311–312. See also specific infection, e.g., *Pneumonia.*
  and wound healing, 245–246
  as complication of biopsy, 22, 26
  as complication of burns, 261
  diagnosis of, sample collection in, 17–20
  management of, *312*
  pediatric, 333–334, 334t
Infectious anemia, 265, 290–291
Inflammation, eosinophilic, 562
  suppurative, of lower respiratory tract, 561
  peritoneal fluid in, 555–556
Inflammatory phase, of wound healing, 240–241

Influenza, vaccination schedule for, 701
Infusion technique, intraosseous, 15–16
Inguinal herniation, 182–183
Inhalation, smoke, 447–448, 562
Injured horse, nutritional guidelines for, 658–663
Inotropes, potency of, 527t
Insecticide poisoning, 605–606
Insulin, 586–587
  dosage of, 672
  for hyperlipidemia, 279
  toxicity of, 611
Insulin with dextrose, for hyperkalemia, 130
Intestinal causes, of sudden and unexpected death, 634
Intestine(s), borborygmi in, auscultation for, 158–159
  incarceration of, 156
  large. See *Large intestine.*
  small. See *Small intestine.*
Intoxication. See also *Toxicity.*
  ammonia, 608
  cantharidin, 223–225
Intra-articular disorder(s), correlation of synovial fluid parameters and, 79t
Intracardiac drugs, injection of, complications of, 517
Intracarotid drugs, inadvertent injection of, hyperexcitability due to, 370–371
  oil-based, adverse reactions to, 589
  water-soluble, adverse reactions to, 588–589
Intramuscular administration, of medications, 7, *8, 9*
Intraosseous infusion technique, 15–16
Intrasynovial administration, of medications, 11
Intrasynovial anesthesia, complications of, 76
  for diagnosis of lameness, 65, *70–75,* 76
  of coxofemoral joint, 75, *75*
  of distal limb, 70, *70*
  of elbow joint, 72, *72*
  of proximal forelimb, 70, *71*
  of proximal hindlimb, 73, *73*
  of scapulohumeral joint, 72, *72*
  of stifle joint, 74, *74*
Intrathecal administration, of medications, 11
Intravenous catheter placement. See *Catheter(s), intravenous placement of.*
Intravenous fluid therapy, 578–580
Intubation, complications of, 36

Intubation *(Continued)*
    nasogastric, for grain overload, 172
        in abdominal pain, 159
        of newborn foal, 477
    nasotracheal, 34–35
    orotracheal, 35–36
Intussusception, cecocolic, 196
    colic due to, in newborn foal, 501
    small intestinal, 175–177
Intussusceptum, 175
Intussuscipiens, 175
Ionophore toxicity, 148–151, 624–626
    clinical signs of, 149, 624–625
    diagnosis of, 149–151, *150,* 625
    treatment of, 151, 151t, 625–626
Ipratropium bromide, dosage of, 672
Iron, overdose of, treatment for, 594t
    serum, parameters of, 692
    toxicity of, causing liver failure, 283,
        617–618
Ischemia-reperfusion injury, treatment of,
    164
Isoerythrolysis, neonatal, 288–289
Isoflurane, overdose of, treatment for, 594t
Isoproterenol, 580
    dosage of, 672
    for sinus bradycardia, 106
    for third-degree AV block, 103
Isoxsuprine, 582
    for laminitis, 326
    overdose of, treatment for, 594t
Itraconazole, 569–570
    dosage of, 672
    for fungal meningitis, 363
Ivermectin, dosage of, 672, 686
    overdose of, treatment for, 595t

Japanese yew poisoning, 626–627
Jaundice (icterus), 273, *274,* 275
    diagnostic tests for, 275
Jaw, fracture of, 373
Jejunitis, 187–189, *188*
Joint(s). See also named joint, e.g., *Carpal
        joint.*
    degenerative and traumatic disease of,
        synovial fluid in, 559
    inflammatory disease of, synovial fluid
        in, 559–560
    lacerations to, 319–320
Jugular catheter(s), broken, 591
Jugular vein(s), external, venipuncture via,
    2
    thrombosed, 442
        euthanasia of patient with, 657

Kaolin, dosage of, 672
Keratitis, eosinophilic, 395–397, Color
    Plate 2
Ketamine, 571–572
    dosage of, 672
    overdose of, treatment for, 595t
    used in field emergencies, 648t, 649
Ketoconazole, 570
Ketoprofen, 575
    dosage of, 672
    for abdominal pain, 158t
    overdose of, treatment for, 595t
Kidney(s). See *Renal* entries.
Kleingrass poisoning, causing liver failure,
    282–283, 618

Laceration(s), 312–320
    blunt trauma to eye without, 381
    causing degloving injuries, 317
    of blood vessels and nerves, 317–318
    of coronary band, 318
    of extensor tendons, *316,* 316–317
    of eyelid, 384–386
    of fibrous coat of globe, 388–390
        full-thickness, 388–389
        partial thickness, 390
        with poor prognosis, 388
    of flexor tendons, 313–315, *314,* 315t
    of hoof wall, 318–319, *319*
    of joints, 319–320
    of penis, 409
    severe, anesthesia for, in field emergen-
        cies, 653
β-Lactam drugs, 565–567
Lactated Ringer's solution, used in field
    emergencies, 648t, 650
Lactating mare, dietary guidelines for,
    661t
Lameness, diagnosis of, local anesthesia
        in, 64–76
        complications of, 76
        equipment for, 64–65
        evaluation of results in, 76
        procedure for, 65, *66–75,* 76
        via intrasynovial route, 65, *70–75,*
            76
        via perineural route, 65, *66–69*
    nonweight-bearing, management of, *312*
Laminitis, 323–328
    acute, 323
    advanced/refractory, 323, 325–328
        diagnosis of, 325–326
        medical treatment of, 326–327
        physical and nutritional therapy for,
            327

Laminitis *(Continued)*
  precipitating factors in, 323, 325
  preventive measures in, 325
  prognosis of, 328
  surgical treatment of, 327
  therapeutic trimming and shoeing for,
    327
  quinidine-induced, 118
Large intestine. See also specific part,
    e.g., *Colon.*
  disorder(s) of, atresia coli as, 203–204
    causing colic, 191–204
    cecal impaction as, 191–192
    cecal perforation as, 192–193
    cecocolic intussusception as, 196
    large colon displacements as, 196–
      198, *198–200,* 201
    large colon impaction as, 193–194
    large colon volvulus as, 201, *202,*
      203
    sand impaction as, 194–195
Laryngeal edema, 435–436
Laryngeal obstruction, 435–441
Laryngeal paralysis, in foals, 438–439
Laryngeal spasms, 437
Lavage, bronchoalveolar, 38–39
    material collected by, microscopic fea-
      tures of, 560–563
  of pericardial sac, 146, 148
  to relieve choke, 167
  wound, 254
    antiseptics for, 246–247
Laxatives, for acute abdominal pain, 163
  for meconium impaction, 499
Laxity, of periarticular structures, in
    angular limb deformity, 336
Lead poisoning, 611–612
  acute, trembling with, 358
Leg-Savr Brace, 302
Lens, luxation of, 400
Lethal white foal disease, 204
Leukocyte counts, 696
  altered, cause of, 684
Leukoencephalomalacia, 281
Lidocaine, 583
  adverse effects of, 125t
  dosage of, 124t, 672
  for acute colitis, 220
  for cardiopulmonary resuscitation, 518t,
    523
  for congestive heart failure, 141
  for duodenitis/jejunitis, 189
  for laminitis, 327
  for quinidine-induced arrhythmias, 113t,
    115
  for renal failure, in peripartum
    asphyxia, 494

Lidocaine *(Continued)*
  for ventricular arrhythmia, 123
  indications for, 124t
  overdose of, treatment for, 595t
  used in field emergencies, 648t, 650–
    651
Limb(s). See also *Forelimb; Hindlimb.*
  angular deformity of, as pediatric ortho-
    pedic emergency, 334, *335,* 336,
    497, 498
  contracture of, in newborn foal, 481
  distal, dermatitis of, 620
    intrasynovial anesthesia of, 70, *70*
    perineural anesthesia of, sequential
      sites for, 66, *66*
  edema of, acute onset of, 264
Limb reflexes, in newborn foal, 479
Lipizzaner horse, registry information for,
    716
Lipoma, pedunculated, of small intestine,
    184–185
Liver. See also *Hepatic; Hepato-* entries.
  biopsy of, 25–26, 283
  toxins affecting, 616–619
  ultrasound study of, 283
Liver failure, 273–284
  Alsike clover causing, 283
  bile duct obstruction causing, 281–282
  cholangiohepatitis and cholelithiasis
    causing, 277–278
  fulminant, management of, 283–284
  hyperammonemia causing, 282
  hyperlipemia causing, 278–280
  iron intoxication causing, 283
  jaundice in, 273, *274,* 275
  Kleingrass and fall panicum causing,
    282–283
  portocaval shunts causing, 282
  pyrollizidine toxicosis causing, 280
  Theiler's disease causing, 276–277
  Tyzzer's disease causing, 281
Local anesthesia, in diagnosis of
    lameness, 64–76
  complications of, 76
  equipment in, 64–65
  evaluation of results in, 76
  procedure in, 65, *66–75,* 76
  via intrasynovial route, 65, *70–75,*
    76
  via perineural route, 65, *66–69*
Locoweed poisoning, 612, *613*
Locust poisoning, 602
Longus capitis muscle, rupture of, 461
Loperamide, dosage of, 672
  for enteritis, 503
Lumbar nerve, disorders of, 377

Lumbosacral space, cerebrospinal fluid collection from, 87, *88*
Lung(s). See also *Pulmonary; Respiratory* entries.
abnormal sounds of, in congestive heart failure, 136
biopsy of, 26–27
Luxation(s), of joints, 310–311
of lens, 400
of superficial digital flexor tendon, 330
Lyme disease, 265–266
Lymph node(s), biopsy of, 23–24
retropharyngeal, strangles with, in foals, 438
Lymphangitis, 269–270
Lymphocyte count, 696

Magnesium, intravenous administration of, 578
overdose of, treatment for, 595t
Magnesium sulfate, 583
dosage of, 124t, 672
for acute abdominal pain, 163
for cardiopulmonary resuscitation, 518t, 524
for grain overload, 171
for hypomagnesemia, 132
for quinidine-induced arrhythmias, 113t
for quinidine-induced torsades de pointes, 115
for ventricular tachycardia, 125
indications for, 124t
Maladjustment syndrome, neonatal. See *Asphyxia, peripartum.*
Malicious death, causes of, 635
Malnutrition. See also *Nutritional* entries.
and wound healing, 243
Mandible, fracture of, 305, 307
Mannitol, 585
dosage of, 673
for CNS disturbances, in peripartum asphyxia, 493
for cranial trauma, 365
Maple, red, *628*
toxicity of, 285, 628–629, 632
Mare, agalactia in, treatment of, 431
lactating, dietary guidelines for, 661t
late-term pregnant, colic in, 211–215
pregnant, dietary guidelines for, 661t
late-term, colic in, 211–215
Marijuana poisoning, 612
Mastitis, 429–430
Maturation phase, of wound healing, 242–243

Maxillary sinus, trephination of, 46–47. See also *Paranasal sinus trephination.*
Mebendazole, dosage of, 673
Mebezonium, overdose of, treatment for, 593t
Mechanical positive-pressure ventilation, as respiratory support for septicemia, 488
Meclofenamic acid, 575
Meconium, aspiration of, in foals, 459–460
impaction of, colic due to, 498–499
treatment of, 499
in newborn foal, 476
retention of, in small colon, 206–207, *207*
Medial antebrachial nerve block, of proximal forelimb, 68, *68*
Median antebrachial nerve block, of proximal forelimb, 68, *68*
Medication(s). See also named drug or drug group.
administration of, 6–12
epidural, 11–12
intramuscular, 7, *8, 9*
intrasynovial, 11
intrathecal, 11
intravenous, 9–10
oral, 6–7
rectal, 10
topical, 10
transdermal/cutaneous, 11
adverse reactions to, 588–598
recommended treatment for, 592t–598t
reference information for, 588
anaphylaxis with, 590
emergency, dosages of, 666–677
overdose of, 591
recommended treatment for, 592t–598t
Membrane atresia, of intestines, 203
Meningitis, fungal, 363
in newborn foal, 480
Mentation, change in, 358–363
cerebral abscess causing, 361–363
encephalopathy causing, 358–360
fungal meningitis causing, 363
self-mutilation causing, 363
viral encephalitides causing, 360–361
Meperidine hydrochloride, 570
dosage of, 673
for abdominal pain, 158t
overdose of, treatment for, 595t
Mercury poisoning, 608, 630–631

Mesenteric herniation, 180–181
Mesocolic rupture, of small colon, 207–208
Metamucil, dosage of, 673
Metaphysis, disproportionate growth of, in angular limb deformity, 336
Metatarsal artery, dorsal, puncture of, 6
L-Methionine, dosage of, 673
Methocarbamol, 585
  overdose of, treatment for, 595t
Methylene blue, dosage of, 673
  for necrotizing enterocolitis, 228
  for sepsis-induced hypotension, 487
Metoclopramide, dosage of, 673
  for gastrointestinal dysmotility, in peri-partum asphyxia, 494
  for ileus, 500
  for ulcers, 574
  overdose of, treatment for, 595t
Metritis, septic, 426–428
  treatment of, 427–428
Metronidazole, 568
  dosage of, 673
  for antibiotic-induced diarrhea, 222, 236
  for aspiration pneumonia, 459
  for bacterial pneumonia, 454
  for cellulitis, 268
  for clostridial myositis, 269
  for esophageal perforation, 169
  for necrotizing enterocolitis, 228
  for peritonitis, 217
  for pleuropneumonia, 457
  for smoke inhalation, 448
  for snake bites, 443
  prophylactic, for choke, 167
Microorganism(s), in wounds, virulence of, 252
"Milk feces," 476
Milk of magnesia, dosage of, 673
  for meconium impaction, 499
Milrinone, dosage of, 673
  for heart disease, 119t
Mineral oil, dosage of, 673
  for acute abdominal pain, 163
Miniature horse, registry information for, 716
Misoprostol, dosage of, 673
  for NSAID toxicity, 222
  for ulcers, 573
Mitral valve, regurgitation of, clinical signs of, 135t
  ruptured chordae tendineae of, echocar-diogram of, *138, 140*
Moldy corn poisoning, 358–360
Moldy sweet clover poisoning, 627–628
Monensin, overdose of, treatment for, 595t

Monobactams, 567
Monocyte count, 696
Morab horse, registry information for, 716
Morgan horse, registry information for, 716
Morphine sulfate, 570
  dosage of, 673
  for abdominal pain, 158t
  overdose of, treatment for, 595t
Motor neuron disease, 350–351
Mouth, disorders of, 164–166
  localized causes of, 165
  systemic causes of, 166
  treatment of, 165
Mouth ulcers, quinidine-induced, 118
Mouth-to-nose ventilation, in foals, 510, 511
Moxidectin, dosage of, 673
  for cyathostomiasis, 222
Mucomyst, dosage of, 673
Mucous membranes, of newborn foal, 474
Murmurs, cardiac, characterization of, 97t
  duration of, 95, 97
  grading of, 95
  in congestive heart failure, 136
  in newborn foal, 475
  intensity of, 94–95
    point of maximal, 97
  quality of, 97
  radiation of, 97–98
  shape of, 97
  timing of, 95
Muscle biopsy, 28–29
Muscle disorder(s), drug therapy for, 585
Muscle soreness, as complication of intramuscular drug administration, 9
Muscle spasms, trembling with, 358
Musculoskeletal system, injuries to, 297–336. See also *Orthopedic emergency(ies).*
  of newborn foal, 480–481
  toxins affecting, 622–624
Mutilation, self, 363
Mycosis, guttural pouch, 460–461
Mycotoxic encephalopathy, 358–360
Myelitis, protozoal, 338–339
Myeloencephalitis, equine herpes virus–1, 340–342
Myelopathy, cervical stenotic, 339–340
Myocardial heart disease, drug therapy for, 119t
Myopathy, nutritional, 270–271
  polysaccharide storage, 357
  trembling with, 356–357
Myositis, clostridial, 268–269
  trembling with, 356–357

Naloxone, administration of, 587
  dosage of, 673
Narcotics, 570–572
Nasal cavity, trauma to, 441–442
Nasal hemorrhage. See *Epistaxis.*
Nasal mass(es), 462
Nasal obstruction, 441–443
Nasal oxygen insufflation, 40–41
Nasofacial fracture, 309–310
Nasogastric intubation, for grain overload, 172
  in abdominal pain, 159
  of newborn foal, 477
Nasogastric tube, and demand valve, ventilation with, 43
  placement of, 53–55
    complications of, 55
Nasolacrimal duct, cannulation of, 82
Nasotracheal intubation, 34–35
National Poison Control Center hotlines, 600
Nebulization, for COPD, 450
Necropsy, samples taken at, 19
Necrotizing enterocolitis, in nursing foals, 225–229
  clinical signs of, 226
  diagnosis of, 226–227, *226–227*
  prognosis of, 228–229
  treatment of, 228
Needle(s), placement of, for centesis, 321, *321*
Needle breakage, as complication of local anesthesia, 76
Neomycin, dosage of, 673
Neonatal hypercapnia, birth resuscitation in, 536
Neonatal hypoxia, birth resuscitation in, 535–536
Neonatal isoerythrolysis, 288–289
Neonatal maladjustment syndrome. See *Asphyxia, peripartum.*
Neoplasia, diagnosis of, by bronchoalveolar lavage, 563
  peritoneal fluid in, 557
Neostigmine, dosage of, 674
  for necrotizing enterocolitis, 228
  for ulcers, 574
  overdose of, treatment for, 596t
Nephritis, septic, acute, 465
Nephropathy, pigment, 463–464
  vasomotor, 464
Nerve(s). See also named nerve, e.g., *Facial nerve.*
  peripheral, diseases of, 374–378
Nerve block(s), auriculopalpebral, 83, *84*, 379

Nerve block(s) *(Continued)*
  frontal, 379–380
  incomplete, as complication of epidural anesthesia, 12
  of distal limb, abaxial sesamoid, 66, *66*
    palmar digital, 66, *66*
    palmar metacarpal, 66, *66*
  of proximal forelimb, antebrachial, 68, *68*
    palmar metacarpal, 67, *67*
  of proximal hindlimb, dorsal metatarsal, 68, *69*
    peroneal, 68, *69*
    plantar metatarsal, 68, *69*
    tibial, 68, *69*
    supraorbital, 83, *84*
Nervous system, central. See *Central nervous system.*
  disorder(s) of, 337–378
    acute ataxia as, 337–348
    change in mentation as, 358–363
    dysphagia as, 372–374
    peripheral nerve disease as, 374–378, 380
    sudden collapse as, 363–372
    trembling as, 348–358
    toxins affecting, 608–616
Nettles, stinging, 621
Neurologic causes, of sudden and unexpected death, 633–634
Neurologic evaluation, of newborn foal, 479–480
Neuromuscular blocking agents, 585–586
Neutrophil counts, 696
Newborn foal, 473–503
  abdominal examination of, 476–478
  asphyxia in, 530
  atresia coli in, 203–204
  cardiovascular system of, 475
  colic in, 498–503
    enteritis causing, 225–234, 501–503
    ileus causing, 499–501
    intussusception causing, 501
    meconium impaction causing, 498–499
  congenital hernia in, 182
  diarrhea in, 233–234
  drug therapy in, consideration of, 587
  meconium impaction in, 206, 207
  modified Apgar score for, 532t
  mucous membranes and sclera of, 474–475
  musculoskeletal system of, 334–336, 480–481
  nephrosplenic displacement in, 196–201
  neurologic evaluation of, 479–480

Newborn foal *(Continued)*
  nursing behavior of, 481–482
  ophthalmic examination of, 479
  physical examination of, 473–482
  placenta of, 474
  rejection of, 431
  respiratory system of, 475–476, 494–496
  resuscitation of, 528–537. See also *Birth resuscitation.*
  urogenital system of, 469, 470, 478–479, 493
  vital signs in, 473t
  weakness and loss of suckle in, 482–498
    peripartum asphyxia causing, 491–496
    prematurity/dysmaturity causing, 496–498
    septicemia causing, 482–491
Nitric oxide, dosage of, 674
  for pulmonary vasoconstriction, in peripartum asphyxia, 494
Nitric oxide–nitroglycerine patches, for laminitis, 327
Nitroglycerin, 582
  overdose of, treatment for, 596t
Nitroglycerin cream, 674
Nitroprusside, 582
Nodule, biopsy of, 22–23
Nonselenium-deficient tying-up syndrome, 356
Nonsteroidal anti-inflammatory drugs (NSAIDs), 574–576
  for enteritis, 503
  for limb edema, 264
  for paraphimosis, 405–406
  for penile hematoma, 407
  for uveitis, 402
  in wound healing, 244
  toxicity of, 218
  treatment for, 222
Nonstrangulating infarction, of small intestine, 189–191
Nonstrangulating obstruction, of gastrointestinal tract, 156
Nonweight-bearing lameness, infection in, 311
  management of, *312*
Norepinephrine, dosage of, 674
  for sepsis-induced hypotension, 487
  potency of, 527t
NSAIDs. See *Nonsteroidal anti-inflammatory drugs (NSAIDs).*
Nursemare directory, 432–433
Nursing foal, behavior of, 481–482

Nursing foal *(Continued)*
  diarrhea in, 225–234. See also *Diarrhea, in nursing foals.*
  nutrition for, 658, 660–662
Nutritional guidelines, for injured horse, 658–663
Nutritional myopathy, 270–271
Nutritional support, by tube, 662t, 662–663
  for acute abdominal pain, 164
  for hyperlipidemia, 279
  for laminitis, 327
  for neonatal isoerythrolysis, 289
  for nursing foals, 658, 660–662
  for physiologic stress, 658, 661t
  for septicemia, 488–490
  for sick horse, 658, 659t–660t

Oak poisoning, 604–605
Obstruction, bile duct, 281–282
  esophageal, 166–168
  gastrointestinal, functional, 156
    nonstrangulating and strangulating, 156
    persistence of, 156–157
  laryngeal, 435–441
  nasal, 441–443
  of lower urinary tract, 468–469
Ocular emergency(ies), 379
  acute hyphema as, 399
  corneal abrasions and ulcers as, 390–395
  corneal edema as, 398–399
  corneal foreign bodies as, 397–398
  eosinophilic keratitis as, 395–397
  fungal ulcers as, 395
  glaucoma as, 403–404
  involving eyelids, 382–386
  involving globe, 386–390
  involving head, 380–382
  lens luxation as, 400
  treatment of, diagnostic and therapeutic aids in, 379–380
  uveitis as, 400–403
Oil-based intracarotid drugs, adverse reactions to, 589
Oleander poisoning, 627
Omental herniation, as complication of abdominocentesis, 59
Omeprazole, dosage of, 674
  for gastric ulcers, in foals, 174
  for ulcers, 573
Onchocerca, 266
Onion poisoning, 630

Ophthalmic examination, of newborn foal, 479
Oral administration, of medications, 6–7
Orbital fracture, 308–309
Organic molecules, small, serum chemistry concentrations of, 699
Organophosphate(s), 687
  toxicity of, 605–606
Oropharyngeal cavity, contamination of, 561
Orthopedic emergency(ies), 297–323. See also specific emergency, e.g., *Fracture(s)*.
  common, 298
  fractures as, 298–310
  infections as, 311–312
  lacerations as, 312–320
  luxations as, 310–311
  pediatric, 328–336
    angular limb deformity as, 334, *335,* 336
    fractures as, 330–333, *331–332*
    infection as, 333–334, 334t
    luxation of superficial digital flexor tendon as, 330
    splints and casts for, 328–329
    tendon rupture as, 329–330
    puncture wounds as, 320–323
  steps in, 297
  tranquilization, sedation, and pain relief in, 29, 298t
  weight-bearing, algorithm for management of, *324*
Ossification, incomplete, in angular limb deformity, *335,* 336
Osteomyelitis, septic, in newborn foal, 481
Otitis, with vestibular syndrome, 343–344
Overdose, drug, 591
  recommended treatment for, 592t–598t
Oxfendazole, dosage of, 674
Oxibendazole, dosage of, 674
Oxygen insufflation, nasal, 40–41
Oxygen tension, and wound healing, 250
Oxygen therapy, as respiratory support for septicemia, 487–488
  for septic shock and SIRS, 540–541
  for traumatic pneumothorax, 444
Oxymorphone, 570
  overdose of, treatment for, 595t
Oxytetracycline, 568
  overdose of, treatment for, 596t
Oxytocin, dosage of, 674
  for retained placenta, 426
  induction of parturition with, 422

Oxytocin (*Continued*)
  overdose of, treatment for, 596t

Pacemaker. See *Cardiac pacemaker.*
Packed cell volume, in assessment of dehydration, 160
Pain, abdominal. See *Abdominal pain.*
Pain relief, for orthopedic emergencies, 297, 298t
Palmar digital nerve block, of distal limb, 66, *66*
Palmar metacarpal nerve block, of distal limb, 66, *66*
  of proximal forelimb, 67, *67*
Palomino horse, registry information for, 717
Paralysis, hyperkalemic periodic. See *Hyperkalemic periodic paralysis.*
  laryngeal, in foals, 438–439
  of facial nerve, 383–384
  of retractor muscle, following tranquilization, 407
  peroneal, 376
  tibial, 376–377
Paranasal sinus trephination, 46–49
  complications of, 49
  equipment for, 44
  procedure for, 47–49, *48*
  sites for, *48*
Paraphimosis, 405–408
  quinidine-induced, 117
  secondary to inanition or debility, 408
  treatment of, 405–406
Parascaris equorum infestation, 186
Parenteral nutrition, total, components of, 488–489
  for hyperlipidemia, 279
Paresis, laryngeal, temporary, 437
Paromomycin, dosage of, 674
  for *Cryptosporidium parvum*–associated diarrhea, 232
Parturition, induced, for hydrops of fetal membranes, 421–422
  complications of, 422
  premature, 211
Paso Fino horse, registry information for, 717
Pastern joint, anesthesia of, 70, *70*
Patella, luxation of, 311
Pectin, dosage of, 674
Pediatric orthopedic emergency(ies), 328–336
  angular limb deformity as, 334, *335,* 336, 497, 498

Pediatric orthopedic emergency(ies) (*Continued*)
   fractures as, 330–333, *331–332*
   infection as, 333–334, 334t
   luxation of superficial digital flexor tendon as, 330
   splints and casts for, 328–329
   tendon rupture as, 329–330
Pedunculated lipoma, of small intestine, 184–185
Pelleted feed, 662
   treatment of, 497–498
Penicillin, dosage of, 674
   for acute abdominal pain, 164
   for aspiration pneumonia, 459
   for botulism, 349
   for cellulitis, 268
   for cerebral abscess, 362
   for clostridial myositis, 269
   for duodenitis/jejunitis, 189
   for esophageal perforation, 169
   for lacerations, 315t
   for necrotizing enterocolitis, 228
   for nonstrangulation infarction, 190
   for paraphimosis, 406
   for penile hematoma, 407
   for pericarditis, 148
   for peritonitis, 217
   for pleuropneumonia, 457
   for purpura hemorrhagica, 263
   for septicemia, 489
   for smoke inhalation, 448
   for snake bites, 443
   for testicular trauma, 410
   for tetanus, 355
   for Tyzzer's disease, 281
   for vaginal hemorrhage, 423
   overdose of, treatment for, 596t
   postdystocia, 415
Penicillin G, for infections, in newborns and foals, 334t
   prophylactic, for choke, 167
Penis, abrasions and lacerations of, 409
   corpus spongiosum of, ruptured, 408–409
   hematoma of, 406–407
   paralysis of, 407
   support for, 406, *406*
Pentazocine, dosage of, 674
   for abdominal pain, 158t
   overdose of, treatment for, 595t
Pentobarbital, dosage of, 674
Pentoxifylline, dosage of, 674
   for acute colitis, 221
   for grain overload, 172
   for lymphangitis, 269

Pentoxifylline (*Continued*)
   for pulmonary edema, 446
   for septic shock and SIRS, 541
   for Tyzzer's disease, 281
Percheron horse, registry information for, 717
Perforation(s), cecal, 192–193
   duodenal, 175
   esophageal, 168–169
   gastric, 175
   rectal, 208–209, *210*
Pergolide, dosage of, 674
   for hyperlipidemia, 279
   overdose of, treatment for, 597t
Pericardial effusion, 142–148
   echocardiogram for, 142–144, *143–145*
   etiology of, 147t
   treatment of, 144, 146, 148
Pericardial sac, lavage of, 146, 148
Pericardiocentesis, for pericarditis, 144, 146
Pericarditis, 142–148
   echocardiogram for, 142–144, *143–145*
   treatment of, 144, 146, 148
Perineural anesthesia, complications of, 76
   for diagnosis of lameness, 65, *66–69*
   sequential sites for, of distal limb, 66, *66*
      of proximal forelimb, 67–68, *67–68*
      of proximal hindlimb, 68, *69*
Periorbital fracture, 308–309
Peripheral nerve disease, 374–378
Peritoneal fluid, 553–557
   abnormalities in, 161
   analysis of, 57, 58t
   biochemistry reference values for, 682
   cell counts and cytologic examination of, 554–555
   interpretation of, in enterocentesis, 555
      in gastrointestinal rupture, 555
      in hemorrhagic effusions, 556
      in neoplasia, 557
      in seminoperitoneum, 556
      in suppurative inflammation, 555–556
      in uroperitoneum, 556–557
      incidental findings in, 557
Peritonitis, 215–217
   as complication of cecal trocharization, 60
   as complication of renal biopsy, 25
   treatment of, 216–217
Peroneal nerve, paralysis of, 376
Peroneal nerve block, of proximal hindlimb, 68, *69*
Perphenazine, dosage of, 674
Persistent fetal circulation pulmonary vasoconstriction, in peripartum asphyxia, treatment of, 494–495

pH, and wound healing, 250–251
Phenobarbital, dosage of, 674
  for cerebral abscess, 362
  for CNS disturbances, in peripartum
      asphyxia, 492
  for cranial trauma, 365
  for hyperexcitability, 371
  for seizures, 370
  for tetanus, 355
  for viral encephalitis, 361
Phenoxybenzamine, 582
  dosage of, 674
  for laminitis, 326
  for urinary incontinence, 472
  overdose of, treatment for, 596t
Phenylbutazone, 575
  dosage of, 674
  for abdominal pain, 158t
  for corneal ulcers, 394
  for duodenitis/jejunitis, 189
  for eyelid lacerations, 386
  for hematoma, 270
  for laminitis, 326
  for lymphangitis, 269
  for nutritional myopathy, 271
  for paraphimosis, 405
  for penile hematoma, 407
  for uveitis, 402
  for vestibular disease, 344
  for viral encephalitis, 361
Phenylephrine, 581
  dosage of, 124t, 674
  for quinidine-induced arrhythmias, 113t
  for quinidine-induced hypotension, 116
  for sepsis-induced hypotension, 487
  indications for, 124t
  potency of, 527t
Phenylguanidine, 687
Phenylpropanolamine, 581
  dosage of, 675
  for urinary incontinence, 472
  overdose of, treatment for, 597t
Phenytoin, 583
  adverse effects of, 125t
  dosage of, 124t, 675
  for congestive heart failure, 141
  indications for, 124t
  overdose of, treatment for, 597t
PHF (Potomac horse fever), 217, 218
  tetracycline for, 222
  vaccination schedule for, 702
Phlebitis, as complication of intravenous
      catheters, 15
Phosphorus, intravenous administration of,
      579
Physeal fracture(s), in foals, 331–332, *332*

Physical therapy, for laminitis, 327
Physiologic stress, nutrition for, 658, 661t
Physis, fracture of, 331–332, *332*
Pigment nephropathy, 463–464
Pinto horse, registry information for,
      717–718
Piperazine, 687
  dosage of, 675
  overdose of, treatment for, 597t
Piroplasmosis *(Babesia),* 289–290
Placenta, examination of, in newborn foal,
      474
  retained, 425–426
Plantar metatarsal nerve block, of
      proximal hindlimb, 68, *69*
Plant-induced ataxia, 347–348
Plasma, equine, intravenous administration
      of, 578–579
  for grain overload, 172
  for septic shock and SIRS, 540
Plasma exchange, for purpura
      hemorrhagica, 263
Plasma protein, normal, in foals, 693
Plasma transfusion, for septicemia, 490
Platelets, normal, in foals, 693
Pleural fluid, analysis if, 52
  reference values for, 681
Pleuritis, 456–458
Pleuropneumonia, 456–458
  clinical signs and physical changes of,
      456t
  treatment of, 457–458
  with toxemia, 458
Pneumomediastinum, 445
Pneumonia, aspiration, 458–460
  bacterial, in foals, 453–454, 485
  bronchointerstitial, in foals, 454–455
  pneumothorax secondary to, 444
  Rhodococcus equi, in foals, 452–453
Pneumothorax, 443–445
  as complication of thoracocentesis, 52
  secondary to pneumonia, 444
  traumatic, 444
Poisoning. See *Toxicity.*
Polymyxin, dosage of, 675
  for acute colitis, 221
Polysaccharide storage myopathy, 357
Polyvinylchloride splint, wired, for
      extensor tendon lacerations, 316, *316*
Pony of the Americas, registry
      information for, 718
Portocaval shunts, causing liver failure,
      282
Postcastration, complications following,
      410–411
Postfoaling colic, 415

Potassium, for congestive heart failure, 141
  fractional excretion of, calculation of, 108
Potassium chloride, dosage of, 675
  for hypokalemia, 131–132
  for ventricular fibrillation, 128t
Potomac horse fever (PHF), 217, 218
  tetracycline for, 222
  vaccination schedule for, 702
Pouch mycosis, guttural, 460–461
Povidone-iodine solution, for wound lavage, 247
Pralidoxime, dosage of, 675
Prednisolone, 577
  dosage of, 675
  used in field emergencies, 648t, 651
Prednisone, 577
  dosage of, 675
  for heaves, 449
  for limb edema, 264
  for motor neuron disease, 351
  for pruritus, 272
  for urticaria, 267
Pregnant mare, dietary guidelines for, 661t
  late-term, colic in, 211–215
Premature parturition, 211
Prematurity/dysmaturity, clinical signs of, 496
  in foals, 474
  musculoskeletal signs of, 481
  treatment of, 497–498
  weakness due to, 496–498
Premaxilla, fracture of, 305, 307
Prepubic tendon, rupture of, 428–429
  in pregnant mare, 214–215
Procainamide, adverse effects of, 125t
  dosage of, 124t, 675
  for quinidine-induced arrhythmias, 113t
  for ventricular tachycardia, 123, 125
  indications for, 124t
  overdose of, treatment for, 597t
Procaine penicillin, 566
  adverse reaction to, hyperexcitability as, 371
  for dysphagia, 373
Product manufacturers, 704–710
Progesterone, dosage of, 675
Prolapse, bladder, 471
  rectal, 209–211
  uterine, 429
Promazine, overdose of, treatment for, 597t
Propafenone, adverse effects of, 125t
  dosage of, 124t, 675
  for quinidine-induced arrhythmias, 113t

Propafenone (Continued)
  for ventricular tachycardia, 123, 125
  indications for, 124t
Propantheline bromide, overdose of, treatment for, 597t
Propofol, dosage of, 676
Propranolol, 583
  adverse effects of, 125t
  dosage of, 124t, 676
  for atrial fibrillation, with congestive heart failure, 119
  for quinidine-induced arrhythmias, 113t
  for ventricular tachycardia, 125
  indications for, 124t
  overdose of, treatment for, 597t
Prostaglandin E₁, dosage of, 676
Prostanoic inhibitors, for septic shock and SIRS, 541
Protein deficiency, and wound healing, 243
Protocols, for anesthesia, in field emergencies, 654, 656
Protozoal myelitis, 338–339
Proximal forelimb, intrasynovial anesthesia of, 70, 71
  perineural anesthesia of, sequential sites for, 67–68, 67–68
Proximal hindlimb, intrasynovial anesthesia of, 73, 73
  perineural anesthesia of, sequential sites for, 68, 69
Pruritus, acute, 272
  as complication of burns, 262
Pseudotuberculosis, Corynebacterium, 270
Psyllium hydrophilic mucilloid, dosage of, 676
  for acute abdominal pain, 163
  for sand impaction, 195
Ptyalism, 164–166
Pulmonary. See also Lung(s).
Pulmonary edema, 445–447
  treatment of, 136
Pulmonary hemorrhage, exercise-induced, 461
Pulmonary hypertension, persistent, birth resuscitation in, 535
Pulmonary vasoconstriction, in peripartum asphyxia, treatment of, 494–495
Pulse(s), arterial, during resuscitation, of foals, 515–516
  peripheral, in newborn foal, 475
Puncture wounds, 320–323, 321–322
Pupil size, during resuscitation, of foals, 516
Pupillary light response, in newborn foal, 479

Purpura hemorrhagica, 262–263
  treatment of, 263
Pyrantel, dosage of, 676
Pyrimethamine, 568
  dosage of, 676
  for equine protozoal myelitis, 339
Pyrimidine, 687
Pyrrolizidine alkaloid toxicity, 280, 438,
  618–619, *619*

QRS complex, prolonged, as sign of
  quinidine toxicity, quinidine-induced,
  12, *114*
Quarab horses, registry information for,
  718
Quarter horses, registry information for,
  718
Quinidine, 583
  adverse effects of, 125t
  overdose of, treatment for, 598t
  toxicity of, 111t, 112
    electrocardiographic monitoring of,
      112–113, *114*
    rapid supraventricular tachycardia due
      to, 112–113, *114–115*
    ventricular arrhythmias associated with,
      113, 115, *116*
    treatment of, 113t
Quinidine gluconate, adverse reaction and
    toxic side effects of, 111t, 112
  dosage of, 124t, 676
  for atrial fibrillation, 110
  for ventricular tachycardia, 123
  indications for, 124t
Quinidine sulfate, adverse reaction and
    toxic side effects of, 111t, 112
  dosage of, 124t, 676
  for atrial fibrillation, 110
  indications for, 124t

Rabies, 344–346
  clinical signs of, 345, 345t
  precautions in dealing with, 345–346
  submission of tissue samples to labora-
    tories, 346
  vaccination schedule for, 702
Radial nerve, disorders of, 374–375
Radiography, abdominal, of newborn foal,
  477
  contrast, of newborn foal, 477–478
  thoracic, of bronchopneumonia, *484–
    486,* 485

Ranitidine, dosage of, 676
  for gastric ulcers, 173
    in foals, 173
  for gastrointestinal dysmotility, in peri-
    partum asphyxia, 494
  for ileus, 500
  for ulcers, 573
    in bronchointerstitial pneumonia, 455
    in enteritis, 503
Rectal disorder(s), 208–211
  prolapse as, 209–211
  tears as, 208–209, *210*
Rectal drug administration, 10
Rectal examination, findings in, abdominal
  pain and, 159
Rectal surgery, dietary guidelines for, 660t
Red clover poisoning, 606–607
Red maple, *628*
  toxicity of, 285, 628–629, 632
Reflexes, limb, in newborn foal, 479
Reflux, in newborn foal, 477
Registry information, for breeds of horses,
  711–720
Renal biopsy, 24–25
Renal disease, dietary guidelines for, 660t
Renal failure, acute, 462–465
  nephropathy in, 463–464
  nephrotoxic causes of, 462–463
  treatment of, 464–465
  in peripartum asphyxia, treatment of,
    493–494
Renal function, 694
Renosplenic displacement, 196–201
Repair phase, of wound healing, 241–242
Reproductive emergency(ies), 405–434
  agalactia as, 430–431
  arterial ruptures as, 424–428
  dystocia as, 411–415
  foal rejection as, 431–434
  hydrops of fetal membranes as, 419–
    422
  mastitis as, 429–430
  postcastration complications as, 410–
    411
  stallion breeding injuries as, 405–410
  uterine torsion as, 415–419
  vaginal/vestibular hemorrhages as, 422–
    424
  ventral ruptures as, 428–429
Respiratory causes, of sudden and
  unexpected death, 634–635
Respiratory compromise, in peripartum
  asphyxia, treatment of, 495–496
Respiratory distress, after anthelmintic
  therapy, in foals, 455–456
  in newborn foal, 476, 495–496

Respiratory distress *(Continued)*
  with noise, 435–443
    laryngeal obstruction in, 435–441
    nasal obstruction in, 441–443
  without noise, 443–455
    bacterial pneumonia in, 453–454
    bronchointerstitial pneumonia in,
      454–455
    heaves in, 449–451
    pneumothorax in, 443–445
    pulmonary edema in, 445–447
    Rhodococcus equi infection in, 452–
      453
    smoke inhalation in, 447–448
    viral, 451–452
Respiratory fluid analysis, 39–40
Respiratory rate, in newborn foal, 475
Respiratory support, during birth
    resuscitation, 533
  in birth resuscitation, during dystocia,
    536–537
  in field emergencies, 651–652
Respiratory tract, emergency(ies) of,
    434–462
    after anthelmintic treatment, in foals,
      455–456
    aspiration pneumonia as, 458–460
    drugs for, 576–577
    epistaxis as, 460–462
    pleuropneumonia/septic pleuritis as,
      456–458
    with noise, 435–443
    without noise, 443–455
  lower, suppurative inflammation of, 561
  of newborn foal, 475–476
  upper, obstruction of, quinidine-induced,
    117
Restraint drugs, in field emergencies,
    647–650, 648t
Resuscitation, cardiopulmonary. See
    *Cardiopulmonary resuscitation
    (CPR).*
  of foal at birth, 528–537. See also *Birth
    resuscitation.*
Resuscitation drugs, in field emergencies,
    648t, 650–651
Retractor muscle, paralysis of, following
    tranquilization, 407
Retropharyngeal lymph node, strangles
    with, in foals, 438
Rhinopneumonitis, vaccination schedule
    for, 703
Rhodococcus equi pneumonia, in foals,
    452–453
Rhodococcus equi–associated diarrhea, in
    weanlings and yearlings, 233–235

Rib fracture(s), 293
  during chest compression, 515
Rifampin, 569
  dosage of, 676
  for *Rhodococcus equi* pneumonia, 452
  for *Rhodococcus equi*–associated diar-
    rhea, 234
Ringer's solution, lactated, used in field
    emergencies, 648t, 650
Robert Jones bandage, for forelimb or
    hindlimb fractures, at level 2, 302
  plus splint, at level 3, 302–303, *303–
    304*
  material for, 302
Rotavirus diarrhea, in foals, 231–232
Rupture, of abdominal muscles, 428–429
  of aorta, 293
  of aortic root, 152–155, *153–155*
  of bladder, 469–471
    in foals, 469–470
  of chordae tendineae of mitral valve,
    138, 140
  of iliac artery, 424–428
  of longus capitis muscle, 461
  of middle uterine artery, 293
  of prepubic tendon, 428–429
    in pregnant mare, 214–215
  of tendons, as pediatric orthopedic emer-
    gency, 329–330
  of uterine artery, 424–428
  of uterus, 418–419
    in pregnant mare, 213–214
Ryegrass poisoning, 613

S1 heart sound, 95t
S2 heart sound, 95t
S3 heart sound, 95t
S4 heart sound, 95t
Sacral nerve, disorders of, 377
Saddle thrombus, trembling with, 358
Saddlebred horse, registry information for,
    718
Saline, dosage of, 676
  hypertonic, intravenous administration
    of, 579
  used in field emergencies, 648t, 650
Salivation, excessive, 164–166
Salmonella, diarrhea caused by, 217, 218,
    219
Salmonellosis, in foals, 229–231
    clinical findings of, 229
    diagnosis of, 229–230
    treatment of, 230–231
  in weanlings and yearlings, 236

Salt, toxicity of, 607–608
Salter-Harris classification, of fractures, *332*
Sand impaction, 194–195
  in large colon, 194–195
Scapulohumeral joint, anesthesia of, 72, *72*
  luxation of, 310–311
Schiff-Sherrington syndrome, 367
Sciatic nerve, disorders of, 376
Sclera, of newborn foal, 475
Second-degree AV block, 105, *105–106*
Sedation, for orthopedic emergencies, 297, 298t
Sedatives, 570–572
Seizure(s), 368–370
  anesthesia for, in field emergencies, 653
  drug-induced, 370–372
  generalized, 368
  idiopathic, 369
  in newborn foal, causes of, 480
  metabolic disease in, 369
  partial, 368
  quinidine-induced, 118
  rules out for, 369
  structural brain disease in, 368–369
  treatment of, 370
Selenium, deficiency of, 440
  dosage of, 676
  for nutritional myopathy, 271
  overdose of, treatment for, 598t
  toxicity of, 613–614
Selenium-deficient tying-up syndrome, 356
Selle Français horses, registry information for, 719
Seminoperitoneum, peritoneal fluid in, 556
Sensitive fern poisoning, 619
Sepsis. See also *Septicemia.*
  early signs of, 482
Septic arthritis, in newborn foal, 481
Septic metritis, 426–428
  treatment of, 427–428
Septic nephritis, acute, 465
Septic osteomyelitis, in newborn foal, 481
Septic shock, 538. See also *Septicemia.*
  signs of, 483
  treatment of, 539–542
    antimicrobial, 541
    monitoring during, 542
    prostanoic inhibitors in, 541
    pump support in, 540–541
    volume support in, 539–540
Septic thrombophlebitis, as complication of venipuncture, 4
Septicemia, causing sudden and unexpected death, 634

Septicemia *(Continued)*
  in newborn foal, 482–491
    cardiovascular support for, 486–487
    clinical pathology of, 483–484
    clinical signs of, 482–483
    diagnostic cultures for, 484
    diagnostic radiographs for, *484–486,* 485
    immune system support for, 490
    nursing care for, 490–491
    nutritional support for, 488–490
    plasma transfusion for, 490
    respiratory support for, 487–488
    treatment of, 486–490
Seroma, and wound healing, 248
Serum, hyperimmune, intravenous administration of, 578
Serum chemistry concentrations, of small organic molecules, 699
Serum electrolyte concentrations, in foals, 691
Serum enzyme activities, 695
Serum iron, parameters of, 692
Serum protein values, 697
Sesamoid bone, biaxial fracture of, 331, *331*
Shetland pony, registry information for, 719
Shock, 538
  burn, life-threatening, 260–261
  pulmonary edema secondary to, 446
  septic. See *Septic shock.*
Shoulder, luxation of, 310–311
Shunt(s), portocaval, causing liver failure, 282
Sick horse, nutrition for, 658, 659t–660t
Sick sinus syndrome, 107
Silicosis, 563
Sinoatrial arrest, 106–107
  treatment of, 107
Sinoatrial block, 105–106
  treatment of, 106
Sinus arrhythmia, 105–106
  treatment of, 106
Sinus bradycardia, 105–106
  treatment of, 106
Sinus of Valsalva aneurysm, ruptured, *154–155*
Sinus trephination, 46–49
SIRS. See *Systemic inflammatory response syndrome (SIRS).*
Skin, anatomy of, 238–239, *239–240*
  biopsy of, 21–22
  collection of fungal samples from, 20
  preparation of, antiseptics for, 246
  toxins affecting, 620–621

Slaframine toxicity (slobber syndrome), 166
"Slipper" cast, for hoof wall lacerations, 319, *319*
Slobber syndrome (slaframine toxicity), 166
Small intestine. See also specific part, e.g., *Duodenum.*
  disorder(s) of, ascarid impaction as, 186–187
    causing colic, 175–191
    duodenitis/jejunitis as, 187–189, *188*
    herniation as, 178–184, *183*
    ileal impaction as, 185–186
    intussusception as, 175–177
    nonstrangulating infarction as, 189–191
    pedunculated lipoma as, 184–185
    volvulus as, 177–178
  resection of, dietary guidelines for, 659t
Smoke inhalation, 447–448, 562
Snake bites, 271–272, 442–443
Snow-on-the-mountain poisoning, 620, *620*
Sodium bicarbonate, dosage of, 124t, 676
  for antibiotic-induced diarrhea, 235–236
  for cardiopulmonary resuscitation, 518t, 520–521
  for hyperkalemia, 130
  for quinidine-induced arrhythmias, 113t
  for supraventricular tachycardia, 112
  indications for, 124t
  intravenous administration of, 579
  overdose of, treatment for, 598t
Sodium chloride, for hypercalcemia, 134
Sodium nitrate, dosage of, 676
Sodium thiosulfate, dosage of, 676
Solid tissue samples, collection and transport of, 19
Soreness, muscle, as complication of intramuscular drug administration, 9
Spanish barb horse, registry information for, 719
Spasms, laryngeal, 437
  muscle, trembling with, 358
Specific gravity, of urine, in newborn foal, 478
Spectinomycin, 569
Spider bites, 271–272
Spinal cord trauma, 366–368
  as complication of cerebrospinal fluid collection, 91
  localizing lesion in, 367
Splenic aspiration, as complication of abdominocentesis, 59

Splint(s), board, for flexor tendon lacerations, application of, *314,* 314–315
  materials for, 314
  for pediatric orthopedic emergencies, 328–329
  Robert Jones bandage plus, for forelimb or hindlimb fractures, at level 3, 302–303, *303–304*
  wired polyvinylchloride, for extensor tendon lacerations, 316, *316*
Splint-cast, for forelimb or hindlimb fractures, at level 1, 299–300, *300–301,* 302
  materials for, 299
Saint John's wort, toxicity of, 621
Staining, of cytologic specimens, 550–551
Stallion breeding injury(ies), paraphimosis as, 405–408
  penile abrasions and lacerations as, 409
  ruptured corpus spongiosum penis as, 408–409
  testicular trauma as, 410
Standardbred horse, registry information for, 719
Stifle joint, anesthesia of, 74, *74*
  luxation of, 311
Sting(s), bee, 271–272, 442
Stinging nettles, 621
Stomach, acute dilation of, 169–170
  disorders of, 169–175
  grain overload of, emergency, 171
    symptomatic, 171–172
  impaction of, 170–171
  perforation of, 175
  ulcers of, 172–173
    in foals, 173–175
Strangles, vaccination schedule for, 703
  with retropharyngeal lymph node involvement, in foals, 438
Strangulating obstruction, of gastrointestinal tract, 156
Stratum basale, of epidermis, 238, *239*
Stratum corneum, of epidermis, 238, *239*
Stratum granulosum, of epidermis, 238, *239*
Stratum lucidum, of epidermis, 238, *239*
Stratum spinosum, of epidermis, 238, *239*
Stress, physiologic, nutrition for, 658, 661t
Strongylus vulgaris larvae, 190
Styloid bone, fracture of, 373
Subpalpebral catheter placement. See *Catheter(s), subpalpebral placement of.*
Succinylcholine, 585–586
  overdose of, treatment for, 598t

Suckle, loss of, in newborn foal, 482–498
Sucralfate, dosage of, 677
    for enteritis, 503
    for gastric ulcers, in foals, 174
    for gastrointestinal dysmotility, in peripartum asphyxia, 494
    for ileus, 500
    for NSAID toxicity, 218
    for ulcers, 573
Sudan grass poisoning, 614
Sudden death. See *Death, sudden and unexpected.*
Sulfadiazine, for equine protozoal myelitis, 339
Supraorbital nerve block, needle placement for, 83, *84*
Suprascapular nerve, disorders of, 374
Supraventricular tachycardia, quinidine toxicity causing, 112–113, *114–115*
Sutures (suturing), in eyelid laceration repair, 385
    in wound closure, *249,* 255
    in wound healing, 248, *249*
Swallowing, difficulty in (dysphagia), 372–374
Swelling, acute. See *Edema.*
Sympathomimetic drugs, for third-degree AV block, 103
Synovial fluid, 558–560
    analysis of, 78, 79t, 80
    cell counts and cytologic examination of, 558
    interpretation of, in degenerative and traumatic joint disease, 559
        in inflammatory joint disease, 559–560
Systemic inflammatory response syndrome (SIRS), 538–539
    treatment of, 539–542
        antimicrobial, 541
        monitoring during, 542
        prostanoic inhibitors in, 541
        pump support in, 540–541
        volume support in, 539–540

Tachyarrhythmia(s), 107–125
    atrial fibrillation as, 107–119
    ventricular tachycardia as, 119–125
Tachycardia, supraventricular, quinidine toxicity causing, 112–113, *114–115*
    ventricular, 119–125
        causing congestive heart failure, 137
        echocardiogram of, 120, *123*
        electrocardiogram of, 120, *121–122*

Tachycardia *(Continued)*
    treatment of, 120, 122–126
        antiarrhythmics in, 123, 124t, 125
            adverse effects of, 126t
            indications for, 122t
Tackle box, analgesic, anesthetic, and restraint drugs for, 647–650, 648t
    resuscitation drugs for, 648t, 650–651
Tactile stimulation, during birth resuscitation, 532
Tarpan horse, registry information for, 720
Tarsal joints, anesthesia of, 73, *73*
Tarsorrhaphy, temporary, 383
Temperature, and wound healing, 250–251
Temporomandibular joint, fracture of, 307
Tendon(s). See also named tendon, e.g., *Flexor tendon(s).*
    ruptured, as pediatric orthopedic emergency, 329–330
Tennessee walking horse, registry information for, 720
Tension suture(s), in wound closure, *249,* 255
Terbutaline challenge, in anhydrosis, 544
Terbutaline overdose, treatment for, 598t
Testicular trauma, 410
Tetanic hypocalcemia, 351–353
Tetanus, 354–356
    vaccination schedule for, 703
Tetanus antitoxin, 355
Tetanus prophylaxis, for lacerations, 313
Tetracaine overdose, treatment for, 593t
Tetracycline, 568
    dosage of, 677
    for lymphangitis, 269
    for Potomac horse fever, 222
Theiler's disease, 276–277
Theophylline, dosage of, 677
    for respiratory compromise, in peripartum asphyxia, 495
Thermal injury. See *Burn(s).*
Thermal management, during birth resuscitation, 533–534
Thiabendazole, dosage of, 677
Thiamine, dosage of, 677
    for mycotoxic encephalopathy, 359
Thiopental, dosage of, 677
    used in field emergencies, 648t, 649
Third eyelid flap(s), for corneal ulcers, 395
Third-degree AV block, 102–105
    electrocardiogram of, 102–103, *102–103*
    treatment of, 103–105, *104*
Thistle poisoning, 373, 615–616, *616*
Thoracic fluid, cytologic analysis of, 557–558

Thoracic radiography, of
  bronchopneumonia, *484–486,* 485
Thoracocentesis, 50–52
  complications of, 52
  equipment for, 50
  fluid analysis following, 52
  procedure for, 51–52
Thoroughbred horse, registry information
  for, 720
Thrombocytopenia, epistaxis due to, 461
Thrombophlebitis, as complication of
  intravenous catheters, 15
Thrombosis, aortic-iliac, trembling with,
  358
  as complication of venipuncture, 4
  of jugular veins, 442
Tibial nerve, paralysis of, 376–377
Tibial nerve block, of proximal hindlimb,
  68, *69*
Ticarcillin/clavulanic acid, 566
  dosage of, 668, 677
  for bacterial pneumonia, 454
  for infections, in newborns and foals,
    334t
  for lacerations, 315t
  for salmonellosis, 230
  for septicemia, 489
Tobacco, toxicity of, 607
Tolazine, 572
  dosage of, 677
Tolazoline, dosage of, 677
  for pulmonary vasoconstriction, in peri-
    partum asphyxia, 494
Topical administration, of medications, 10
Topical anesthesia, for ocular emergencies,
  380
Torbugesic tartrate, dosage of, 677
Torsades de pointes, quinidine-induced,
  115
  ventricular tachycardia, 120, *122*
Torsion, uterine, 415–418
  in pregnant mare, 211–213
Total parenteral nutrition, components of,
  488–489
  for hyperlipidemia, 279
Total plasma protein, in assessment of
  dehydration, 160
Toxemia, pleuropneumonia with, 458
Toxic anemia, 285, 287
Toxicity, algae, 631–632
  Alsike clover, causing liver failure, 283,
    617
  aminoglycoside, 630
  amitraz, 601–602
  arsenic, 608
  atropine, 602

Toxicity *(Continued)*
  Australian dandelion, 608
  avocado, 609
  black locust, 602
  black walnut, 622
  blister beetle, 223–225, 602–603
  bracken fern, 609–610, *610*
  buckeye, 604
  buttercup, 603–604
  castor bean, 604
  cyanide, 632
  day-blooming jessamine, 622–623
  digoxin, 110, *112,* 141
  fall panicum, causing liver failure, 282–
    283, 618
  fumonisin, 610–611
  Hoary alyssum, limb edema due to,
    264, *623,* 623–624
  horsetail, 611
  insecticide, 605–606
  insulin, 611
  ionophore, 148–151, 624–626
  iron, causing liver failure, 283, 617–618
  Japanese yew, 626–627
  kleingrass, causing liver failure, 282–
    283, 618
  laboratories testing for, 600–601
  lead, 611–612
    trembling with, 358
  locoweed, 612, *613*
  marijuana, 612
  mercury, 608, 630–631
  moldy white sweet clover, 627–628
  moldy yellow sweet clover, 627–628
  NSAID, 218
    treatment of, 218
  oak, 604–605
  oleander, 627
  onion, 630
  pyrrolizidine alkaloid, 280, 438, 618–
    619, *619*
  quinidine, 111t, 112
    electrocardiographic monitoring of,
      112–113, *114*
  red clover, 606–607
  red maple, 285, *628,* 628–629, 632
  ryegrass, 613
  salt, 607–608
  selenium, 613–614
  sensitive fern, 619
  slaframine (slobber syndrome), 166
  snow-on-the-mountain, 620, *620*
  Saint John's wort, 621
  stinging nettle, 621
  sudan grass, 614
  suspicion of, 599

Toxicity *(Continued)*
tobacco, 607
vitamin K₃, 631
warfarin, 629–630
white snakeroot, 614–615, *615*
trembling with, 357
yellow star thistle, 373, 615–616, *616*
Toxin(s), affecting cardiovascular system, 624–627
affecting gastrointestinal tract, 601–608
affecting liver, 616–619
affecting musculoskeletal system, 622–624
affecting nervous system, 608–616
affecting skin, 620–621
affecting urinary system, 630–631
causing hemolysis, 627–630
causing sudden and unexpected death, 631–635
Tracheal collapse, 440
Tracheal foreign bodies, 441
Tracheotomy, 44–46
complications of, 46
equipment for, 44
technique of, 44–45, *45*
Trakehner horse, registry information for, 720
Tranquilization, for orthopedic emergencies, 297, 298t
paralysis of retractor muscle following, 407
Tranquilizers, 570–572
Transdermal/cutaneous administration, of medications, 11
Transfusion(s), blood. See *Blood transfusion(s)*.
plasma, for septicemia, 490
Transtracheal aspiration, 36–37, *38*
complications of, 37–38
material collected by, microscopic features of, 560–563
Trauma. See also specific type, e.g., *Burn(s)*.
and wound healing, 244–245
breeding, 405–410. See also *Breeding injury(ies)*.
cranial, 363–366
head, 380–382
in newborn foal, 480
hemorrhage with, 292
musculoskeletal, 297–336. See also *Orthopedic emergency(ies)*.
nasal cavity, 441–442
ocular, 381
spinal cord, 366–368
Trembling, 348–358

Trembling *(Continued)*
botulism causing, 348–350
hyperkalemic periodic paralysis causing, 353–354
motor neuron disease causing, 350–351
myopathy/myositis causing, 356–357
other causes of, 357–358
tetanic hypocalcemia causing, 351–353
tetanus causing, 354–356
Trephination, paranasal sinus, 46–49
complications of, 49
equipment for, 44
procedure for, 47–49, *48*
sites for, *48*
Triamcinolone, 578
Trichlormethiazide/dexamethasone, dosage of, 677
Trichlorofon overdose, treatment for, 596t
Triglycerides, serum concentration of, 699
Trimethoprim-sulfa, dosage of, 677
for cerebral abscess, 362
for cholangiohepatitis, 277
for dysphagia, 373
for equine herpes virus–1 myeloencephalitis, 342
for lymphangitis, 269
for *Rhodococcus equi* pneumonia, 453
for septicemia, 489
overdose of, treatment for, 598t
prophylactic, for choke, 167
Trimethoprim-sulfadiazine, for lacerations, 315t
Trimethoprim-sulfonamides, 567–568
Trimming and shoeing, for laminitis, 327
Trocharization, cecal, 59–60
Tube feeding, 662t, 662–663
comments on, 663
Tumor, biopsy of, 22–23
Tyzzer's disease, 281

Ulcer (ulceration), corneal. See *Corneal ulcer(s)*.
drug therapy for, 573–574
duodenal, 173–175
fungal, ocular, 395
gastric, in adults, 172–173
in foals, 173–175
prophylaxis for, 228
oral, quinidine-induced, 118
Ulnar antebrachial nerve block, of proximal forelimb, 68, *68*
Ultrasonography, of liver, 283
transabdominal, of newborn foal, 478
Ultrasound-guided biopsy, of kidney, 24–25

Umbilicus stump, in newborn foal, 479
Urinalysis, 62–63
Urinary emergency(ies), 462–472
    acute renal failure as, 462–465
    acute septic nephritis as, 465
    discolored urine in, 465, 466t, 467–468
    incontinence associated with foaling as,
      472
    lower urinary tract obstruction as, 468–
      469
    prolapsed bladder as, 471
    ruptured bladder as, 469–471
Urinary incontinence, associated with
    foaling, 472
Urinary tract, catheterization of, 61–63
    complications of, 63
    in females, 62
    in males, 61–62
    endoscopic examination of, 33
    lower, obstruction of, 468–469
    toxins affecting, 630–631
Urination, in newborn foal, 478–479
Urine, discolored, 465–468
    blood causing, 467–468
    differential diagnosis of, 466t
    specific gravity of, in newborn foal, 478
Urine chemistry, reference values for, 680
Urine samples, collection and transport of,
    19
Urogenital system, of newborn foal,
    478–479
Uroperitoneum, peritoneal fluid in,
    556–557
Urticaria, idiopathic, 267
    quinidine-induced, 117
Uterine artery, middle, rupture of, 293
    rupture of, 424–428
Uterine cultures, collection and transport
    of, 19
Uterine prolapse, 429
Uterine rupture, 218–219, 418–419
    in pregnant mare, 213–214
Uterine torsion, 415–418
    diagnosis of, 415–416
    in pregnant mare, 211–213
    prognosis of, 418
    treatment of, 212–213, 416–418, *417*
Uveitis, 400–403
    acute, 401
    chronic, 401–402
    treatment of, 402–403

Vaccination schedule, 700–703
Vagina, manipulation of, at term, 416

Vaginal hemorrhage, during late
    pregnancy, 423
    following natural service delivery, 423
    postpartum, 422
    treatment of, 423–424
Vaginal surgery, dietary guidelines for,
    660t
Vagolytic drugs, for third-degree AV
    block, 103
Valvular heart disease, drug therapy for,
    119t
Vancomycin, 569
    dosage of, 677
    for *Rhodococcus equi* pneumonia, 453
    for *Rhodococcus equi*–associated diar-
      rhea, 234
Vascular access, establishing, during
    resuscitation, 516–517
Vasodilators, 582–583
Vasomotor nephropathy, 464
Vasopressin overdose, treatment for, 598t
Vein(s). See named vein, e.g., *Jugular
    vein(s)*.
Venipuncture, 2–4, *5*
    complications of, 4
Ventilation, assisted, 41–43
    complications of, 43
      nasogastric tube and demand valve,
        43
    using ambu bag, in foals, 43, 513
    with demand valve, 42–43, 513
    during resuscitation, in foals, 513–514
    mouth-to-nose, in foals, 510, *511*
Ventilatory aids, for foals, 513
Ventral midline celiotomy, for uterine
    torsion, 213
Ventricular fibrillation, cardiopulmonary
    resuscitation of patient with, 127,
    128t, 129
Ventricular tachycardia, 119–125
    causing congestive heart failure, 137
    echocardiogram of, 120, *123*
    electrocardiogram of, 120, *121–122*
    treatment of, 120, 122–126
      antiarrhythmics in, 123, 124t, 125
        adverse effects of, 126t
      indications for, 122t
Verapamil, adverse effects of, 125t
    dosage of, 124t, 677
    for quinidine-induced arrhythmias, 113t
    indications for, 124t
Vertebral malformation, cervical, dietary
    guidelines for, 659t
Vestibular disease, 343–344
Viral arteritis, vaccination schedule for,
    702

Viral encephalitis, 360–361
Viral respiratory distress syndrome, 451–452
Viral samples, collection of, equipment in, 18
   procedure for, 20
Vital signs, in newborn foal, 473t
Vitamin(s), dosage of, 677
Vitamin E, for cranial trauma, 365
   for ionophore toxicity, 151
   for motor neuron disease, 351
Vitamin K₃, toxicity of, 631
Volvulus, large colon, 201, *202, 203*
   small intestinal, 177–178

Walnut, black, toxicity of, 622
Warfarin, overdose of, treatment for, 598t
   toxicity of, 629–630
Water-soluble intracarotid drugs, adverse reactions to, 588–589
Weakness, in newborn foal, 482–498
   peripartum asphyxia causing, 491–496
   prematurity/dysmaturity causing, 496–498
   septicemia causing, 482–491
Weanling(s), diarrhea in, 234–236
   salmonellosis in, 236
Welsh pony and cob, registry information for, 720
Wheals, quinidine-induced, 117
White muscle disease, 356–357
White snakeroot poisoning, 614–615, *615*
   trembling with, 357
Wild onion poisoning, 630
Wound(s), puncture, 320–323, *321–322*
Wound closure, 254–258
   primary, *249,* 255–256
      delayed, 256
   secondary, 256–257
   secondary intention healing in, 257–258
Wound debridement, 247–248
Wound healing, 239–243
   debridement phase of, 241
   factor(s) affecting, 243–251
      anemia and blood loss as, 243
      antiseptics as, 246–247
      bandaging and dressings as, 248–250
      blood supply and oxygen tension as, 250

Wound healing *(Continued)*
      corticosteroids as, 244
      debridement as, 247–248
      dehydration and edema as, 250
      hematoma and seroma as, 248
      infection as, 245–246
      malnutrition and protein deficiency as, 243
      NSAIDs as, 244
      sutures and suturing as, 248, *249*
      trauma as, 244–245
   inflammatory phase of, 240–241
   maturation phase of, 242–243
   repair phase of, 241–242
Wound infection, as complication of paranasal trephination, 49
Wound lavage, antiseptics for, 246–247
Wound management, 251–254
   historical features of injury in, 251
   initial examination in, 253
   lavage in, 254
   mechanism of injury in, 252
   preparation in, 253
   type of contamination in, 252
   virulence of microorganism in, 252
Wound supports, selection of, 258

Xylazine, 571
   dosage of, 677
   for abdominal pain, 158t
   for antibiotic-induced diarrhea, 235
   for cranial trauma, 365
   for meconium impaction, 499
   for orthopedic emergencies, 298t
   for seizures, 370
   overdose of, treatment for, 598t
   used in field emergencies, 648t, 649–650

Yearling(s), diarrhea in, 233–234
   salmonellosis in, 236
Yellow star thistle poisoning, 373, 615–616, *616*
Yew, Japanese, toxicity of, 626–627
Yohimbine, dosage of, 677
   used in field emergencies, 648t, 651

ORSINI

ISBN 0-7216-2425-1

Cough-
Robbutussin CM:
1000 Lb horse = 20-25 ccs 2x a day